Surgery of the Lumbar Spine

Ali A. Baaj • Yu-Mi Ryang
Sameh Abolfotouh • Nader S. Dahdaleh
Avelino Parajón
Editors

Surgery of the Lumbar Spine

Principles and Techniques

Springer

Editors
Ali A. Baaj
Department of Neurological Surgery
Northwestern Medicine
Chicago, IL, USA

Sameh Abolfotouh
Medcare Orthopedics and Spine Hospital
Dubai, United Arab Emirates

Avelino Parajón
Neurosurgery
Hospital Universitario Ramón y Cajal
Madrid, Spain

Yu-Mi Ryang
Department of Neurosurgery & Centre for Spine Therapy
Helios Hospital Berlin-Buch
Berlin, Germany

Nader S. Dahdaleh
Neurological Surgery
Northwestern Medicine
Chicago, IL, USA

ISBN 978-3-032-18096-4 ISBN 978-3-032-18097-1 (eBook)
https://doi.org/10.1007/978-3-032-18097-1

This Springer imprint is published by the registered company Springer Nature Switzerland AG
The registered company address is: Gewerbestrasse 11, 6330 Cham, Switzerland

Baaj
To my wife, Gabriela, and my children, Hannah and Joseph. I'm blessed to have you in my life. Thank you for the unconditional love and support.

Prof. Dr. med. Yu-Mi Ryang
Dedicated to my parents who taught me to always strive for excellence.
"Learning is not attained by chance, it must be sought for with ardor and attended to with diligence." Abigail Adams
To those who gave me the opportunity to learn and grow and teach others what I learned.

Sameh Abolfotouh
To my parents, for their lifelong support and for teaching me the value of dedication.

Nader S. Dahdaleh, MD, MS
This book is dedicated to my mentees—neurosurgeons who care deeply for their patients and whose work saves lives every day.

Avelino Parajón
"To my father, who taught me to see wonder in nature and to seek understanding through science"

Foreword

Lumbar spine surgery accounts for the majority of all spinal surgery.

The peculiarity of this book is that it deals with all aspects of lumbar vertebral pathologies with extreme scientific competence. The authors of each chapter have elaborated in a very in-depth way the lumbar vertebral pathologies, starting from the causes, pathophysiology, biomechanics to offer a complete and comprehensive panorama of how to deal with this problem.

It is known that back pain is the main cause of medical consultation, and precise knowledge of the origin of the problem leads to the most effective treatment.

This text comprehensively encompasses all the topics of spinal surgery of the lumbar area, thoroughly dissecting every possible solution.

The reader will therefore be able to find in this text all the answers to the questions that doctors ask themselves in dealing with lumbar vertebral diseases.

It was a superlative work by the authors and I congratulate Ali Baaj for having collected in a single text every detail of lumbar spinal surgery, both from diagnosis to end with postoperative rehabilitation.

This text therefore represents a valid growth opportunity for young surgeons, but also a valid support for experienced surgeons.

In addition this book is intended for clinicians as well as researchers in many field of lumbar spinal disorders, and its use to orthopedic and neurosurgeons, as well as rheumatologists, neurologists, physiatrists, and physical therapists.

Spinal Department, UOC Orthopedic Spinal Surgery — Massimo Balsano
University and Hospital Trust
AOUI Verona
Verona, Italy

Preface

We're excited to present this new work dedicated to the principles and techniques involved in lumbar spine surgery. As lumbar spine disease is among the commonest conditions treated by spine specialists, we felt the literature needed such a textbook that dives deep into diagnoses, treatments, as well as surgical and nonsurgical strategies. We were keen on including the traditional, core topics like degenerative disease, trauma, and oncology. However, we also were mindful to present new and innovative topics like minimally invasive spine surgery, endoscopy, and robotic spine surgery. We are grateful to the many contributors who provided invaluable content, and we are hopeful that clinicians in various stages of their training or practices find this textbook helpful.

Chicago, IL, USA	Ali A. Baaj
Berlin, Germany	Yu-Mi Ryang
Dubai, United Arab Emirates	Sameh Abolfotouh
Chicago, IL, USA	Nader S. Dahdaleh
Madrid, Spain	Avelino Parajón

Contents

1 **Anatomy of the Lumbar Spine** 1
Faith C. Robertson, Tariq Parker, Stephanie M. Cohen, and Jean-Valery C. E. Coumans

2 **Biomechanics of the Lumbar Spine** 11
Ali Haider Bangash, Reza Yassari, and Rafael De la Garza Ramos

3 **Epidemiology and Healthcare Burden of Lumbar Degenerative Spine Disease** 25
Abraham Dada, Vivian Kwok, and Anthony DiGiorgio

4 **Physical Examination in Lumbar Spine Disease** 33
Ebtesam Abdulla, Mohammad Almalki, Ibrahim A. Alhalal, and Saleh S. Baeesa

5 **Radiological Assessment of the Lumbar Spine** 39
Joshua Chalif, James Tanner McMahon, David Liu, and Hasan Zaidi

6 **Intraoperative Neuromonitoring in Lumbar Spine Surgery** . . . 49
Sarah Bin Abdulqader, Muhammad Tariq Imtiaz, and Sultan Aldebeyan

7 **Bone Health Optimization** 57
Zach Pennington, Anthony L. Mikula, and Benjamin D. Elder

8 **Interventional Pain Techniques in the Lumbar Spine** 69
Andrew Lederman

9 **Physiotherapy for Degenerative Lumbar Spine Disease** 77
Hana Alsobayel and Dalia Alimam

10 **Lumbar Spine Trauma** 85
Warren Roth, Jason Silvestre, James P. Lawrence, and Robert A. Ravinsky

11 **Sacral Trauma** 95
Kyle J. Holmberg, Michael T. Quinet, and John C. France

12 Lumbar Disc Herniations 103
Michael Prim

13 Lumbar Spinal Stenosis 109
Stefan Motov, Felix C. Stengel, and Martin N. Stienen

14 Intradural Lumbar Spinal Tumors 117
Victor M. Lu and Allan D. Levi

15 Metastatic Disease to the Lumbar Spine 127
Puya Alikhani, Carballo-Cuello Cesar, Kumar Jay, and Soto-Rubio Diego

16 Lumbo-Sacral Primary Tumors 135
Zach Pennington, Daniel Schneider, Sheng-Fu Larry Lo, and Daniel M. Sciubba

17 Lumbar Synovial Cysts 145
Patrick Kramer, Tej Azad, and Ali Bydon

18 Degenerative Spondylolisthesis and Spondylolysis 155
Marisa Gandía, Diego Gordon, and Mario Taravilla-Loma

19 Decompression Without Fusion for Lumbar Degenerative Lumber Spondylolisthesis (DLS) Decompression Without Fusion: Evidence and Technique 163
Clemens Weber and Ivar Magne Austevoll

20 Decompression and Fusion for Lumbar Degenerative Spondylolisthesis: Evidence-Based Medicine and Technique . . . 171
Evgenii Belykh, Vadim A. Byvaltsev, Subu Magge, and Zoher Ghogawala

21 Lumbar Degenerative Deformity 185
Luis Felipe Colón and Han Jo Kim

22 High-Grade Spondylolisthesis 197
Maile Curbo and Eric Klineberg

23 Lumbar Spondylodiscitis 205
Marc Khalifé, Jean-Baptiste Odent, Thomas Volpé, and Michaël Thy

24 Postoperative Spinal Infections 211
Vincent Raymaekers, Maarten Wissels, and Sven Bamps

25 Lumbar Open and Tubular Microdiscectomy 221
Yazid Maghrabi, Fatimah A. Alghabban, and Saleh S. Baeesa

26 Lumbar Endoscopic Decompression 227
Abhinav K. Sharma, Don Young Park, and Peter B. Derman

27 Lumbar Endoscopy, Beyond Degenerative Decompression 237
Vincent Hagel and Kai-Uwe Lewandrowski

28 Complication Management in Lumbar Endoscopy 247
Alexandre Simonin

29 Open Transforaminal Lumbar Interbody Fusion (TLIF) 253
Fernando Padilla-Lichtenberger, A. Guiroy, F. Landriel, and J. Emmerich

30 Posterior Lumbar Interbody Fusion: MIS 261
Avelino Parajón, Angela Carrascosa, and Jose Antonio Gutiérrez

31 Lateral Lumbar Interbody Fusion 269
Rodrigo Amaral, Gabriel Pokorny, Jullyene Pokorny, Fernando Marcelino, Igor Barreira, Rafael Moriguchi, and Luiz Pimenta

32 Prone Lateral Lumbar Spine Surgery 275
Luiz Pimenta, Gabriel Pokorny, Jullyene Pokorny, Fernando Marcelino, Igor Barreira, Rafael Moriguchi, and Rodrigo Amaral

33 Anterior Lumbar Interbody Fusion (ALIF) 281
Alfredo Guiroy, Matías Orellana, Alfredo Sícoli, and Cristiano Menezes

34 Sacropelvic Fixation Strategies 287
Justin L. Reyes, Prerana Katiyar, Josephine R. Coury, and Zeeshan M. Sardar

35 Osteotomies in the Lumbar Spine 297
Allie Harbert and Cheerag Upadhyaya

36 Navigation and Robotics in Lumbar Spine Surgery 301
Abdurrahman F. Kharbat, Hakeem J. Shakir, Chao Li, and Zachary A. Smith

37 Awake Lumbar Spine Surgery 307
Daivik B. Vyas, Brian J. Park, and Michael Y. Wang

38 Current Applications of Artificial Intelligence and Machine Learning in Lumbar Spine Surgery 313
Zach Pennington, Karim Rizwan Nathani, and Mohamad Bydon

Index 321

Contributors

Ebtesam Abdulla Department of Neurosurgery, Government Hospitals, Manama, Bahrain

Sarah Bin Abdulqader Department of Neurosurgery, National Neuroscience Institute, King Fahad Medical City, Riyadh, Saudi Arabia

Sultan Aldebeyan Department of Spine Surgery, National Neuroscience Institute, King Fahad Medical City, Riyadh, Saudi Arabia

Fatimah A. Alghabban, MBBS Neurosurgery Department, King Abdulaziz Speciality Hospital, Taif, Saudi Arabia

Ibrahim A. Alhalal Department of Spine Surgery, Banner University Medical Centre, University of Arizona, Tucson, AZ, USA

Puya Alikhani Department of Neurosurgery and Brain Repair, University of South Florida, Morsani College of Medicine, Tampa, FL, USA

Dalia Alimam Department of Rehabilitation Sciences, College of Applied Medical Sciences, King Saud University, Riyadh, Saudi Arabia

Mohammad Almalki Department of Spine Surgery, Prince Sultan Military Medical City, Riyadh, Kingdom of Saudi Arabia

Hana Alsobayel Department of Rehabilitation Sciences, College of Applied Medical Sciences, King Saud University, Riyadh, Saudi Arabia

Rodrigo Amaral Instituto de Patologia da Coluna, São Paulo, Brazil

Ivar Magne Austevoll Department of Orthopedic Surgery, Haukeland University Hospital, Bergen, Norway

Tej Azad Department of Neurosurgery, Johns Hopkins University School of Medicine, Baltimore, MD, USA

Saleh S. Baeesa, MD, FRCSC Department of Neurosciences, King Faisal Specialist Hospital and Research Centre, Jeddah, Saudi Arabia

Sven Bamps Department of Neurosurgery Jessa Hospital, Hasselt, Belgium
Faculty of Medicine and Life Sciences, Hasselt University, Hasselt, Belgium
Study and Research Center Neurosurgery Virga Jesse, Hasselt, Belgium

Ali Haider Bangash Spine Tumor Mechanics and Outcomes Research Lab, Montefiore Medical Center, Albert Einstein College of Medicine, Bronx, NY, USA
Department of Neurosurgery, Montefiore Medical Center, Albert Einstein College of Medicine, Bronx, NY, USA

Igor Barreira Instituto de Patologia da Coluna, São Paulo, Brazil

Evgenii Belykh Department of Neurosurgery, Lahey Hospital and Medical Center, Burlington, MA, USA
Department of Neurosurgery, Rutgers New Jersey Medical School, Newark, NJ, USA

Ali Bydon Department of Neurosurgery, Johns Hopkins University School of Medicine, Baltimore, MD, USA

Mohamad Bydon Mayo Clinic Neuro-Informatics Laboratory, Department of Neurologic Surgery, Mayo Clinic, Rochester, MN, USA
Department of Neurologic Surgery, Mayo Clinic, Rochester, MN, USA

Vadim A. Byvaltsev Department of Neurosurgery, Irkutsk State Medical University, Irkutsk, Russia

Angela Carrascosa Department of Neurosurgery, Hospital Universitario San Carlos, Madrid, Spain

Carballo-Cuello Cesar Department of Neurosurgery and Brain Repair, University of South Florida, Morsani College of Medicine, Tampa, FL, USA

Joshua Chalif Department of Neurosurgery, Brigham and Women's Hospital, Boston, MA, USA

Stephanie M. Cohen Department of General Surgery, Beth Israel Deaconess Medical Center, Boston, MA, USA

Luis Felipe Colón Complex Spine and Scoliosis Center, Hospital for Special Surgery, New York, NY, USA

Jean-Valery C. E. Coumans Department of Neurosurgery, Massachusetts General Hospital, Boston, MA, USA

Josephine R. Coury Columbia University Orthopedics, New York, NY, USA
NewYork-Presbyterian Och Spine Hospital, New York, NY, USA

Maile Curbo UTHealth Houston, McGovern Medical School, Department of Orthopaedic Surgery, Houston, TX, USA

Abraham Dada University of California, San Francisco, Department of Neurological Surgery, San Francisco, CA, USA

Rafael De la Garza Ramos Spine Tumor Mechanics and Outcomes Research Lab, Montefiore Medical Center, Albert Einstein College of Medicine, Bronx, NY, USA
Department of Neurosurgery, Montefiore Medical Center, Albert Einstein College of Medicine, Bronx, NY, USA

Peter B. Derman Texas Back Institute, Plano, TX, USA

Soto-Rubio Diego Department of Neurosurgery and Brain Repair, University of South Florida, Morsani College of Medicine, Tampa, FL, USA

Anthony DiGiorgio University of California, San Francisco, Department of Neurological Surgery, San Francisco, CA, USA
University of California, San Francisco, Philip R Lee Institute for Health Policy Studies, San Francisco, CA, USA

Benjamin D. Elder Department of Neurologic Surgery, Mayo Clinic, Rochester, MN, USA

J. Emmerich Department of Neurological Surgery, Children's Hospital La Plata, La Plata, Argentina

John C. France West Virginia University Department of Orthopaedic Surgery, Morgantown, WV, USA

Marisa Gandía University Hospital La Paz, Department of Neurosurgery, Madrid, Spain

Zoher Ghogawala Department of Neurosurgery, Lahey Hospital and Medical Center, Burlington, MA, USA

Diego Gordon University Hospital La Paz, Department of Neurosurgery, Madrid, Spain

A. Guiroy Spine Surgery Department, Clínica de Cuyo, Mendoza, Argentina

Alfredo Guiroy Clínica de Cuyo, Mendoza, Argentina

Jose Antonio Gutiérrez Department of Neurosurgery, Hospital Universitario Ramón y Cajal, Madrid, Spain

Vincent Hagel Asklepios Hospital Lindau, Spine Center, Lindau, Germany

Allie Harbert Department of Neurosurgery, University of North Carolina, Chapel Hill, NC, USA

Kyle J. Holmberg West Virginia University Department of Orthopaedic Surgery, Morgantown, WV, USA

Muhammad Tariq Imtiaz Department of Neurophysiology, National Neuroscience Institute, King Fahad Medical City, Riyadh, Saudi Arabia

Kumar Jay Department of Neurosurgery and Brain Repair, University of South Florida, Morsani College of Medicine, Tampa, FL, USA

Prerana Katiyar Hospital for Special Surgery, New York, NY, USA

Marc Khalifé Department of Orthopaedic Surgery, Hôpital Européen Georges-Pompidou, AP-HP, Paris, France
Université Paris-Cité, Paris, France

Abdurrahman F. Kharbat Department of Neurosurgery, University of Oklahoma Health Sciences Center, Oklahoma City, OK, USA

Han Jo Kim Complex Spine and Scoliosis Center, Hospital for Special Surgery, New York, NY, USA

Eric Klineberg UTHealth Houston, McGovern Medical School, Department of Orthopaedic Surgery, Houston, TX, USA

Patrick Kramer Department of Neurosurgery, Johns Hopkins University School of Medicine, Baltimore, MD, USA

Vivian Kwok University of California, San Francisco, Department of Neurological Surgery, San Francisco, CA, USA

F. Landriel Department of Neurological Surgery, Hospital Italiano de Buenos Aires, Buenos Aires, Argentina

James P. Lawrence Department of Orthopaedics and Physical Medicine, Medical University of South Carolina, Charleston, SC, USA

Andrew Lederman Department of Orthopedic Surgery, New England Baptist Hospital, Boston, MA, USA

Allan D. Levi Department of Neurological Surgery, University of Miami Miller School of Medicine, Miami, FL, USA

Kai-Uwe Lewandrowski Division Personalized Pain Research and Education, Center for Advanced Spine Care of Southern Arizona, Tucson, AZ, USA
Department of Orthopaedic Surgery, University of Arizona, Banner Medical Center, Tucson, AZ, USA
Department of Orthopaedics, Fundación Universitaria Sanitas, Bogotá D.C., Colombia
Department of Orthopedics at Hospital Universitário Gaffree Guinle, Universidade Federal do Estado do Rio de Janeiro, Rio de Janeiro, Brazil

Chao Li Department of Neurosurgery, University of Oklahoma Health Sciences Center, Oklahoma City, OK, USA

David Liu Department of Neurosurgery, Brigham and Women's Hospital, Boston, MA, USA

Sheng-Fu Larry Lo Department of Neurosurgery, Donald and Barbara Zucker School of Medicine at Hofstra/Northwell Health, Manhasset, NY, USA

Victor M. Lu Department of Neurological Surgery, University of Miami Miller School of Medicine, Miami, FL, USA

Subu Magge Department of Neurosurgery, Lahey Hospital and Medical Center, Burlington, MA, USA

Yazid Maghrabi, MBBS Neurosciences Department, King Abdulaziz Medical City, Ministry of the National Guard-Health Affairs, Jeddah, Saudi Arabia

Fernando Marcelino Instituto de Patologia da Coluna, São Paulo, Brazil

James Tanner McMahon Department of Neurosurgery, Brigham and Women's Hospital, Boston, MA, USA

Cristiano Menezes Federal University of Minas Gerais (UFMG), Belo Horizonte, Brazil

Anthony L. Mikula Department of Neurologic Surgery, Mayo Clinic, Rochester, MN, USA

Rafael Moriguchi Instituto de Patologia da Coluna, São Paulo, Brazil

Stefan Motov H-OCH Health Ostschweiz, Interdisciplinary Spine Center & Department of Neurosurgery, Kantonsspital St.Gallen & School of Medicine, University of St. Gallen, St. Gallen, Switzerland

Karim Rizwan Nathani Mayo Clinic Neuro-Informatics Laboratory, Department of Neurologic Surgery, Mayo Clinic, Rochester, MN, USA
Department of Neurologic Surgery, Mayo Clinic, Rochester, MN, USA

Jean-Baptiste Odent Department of Orthopaedic Surgery, Hôpital Européen Georges-Pompidou, AP-, HP, Paris, France
Université Paris-Cité, Paris, France

Matías Orellana Clínica de Cuyo, Mendoza, Argentina

Fernando Padilla-Lichtenberger Spine Surgery Department, Université de Montréal, Montreal, QC, Canada

Avelino Parajón Department of Neurosurgery, Hospital Universitario Ramón y Cajal, Madrid, Spain

Brian J. Park Department of Neurological Surgery, University of Miami, Miami, FL, USA

Don Young Park Department of Orthopaedic Surgery, University of California, Irvine, Orange, CA, USA

Tariq Parker Department of Neurosurgery, Massachusetts General Hospital, Boston, MA, USA

Zach Pennington Department of Neurologic Surgery, Mayo Clinic, Rochester, MN, USA
Mayo Clinic Neuro-Informatics Laboratory, Department of Neurologic Surgery, Mayo Clinic, Rochester, MN, USA

Luiz Pimenta Instituto de Patologia da Coluna, São Paulo, Brazil

Gabriel Pokorny Instituto de Patologia da Coluna, São Paulo, Brazil

Jullyene Pokorny Instituto de Patologia da Coluna, São Paulo, Brazil

Michael Prim Department of Neurosurgery, Banner University Medical Center, University of Arizona College of Medicine, Phoenix, AZ, USA

Michael T. Quinet West Virginia University Department of Orthopaedic Surgery, Morgantown, WV, USA

Robert A. Ravinsky Department of Orthopaedics and Physical Medicine, Medical University of South Carolina, Charleston, SC, USA

Vincent Raymaekers Department of Neurosurgery Jessa Hospital, Hasselt, Belgium
Faculty of Medicine and Life Sciences, Hasselt University, Hasselt, Belgium
Faculty of Medicine and Health Sciences, University of Antwerp, Antwerp, Belgium

Justin L. Reyes Columbia University Orthopedics, New York, NY, USA
NewYork-Presbyterian Och Spine Hospital, New York, NY, USA

Faith C. Robertson Department of Neurosurgery, Massachusetts General Hospital, Boston, MA, USA

Warren Roth Department of Orthopaedics and Physical Medicine, Medical University of South Carolina, Charleston, SC, USA

Zeeshan M. Sardar Columbia University Orthopedics, New York, NY, USA
NewYork-Presbyterian Och Spine Hospital, New York, NY, USA

Daniel Schneider Department of Neurosurgery, Donald and Barbara Zucker School of Medicine at Hofstra/Northwell Health, Manhasset, NY, USA

Daniel M. Sciubba Department of Neurosurgery, Donald and Barbara Zucker School of Medicine at Hofstra/Northwell Health, Manhasset, NY, USA

Hakeem J. Shakir Department of Neurosurgery, University of Oklahoma Health Sciences Center, Oklahoma City, OK, USA

Abhinav K. Sharma Department of Orthopaedic Surgery, University of California, Irvine, Orange, CA, USA

Alfredo Sícoli Clínica de Cuyo, Mendoza, Argentina

Jason Silvestre Department of Orthopaedics and Physical Medicine, Medical University of South Carolina, Charleston, SC, USA

Alexandre Simonin Sion Cantonal Hospital, Sion, Switzerland

Zachary A. Smith Department of Neurosurgery, University of Oklahoma Health Sciences Center, Oklahoma City, OK, USA

Felix C. Stengel H-OCH Health Ostschweiz, Interdisciplinary Spine Center & Department of Neurosurgery, Kantonsspital St.Gallen & School of Medicine, University of St. Gallen, St. Gallen, Switzerland

Martin N. Stienen H-OCH Health Ostschweiz, Interdisciplinary Spine Center & Department of Neurosurgery, Kantonsspital St.Gallen & School of Medicine, University of St. Gallen, St. Gallen, Switzerland

Mario Taravilla-Loma Department of Neurosurgery, University Hospital La Paz, Madrid, Spain

Michaël Thy Université Paris-Cité, Paris, France
Department of Infectious and Tropical Diseases, Bichat-Claude Bernard Hospital, AP-HP, Paris, France

Cheerag Upadhyaya Department of Neurosurgery, University of North Carolina, Chapel Hill, NC, USA

Thomas Volpé Université Paris-Cité, Paris, France
Department of Infectious and Tropical Diseases, Bichat-Claude Bernard Hospital, AP-HP, Paris, France

Daivik B. Vyas Department of Neurological Surgery, University of Miami, Miami, FL, USA

Michael Y. Wang Department of Neurological Surgery, University of Miami, Miami, FL, USA

Clemens Weber Department of Neurosurgery, Stavanger University Hospital, Stavanger, Norway

Maarten Wissels Department of Neurosurgery Jessa Hospital, Hasselt, Belgium
Study and Research Center Neurosurgery Virga Jesse, Hasselt, Belgium

Reza Yassari Spine Tumor Mechanics and Outcomes Research Lab, Montefiore Medical Center, Albert Einstein College of Medicine, Bronx, NY, USA
Department of Neurosurgery, Montefiore Medical Center, Albert Einstein College of Medicine, Bronx, NY, USA

Hasan Zaidi Department of Neurosurgery, Brigham and Women's Hospital, Boston, MA, USA

Anatomy of the Lumbar Spine

1

Faith C. Robertson, Tariq Parker, Stephanie M. Cohen, and Jean-Valery C. E. Coumans

Introduction

Low back pain (LBP), often stemming from degenerative lumbar spine conditions, is one of the most common reasons for patient visits to healthcare providers and is the leading cause of years lived with disability worldwide [1]. In 2020, LBP affected 619 million people globally, with projected increases to 843 million by 2050 [2]. In a 2021 study of patients aged over 65, the overall prevalence of diagnosed spinal degenerative disease was 27.3% [3]. With a globally aging population, proper diagnosis and management of spine pathology is paramount.

The lumbar spine, which bears the weight of the upper body while permitting a wide range of motion, is uniquely susceptible to mechanical stress and degenerative changes. Conditions such as lumbar disc herniation, spinal stenosis, and spondylolisthesis frequently arise from structural alterations in the vertebrae, intervertebral discs, ligaments, and neural elements. A foundational understanding of the intricate anatomy of the lumbar spine is key to diagnosing and treating these conditions.

This chapter provides a detailed examination of the bony, ligamentous, neural, and vascular structures of the lumbar spine, focusing on their clinical relevance in common pathologies. The bony elements, including the vertebral bodies, pedicles, and facet joints, along with ligamentous structures that contribute to spinal stability, are explored in the context of spinal biomechanics and their role in degenerative disease. Neural structures, including the spinal cord, conus medullaris, cauda equina, and nerve roots, are discussed with emphasis on their anatomical relationships and vulnerability to compression syndromes. Additionally, the vascular anatomy of the lumbar spine, which is critical in avoiding complications during surgery, is reviewed. By presenting an in-depth anatomical framework, this chapter aims to equip the reader with the knowledge required for effective clinical decision-making and surgical intervention in lumbar spine disorders.

Bony Anatomy

The typical human spine is comprised of 33 vertebrae with 7 cervical, 12 thoracic, 5 lumbar, 5 fused sacral vertebrae, and 4 ossicles of the coccyx. Given humans' upright posture for bipedal ambulation, there are additional biomechanical

F. C. Robertson (✉) · T. Parker · J.-V. C. E. Coumans
Department of Neurosurgery, Massachusetts General Hospital, Boston, MA, USA
e-mail: ROBERTSON@MGH.HARVARD.EDU; tparker3@mgh.harvard.edu; JCOUMANS@mgh.harvard.edu

S. M. Cohen
Department of General Surgery, Beth Israel Deaconess Medical Center, Boston, MA, USA
e-mail: scohen10@bidmc.harvard.edu

A. A. Baaj et al. (eds.), *Surgery of the Lumbar Spine*, https://doi.org/10.1007/978-3-032-18097-1_1

stresses and axial loading on the inferior segments of the spinal column. The lumbar spine is unique in that it must support diverse types of truncal motion, including flexion, extension, rotation, and side bending. We see a substantial increase in robustness of the bony morphology, joints, and ligamentous structures in the lower portions of the spine to improve structural support at the caudal elements, even within the lumbar spine itself (see Fig. 1.1 for differences between L2 and L5 vertebra) [4]. Of note, there are also anatomic variants such as transitional lumbar spine anatomy with a lumbarized S1, sacralized L5, or Bertolotti's syndrome, which may predispose individuals to the development of back pain and pose unique challenges to healthcare professionals [5].

Vertebral Body

In the axial view, the vertebral body in the upper lumbar spine is more rounded and progresses to a kidney shape at L4 and a more oval shape at L5 with a broader base. The increased bony width adds to its cross-sectional area and improves the biomechanical compression strength, from nearly 4000 newtons at L1 to 8000 newtons at L4 (roughly 6000 at L5) [4]. In the sagittal view, the lumbar height is generally comparable ventrally and dorsally through L1-L4, which differs from the thoracic spine where vertebral bodies are shorter ventrally, adding to the natural kyphosis of the thorax. At L4-L5, some reverse wedging can occur (greater height ventrally than dorsally) to contribute to the lumbar lordosis. Notably, it is predominantly disc shape rather than vertebral body shape that preserves the lordotic curvature in the lumbar spine; the anterior disc is thicker than the posterior portion, which elevates the vertebrae ventrally more than dorsally [6]. This principle is key, as disc degeneration or disc removal can lead to loss of lordosis, and correction of lordosis can often be obtained with interbody implants that are lordotically shaped.

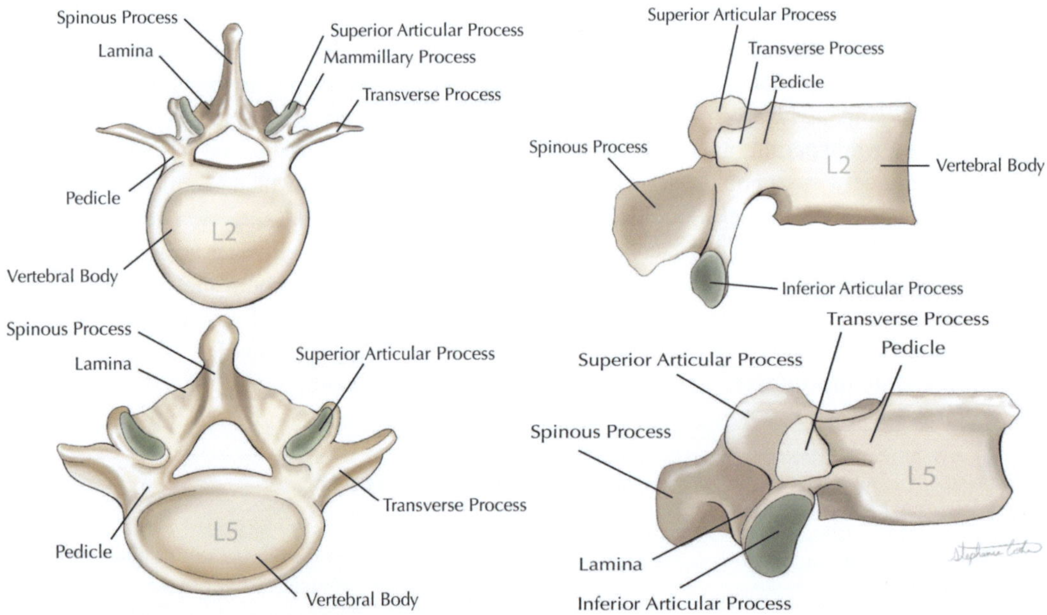

Fig. 1.1 Lumbar vertebrae bony anatomy: Superior and lateral views of L2 and L5. The bone structures become progressively more robust as one moves caudal in the lumbar spine to reflect the need for supporting greater axial loading forces

Vertebral Canal

Other key bony features in the lumbar spine include the spinous processes, which are often described as "hatchet-shaped" and become slightly shorter and less shingled downward as you move rostral to caudal. The spinous process merges with the lamina ventrally and forms the roof of the triangular vertebral foramen (or canal), which is larger in the lumbar spine than in the thoracic, but smaller than in the cervical. Forming the lateral borders of the vertebral foramen are the pedicles (Latin for *small foot*). Pedicles generally become shorter, broader, and more lateral from L1 to L5; this narrows the canal's anteroposterior (AP) diameter and widens the transverse diameter (Fig. 1.1).

As transpedicular fixation with pedicle screws is a foundational procedure within spine surgery, special attention to pedicle anatomy is warranted. In the lumbar spine, the pedicle-axis orientation in an AP view is essentially co-planar with the vertebral body (parallel to the endplates). In the superior-inferior plane, the pedicle attaches to the vertebral body just below the apophyseal ring of the superior endplate. Below the pedicle is the intervertebral foramen where the nerve exits. Transverse pedicle width—which is a key measurement in screw sizing—typically increases from L1 to L5 with an average of approximately 7 mm for L1 and 17 mm for L5 [7, 8]. Sagittal pedicle width (height) varies but generally decreases slightly from L1 to L5 (from 14–15 mm to 12–14 mm) [7, 8]. Regarding pedicle-axis angulation, lumbar pedicles travel lateral to medial as they move ventrally toward the vertebral body. Thus, the start point for a pedicle screw becomes more lateral toward L5, and the pedicle-axis trajectory becomes more medialized.

Joints

While different from joints in the appendicular skeleton such as the hip and knee, the spinal column is indeed a series of mobile joints. The functional unit of the spine, or the spinal motion segment, includes the intervertebral discs and a facet joint (FJ) above and below each vertebral body. This "three-joint complex" enables controlled movement, load distribution, and stability across each vertebral level, supporting 33% of the dynamic compressive load and 35% of the static load of the spine [9, 10].

The FJ, or zygapophysial joint, includes the superior articular process (SAP) of the vertebra with the inferior articular process (IAP) of the vertebra above (Fig. 1.2). The thin bridge of bone between the superior and inferior facets is called the pars interarticularis. The FJ is a synovial joint with a true capsule, comprised of an outer layer of collagenous fibers and an inner elastic layer, with synovial fluid between cartilaginous surfaces.

The orientation of the SAP and IAP varies across patients and has been linked to pathologic processes. Facet joint angulation is the angle between a line that bisects the facet joint process and a line drawn in the sagittal plane through the middle of the vertebral body and the spinous process [11]. Studies have shown that patients with more sagittally oriented facets have a higher propensity for degenerative spondylolisthesis and lumbar disc herniation [10–13]. As noted in the SLIP clinical trial, patients with motion at spondylolisthesis >1.25 mm, disc height >6.5 mm, and facet angle >50° are more likely to experience instability following decompression surgery for Grade I lumbar spondylolisthesis [11, 14]. FJ osteoarthritis is another common spine pathology widely prevalent in older adults and a common cause of back and neck pain. Although often viewed as a disease of articular cartilage loss and bony hypertrophy, the process of joint failure is suspected to include the whole joint, including the subchondral bone, cartilage, ligaments, capsule, synovium, and periarticular paraspinal muscles and soft tissues [15]. Juxtafacet cysts include both synovial cysts (those having a synovial lining membrane) and ganglion cysts (those lacking synovial lining) [16]. These occur most often at L4–5 and can cause compression of the adjacent nerve roots [17].

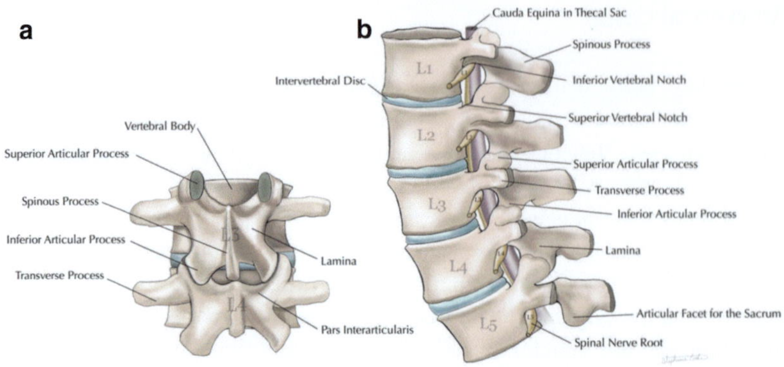

Fig. 1.2 Lumbar vertebrae bony anatomy. (**a**) Posteroanterior view of a lumbovertebral joint. (**b**) Sagittal view of the lumbar column

Additional Bony Landmarks

The mammillary process is the bony prominence on the superior articular process of the lumbar vertebrae. The mammillary process is a small, rounded mound that can vary in size. It's unique to the lumbar spine and serves as an attachment site for the multifidi lumborum muscles which have recently become a neuromodulation target for refractory low back pain [18].

The transverse processes (TPs) in the lumbar spine are long and thin lateral projections with accessory processes on the posterior surface at the base of each process. TPs are used as lever arms by the deep spinal muscles to maintain posture and to induce rotation and lateral bending. Additionally, the midpoint of the TP is a key anatomical landmark for the entry point of a pedicle screw in the lumbar spine. The optimal entry point is at the junction of the midpoint of the TP, the pars interarticularis, and the inferior point of the SAP [19].

The lateral recess, or subarticular zone, is the area where the nerve root exits the central canal and extends caudally and laterally. It is the corner formed by the pedicle, vertebral body, and superior articular facet. Lateral recess stenosis or narrowing is one of the most common sites of nerve root compression that causes radicular pain, and it arises from facet joint arthrosis and SAP overgrowth as well as ligament hypertrophy.

Ligamentous Anatomy

The lumbar spine's bony infrastructure is supported by a network of ligaments that help limit excessive movement and maintain structural integrity (Fig. 1.3). The anterior longitudinal ligament (ALL) runs anterior to the vertebral bodies, preventing hyperextension and providing stability during flexion. The posterior longitudinal ligament (PLL) is narrower and resists hyperflexion, though it is less motion-restricting than the ALL. The interspinous ligaments span the spinous processes, resisting flexion forces, while the supraspinous ligament runs along the tips of the spinous processes, providing additional stability to prevent excessive forward bending.

The ligamentum flavum is dorsolateral to the thecal sac and provides stability between laminae, resisting excessive separation of the adjacent vertebral lamina during flexion. It is also known as the yellow ligament because its composition of 80% elastin and 20% collagen fibers provides its yellow color and flexibility. The ligamentum flavum is a paired structure that is represented symmetrically on the right and left of midline. The medial segment arises from the lower half of the anterior surface of the superior lamina and attaches with a cup-like grasp to the posterior superior margin of the inferior lamina and fuses with the interspinous ligament [20]. The lateral segment passes ventral to the facet, attaching to

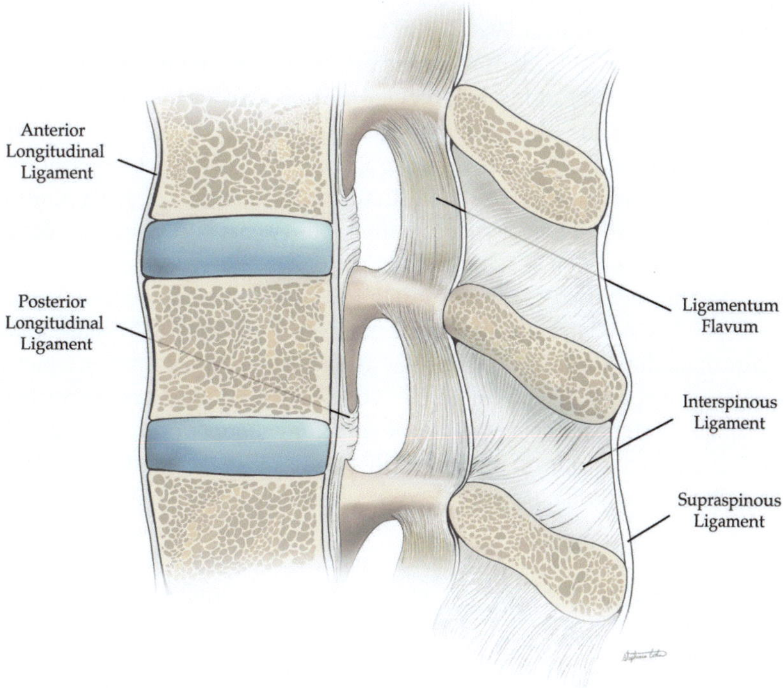

Fig. 1.3 Lumbar ligamentous anatomy

the anterior IAP and SAP and forming the anterior joint capsule. The most lateral fibers extend beyond the SAP to the pedicle below.

Hypertrophy of the ligamentum flavum is often a cause of spinal stenosis. With age, there is a loss of elastic fibers and an increase in collagen fibers that can cause the ligament to thicken and buckle. Furthermore, stress over time can cause the ligament to calcify and become more rigid. These changes in turn can narrow the spinal canal centrally, causing central stenosis, or can cause compression in the lateral recess leading to radiculopathy. Consequently, ligamentum flavectomy is often an essential step in lumbar surgical decompressions.

Together, these ligaments contribute to the controlled mobility and robustness of the lumbar spine, playing essential roles in spinal biomechanics and are frequently implicated in degenerative changes and clinical pathologies like spinal stenosis.

Common Pathology

Lumbar spinal stenosis is characterized by a narrowing of the spinal canal, neuroforamina, and/or lateral recesses. The etiology of lumbar stenosis is most commonly degenerative and may include hypertrophic changes in the facet joints, thickening of the ligamentum flavum, bulging of intervertebral discs, osteophyte and synovial cyst formation, which may eventually result in vertebral misalignment. Symptomatic lumbar stenosis most frequently affects the L4-L5 level [21]. These anatomical alterations lead to nerve root compression, often resulting in lower back pain, leg pain, or neurogenic claudication, particularly during physical activity.

Degenerative disc disease (DDD) is another common lumbar spine pathology, primarily attributed to progressive changes within the intervertebral discs. Age-related degeneration involves a decline in proteoglycan content, leading to disc desiccation which compromises the disc's capacity to absorb mechanical loads. Over time, tears develop in the annulus fibrosus, the outer fibrous layer of the disc, resulting in structural disruption. This can allow the nucleus pulposus, the inner portion of the disc, to herniate and exert pressure on adjacent neural structures. Advanced DDD stages involve mucoid degeneration, fibrosis, and disc resorption, resulting in a reduction in disc height, increased segmental instability, and susceptibility to injury. Osteophytes may also form along the vertebral body margins as a compensatory response, which can further contribute to spinal rigidity and pain. Additional pathology and associated treatment options will be discussed in subsequent chapters.

Neural Anatomy

In the typical adult, the spinal cord terminates as the conus medullaris around the L1 vertebra (with variations ranging from T11 to L3). Below the conus lie the remaining nerve roots free floating within the thecal sac [22]. Sacral roots are more centralized within the thecal sac, whereas the lumbar roots are more lateral [4]. A summary of nerve roots in the lumbar and upper sacral spine and their corresponding peripheral nerves and functions can be seen in Fig. 1.4 and Table 1.1. Each lumbar spinal nerve exits below its corresponding vertebra—for example, the L4 nerve exits below the L4 vertebra and pedicle through the L4-L5 neural foramen (Fig. 1.2). The lateral and caudal trajectory of the paired nerve roots resembles a pair of arms on a body, which inspired descriptions of the nerve root "shoulder" superiorly, and "axilla" inferiorly. The shoulder of the nerve root is located in the lateral recess of the canal just before the nerve root exits through the foramen. Typically, the corresponding intervertebral disc is just inferior to the nerve root axilla.

Most lumbar disc herniations occur centrally and do not compress the exiting nerve root at the level of the disc. The nerve root most commonly affected by a central disc herniation exits one level below the herniated disc. For example, an

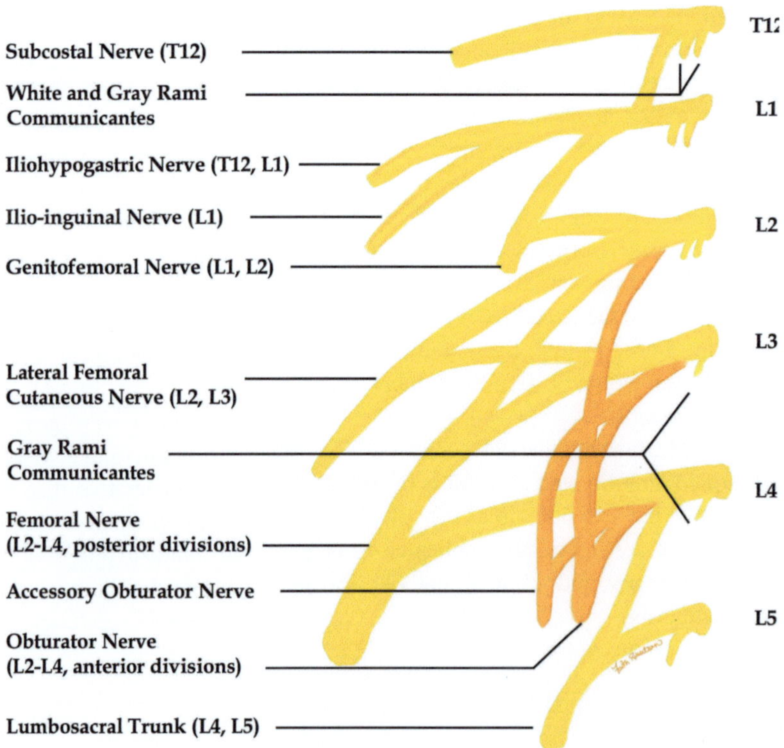

Fig. 1.4 Lumbar plexus nerve anatomy

Table 1.1 Summary of nerve roots in the lumbar and upper sacral spine and their corresponding peripheral nerves and functions

Lumbar nerve root	Peripheral nerve	Muscle innervated	Primary motion/exam test
L1	Iliohypogastric nerve (with contributions from T12), ilioinguinal nerve, genitofemoral nerve	Iliopsoas	Hip flexion
L2	Genitofemoral nerve, lateral femoral cutaneous nerve, femoral nerve, obturator nerve	Iliopsoas, quadriceps	Hip flexion, knee extension
L3	Lateral femoral cutaneous nerve, femoral nerve, obturator nerve	Quadriceps, hip adductors	Knee extension, hip adduction
L4	Deep peroneal nerve, obturator nerve	Quadriceps, tibialis anterior	Knee extension, ankle dorsiflexion
L5	Deep peroneal nerve, superior gluteal nerve	Extensor Hallucis longus, gluteus Medius	Great toe extension, hip abduction
S1	Tibial nerve	Semitendinosus, gastrocnemius, soleus	Knee flexion, ankle plantarflexion

L4-L5 central disc herniation will most commonly compress the L5 nerve root in the lateral recess of the spinal canal. However, in the setting of a far lateral disc herniation, the L4 nerve root may be compressed [23]. This difference is due to the more central position of the traversing spinal nerves compared to the more lateral position of the exiting spinal nerves.

An important anatomical structure when considering far lateral disc herniations is Kambin's Triangle, first introduced in 1973 by Dr. Parviz Kambin [24]. This working zone is bordered anteriorly by the exiting root (the hypotenuse of the triangle), inferiorly by the superior endplate of the lumbar vertebral body below (base of triangle), the superior articulating facet (the height of the triangle), and medially by the traversing nerve root and dural sac (location in space) [25, 26]. More recently, Kambin's prism has been described to recognize the three-dimensional nature of the corridor [26]. Today, this corridor is leveraged for posterolateral nerve root steroid injections, diagnostic discograms, and endoscopic spinal discectomy and fusion surgeries [26].

Vascular Anatomy

The lumbar spine blood supply is primarily provided by four paired lumbar arteries that originate from the abdominal aorta and travel dorsolaterally around the vertebral body and provide the vertebral body blood supply at vertebral levels L1-L4, below which the aorta typically bifurcates into the common iliac arteries [27]. These lumbar arteries subdivide into three branches at the level of the intervertebral foramen: medial, middle, and lateral divisions. The medial branch supplies the lumbar segments of the spinal cord and regional sympathetic ganglia, the middle branch supplies the lumbar joints and spinal muscles, and the lateral branch supplies the abdominal muscles [27].

The artery of Adamkiewicz (AA) is comparable in size and function to the more rostral anterior spinal artery (ASA) (0.5–0.8 mm diameter), making it the largest radiculomedullary artery [4]. The AA generally originates between T8 and L2, predominantly from the left side, and ascends within the spinal canal and forms a characteristic hairpin loop before joining the anterior spinal artery to provide critical blood flow to the anterior two-thirds of the spinal cord. The lumbar plexus is supplied by the iliolumbar artery, which is a branch of the internal iliac artery.

The venous drainage system of the lumbar spine, also commonly referred to as the venous plexus of Batson [28], has a unique quality of valveless veins allowing for pressure gradients to move blood bidirectionally. This quality is important in its function in regulating intraspinal pressure during changes in position, but also has pathologic significance in providing a pathway for hematogenous spread of pelvic metastases and the hematogenous spread of infection, particularly from the prostate, to the spine. Intradural drainage of the spinal cord occurs via retrograde flow through anterior and posterior central veins. This venous outflow exits the dura via anterior and posterior segmental radiculomedullary veins which communicate with the internal vertebral venous plexus in the epidural space.

The internal vertebral venous plexus is a longitudinal network of veins located anteriorly and posteriorly within the epidural space, and communicates with the basivertebral plexus that tunnels horizontally through the vertebral bodies. The external venous plexus includes anterior veins, located anterior to the vertebral bodies, and posterior veins, which are found along the posterior surface of the vertebral arches. Venous drainage from the external vertebral venous plexus largely empties into the ascending lumbar veins and the azygous vein. Lymphatic drainage from the lumbar spine passes through the lumbar lymph nodes, which receive lymph from the common iliac nodes and eventually drain into the thoracic trunk. Less well-studied is the glymphatic system of the spinal cord, which describes the circulation of CSF and waste materials along periarteriolar and venular pathways, and likely contributes to the neuroimmune adaptations of the spinal cord to injury [29].

Attention to the aortic and iliac vasculature is particularly important when considering anterior retroperitoneal spinal surgery. Patients have variable anatomy regarding the position of vessel bifurcation and their tortuosity. Compared to the arterial system the venous system is much more susceptible to variations and congenital malformations, and consequent injury during surgery, so preoperative computed tomography angiography or magnetic resonance imaging can be useful when considering anterior spinal approaches [30].

Conclusion

Lumbar spine anatomy is vulnerable to degenerative changes and mechanical stress, which frequently lead to debilitating conditions like low back pain, lumbar disc herniation, and spinal stenosis. A detailed analysis of lumbar anatomical structures underscores the spine's complex biomechanical demands and highlights the potential for complications in surgical interventions, emphasizing the need for careful preoperative planning. Recognizing anatomical variations and common degenerative changes aids clinicians in making precise clinical decisions, optimizing surgical outcomes, and minimizing risks in treating lumbar spine disorders. Given the increasing prevalence of these issues globally, particularly among the aging population, an understanding of lumbar anatomy is not only essential for surgeons and rehabilitation specialists, but also for all healthcare providers. An appreciation of the lumbar spine's bony, ligamentous, neural, and vascular structures, with a focus on their clinical relevance, is critical to accurately diagnose spinal pathologies and counsel patients on appropriate surgical or non-surgical treatments to alleviate symptoms and restore function.

References

1. Ravindra VM, Senglaub SS, Rattani A, Dewan MC, Härtl R, Bisson E, et al. Degenerative lumbar spine disease: estimating global incidence and worldwide volume. Global Spine J. 2018;8(8):784–94. https://doi.org/10.1177/2192568218770769.
2. Ferreira ML, de Luca K, Haile LM, Steinmetz JD, Culbreth GT, Cross M, et al. Global, regional, and national burden of low back pain, 1990–2013; 2020, its attributable risk factors, and projections to 2050: a systematic analysis of the Global Burden of Disease Study 2021. Lancet Rheumatol. 2023;5(6):e316–e29. https://doi.org/10.1016/S2665-9913(23)00098-X.
3. Parenteau CS, Lau EC, Campbell IC, Courtney A. Prevalence of spine degeneration diagnosis by type, age, gender, and obesity using Medicare data. Sci Rep. 2021;11(1):5389. https://doi.org/10.1038/s41598-021-84724-6.
4. Lollis SS. Chapter 9 – Applied anatomy of the thoracic and lumbar spine. In: Steinmetz MP, Benzel EC, editors. Benzel's spine surgery, 2-volume set (fourth edition). Philadelphia: Elsevier; 2017. p. 95–113.e1.
5. Konin GP, Walz DM. Lumbosacral transitional vertebrae: classification, imaging findings, and clinical relevance. AJNR Am J Neuroradiol. 2010;31(10):1778–86. https://doi.org/10.3174/ajnr.A2036.

6. Witek AM, Khalil A, Krishnaney AA. Chapter 3 – Relevant surgical anatomy of the dorsal lumbar spine. In: Manjila SV, Mroz TE, Steinmetz MP, editors. Lumbar interbody fusions. Elsevier; 2019. p. 19–25.
7. Verma V, Agrawal U Sr. Lumbar pedicle morphometry of dry vertebral columns in relation to transpedicular fixation: a cross-sectional study from Central India. Cureus. 2023;15(4):e38108. https://doi.org/10.7759/cureus.38108.
8. Benzel EC. Biomechanics of spine stabilization. 3rd ed. Thieme/AANS; 2015.
9. Lorenz M, Patwardhan A, Vanderby R Jr. Load-bearing characteristics of lumbar facets in normal and surgically altered spinal segments. Spine (Phila Pa 1976). 1983;8(2):122–30. https://doi.org/10.1097/00007632-198303000-00002.
10. Samartzis D, Cheung JP, Rajasekaran S, Kawaguchi Y, Acharya S, Kawakami M, et al. Critical values of facet joint angulation and tropism in the development of lumbar degenerative spondylolisthesis: an international, large-scale multicenter study by the AOSpine Asia Pacific Research Collaboration Consortium. Global Spine J. 2016;6(5):414–21. https://doi.org/10.1055/s-0035-1564417.
11. Ghogawala Z, Dziura J, Butler WE, Dai F, Terrin N, Magge SN, et al. Laminectomy plus fusion versus laminectomy alone for lumbar spondylolisthesis. N Engl J Med. 2016;374(15):1424–34. https://doi.org/10.1056/NEJMoa1508788.
12. Dai LY. Orientation and tropism of lumbar facet joints in degenerative spondylolisthesis. Int Orthop. 2001;25(1):40–2. https://doi.org/10.1007/s002640000201.
13. Degulmadi D, Dave B, Krishnan A, Patel D. The relationship of facet joint orientation and tropism with lumbar disc herniation and degenerative spondylolisthesis in the lower lumbar spine. Asian Spine J. 2019;13(1):22–8. https://doi.org/10.31616/asj.2018.0116.
14. Blumenthal C, Curran J, Benzel EC, Potter R, Magge SN, Harrington JF Jr, et al. Radiographic predictors of delayed instability following decompression without fusion for degenerative grade I lumbar spondylolisthesis. J Neurosurg Spine. 2013;18(4):340–6. https://doi.org/10.3171/2013.1.Spine12537.
15. Gellhorn AC, Katz JN, Suri P. Osteoarthritis of the spine: the facet joints. Nat Rev Rheumatol. 2013;9(4):216–24. https://doi.org/10.1038/nrrheum.2012.199.
16. Kao CC, Winkler SS, Turner JH. Synovial cyst of spinal facet. Case report. J Neurosurg. 1974;41(3):372–6. https://doi.org/10.3171/jns.1974.41.3.0372.
17. Sabo RA, Tracy PT, Weinger JM. A series of 60 juxtafacet cysts: clinical presentation, the role of spinal instability, and treatment. J Neurosurg. 1996;85(4):560–5. https://doi.org/10.3171/jns.1996.85.4.0560.
18. Deckers K, De Smedt K, Mitchell B, Vivian D, Russo M, Georgius P, et al. New therapy for refractory chronic mechanical low back pain-restorative neurostimulation to activate the lumbar multifidus: one year results of a prospective multicenter clinical trial. Neuromodulation. 2018;21(1):48–55. https://doi.org/10.1111/ner.12741.
19. Alex Vaccaro FK, Fehlings M, Shanmughanathan R. Pedicle screw insertion in the thoracolumbar spine. https://surgeryreference.aofoundation.org/spine/trauma/thoracolumbar/basic-technique/pedicle-screw-insertion (2024). Accessed Sept 2024.
20. Iwanaga J, Ishak B, Saga T, Singla A, Impastato D, Chapman JR, et al. The lumbar Ligamentum Flavum does not have two layers and is confluent with the Interspinous ligament: anatomical study with application to surgical and interventional pain procedures. Clin Anat. 2020;33(1):34–40. https://doi.org/10.1002/ca.23437.
21. Wu L, Munakomi S, Cruz R. Lumbar spinal stenosis. In: StatPearls [Internet]. Treasure Island (FL): StatPearls Publishing; 2024.
22. Soleiman J, Demaerel P, Rocher S, Maes F, Marchal G. Magnetic resonance imaging study of the level of termination of the conus medullaris and the thecal sac: influence of age and gender. Spine (Phila Pa 1976). 2005;30(16):1875–80. https://doi.org/10.1097/01.brs.0000174116.74775.2e.
23. Basit H, Reddy V, Varacallo M. Anatomy, Back, Spinal Nerve-Muscle Innervation. In: StatPearls. Treasure Island (FL): ineligible companies. StatPearls Publishing Copyright © 2024, StatPearls Publishing LLC; 2024.
24. Kambin P, Sampson S. Posterolateral percutaneous suction-excision of herniated lumbar intervertebral discs. Report of interim results. Clin Orthop Relat Res. 1986;207:37–43.
25. Kambin P, Zhou L. History and current status of percutaneous arthroscopic disc surgery. Spine (Phila Pa 1976). 1996;21(24 Suppl):57s–61s. https://doi.org/10.1097/00007632-199612151-00006.
26. Fanous AA, Tumialán LM, Wang MY. Kambin's triangle: definition and new classification schema. J Neurosurg Spine. 2020;32(3):390–8. https://doi.org/10.3171/2019.8.Spine181475.
27. Baaj AA, Mummaneni P, Uribe JS, Vaccaro AR, Greenberg MS. Handbook of Spine Surgery 3 2025 ed. MedOne: Thieme; 2024.
28. Carpenter K, Decater T, Iwanaga J, Maulucci CM, Bui CJ, Dumont AS, et al. Revisiting the vertebral venous plexus-a comprehensive review of the literature. World Neurosurg. 2021;145:381–95. https://doi.org/10.1016/j.wneu.2020.10.004.
29. Gonuguntla S, Herz J. Unraveling the lymphatic system in the spinal cord meninges: a critical element in protecting the central nervous system. Cell Mol Life Sci. 2023;80(12):366. https://doi.org/10.1007/s00018-023-05013-1.
30. Serratrice N, Manchon A, Prost S, Farah K, Bartoli JM, Tropiano P, et al. An updated classification of the anatomical variations of the internal iliac venous drainage system: surgical implications for anterior lumbar spinal approaches. Neurochirurgie. 2024;70(4):101558. https://doi.org/10.1016/j.neuchi.2024.101558.

Biomechanics of the Lumbar Spine

2

Ali Haider Bangash, Reza Yassari,
and Rafael De la Garza Ramos

Biomechanically Relevant Anatomy of the Lumbar Spine

The lowest part of the mobile spine, the lumbar spine, is a location of major biomechanical stress and clinical significance. It is an important area that transitions from the permanent kyphosis of the sacrum to the lordotic curvature of the lumbar region, which then changes to kyphosis in the thoracic spine. Because of its unique location, as well as its function in sustaining the weight of the upper body and allowing for trunk movement, the lumbar spine is subject to significant mechanical stresses. Consequently, it is a region that is especially vulnerable to pathological diseases and degenerative changes. As such, a comprehensive knowledge of its anatomical and biomechanical features is crucial for effective clinical management.

A. H. Bangash · R. Yassari
R. De la Garza Ramos (✉)
Spine Tumor Mechanics and Outcomes Research Lab, Montefiore Medical Center, Albert Einstein College of Medicine, Bronx, NY, USA

Department of Neurosurgery, Montefiore Medical Center, Albert Einstein College of Medicine, Bronx, NY, USA
e-mail: alhaider@montefiore.org; RYASSARI@montefiore.org; rdelag@montefiore.org

Vertebral Body

In relation to other spinal regions, the lumbar vertebral bodies are the largest in size. As one moves from the upper to the lower lumbar levels, their dimensions increase progressively. Table 2.1 provides an overview of the average dimensions of lumbar vertebral bodies [1–3]. The ventral and dorsal heights of the vertebral bodies vary only in the lumbar spine, with the former being higher than the latter [4]. The greater strength and capacity of lumbar vertebral bodies to support weight are correlated with their larger size and volume.

Facet Joints

When an individual is upright, their lumbar facet joints, also known as zygapophyseal joints, can support between 16% and 25% of the compressive stress that passes through the lumbar spine [5]. Especially in flexion, extension, and axial rotation motions, the facet joints are essential for controlling and regulating the range of motion. From L1 to L5, the facet joints' angle with respect to the midline gradually increases [6].

Lamina and Spinal Canal

The laminae create the posterior bony arches of the spinal canal. In order to guarantee appropriate

A. A. Baaj et al. (eds.), *Surgery of the Lumbar Spine*, https://doi.org/10.1007/978-3-032-18097-1_2

neural function and avoid compression or impingement, the dimensions and shape of the lumbar spinal canal are biomechanically significant. From upper to lower lumbar levels, the canal width widens while the depth essentially stays constant [7].

Pedicle

The pedicles are short, cylindrical bony projections that attach the lumbar spine's posterior components (facet joints and laminae) to the vertebral body located anteriorly. Table 2.1 provides an overview of the average dimensions of lumbar pedicles [8, 9]. These dimensions are significant to biomechanics [10]. The lumbar spine's transverse pedicle angle, or the angle formed between the pedicle and the midline in the transverse plane, rises caudally [11]. The pedicles add to the overall stability of the vertebral column by acting as attachment places for a variety of spinal muscles and ligaments.

Intervertebral Disc

In the lumbar spine, the fibrocartilaginous intervertebral discs are situated in between neighboring vertebral bodies. They comprise an annulus fibrosus around the core nucleus pulposus. Concentric layers of fibrous tissue that are positioned at a slight angle of approximately 30° to the vertebral endplates make up the annulus. The inclined orientation of annulus fibers provides them more resistance against rotational loads but poorer resistance against compressive stresses [12]. The discs transfer compressive stresses uniformly over the vertebral endplates, serve as shock absorbers, and provide limited mobility. They have a significant resistance to axial loads, although that decreases with age. The lumbar spine has higher load-bearing requirements than other spinal areas, which is reflected in their larger dimensions [13].

Transverse and Spinous Process

The lumbar vertebrae are characterized by thick, horizontally oriented spinous processes protruding posteriorly and broad, flat transverse processes extending laterally. While spinous processes extend from the laminae junction, transverse processes emerge anteriorly from the lamina-pedicle junction. The quadratus lumborum and interspinous ligaments are two examples of the spinal muscles and ligaments that adhere to these processes. The transverse processes offer leverage for lateral bending, but under heavy loads, they are susceptible to fracture due to limited vascularization [14]. Through their attachments to muscles and ligaments, these mechanisms work together to promote mobility and enhance the stability of the lumbar spine as a whole [14, 15].

Ligaments and Muscles

The ligamentum flavum, longitudinal ligaments, capsular ligaments, and interspinous ligaments are among the ligaments that promote stability to the lumbar spine. The anterior and posterior longitudinal ligaments primarily oppose extension and flexion, respectively, whereas ligaments with longer moment arms, such as the interspinous ligament, offer higher mechanical advantage and flexion resistance [16]. The torso muscles contribute both directly and indirectly to lumbar biomechanics: the erector spinae facilitate extension and lateral bending, the psoas aids in flexion [17], and the rectus abdominis, despite lacking direct spinal attachments, functions as a strong flexor because of its long moment arm from the anterior abdominal wall to the instantaneous axis of rotation (IAR) [18].

Table 2.1 Reported dimensions of lumbar vertebral bodies and pedicles [1–9]

	Vertebral body [1–3]										Pedicle [8, 9]			
Vertebra	Superior Width (M/F) (mm)	Inferior Width (M/F) (mm)	Superior Length (M/F) (mm)	Inferior Length (M/F) (mm)	Anterior Height (M/F) (mm)	Posterior Height (M/F) (mm)	Mean Height (mm)	Mean Width (mm)	Mean Diameter (mm)	Area (mm^2)	Pedicle Width (mm)	Pedicle Height (mm)	Transverse Pedicle Angle (°)	Pedicle axis length (mm)
L1	38.7/32.7	39.7/36.0	29.0/26.6	29.7/25.3	25.0/24.5[a]	26.5/24.5[a]	–	–	–	–	8.2 - 9.2 M/F: 8.4 (±1.8) / 6.5 (±1.6)	15.35–18.2 M/F: 16.7 (±1.6) / 14.8 (±1.3)	M/F: 10.7 (±3.5) / 11.1 (±3.8)	M/F: 54.6 (±4.1) / 49.1 (±3.9)
L2	38.1/33.0	41.1/32.7	28.9/27.1	29.0/26.0	26.5/25.8[a]	27.5/25.3[a]	26.6[b]	49.0[b]	43.6[b]	4010[b]	8.3 - 8.9 M/F: 8.9 (±1.8) / 6.8 (±1.5)	14.71–17.2 M/F: 15.8 (±1.7) / 14.0 (±1.3)	M/F: 11.9 (±4.2) / 10.6 (±3.3)	M/F: 55.4 (±4.4) / 49.4 (±3.4)
L3	40.2/34.7	40.6/37.9	29.7/26.3	30.4/25.4	27.8/27.1	28.4/26.0	35.9	47.2	43.6[b]	1368	10.0 - 10.73 M/F: 10.7 (±2.0) / 8.2 (±1.8)	14.3–16.9 M/F: 15.5 (±1.8) / 13.7 (±1.5)	M/F: 14.2 (±3.8) / 14.0 (±4.1)	M/F: 56.5 (±4.6) / 50.8 (±3.5)
L4	42.4/37.7	48.9/41.1	28.9/26.1	30.6/28.1	30.27 ± 1.17	28.73 ± 0.99	26.6[b]	50.3 ± 0.26	43.6[b]	4010[b]	12.5–14.7 M/F: 12.5 (±2.0) / 10.3 (±1.7)	13.55–15.6 M/F: 14.2 (±2.0) / 12.7 (±1.6)	M/F: 16.0 (±4.2) / 16.9 (±4.7)	M/F: 56.0 (±4.4) / 51.1 (±3.6)
L5	43.9/38.1	46.6/41.8	27.6/27.7	27.4/25.1	27.5/27.0[a]	27.0/25.0[a]	–	–	–	–	17.32 - 20.1 M/F: 16.4 (±2.6) / 14.1 (±2.1)	13.49–16.2 M/F: 13.3 (±1.8) / 12.1 (±1.6)	M/F: 25.4 (±5.6) / 27.4 (±6.3)	M/F: 54.0 (±5.1) / 50.5 (±3.9)

Values provided as mean (with standard deviations, where reported)
[a]Estimated values based on trends and available data
[b]Mean values for L2-L4

Bone

The primary weight-bearing elements of the lower spine are the lumbar vertebral bodies, with their dimensions proportional to the loads they support. The weight-bearing capacity is influenced by the ratio of cortical to cancellous bone, which is higher in the pedicles than in the vertebral bodies [19].

Basics of Physics and Kinematic Principles in Lumbar Spine Biomechanics

Fundamental Physical Concepts

Several basic physical principles influence the biomechanics of the lumbar spine. External stresses on the lumbar spine include shear, tension, and compression forces. These forces may be shown as vectors in three dimensions, with fixed orientations (Fig. 2.1). Moments indicate rotational forces operating on lumbar vertebrae, frequently as a result of muscle activity or external pressures, and are an important concept in lumbar spine biomechanics [20].

Moment arms, which are closely associated with moments, are the perpendicular distances between a point and a force's line of action (Fig. 2.1). If a force is applied at a given distance from a fulcrum, a bending moment is created. The bending moment applied to a point in space causes rotation, or a tendency to rotate, about an axis, called the IAR [21]. The IAR moves depending on the loads and forces applied. At every instant, there is a hypothetical line in the human body that does not move, and around which all other movement occurs. In the lumbar spine, the IAR usually passes through or at least close to the vertebral body (Fig. 2.2). It is imperative to note that the IAR can change because of movement, disease (degenerative disease, trauma, infection, tumor, etc.), or instrumentation (Fig. 2.3).

Kinematics of the Lumbar Spine

With six degrees of freedom—three translational (anterior-posterior, medial-lateral, superior-inferior) and three rotational (flexion-extension, lateral bending, axial rotation)—the lumbar spine has complex kinematics. The idea of IAR is essential to understand lumbar spine kinematics. At any one time, every lumbar vertebral segment rotates around the IAR [22]. Its dynamic placement affects phenomena including neuroforaminal compression or decompression during spinal motions, which has important consequences for spinal function.

The lumbar spine exhibits two significant kinematic phenomena: coupling and paradoxical motion. Unexpected segmental movement that can occur while implementing specific stabilizing procedures or in cases of lumbar instability is referred to as "paradoxical motion" [22]. Coupling, specific to the lumbar region, describes how spinous processes rotate in tandem with the concave side of the bend during lateral bending [4]. These ideas are essential to comprehending both typical lumbar spine function and pathological conditions.

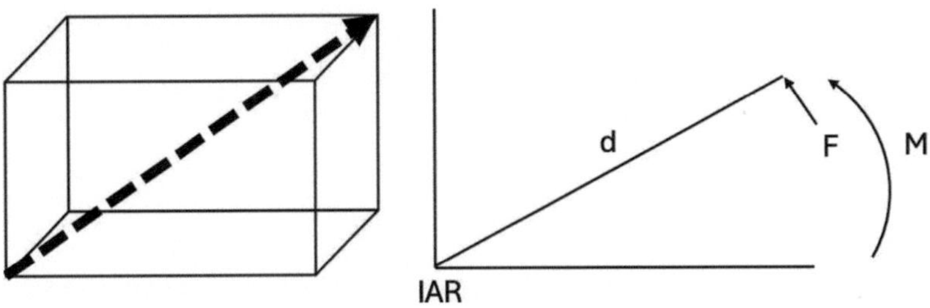

Fig. 2.1 Left: A force is a vector in three-dimensional space. Right: A bending moment (M) is created by applying a force (F) at a distance (d) from a fulcrum, in this case called an Instantaneous Axis of Rotation. (Images copyright of Rafael De la Garza Ramos)

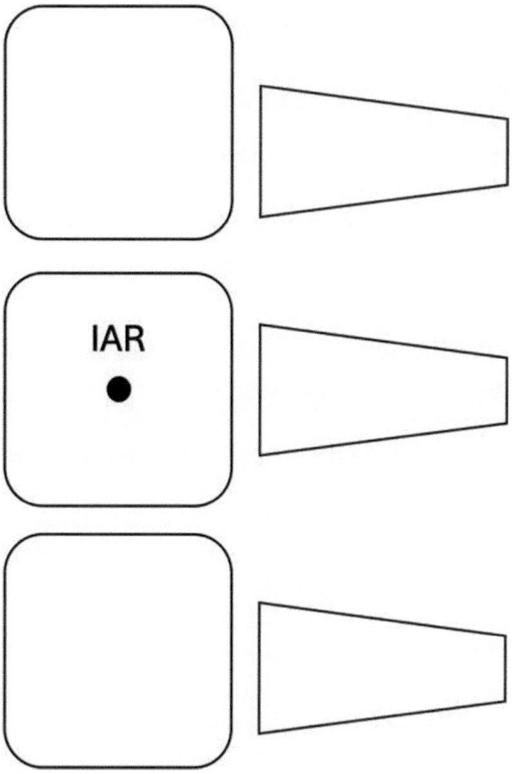

Fig. 2.2 The Instantaneous Axis of Rotation is usually found in the vertebral body when standing. (Images copyright of Rafael De la Garza Ramos)

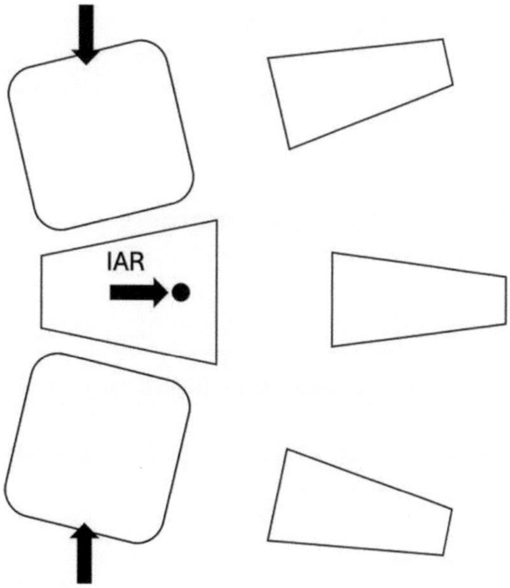

Fig. 2.3 The Instantaneous Axis of Rotation moves dorsally when a compressive force is applied in the ventral vertebral body, as is the case in a compression fracture. As a general rule of thumb, the IAR moves in the direction of the non-pathologic tissue. (Images copyright of Rafael De la Garza Ramos)

Biomechanical Principles

The lumbar spine behaves in accordance with several basic biomechanical principles. The basis for comprehending how the lumbar spine reacts to outside pressures and collisions is provided by Newton's Laws of Motion. For the analysis of load distribution, the idea of force pairs—equal and opposing forces acting on the lumbar spine—is essential. Similarly, couples play a part in the biomechanics of the lumbar spine. Couples are pairings of equal and opposing pressures that produce rotation without translation [23].

The load-deformation curve and Hooke's Law are crucial for comprehending the mechanical behavior of lumbar spine structures. The neutral zone—where tiny pressures produce huge displacements—has special significance for the flexibility of the lumbar spine. The elastic limit denotes the point beyond which spinal tissues permanently deform, whereas the elastic zone denotes the area where lumbar structural deformation is reversible. The lumbar spine tissues and implant materials may both be measured for stiffness using the elastic modulus [24].

The Functional Spinal Unit in the Lumbar Spine

A key idea in lumbar spine biomechanics is the Functional Spinal Unit (FSU). It is made up of the intervertebral disc that sits between two neighboring lumbar vertebrae, as well as the associated ligaments. The FSU includes several key components: vertebral bodies, intervertebral disc, facet joints, and ligaments. Comprehending the FSU is essential as it provides the foundation for understanding localized lumbar spine mechanics and acts as a building block for delving into more intricate, multi-segment lumbar spine biomechanics [25].

Gaining knowledge of these concepts offers a thorough foundation for examining the biomechanics of the lumbar spine in both healthy and pathological states.

Spinal Instability in Disorders of the Lumbar Spine

A key idea in lumbar spine biomechanics is spinal instability, which is frequently brought on by a variety of clinical diseases. It's crucial to understand that spinal stability is not an absolute condition, but rather a continuum. With an emphasis on biomechanical data, this section examines the roles that disc degeneration, spinal stenosis, trauma, and tumors play in lumbar spine instability.

Simply put, spinal instability has been defined as "the inability to limit excessive or abnormal spinal displacement that would cause neurologic deficits, deformity, or pain under normal physiologic loads" [26]. Four kinds of instability may be distinguished: overt instability and restricted instability (both acute); as well as glacial instability and instability linked to maladaptive segmental motion (both chronic) [27]. These categories are not distinct from each other and may overlap in clinical presentations [26, 27] (Table 2.2). Comprehending these classifications is essential for appropriate clinical decision-making and management planning.

Chronic instability caused by disc degeneration frequently takes the form of either glacial instability or abnormal segmental motion in the lumbar spine. Discs lose height and hydration when they degenerate, which modifies the biomechanics of FSU [26, 28, 29] (Table 2.3). An extended applied moment arm in cases of glacial instability may promote the evolution of deformity by an increased length of an applied moment arm, exacerbated by dorsal ligamentous laxity. Due to this biomechanical disadvantage, there may be a "deformity begets deformity" situation. For instance, if axial loading causes a kyphotic deformity, the stress concentration in the ventral vertebral body area may increase the deformity [31].

Table 2.2 Types of spinal instability in the lumbar spine [26, 27]

Type	Timeframe	Description	Key characteristics
Overt instability	Acute	Severe loss of spinal integrity	Immediate risk of neurological injury or deformity Often traumatic in origin Requires urgent intervention
Limited instability	Acute	Loss of either ventral or dorsal spinal integrity with preservation of the other	Ventral: Isolated endplate or vertebral body fractures, true burst fractures Dorsal: Ligamentous (spinal strain) or bony (laminar or facet fracture) Score of 5 or more points on instability scale
Glacial instability	Chronic	Gradual progression of deformity over time	Not overt, but progresses over months or years Can manifest as progressive translational, rotational, or angular deformity Often associated with spondylolisthesis Causes: Spondylosis, trauma, tumor, congenital defects, infection
Dysfunctional segmental motion	Chronic	Abnormal motion patterns at specific spinal segments	Often associated with disc degeneration or spinal stenosis May present with mechanical back pain Can lead to accelerated degenerative changes May not be apparent on static imaging

Note: These categories are not mutually exclusive and may overlap in clinical presentations. Assessment should consider both biomechanical data and clinical judgment

Table 2.3 Biomechanical changes in common lumbar spine pathologies [26, 28–30]

Pathology	Biomechanical changes	Quantitative data
Disc degeneration	Increased range of motion Altered load distribution Reduced nuclear pressure Increased facet joint loading	Disc height loss: Up to 3–4 mm Flexion-extension increase: 59% Lateral bending increase: 43% Axial rotation increase: 31% Nuclear pressure reduction: 0.5 MPa to 0.1 MPa Facet joint load increase: Up to 70%
Spinal stenosis	Reduced spinal canal area Increased facet joint forces Ligamentum flavum hypertrophy Potential for reduced intersegmental motion	Spinal canal area reduction: 30–50% Facet joint force increase: Up to 2.5 times normal in extension Ligamentum flavum thickness increase: From 3 mm to 6–8 mm Flexion-extension decrease: Up to 40%
Traumatic injuries	Loss of anterior column height Increased range of motion in all planes Ligamentous disruption leading to abnormal movement	Anterior column height loss (burst fractures): Up to 50% Range of motion increase: 200–300% in all planes Posterior ligament complex disruption: Flexion increase by avg. 18° Anterior longitudinal ligament rupture: Extension increase by avg. 2.5°
Spinal tumors	Weakened vertebral body structure Reduced compression strength Compromised torsional strength with pedicle involvement	25–50% vertebral body involvement: Compression strength reduced by 55–70% >50% involvement: Significantly increased risk of pathological fracture Unilateral pedicle destruction: Torsional strength reduced by 21.9% Bilateral pedicle destruction: Torsional strength reduced by 54.3%

Note: These biomechanical changes can vary based on the severity of the pathology and individual patient factors. The quantitative data presented represents typical findings from biomechanical studies

This idea is illustrated biomechanically by the longer moment arm that develops with increasing deformity. Axial loads exert an increasingly greater bending moment as the deformity grows, which causes the spine to be eccentrically loaded which accentuates the deformity even further. As a result, stress is concentrated on the concave side of the curve, which may hasten instability and degenerative processes [32]. The Cobb angle measurement can be used to quantify the degree of angular deformities. This idea may be used to lumbar spine anomalies in the sagittal plane, albeit it is mostly employed for scoliosis [33]. The moment arm length applied to the spine increases with the Cobb angle, potentially exacerbating instability. It's crucial to note that due to differences in the radius of curvature, equivalent Cobb angles may indicate varying degrees of instability at the segmental level.

Apart from these modifications, variations in the IAR and Center of Rotation may also be indicative of instability in the lumbar segments [34]. Unusual fluctuations in these metrics indicate modified biomechanics and possible instability, even in cases when overall motion seems normal through routine imaging. These changes in biomechanics frequently result in mechanical instability, which is typified by pain that worsens when standing or moving, caused by spinal loading. The inability of the spine to withstand typical physiological pressures because of instability is reflected in this pattern of pain [26]. It is noteworthy that the existence of notable lumbar degenerative changes may indicate a history of improper segmental mobility. Even if the current imaging reveals restricted mobility because of severe degeneration, the high stressors or motion that caused these degenerative alterations point to a history of instability [35].

Chronic instability can result from spinal stenosis, which narrows the spinal canal or neural foramina and changes the spine's biomechanics.

Frequently, this shows up as dysfunctional segmental motion [26, 30] (Table 2.3). When diagnosing defective motion segments linked to spinal stenosis or other types of instability, dynamic radiographs (flexion and extension) may be helpful. Although no universal consensus exists, movement of ≥4 mm is typically indicative of radiographic instability. It is imperative to understand that while pain and muscular guarding might conceal underlying instability, the lack of excessive movement on these imaging does not always rule out instability. Even while MRI is essential for stenosis diagnosis, it is not always reliable for identifying instability, particularly in chronic cases [36]. Because of its high sensitivity to degenerative changes, MRI can occasionally cause instability to be overestimated. For a thorough evaluation of lumbar instability, flexion-extension radiographs are among the imaging modalities that are frequently required [37].

The body frequently adjusts to instability by inducing an amplification of the reflex muscle reaction, which enhances stability. Although this might improve stability momentarily, over time it can also cause muscular fatigue and worsen discomfort. A key component of spinal stability is muscle. Due to their attachment to structures ventral to the spinal column, the rectus abdominis and related ventral abdominal wall muscles significantly stabilize the lumbar spine [38]. When degeneration or injury weakens the passive stabilizing systems, the muscle support becomes even more crucial. Additionally, opposing muscle groups including the rectus abdominis and erector spinae can work in harmony to greatly improve spinal stability. Acting as dynamic stabilizers of the spine, these muscles produce a stabilizing effect without causing motion when they contract concurrently with a comparable force.

Since they disturb the osteoligamentous components, traumatic lesions to the lumbar spine might result in acute overt instability or limited instability [26] (Table 2.3). Traumatic instability can also present as aberrant pivoting motions in addition to translational movements. For an accurate diagnosis, these intricate motion patterns may be difficult to identify with conventional imaging and may require advanced biomechanical analysis. Furthermore, spinal tumors provide a unique challenge as they can damage the structure of the vertebral body and change the biomechanics of the afflicted spinal segment, which can result in either acute or chronic instability. The extent of instability depends on the degree of vertebral body involvement [26] (Table 2.3).

It is challenging to assess lumbar spine instability in spite of these biomechanical findings. The capacity of spine to correct for instability and the complex interplay of static and dynamic stabilizers make objective measurement challenging. This difficulty emphasizes how crucial it is to match clinical presentation with biomechanical data for accurate diagnosis and management planning in cases of lumbar spine instability [37].

Surgical Considerations and Instrumentation of the Lumbar Spine

Decompression Procedures

The biomechanics of the spine can be dramatically changed by surgical intervention. Although decompression procedures including laminectomy and laminotomy are frequently used to relieve neural compression, they can have variable effects on spinal stability.

By reducing the posterior tension band during a laminectomy procedure, for example, the IAR may move ventrally and cause greater flexion [26]. There is a risk of postoperative instability and increased segmental mobility, especially in flexion-extension, particularly if more than 50% of the facet joints are removed [26]. A laminotomy, on the other hand, which entails removing part of the lamina, usually has less of an effect on spinal biomechanics. It has a lesser risk of postoperative instability and retains more of the posterior tension band [26]. Though not as much as laminectomy, it can nonetheless result in modest increases in segmental mobility.

Facetectomy can have a significant effect on spinal stability, especially if it is done bilaterally. While unilateral facetectomy has less of an effect, it can still result in unequal loading and possible instability. Bilateral facetectomy can increase range of motion between flexion and extension by up to 300% [26]. These biomechanical changes highlight the significance of meticulous surgical planning and may necessitate stabilizing techniques in addition to decompression.

Spinal Fixation Procedures

Lumbar spine instrumentation may be required if instability is evident or expected after decompression. The gold standard for lumbar fixation is a pedicle screw, which connects the posterior parts to the vertebral body with a strong anchor point. Comprehending the lumbar vertebral architecture in detail is essential for comprehending the surgical anatomy involved in screw insertion. The pedicle creates a natural corridor for screw placement by acting as a cylindrical bridge between the anterior and posterior columns of spine [26, 39, 40] (Table 2.4).

Certain advanced principles become pertinent in the setting of instrumentation for the lumbar spine. An indicator of the strength of lumbar implants, such as screws and rods, is the section modulus (Z). The moment of inertia (I) characterizes the stiffness of lumbar spine implants, whereas stress (θ) is essential for forecasting lumbar implant failure. These ideas influence the selection and design of lumbar instrumentation and aid in the prediction and prevention of lumbar implant failure [41]. In order to maximize biomechanical stability and minimize complications, screw design has undergone tremendous evolution. The majority of contemporary pedicle screws are, therefore, composed of titanium or stainless steel with several key design features [26, 42–44] (Table 2.5).

Enhancing spinal stability is a major function of spinal instrumentation, with its application guided by biomechanical principles and the specific type of instability encountered. The concept of IAR is central to comprehend the biomechanical implications of instrumentation and spinal disease. Studies have indicated that a dorsal shift of the IAR is usually caused by a loss of ventral axial load-bearing capacity, whereas a ventral IAR shift is caused by a reduced dorsal axial load-bearing ability. These shifts are predictable; in general, the IAR moves in the direction of the non-pathologic neutral axis [26]. To

Table 2.4 Key anatomical considerations of lumbar vertebral pedicles [26, 39, 40]

Anatomical features	Key considerations
Pedicle dimensions	The pedicle width and height vary across lumbar levels, typically being narrowest at L5. Accurate preoperative measurement is crucial to select appropriate screw sizes
Pedicle angle	The medial angulation of pedicles increases in the lower lumbar levels. At L1, the angle is approximately 0–10 degrees, increasing to 20–30 degrees at L5. This requires careful adjustment of the trajectory during screw insertion
Proximity to neural structures	The exiting nerve root lies in close proximity to the pedicle, especially at L5. The medial wall of the pedicle borders the spinal canal, emphasizing the need for precise screw placement to avoid neurological injury
Cortical thickness	The lateral wall of the pedicle is typically thicker than the medial wall, influencing the preferred direction of any breach

Table 2.5 Key design factors of lumbar pedicle screws [26, 42–44]

Screw design features	Specifications
Thread design	Dual-lead threads increase the bone-screw interface, enhancing pullout strength. Variable thread pitch can improve purchase in different bone densities
Core diameter	A larger core diameter increases bending and torsional strength but may decrease pullout strength. A balance is necessary based on bone quality and loading expectations
Head design	Polyaxial heads allow for easier rod seating and can accommodate minor misalignments, while monoaxial screws provide more rigidity and may be preferred in deformity correction
Cannulation	Cannulated screws facilitate placement over a guidewire, which can be particularly useful in minimally invasive techniques or in revision surgeries

properly restore stability, these biomechanical alterations must be considered in the choice and configuration of spinal instrumentation. Critical considerations in this process are the load-bearing and load-sharing characteristics. For instance, posterior instrumentation may be required to sustain a larger amount of the axial stress in situations with anterior column deficit. This may require more robust constructs or additional points of fixation. On the other hand, anterior column support can be required in situations of posterior element deficiency in order to avoid placing undue strain on posterior instrumentation [26]. By utilizing these biomechanical concepts, surgeons may customize instrumentation tactics to particular pathologies, maximizing stability and lowering the risk of neighboring segment degeneration or construct failure [45] (Fig. 2.3).

In lumbar fusion surgery, pseudoarthrosis—failure of solid bony fusion—remains a significant concern. Smoking, osteoporosis, multi-level fusions, and inadequate stabilizations are risk factors [46]. From a biomechanical perspective, bone production may be hampered by micromotion at the fusion site. Both adequate load sharing between the anterior and posterior columns and adequate compression over the fusion site are critical. Careful endplate preparation is one strategy to reduce the likelihood of pseudoarthrosis. A delicate balance is required because excessive micromotion (usually >150 μm) at the fusion site might encourage the production of fibrous tissue rather than bone, whereas some micromotion (<60 μm) may actually induce bone formation [26]. By promoting osteoblast activity and improving bone-to-bone contact, appropriate compression promotes osteogenesis. By appropriate load sharing between the anterior and posterior columns, it is ensured that neither the implants nor the developing fusion mass experiences undue stress.

Arthrodesis

A favorable biological environment for fusion is promoted by thorough decortication of endplates, which enhances the surface area for fusion and exposes the vascular subchondral bone [47]. Optimal implant selection, biological augmentation, smoking cessation, osteoporosis management, and nutritional optimization are additional strategies to reduce pseudoarthrosis risk. Selecting implants—such as dynamic stabilization devices or interbody cages with the right amount of stiffness—that offer sufficient stability while permitting some advantageous micromotion might be helpful [43]. In individuals who are at high risk, the administration of growth hormones including BMP-2 or use of bone graft substitutes can improve the rate of fusion [48]. Taking into account augmentation methods such as cement augmentation or larger diameter screws ensures proper fixation in patients with low bone quality [49].

Segmental Alignment

The natural lordosis of the lumbar spine is important for preserving overall sagittal alignment and balance, which is necessary for effective, pain-free walking and posture. Loss of lumbar lordosis may result in compensatory processes that impair function and produce discomfort, such as thoracic hypokyphosis or pelvic retroversion [50]. Moreover, correct alignment reduces the energy expenditure during standing and walking by enabling optimal function of the paraspinal musculature. Currently, some research efforts have gone into better understanding the importance of segmental (i.e., level by level) alignment. For example, it is agreed upon that most of the lumbar lordosis happens between L4 and S1. Although this is an area of ongoing research, early evidence suggests that insufficient sagittal segmental correction may increase the risk of adjacent segment disease, particularly in cases in which the lordosis between L4 and L5 or between L5 and S1 is suboptimal [51, 52]. This is likely due to altered spinal biomechanics and stress concentration at the adjacent disk segments [52].

Individuals who have their sagittal equilibrium restored have improved functional outcomes, including walking distance and daily living activity performance [53]. The sense of self and general mental health of patients might be positively impacted by improved posture and reduced pain [54]. These elements work together to improve the quality of life for lumbar spine surgery patients, highlighting the significance of achieving and maintaining optimal alignment.

References

1. Masharawi Y, Salame K, Mirovsky Y, Peleg S, Dar G, Steinberg N, et al. Vertebral body shape variation in the thoracic and lumbar spine: characterization of its asymmetry and wedging. Clin Anat N Y N. 2008;21(1):46–54.
2. Ruyssen-Witrand A, Gossec L, Kolta S, Dougados M, Roux C. Vertebral dimensions as risk factor of vertebral fracture in osteoporotic patients: a systematic literature review. Osteoporos Int J Establ Result Coop Eur Found Osteoporos Natl Osteoporos Found USA. 2007;18(9):1271–8.
3. van der Houwen EB, Baron P, Veldhuizen AG, Burgerhof JGM, van Ooijen PMA, Verkerke GJ. Geometry of the intervertebral volume and vertebral endplates of the human spine. Ann Biomed Eng. 2010;38(1):33–40.
4. Galbusera F. Chapter 14 – Biomechanics of the spine. In: Innocenti B, Galbusera F, editors. Human Orthopaedic Biomechanics [Internet]. Academic; 2022 [cited 2024 Aug 26]. pp 265–83. Available from: https://www.sciencedirect.com/science/article/pii/B9780128244814000196.
5. Kapetanakis S, Gkantsinikoudis N. Anatomy of lumbar facet joint: a comprehensive review. Folia Morphol (Warsz). 2021;80(4):799–805.
6. Van den Heuvel SAS, Cohen SPC, de Andrès AJ, Van Boxem K, Kallewaard JW, Van Zundert J. 3. Pain originating from the lumbar facet joints. Pain Pract Off J World Inst Pain. 2024;24(1):160–76.
7. Griffith JF. Advanced quantitative spine imaging. Semin Musculoskelet Radiol. 2020;24:413–27.
8. Morita K, Ohashi H, Kawamura D, Tani S, Karagiozov K, Murayama Y. Thoracic and lumbar spine pedicle morphology in Japanese patients. Surg Radiol Anat SRA. 2021;43(6):833–42.
9. Wang Y, Kahaer A, Shi W, Guo H, Rexiti P. Morphometric measurement of lumbar pedicle in different regions: a systematic review. J Orthop Surg [Internet]. 2023 [cited 2024 Oct 20];18(1). Available from: https://pubmed.ncbi.nlm.nih.gov/36631862/.
10. Hashmi SS, Seifert KD, Massoud TF. Thoracic and lumbosacral spine anatomy. Neuroimaging Clin N Am. 2022;32(4):889–902.
11. Upendra B, Raghavendra R. Techniques of cervical pedicle screw insertion in lower cervical spine – a review. J Clin Orthop Trauma. 2020;11(5):794–801.
12. Guardado AA, Baker A, Weightman A, Hoyland JA, Cooper G. Lumbar intervertebral disc herniation: annular closure devices and key design requirements. Bioeng Basel Switz. 2022;9(2):47.
13. McMorran JG, Gregory DE. The influence of axial compression on the cellular and mechanical function of spinal tissues; emphasis on the nucleus pulposus and annulus fibrosus: a review. J Biomech Eng. 2021;143(5):050802.
14. Ma Q, Miri Z, Haugen HJ, Moghanian A, Loca D. Significance of mechanical loading in bone fracture healing, bone regeneration, and vascularization. J Tissue Eng. 2023;14:20417314231172573.
15. Galbusera F, Bassani T. The spine: a strong, stable, and flexible structure with biomimetics potential. Biomim Basel Switz. 2019;4(3):60.
16. Porrino J, Rao A, Moran J, Wang A, Grauer J, Haims A, et al. Current concepts of spondylosis and posterior spinal motion preservation for radiologists. Skeletal Radiol. 2021;50(11):2169–84.
17. Edwards N, Dickin C, Wang H. Low back pain and golf: a review of biomechanical risk factors. Sports Med Health Sci. 2020;2(1):10–8.
18. Suo M, Zhou L, Wang J, Huang H, Zhang J, Sun T, et al. The application of surface electromyography technology in evaluating paraspinal muscle function. Diagn Basel Switz. 2024;14(11):1086.
19. Chaddha R, Agrawal G, Koirala S, Ruparel S. Osteoporosis and vertebral column. Indian J Orthop. 2023;57(1):163–75.
20. Zhang C, Mannen EM, Sis HL, Cadel ES, Wong BM, Wang W, et al. Moment-rotation behavior of intervertebral joints in flexion-extension, lateral bending, and axial rotation at all levels of the human spine: a structured review and meta-regression analysis. J Biomech. 2020;100:109579.
21. Lerchl T, Nispel K, Baum T, Bodden J, Senner V, Kirschke JS. Multibody models of the thoracolumbar spine: a review on applications, limitations, and challenges. Bioeng Basel Switz. 2023;10(2):202.
22. D'Aprile P, Tarantino A. Biomechanics of the spine. In: D'Aprile P, Tarantino A, editors. MRI of degenerative disease of the spine: a case-based atlas [Internet]. Cham: Springer International Publishing; 2021 [cited 2024 Aug 26]. p. 3–9. Available from: https://doi.org/10.1007/978-3-030-73707-8_1.
23. Alderink GJ, Ashby BM. Lumbopelvic region: chronic low Back pain. In: Alderink GJ, Ashby BM, editors. Clinical kinesiology and biomechanics: a problem-based learning approach [Internet]. Cham: Springer International Publishing; 2023 [cited 2024 Aug 26]. p. 205–43. Available from: https://doi.org/10.1007/978-3-031-25322-5_9.
24. Brill SH, Chong JH, Kim D, Cho W. Spine surgery—part I: biomechanics, materials, and 3-D printing technology: surgical perspective and clinical impact. In: Choi AH, Ben-Nissan B, editors. Innovative bioceramics in translational medicine II: surgical appli-

cations [Internet]. Singapore: Springer; 2022 [cited 2024 Aug 26]. p. 209–29. Available from: https://doi.org/10.1007/978-981-16-7439-6_10.
25. Talukdar RG, Mukhopadhyay KK, Dhara S, Gupta S. Numerical analysis of the mechanical behaviour of intact and implanted lumbar functional spinal units: effects of loading and boundary conditions. Proc Inst Mech Eng [H]. 2021;235(7):792–804.
26. Kehr P, Edward C. Benzel: biomechanics of spine stabilization. Eur J Orthop Surg Traumatol. 2015;25(7):1219.
27. Ko HY. Biomechanics of the spine and spinal cord and pathophysiology of spinal cord injuries. In: Ko HY, editor. A practical guide to care of spinal cord injuries: clinical questions and answers [Internet]. Singapore: Springer Nature; 2023 [cited 2024 Aug 26]. p. 83–100. Available from: https://doi.org/10.1007/978-981-99-4542-9_5.
28. Pradeep K, Pal B. Biomechanical and clinical studies on lumbar spine fusion surgery: a review. Med Biol Eng Comput. 2023;61(3):617–34.
29. Desmoulin GT, Pradhan V, Milner TE. Mechanical aspects of intervertebral disc injury and implications on biomechanics. Spine. 2020;45(8):E457–64.
30. Anderson B, Shahidi B. The impact of spine pathology on posterior ligamentous complex structure and function. Curr Rev Musculoskelet Med. 2023;16(12):616–26.
31. Tempel ZJ, Hlubek RJ, Kachmann MC, Body A, Okonkwo DO, Kanter AS, et al. Novel distributed loading technique using multimaterial, long-segment spinal constructs to prevent proximal junctional pathology in adult spinal deformity correction-operative technique and radiographic findings. World Neurosurg. 2021;155:e264–70.
32. Zhang L, Zhang Q, Zhang Y, Arthur M, Teo EC, Bíró I, et al. The effect of concave-side intertransverse ligament laxity on the stress of ais lumbar spine based on finite element method. Bioeng Basel Switz. 2022;9(12):724.
33. Iii WS, Orías AAE, Shifflett GD, Lee JYB, Siemionow K, Gandhi S, et al. Image-based markers predict dynamic instability in lumbar degenerative spondylolisthesis. Neurospine. 2020;17(1):221–7.
34. Allais R, Capart A, Da Silva A, Boiron O. Biomechanical consequences of the intervertebral disc centre of rotation kinematics during lateral bending and axial rotation. Sci Rep. 2023;13(1):3172.
35. Swanson BT, Creighton D. The degenerative lumbar disc: not a disease, but still an important consideration for OMPT practice: a review of the history and science of discogenic instability. J Man Manip Ther. 2020;28(4):191–200.
36. Kobesova A, Kolar P, Andel R, Kyncl M, Stulik J, Davidek P, et al. Dynamic magnetic resonance imaging assisted diagnosis of occult spinal instability—a new useful approach. J Med Imaging Health Inform. 2020;10(11):2649–53.
37. Wang Y, Huang K. Research progress of diagnosing methodology for lumbar segmental instability: a narrative review. Medicine (Baltimore). 2022;101(1):e28534.
38. Bonnel F, Dimeglio A. Vertebral column: muscles, aponeurosis, and fascia. In: Vital JM, Cawley DT, editors. Spinal anatomy: modern concepts [Internet]. Cham: Springer International Publishing; 2020 [cited 2024 Aug 26]. p. 279–320. Available from: https://doi.org/10.1007/978-3-030-20925-4_20.
39. Rosinski AA, Mittal A, Odeh K, Ungurean V, Leasure J, Telles C, et al. Alternatives to traditional pedicle screws for posterior fixation of the degenerative lumbar spine. JBJS Rev. 2021;9(7)
40. Lopez CD, Boddapati V, Lee NJ, Dyrszka MD, Sardar ZM, Lehman RA, et al. Three-dimensional printing for preoperative planning and pedicle screw placement in adult spinal deformity: a systematic review. Glob Spine J. 2021;11(6):936–49.
41. Ebrahimkhani M, Arjmand N, Shirazi-Adl A. Adjacent segments biomechanics following lumbar fusion surgery: a musculoskeletal finite element model study. Eur Spine J Off Publ Eur Spine Soc Eur Spinal Deform Soc Eur Sect Cerv Spine Res Soc. 2022;31(7):1630–9.
42. Kim KT, Song MG, Park YJ, Lee DY, Kim DH. Cortical trajectory screw fixation in lumbar spine surgery: a review of the existing literature. Asian Spine J. 2022;16(1):127–40.
43. Jain P, Rana M, Biswas JK, Khan MR. Biomechanics of spinal implants-a review. Biomed Phys Eng Express. 2020;6(4):042002.
44. Cheers GM, Weimer LP, Neuerburg C, Arnholdt J, Gilbert F, Thorwächter C, et al. Advances in implants and bone graft types for lumbar spinal fusion surgery. Biomater Sci. 2024;12(19):4875–902.
45. Marciano GF, Simhon ME, Lehman RA, Lenke LG. Strategies to avoid distal junctional pathology. Neurosurg Clin N Am. 2023;34(4):585–97.
46. Veronesi F, Sartori M, Griffoni C, Valacco M, Tedesco G, Davassi PF, et al. Complications in spinal fusion surgery: a systematic review of clinically used cages. J Clin Med. 2022;11(21):6279.
47. Dowling Á, Lewandrowski KU. Endoscopic transforaminal lumbar interbody fusion with a single oblique PEEK cage and posterior supplemental fixation. Int J Spine Surg. 2020;14(s3):S45–55.
48. Feng JT, Yang XG, Wang F, He X, Hu YC. Efficacy and safety of bone substitutes in lumbar spinal fusion: a systematic review and network meta-analysis of randomized controlled trials. Eur Spine J Off Publ Eur Spine Soc Eur Spinal Deform Soc Eur Sect Cerv Spine Res Soc. 2020;29(6):1261–76.
49. Kanno H, Onoda Y, Hashimoto K, Aizawa T, Ozawa H. Innovation of surgical techniques for screw fixation in patients with osteoporotic spine. J Clin Med. 2022;11(9):2577.

50. Cheung JPY. The importance of sagittal balance in adult scoliosis surgery. Ann Transl Med. 2020;8(2):35.
51. Daniels AH, Balmaceno-Criss M, McDonald CL, Singh M, Knebel A, Kuharski MJ, et al. Segmental sagittal alignment in lumbar spinal fusion: a review of evidence-based evaluation of preoperative measurement, surgical planning, intraoperative execution, and postoperative evaluation. Oper Neurosurg Hagerstown Md. 2024;27(5):533–48.
52. Diebo BG, Balmaceno-Criss M, Lafage R, McDonald CL, Alsoof D, Halayqeh S, et al. Sagittal alignment in the degenerative lumbar spine: surgical planning. J Bone Joint Surg Am. 2024;106(5):445–57.
53. Lee BH, Park JO, Kim HS, Suk KS, Lee SY, Lee HM, et al. Spinal sagittal balance status affects postoperative actual falls and quality of life after decompression and fusion in-situ surgery in patients with lumbar spinal stenosis. Clin Neurol Neurosurg. 2016;148:52–9.
54. Sakaguchi T, Gunjotikar S, Tanaka M, Komatsubara T, Latka K, Ekade SJ, et al. Evaluation and rehabilitation after adult lumbar spine surgery. J Clin Med. 2024;13(10):2915.

Epidemiology and Healthcare Burden of Lumbar Degenerative Spine Disease

3

Abraham Dada, Vivian Kwok, and Anthony DiGiorgio

Introduction

Low back pain (LBP) is a global health challenge with profound implications for individuals, healthcare systems, and economies. This chapter examines the multifaceted nature of LBP, emphasizing data from the United States while incorporating global perspectives where relevant. We explore its epidemiology, prevalence trends, and risk factors, analyze the economic burden—including both direct healthcare costs and indirect productivity losses—and discuss treatment strategies, including innovative surgical approaches, that balance clinical efficacy with cost considerations. Finally, we highlight the socioeconomic consequences of LBP, such as its impact on work productivity and healthcare expenditures, underscoring the need for ongoing research and resource optimization.

A. Dada · V. Kwok
University of California, San Francisco, Department of Neurological Surgery, San Francisco, CA, USA
e-mail: Abraham.Dada@ucsf.edu; Vivian.Kwok@ucsf.edu

A. DiGiorgio (✉)
University of California, San Francisco, Department of Neurological Surgery, San Francisco, CA, USA

University of California, San Francisco, Philip R Lee Institute for Health Policy Studies, San Francisco, CA, USA
e-mail: Anthony.Digiorgio@ucsf.edu

Epidemiology and Prevenance

LBP is the leading cause of morbidity worldwide. Currently, LBP affects more than half a billion individuals and its prevalence is estimated to reach 850 million globally by 2050 [1–3]. Since 1990, it has remained among the top causes of DALYs for all adult age groups, further advancing in rank over the last three decades [2]. With a globally aging population and corresponding increase in non-communicable disease and injury-related burdens, LBP has shifted from the 13th to the ninth top cause of DALY for all age groups in 1990 and 2019 respectively [2].

Moreover, LBP affects up to a third of the population at any point [4]. Most people will experience LBP at some point in their life, with an estimated lifetime prevalence of 58 to 84% and a one-month prevalence of about 1 in 4 individuals [5–7]. While LBP is most predominant among occupations requiring physically strenuous labor or low-income workers, it is also prevalent among roles with prolonged sitting [8–10]. Transition to remote work also witnessed a significant increase in LBP compared to in-person work [11].

Consequently, LBP is a major concern across both primary care and emergency department (ED) visits globally. Musculoskeletal (MSK) concerns are the second most common reason for seeking a doctor and comprise up to 20% of primary care consultations in most countries [4].

A. A. Baaj et al. (eds.), *Surgery of the Lumbar Spine*, https://doi.org/10.1007/978-3-032-18097-1_3

Among MSK concerns in the primary care setting, LBP is the most prevalent [12]. In the ED, it is consistently a top presentation for visits around the world, representing up to 17% of ED visits and often with return or repeat visits [13, 14]. Reflecting global trends, LBP represents more than 3% of ED visits in the US [15], with acute presentations often transitioning to chronic LBP [16].

LBP remains a significant public health concern in the United States. There were nearly 50 million cases in 2020 or 10,500 per 100,000 [3]. The three-month prevalence for LBP and/or neck pain is more than 30% [17]. The three-month self-reported prevalence of LBP among workers in the United States was 25.7% in 2010, and 20% were told that their LBP was due to work [18, 19]. In the Medicare population (65 years and older), the overall prevalence of radiographically confirmed spinal disease was 27.3% [20]. Among younger symptomatic adults (20–30 years), more than half showed evidence of lower disc degeneration [21]. In asymptomatic individuals, the prevalence of radiographic disc degeneration increases with age [22]. Nearly100% of 80-year-olds showed evidence of spinal degeneration [22]. Other risk factors for LBP include comorbidities such as obesity, history of smoking, and lifestyle factors, among others [6, 17, 23, 24]. Psychosocial factors in the workplace and job strain are also associated with increased risk for LBP [25].

While work-related ergonomics are one of the top contributing risk factors for LBP, [3] LBP in turn compounds work-related disability. Nearly 20% of workers with severe LBP missed at least one full day of work in the prior three months due to LBP; approximately 17% of workers have any LBP [19]. Up to 10% of workers stopped working, changed jobs, or made a major change in work activities because of LBP. The impact may also be underestimated—one cross-sectional study found that 60% of participants with LBP had work limitations [26].

Economics of Low Back Pain

The impact of LBP on the economy can be understood through both indirect and direct costs, each with distinct implications for healthcare systems and economic productivity. Indirect costs are the value of foregone productivity that could have contributed to other areas of the economy. They arise primarily from the reduced economic productivity of both patients and caregivers. For individuals with LBP, the ability to work or perform at full capacity may be diminished, leading to lost wages, decreased workforce participation, and a broader impact on economic output. This reduction in productivity extends to caregivers, who may need to allocate time and resources away from work to provide care. Direct costs, on the other hand, relate to the resources required to diagnose, manage, and treat LBP. This category includes expenses associated with clinical consultations, imaging studies, therapeutic interventions, medications, and surgical procedures. From an economic perspective, the opportunity cost here lies in the alternative uses that these medical resources could have been applied to. However, accurately measuring these direct costs is challenging due to the complexities and distortions inherent in healthcare pricing.

The distinction between "cost" and "price" in healthcare can be nuanced. In theory, prices should serve as signals that reflect the true costs of resource allocation. In a purely free-market system, prices emerge from the interaction of supply and demand, ideally representing the monetary value of alternatives sacrificed. Prices, in turn, help direct resources toward their most productive uses. We largely use the terms "cost" and "price" interchangeably when performing economic research in healthcare, and we continue that trend in this chapter, but it is worth keeping in mind that "costs" listed here really refer to "prices" and don't reflect the foregone value of alternative resource allocation.

This framework is critical when examining the economic costs of spine care. The true costs extend beyond financial expenditures to include medical resources, human capital, and patient productivity. While this chapter reports financial costs, these figures should prompt reflection on alternative uses for the resources involved. Imaging equipment, operating rooms, therapists, nurses, and physicians are in high demand across healthcare, and their allocation to spine care entails opportunity costs, potentially limiting their availability for other conditions. Those costs must be measured against the gains in patient health. That said, a patient's health should not be valued solely by economic productivity. The intrinsic benefit of alleviating human suffering, though challenging to quantify, must also factor into these considerations.

However, costs are subjective, reflecting the alternatives that are sacrificed when one choice is made over another. In healthcare, government regulations often obscure these true costs. For example, when the Centers for Medicare & Medicaid Services (CMS) sets a reimbursement rate for spine surgery, that rate may not reflect the actual opportunity cost of providing those services. An artificially low reimbursement rate fails to capture the value of resources—both human and technological—that are consumed in delivering spine care. It leads to shortages. Alternatively, large, consolidated health systems routinely inflate prices far above market-clearing levels. These distortions create inefficiencies, obscuring the true economic value of interventions.

Balancing subjective patient preferences with the reality of finite resources remains a complex challenge. The elective nature of spine care positions it well for market forces to play a determining role. Market dynamics, by responding to dispersed knowledge and local conditions, offer an efficient way to balance costs, quality, and innovation. As Friedrich Hayek observed in *The Road to Serfdom*, "The curious task of economics is to demonstrate to men how little they really know about what they imagine they can design." [27]

Lost Income Opportunity

Absenteeism, or time away from work, is a major consequence of LBP, which ranks among the leading causes of work absence globally. A meta-analysis focusing primarily on European populations found that within a six-month period, 15.5% of individuals with LBP took leave from work [28]. In Brazil, lost workdays due to LBP rose from an average of 88 days in 2012 to 100 days in 2016, totaling 59 million days absent from work over the study period [29].

In the United States, the prevalence of work absence due to LBP is similarly high. A US-based study with a 12-month follow-up found that 26% of workers with back pain (prevalence of 17.6%) took leave from work, resulting in a lost-workday prevalence of 4.6%. On average, workers who took leave missed 26.3 days due to back pain [30]. More recent US studies focusing on blue-collar workers reported the prevalence of work leave for back pain to be between 7% and 10%, underscoring the variability in impact depending on job type and industry [31, 32].

Beyond absenteeism, back pain also stifles presenteeism, or productivity while at work. A recent American study demonstrated that LBP impacts lost workdays and on-the-job productivity in equal measure, further amplifying its economic burden [33].

Socioeconomic factors add another layer of complexity to the impact of LBP on employment and income. A retrospective study conducted in Paris revealed that income loss due to LBP was twice as severe for employees in lower-level positions compared to senior leadership, underscoring the disproportionate financial burden on workers with fewer resources and job security [34]. Additionally, patients receiving workers' compensation for LBP often experience worse outcomes following surgery and face protracted recovery times, delaying their return to work compared to non-compensation patients [35, 36].

Preventive strategies remain essential in mitigating work absences associated with back pain. Evidence supports that regular exercise—particularly resistance training and stretching—as well as programs that combine physical activity with patient education are among the most effective measures to reduce LBP-related absenteeism [37].

Treatment Costs

The United States bears the highest economic burden of low back pain (LBP) worldwide, with the costs of managing LBP far surpassing those reported in other regions [38]. In 2013, both LBP and neck pain ranked as the third highest category of healthcare spending in the United States, behind diabetes and ischemic heart disease [39]. These costs encompass a wide range of interventions, vary by payer type, region, intervention used, and treatment setting. They continue to rise despite efforts to curb healthcare expenditures.

For the Medicare population, a large proportion of LBP-related costs are driven by nonsurgical interventions, including chiropractic manipulation, physical therapy, and epidural steroid injections, comprising 72.6% of spending from 2000 to 2021 ($15.2 billion) (Table 3.1) [40]. Over the past decade, inflation-adjusted Medicare reimbursement rates for surgical interventions have declined. However, Medicare patients comprise a significant proportion of patients with surgical pathology; patients with Medicare and Medicaid are more likely to be recommended for spine surgery compared to those with private insurance [41]. Notably, for procedures like lumbar fusion, total prices tend to be higher for privately insured patients than for those with Medicare, highlighting the impact of payer type on resource allocation [42].

Spending of private payors exhibits similar trends to Medicare. Within this population, nonsurgical interventions represented a majority of treatment utilization and thus accounted for 70.8% of cumulative 12-month expenditures after diagnosis spending for LBP ($1.8 billion from 2007 to 2016) [43]. Despite only approximately 1% of patients with LBP undergoing surgery in this population, surgery accounts for nearly 30% of costs [43]. Unnecessary imaging was found to be a key driver of costs among patients who did not receive surgery as this subgroup frequently received care inconsistent with clinical LBP guidelines [43]. More than a third of patients treated nonsurgical received imaging within only 30 days of LBP, a similar proportion of patients underwent imaging prior to a trial of physical therapy [43]. This suggests care pathways that may yield cost-savings for patients with LBP, diverting the need for prescriptions, imaging, ED visits, and overall out-of-pocket expenses.

Work-related injuries requiring lumbar spinal surgery are among the most expensive claims within the Workers' Compensation (WC) system. The cost burden for these injuries primarily comes from indemnity payments—compensations provided to cover lost wages for injured workers—which make up approximately 65% of the total cost per case [44, 45]. This statistic underscores the financial impact of work-related LBP on both the WC system and injured individuals.

Regional disparities further contribute to the variability in LBP treatment costs. A study exam-

Table 3.1 Medicare Part B beneficiaries' cumulative back pain procedure utilization and payments from 2000 to 2021

Back pain procedure group	Utilization	Payments[a]
Chiropractic Manipulation	271,551,290	$8,769,294,802.69
Initial Physical Therapy Consultation	43,355,097	$2,994,495,515.27
Epidural Steroid Injection	17,026,413	$3,451,169,679.12
Lumbar decompression	4,252,629	$2,137,292,205.29
Spinal Fusion	3,496,184	$3,023,078,950.87
SI joint fusion	39,112	$88,056,897.61

[a]Payments are in US 2021 dollars

ining Medicare reimbursement rates for spine procedures found significant geographical differences. In 2021, Alaska had the highest mean reimbursement rate at $1632.95 per procedure, while Nebraska had the lowest at $1133.44. Over the past two decades, reimbursement rates have generally declined across states, with Wisconsin, Michigan, and Hawaii seeing the largest decreases (between 39.6% and 40.8%) [46]. Similarly, Zygourakis et al., using the National Inpatient Sample database, found that spinal surgeries in the Western United States were 23–25% more expensive than in the Northeast, even when accounting for confounding factors. The authors attributed these regional differences to higher labor costs in the West, state policies such as California's nurse-to-patient ratios in acute care hospitals, and cost-containment measures like Massachusetts's healthcare reforms [42].

The prices of LBP treatment also vary by intervention type. For instance, a single-center analysis of single-level lumbar fusions reported an average direct cost of $22,890, with surgical instrumentation as a major cost driver. Circumferential fusion approaches had the highest costs, while posterior spinal fusions without interbody cages had lower upfront costs. The choice of spinal instrumentation accounted for 84.9% of supply costs, with operative time further impacting the overall expense [47]. Decompression procedures alone are less costly than fusion but are associated with higher reoperation rates, making fusion more cost-effective for select pathologies if reoperation rates remain under 43.8% [48].

Minimally invasive surgery (MIS) has emerged as a cost-effective approach for certain spine interventions. Compared to traditional open procedures, MIS techniques offer an average cost savings of 10.4% [49]. When comparing open, MIS, and robotic-assisted surgeries, robotic-assisted procedures are the most expensive, averaging $60,047.01, which is 30% higher than MIS ($41,471.21) and open ($42,538.98) surgeries, after adjusting for complications, revisions, and robot purchasing and operational fees [50].

The setting in which LBP treatments are delivered also affects costs. Outpatient spinal surgeries performed at Ambulatory Surgery Centers (ASCs) have gained popularity due to their cost-effectiveness. A study comparing lumbar laminectomy procedures in hospitals versus ASCs found that ASC-based surgeries resulted in lower initial surgery costs and one-year episode-of-care costs, with similar rates of complications and postoperative resource utilization. Using a Quality-Adjusted Life Year (QALY) analysis, the study found ASC-based laminectomies to be over twice as cost-effective as hospital-based procedures [51]. Similar findings have been reported within the Medicare population, with ASCs offering lower costs for decompression, fusion, and kyphoplasty/vertebroplasty procedures compared to hospital outpatient settings.

Treatment Tradeoffs

In evaluating treatment options for low back pain, particularly surgical interventions, there are essential tradeoffs to consider, including costs, return-to-work (RTW) rates, and patient satisfaction. Prospective, multicenter registries, such as the Quality Outcomes Database (QOD) provides valuable insights into these tradeoffs, assessing outcomes such as return to work, quality-adjusted life years (QALY), and incremental cost-effectiveness ratios (ICER).

For instance, surgery for lumbar spondylolisthesis has demonstrated favorable outcomes in terms of both RTW rates and patient satisfaction. Among patients undergoing surgery for this condition, 76.7% were able to return to work postoperatively. Interestingly, even among those who did not return to work, a substantial proportion (72.1%) still reported satisfaction with their surgical outcome [52]. This finding suggests that surgical interventions may offer benefits that extend beyond work productivity, improving quality of life in ways that are not solely dependent on employment status.

Minimally invasive techniques, such as minimally invasive transforaminal lumbar interbody fusion (MIS-TLIF), have been associated with higher RTW rates compared to traditional open procedures, like the open-TLIF. The reduced tissue disruption and shorter recovery times associated with MIS approaches contribute to quicker rehabilitation and a swifter return to daily activities and work [53]. These benefits underscore the role of minimally invasive techniques in enhancing patient recovery and reducing the socioeconomic burden of prolonged work absences.

Robotic-assisted surgeries represent another technological advancement in spine care, although they come with unique economic considerations. Passias et al. reported that robotic-assisted spine surgeries had a suboptimal one-year cost per QALY when compared to other surgical methods. However, when evaluated over a longer time horizon, extending to life expectancy, the projected cost per QALY fell well within acceptable thresholds, suggesting that the long-term benefits of robotic-assisted surgery may justify its higher initial cost [50]. These findings highlight the importance of evaluating treatment options over an extended timeframe to fully understand their economic and quality-of-life implications.

Conclusion

LBP remains a pervasive health challenge worldwide, imposing an escalating burden on individuals, healthcare systems, and economies. In the United States, where the prevalence and economic impact are particularly pronounced, LBP results in significant healthcare spending and lost income due to absenteeism and reduced work productivity. Treatment options, especially surgical interventions, come with critical tradeoffs involving costs, quality of life improvements, and return-to-work rates. Despite advances in minimally invasive and robotic-assisted surgeries that promise improved outcomes and efficiency, the economic impact of LBP underscores the need for continued efforts in prevention, optimized management, and careful resource allocation. Addressing LBP's challenges calls for a multifaceted approach that balances patient needs, healthcare resources, and societal costs.

References

1. GBD 2017 Disease and Injury Incidence and Prevalence Collaborators. Global, regional, and national incidence, prevalence, and years lived with disability for 354 diseases and injuries for 195 countries and territories, 1990–2017: a systematic analysis for the Global Burden of Disease Study 2017. Lancet. 2018;392(10159):1789–858.
2. GBD 2019 Diseases and Injuries Collaborators. Global burden of 369 diseases and injuries in 204 countries and territories, 1990–2019: a systematic analysis for the Global Burden of Disease Study 2019. Lancet. 2020;396(10258):1204–22.
3. GBD 2021 Low Back Pain Collaborators. Global, regional, and national burden of low back pain, 1990–2020, its attributable risk factors, and projections to 2050: a systematic analysis of the Global Burden of Disease Study 2021. Lancet Rheumatol. 2023;5(6):e316–29.
4. Woolf AD, Pfleger B. Burden of major musculoskeletal conditions. Bull World Health Organ. 2003;81(9):646–56.
5. Hoy D, Brooks P, Blyth F, Buchbinder R. The epidemiology of low back pain. Best Pract Res Clin Rheumatol. 2010;24(6):769–81.
6. Manchikanti L, Singh V, Falco FJE, Benyamin RM, Hirsch JA. Epidemiology of low back pain in adults. Neuromodulation. 2014;17(Suppl 2):3–10.
7. Hoy D, Bain C, Williams G, March L, Brooks P, Blyth F, et al. A systematic review of the global prevalence of low back pain. Arthritis Rheum. 2012;64(6):2028–37.
8. Schneider S, Lipinski S, Schiltenwolf M. Occupations associated with a high risk of self-reported back pain: representative outcomes of a back pain prevalence study in the Federal Republic of Germany. Eur Spine J. 2006;15(6):821–33.
9. Zafar F, Qasim YF, Farooq MU, Shamael I, Khan IU, Khan DH. The frequency of different risk factors for lower back pain in a tertiary care hospital. Cureus. 2018;10(8):e3183.
10. Chowdhury MOSA, Huda N, Alam MdM, Hossain SI, Hossain S, Islam S, et al. Work-related risk factors and the prevalence of low back pain among low-income industrial workers in Bangladesh: results from a cross-sectional study. Bull Fac Phys Ther. 2023;28(1):20.
11. Ambrosio L, Vadalà G, Russo F, Donnici L, Petrucci G, Tecco CD, et al. The effect of transitioning to remote working in patients affected by chronic low back pain: a cross-sectional study. Neurospine. 2023;20(2):692–700.
12. Jordan KP, Kadam UT, Hayward R, Porcheret M, Young C, Croft P. Annual consultation prevalence of regional musculoskeletal problems in primary care: an observational study. BMC Musculoskelet Disord. 2010;11(1):144.
13. Megalla M, Ogedegbe C, Sanders AM, Cox N, DiSanto T, Johnson H, et al. Factors associated with

repeat emergency department visits for low back pain. Cureus. 2022;14(2):e21906.
14. Edwards J, Hayden J, Asbridge M, Gregoire B, Magee K. Prevalence of low back pain in emergency settings: a systematic review and meta-analysis. BMC Musculoskelet Disord. 2017;18(1):143.
15. Waterman BR, Belmont PJ, Schoenfeld AJ. Low back pain in the United States: incidence and risk factors for presentation in the emergency setting. Spine J. 2012;12(1):63–70.
16. Stevans JM, Delitto A, Khoja SS, Patterson CG, Smith CN, Schneider MJ, et al. Risk factors associated with transition from acute to chronic low Back pain in US patients seeking primary care. JAMA Netw Open. 2021;4(2):e2037371.
17. Strine TW, Hootman JM. US national prevalence and correlates of low back and neck pain among adults. Arthritis Rheum. 2007;57(4):656–65.
18. Yang H, Haldeman S, Lu ML, Baker D. Low Back pain prevalence and related workplace psychosocial risk factors: a study using data from the 2010 National Health Interview Survey. J Manip Physiol Ther. 2016;39(7):459–72.
19. Luckhaupt SE, Dahlhamer JM, Gonzales GT, Lu ML, Groenewold M, Sweeney MH, et al. Prevalence, recognition of work-relatedness, and effect on work of low back pain among U.S. workers Ann Intern Med. 2019;171(4):301–4.
20. Parenteau CS, Lau EC, Campbell IC, Courtney A. Prevalence of spine degeneration diagnosis by type, age, gender, and obesity using Medicare data. Sci Rep. 2021;11(1):5389.
21. Berg AJ, Ahmadje U, Jayanna HH, Trégouët P, Sanville P, Kapoor V. The prevalence of lumbar disc degeneration in symptomatic younger patients: a study of MRI scans. J Clin Orthop Trauma. 2020;11(5):932–6.
22. Brinjikji W, Luetmer PH, Comstock B, Bresnahan BW, Chen LE, Deyo RA, et al. Systematic literature review of imaging features of spinal degeneration in asymptomatic populations. AJNR Am J Neuroradiol. 2015;36(4):811–6.
23. Shemory ST, Pfefferle KJ, Gradisar IM. Modifiable risk factors in patients with low back pain. Orthopedics. 2016;39(3):e413–6.
24. Yang H, Haldeman S. Behavior-related factors associated with low back pain in the US adult population. Spine (Phila Pa 1976). 2018;43(1):28–34.
25. Yang H, Lu ML, Haldeman S, Swanson N. Psychosocial risk factors for low back pain in US workers: data from the 2002-2018 quality of work life survey. Am J Ind Med. 2023;66(1):41–53.
26. Feldman DE, Nahin RL. Disability among persons with chronic severe back pain: results from a nationally representative population-based sample. J Pain. 2022;23(12):2144–54.
27. Hayek FA. The road to Serfdom: Text and documents--the definitive edition [Internet]. Caldwell B, editor. Chicago: University of Chicago Press; 2007 [cited 2024 Dec 15]. 304 p. (The Collected Works of F. A. Hayek). Available from: https://press.uchicago.edu/ucp/books/book/chicago/R/bo4138549.html.
28. Wynne-Jones G, Cowen J, Jordan JL, Uthman O, Main CJ, Glozier N, et al. Absence from work and return to work in people with back pain: a systematic review and meta-analysis. Occup Environ Med. 2014;71(6):448–56.
29. Carregaro RL, Tottoli CR, Rodrigues D d S, Bosmans JE, da Silva EN, van Tulder M. Low back pain should be considered a health and research priority in Brazil: lost productivity and healthcare costs between 2012 to 2016. PLoS One. 2020;15(4):e0230902.
30. Guo HR, Tanaka S, Halperin WE, Cameron LL. Back pain prevalence in US industry and estimates of lost workdays. Am J Public Health. 1999;89(7):1029–35.
31. Merlino LA, Rosecrance JC, Anton D, Cook TM. Symptoms of musculoskeletal disorders among apprentice construction workers. Appl Occup Environ Hyg. 2003;18(1):57–64.
32. Shraim M, Cifuentes M, Willetts JL, Marucci-Wellman HR, Pransky G. Regional socioeconomic disparities in outcomes for workers with low back pain in the United States. Am J Ind Med. 2017;60(5):472–83.
33. Fontana MA, Islam W, Richardson MA, Medina CK, Kohilakis EC, Qureshi SA, et al. Presenteeism and absenteeism before and after single-level lumbar spine surgery. Spine J. 2022;22(5):776–86.
34. James-Belin E, Ostertag A, Couzi E, Petrover D, Yelnik A, Orcel P, et al. Economic impact of work disability due to chronic low back pain from the patient perspective. Rev Epidemiol Sante Publique. 2023;71(4):101858.
35. Hani U, Monk SH, Pfortmiller D, Stanley G, Kim PK, Bohl MA, et al. Effect of workers' compensation status on pain, disability, quality of life, and return to work after lumbar spine surgery: a 1-year propensity-matched analysis. J Neurosurg Spine. 2023;39(1):47–57.
36. Monk SH, Hani U, Stanley G, Pfortmiller D, Kim PK, Bohl MA, et al. Mental health comorbidities in workers' compensation patients and the effect on pain, disability, quality of life, and return to work after lumbar spine surgery. J Neurosurg Spine. 2024;40(5):562–9.
37. Ta KNT, Bai CH, Chuang KJ. Prevention of work absence due to back pain: a network meta-analysis. Eur J Investig Health Psychol Educ. 2023;13(12):2891–903.
38. Chang D, Lui A, Matsoyan A, Safaee MM, Aryan H, Ames C. Comparative review of the socioeconomic burden of lower back pain in the United States and globally. Neurospine. 2024;21(2):487–501.
39. Dieleman JL, Baral R, Birger M, Bui AL, Bulchis A, Chapin A, et al. US spending on personal health care and public health, 1996-2013. JAMA. 2016;316(24):2627–46.
40. Dada A, Dalle Ore C, Mummaneni PV, Patel A, Ambati V, Orrico KO, et al. The exponential growth of nonsurgeons performing fusions for low-back pain. J Neurosurg Spine. 2024;41(6):784–91.

41. Benton JA, Weiss BT, Mowrey WB, Yassari N, Wang B, Ramos RDLG, et al. Association of Medicare and Medicaid Insurance Status with increased spine surgery utilization rates. Spine (Phila Pa 1976). 2021;46(17):E939–44.
42. Zygourakis CC, Liu CY, Wakam G, Moriates C, Boscardin C, Ames CP, et al. Geographic and hospital variation in cost of lumbar laminectomy and lumbar fusion for degenerative conditions. Neurosurgery. 2017;81(2):331–40.
43. Kim LH, Vail D, Azad TD, Bentley JP, Zhang Y, Ho AL, et al. Expenditures and health care utilization among adults with newly diagnosed low back and lower extremity pain. JAMA Netw Open. 2019;2(5):e193676.
44. Deyo RA, Mirza SK, Martin BI, Kreuter W, Goodman DC, Jarvik JG. Trends, major medical complications, and charges associated with surgery for lumbar spinal stenosis in older adults. JAMA. 2010;303(13):1259–65.
45. Webster BS, Snook SH. The cost of 1989 workers' compensation low back pain claims. Spine (Phila Pa 1976). 1994;19(10):1111–5; discussion 1116.
46. Haglin JM, Zabat MA, Richter KR, McQuivey KS, Godzik J, Patel NP, et al. Over 20 years of declining Medicare reimbursement for spine surgeons: a temporal and geographic analysis from 2000 to 2021. J Neurosurg Spine. 2022;37(3):452–9.
47. Beckerman D, Esparza M, Lee SI, Berven SH, Bederman SS, Hu SS, et al. Cost analysis of single-level lumbar fusions. Global Spine J. 2020;10(1):39–46.
48. Kaidi AC, Du JY, Subramanian T, Amen T, Asada T, Qureshi SA, et al. Isolated decompression for degenerative spondylolisthesis is less costly than fusion even with high revision rates. Spine J. 2024;24(9):1690–6.
49. Lucio JC, Vanconia RB, Deluzio KJ, Lehmen JA, Rodgers JA, Rodgers W. Economics of less invasive spinal surgery: an analysis of hospital cost differences between open and minimally invasive instrumented spinal fusion procedures during the perioperative period. Risk Manag Healthc Policy. 2012;5:65–74.
50. Passias PG, Brown AE, Alas H, Bortz CA, Pierce KE, Hassanzadeh H, et al. A cost benefit analysis of increasing surgical technology in lumbar spine fusion. Spine J. 2021;21(2):193–201.
51. Rana P, Brennan J, Johnson A, Patton CM, Turcotte JJ. Outcomes and cost-effectiveness of hospital outpatient versus ambulatory surgery center lumbar decompression surgery. Glob Spine J. 2024:21925682241290171.
52. DiGiorgio AM, Mummaneni PV, Park P, Chan AK, Bisson EF, Bydon M, et al. Correlation of return to work with patient satisfaction after surgery for lumbar spondylolisthesis: an analysis of the quality outcomes database. Neurosurg Focus. 2020;48(5):E5.
53. Chan AK, Bisson EF, Bydon M, Foley KT, Glassman SD, Shaffrey CI, et al. A comparison of minimally invasive and open transforaminal lumbar Interbody fusion for grade 1 degenerative lumbar spondylolisthesis: an analysis of the prospective quality outcomes database. Neurosurgery. 2020;87(3):555–62.

4 Physical Examination in Lumbar Spine Disease

Ebtesam Abdulla, Mohammad Almalki,
Ibrahim A. Alhalal, and Saleh S. Baeesa

Key Points

- The lumbar spine examination encompasses motor, sensory, reflex, and specialized tests, in addition to a comprehensive evaluation of regional spine cutaneous alterations, deformities, and other factors.
- A comprehensive survey should be incorporated, while the physical examination is customized based on the patient's history, possible participation, and abnormal findings.
- No protocol can encompass all scenarios; thus, the systematic evaluation must be customized to the individual patient, and the sequence of the examination is adjusted accordingly.

E. Abdulla (✉)
Department of Neurosurgery, Government Hospitals, Manama, Bahrain

M. Almalki
Department of Spine Surgery, Prince Sultan Military Medical City, Riyadh, Kingdom of Saudi Arabia

I. A. Alhalal
Department of Spine Surgery, Banner University Medical Centre, University of Arizona, Tucson, AZ, USA

S. S. Baeesa
Department of Neurosciences, King Faisal Specialist Hospital and Research Centre, Jeddah, Saudi Arabia

Physical Examination of the Lumbar Spine

Inspection [1, 2]

Visual inspection		
	Focus of inspection	Examples of abnormalities
Standing position		
Skin	Pigmentations, dermal markings, tufts of hair, masses, surgical scars	Café-au-lait macules, skin tags, and fibromas in neurofibromatosis Port wine stains, pilose patches, and lipomas are frequently associated with skeletal anomalies such as spina bifida
Back view	Squareness of the shoulders and the pelvis	Asymmetrical shoulder heights are observed in scoliosis Discrepancies in the heights of the iliac crests or pelvic tilt indicate potential variations in leg lengths Listing of the trunk to one side observed with herniated lumbar disc (LDH)
Side view	Cervical, thoracic, and lumbar curves	Loss of lumbar lordosis, hyperlordosis Increased thoracic kyphosis

A. A. Baaj et al. (eds.), *Surgery of the Lumbar Spine*, https://doi.org/10.1007/978-3-032-18097-1_4

Visual inspection		
	Focus of inspection	Examples of abnormalities
Gait	Walk across the room, Heel and toe walk, Tandem gait	Antalgic gait associated with LDH Abnormal heel walking observed in L5 radiculopathy Abnormal toe walking shown in S1 radiculopathy

Palpation [3, 4]

- Palpate the paravertebral muscles for soreness and spasms *(Muscles in spasm seem taut and contorted and may be discernible).*
- Palpate over the spinous processes *(LDH),* greater trochanters *(greater trochanteric bursitis)*, and sacroiliac joints *(sacroiliitis).*
- Palpate for pedal pulses *(arterial insufficiency).*

Range of Motion [4]

Three-Dimensional Assessment (Sagittal, Coronal, Vertical)

- Flexion and extension: The patient must maintain straight knees to touch the toes during flexion.
- Execute lateral flexion bilaterally while sliding the palm down the leg to the maximum extent.
- While the examiner stabilizes the pelvis, rotate to either side.

Neurological Examination

Sensory Examination [1, 3]

- Sensory evaluation is graded (0–2) using the American Spinal Injury Association (ASIA) scale. Each sensory modality is assessed as follows: 0: Absent, 1: Diminished, 2: Normal.
- Major Sensory Types (scored for all patients):
  - Pain (Pinprick): Prick with a sharp object (e.g., neuro-tip).
  - Light Touch: Lightly stroke with cotton wool.
- Minor Sensory Types (scored in focused exams):
  - Vibration: Tested with a 128 Hz tuning fork over bony prominences.
  - Temperature: Use warm and cold stimuli to assess thermal discrimination.
  - Two-Point Discrimination: Assess the ability to differentiate two points on the skin, typically at fingertips.
- General rules in sensory examination.
  - Instruct the patient to close their eyes and respond with "yes" upon perceiving a feeling.
  - Utilize the patient's sternum as a reference point to define the sensation of "normal."
  - Begin distally and go proximally to discern "stocking" sensory loss patterns, frequently observed in peripheral neuropathy.
  - If impaired feeling is observed, proceed proximally until normal sensation is identified, recording any specific "sensory level," which may suggest spinal involvement.

- Inquire whether the experience is the same on both sides, contrasting the left and right.

Motor Examination [1, 2]

- Strength evaluation is graded (0–5) using the Royal Medical Research Council of Great Britain (MRC) scale. Each myotome is assessed as follows: 0: No movement, 1: Flickering of movement, 2: Active movement with gravity eliminated, 3: Active movement against gravity, 4: Active movement against gravity and some resistance (4−: against low resistance; 4+: against high resistance), 5: Normal.

Reflexes [5–10]

- Reflex evaluation is graded (0–4) using the National Institute of Neurological Disorders and Stroke (NINDS) scale. Each deep tension is assessed as follows: 0: Absent reflex, 1: Diminished reflex, 2: Normal reflex, 3: Exaggerated reflex, 4: Exaggerated reflex with clonus.

Clinical presentation of specific nerve root involvement			
Nerve root	Reflex	Motor deficit	Sensory deficit
L1	Cremasteric[a]	–	Iliac crest and groin
L2	Cremasteric[a]	Hip flexion and adduction	Anterior and inner thigh
L3	Hip	Knee extension	Medial thigh-to-knee
L4	Knee	Knee extension and ankle dorsiflexion	Medial leg and foot
L5	Medial hamstring[b]	Foot inversion and toe dorsiflexion Hip extension and abduction	Dorsolateral leg Dorsum of foot, dorsum of Dig. I
S1	Ankle	Foot plantar flexion and eversion	Posterior leg
S2	–	Toe plantar flexion	Sole of the foot
S3, S4	–	Bowel and bladder function	Perineum

[a]*Cremasteric reflex is a superficial reflex in males that lifts the testicle when the inner thigh is stroked. It's supplied by genitofemoral nerve (L1-L2)*

[b]*Medial hamstring reflex is well documented in the literature but hardly mentioned in the clinical notes*

Nerve Root Tension Tests [8–12]

Nerve root tension signs			
Test /sign	Method	Positive finding	Relevance
Lasègue's sign *(straight leg raise (SLR) test)*, Fig. 4.1a	With patient supine, lift affected ankle till pain is felt in the ipsilateral back of leg	The spread of leg pain or paresthesia at <60°. Foot dorsiflexion exacerbates discomfort	Distinguish sciatica from pain resulting from hip disease
Fajersztajin's sign *(crossed straight leg-raising test)*	With patient supine, lift painless ankle until contralateral limb hurts	The spread of leg pain or paresthesia at <60° at contralateral limb	Associate with greater central disc herniation
Cram test	Supine patient, lift symptomatic leg with knee slightly flexed	The spread of leg pain or paresthesia at <60°	Distinguish sciatica from pain resulting from hip disease
Femoral stretch test *(reverse straight leg raising test)*, Fig. 4.1b	Patient prone, examiner's hand near popliteal fossa, knee maximally dorsiflexed	Leg pain or paresthesia along the distribution of pain	L2-L4 nerve root compression, diabetic femoral neuropathy, psoas hematoma
Bowstring sign	Once SLR causes pain, bend the knee and hip to drop the foot to the bed	This maneuver relieves sciatica but not hip pain	Impingement of the sciatic nerve in the hip joint

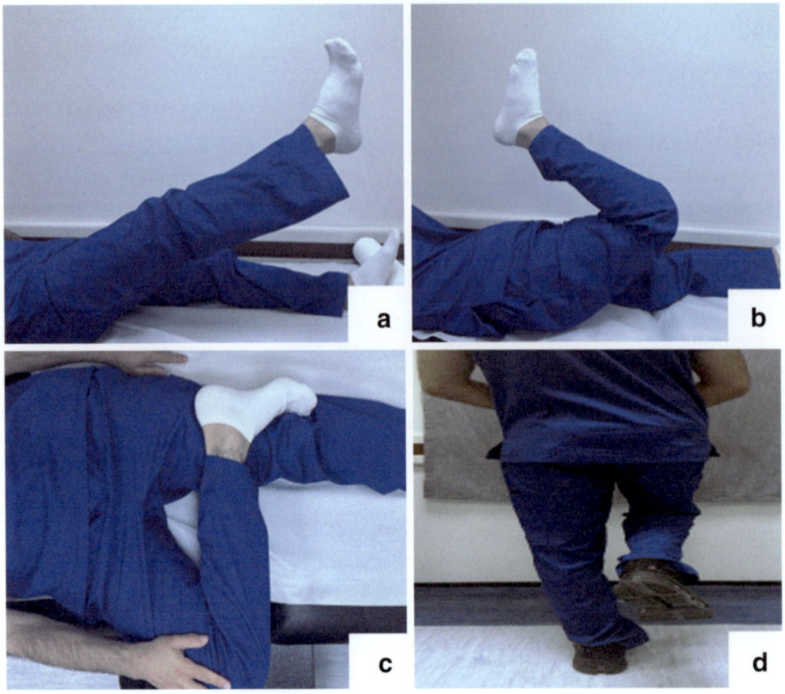

Fig. 4.1 (**a**) Straight leg raise. (**b**) Femoral stretch test, (**c**) FABER test, (**d**) Trendelenburg sign test

Other Tests for Lumbar Radiculopathy [1, 6, 11]

Other tests for lumbar radiculopathy			
Test /sign	Method	Positive finding	Relevance
Trendelenburg sign, Fig. 4.1d	Examiner views pelvis from behind as patient stands and elevates leg	The pelvis tilted toward the elevated leg	Weak contralateral thigh abductors on the stance leg, primarily L5
Faber (Patrick's test), Fig. 4.1c	Hip and knee flexed, lateral malleolus placed on contralateral knee The ipsilateral knee softly descends towards the test table	Presence of hip pain	Hip joint diseases such as sacroiliitis
Crossed adductors	Eliciting patellar reflex contracts contralateral thigh adductors	Hyperactive patellar reflex	Upper motor neuron lesion
Hoover sign	The examiner resists the supine patient lifting one leg off the bed. The examiner gradually raises the leg while placing the palm of the other hand beneath the heel of the unlifted leg	When the patient elevates the normal leg, the paretic leg pulls down harder than on manual testing	Synergetic contraction of the contralateral gluteus Medius distinguishes unilateral functional iliopsoas weakness from pathological weakness
Abductor sign	The examiner touches both legs' sides while the patient is supine. Abduct one leg, then the other, as the examiner provides hand resistance	Hyper adducting contralateral non-abducting limb	Synergetic contraction of the contralateral thigh abductors to identify functional from organic weakness

Differential Diagnosis (Radicular Pain Mimics) [3, 5]

When evaluating radicular pain, it is crucial to examine disorders that may replicate its symptoms. The subsequent differential diagnoses are pertinent:

- *Sacroiliac Joint (SIJ) Arthritis*: Conduct a physical examination focusing on SIJ provocation tests (such as the FABER test) and assess pain response during sacroiliac manipulation.
- *Trochanteric Fasciitis*: Assess tenderness over the greater trochanter and the presence of pain during hip abduction.
- *Hip Osteoarthritis*: Evaluate the range of motion in the hip joint and look for crepitus.
- *Piriformis Syndrome*: Assess the piriformis muscle's tenderness and perform the FAIR test (flexion, adduction, and internal rotation).

Clinical Pearls

- A positive Hoffman and Babinski's sign necessitates additional testing to exclude spinal cord compression (lesion above L1-L2) or cerebral involvement.
- Painless motor deficits in the lower extremities seldomly arise from lumbar nerve compression. Consider diabetic neuropathy, myopathy, and similar conditions.
- Suspect non-organic causes if the patient is overreacting, tenderness is superficial and non-anatomic, sensation is affected in non-dermatomal pattern and if there discrepancy in the examination.

References

1. Greenberg MS. Handbook of neurosurgery. 10th ed. New York: Thieme Medical Publishers, Inc.; 2020. 1990 pages.
2. Pillemer R. A systematic examination of the lumbar spine. In: Handbook of lumbar spine and lower extremity examination. Cham: Springer; 2023.
3. Patton H, Sundsten J, Crill W, et al. Introduction to basic neurology. Philadelphia: W.B. Saunders; 1976.
4. Janka M, Merkel A, Schuh A. Diagnostik an der Lendenwirbelsäule [Clinical examination of the lumbar spine]. MMW Fortschr Med. 2019;161(1):55–8. https://doi.org/10.1007/s15006-019-0069-8.
5. Bateman EA, Fortin CD, Guo M. Musculoskeletal mimics of lumbosacral radiculopathy Muscle Nerve Published online May 10, 2024. https://doi.org/10.1002/mus.28106.
6. van der Windt DA, Simons E, Riphagen II, et al. Physical examination for lumbar radiculopathy due to disc herniation in patients with low-back pain. Cochrane Database Syst Rev. 2010;(2):CD007431. Published 2010 Feb 17. https://doi.org/10.1002/14651858.CD007431.pub2.
7. Litvan I, Mangone CA, Werden W, Bueri JA, Estol CJ, Garcea DO, Rey RC, Sica RE, Hallett M, Bartko JJ. Reliability of the NINDS Myotatic reflex scale. Neurology. 1996;47(4):969–72.
8. Kuris EO, McDonald CL, Palumbo MA, Daniels AH. Evaluation and management of Cauda Equina syndrome. Am J Med. 2021;134(12):1483–9. https://doi.org/10.1016/j.amjmed.2021.07.021.
9. Shahrokhi M, Asuncion RMD. Neurologic Exam. In: StatPearls. Treasure Island (FL): StatPearls Publishing; 2023.
10. de Carvalho Neto EG, Gomes MF, Damiani Monteiro M, Dalla Corte BM, Hoppe AM, Rotta FT. The medial hamstring (L5) reflex. Pract Neurol. 2020;20(6):472–3. https://doi.org/10.1136/practneurol-2020-002595.
11. Hudgins WR. The crossed straight leg raising test: a diagnostic sign of herniated disc. J Occup Med. 1979;21(6):407–8.
12. Supik LF, Broom MJ. Sciatic tension signs and lumbar disc herniation. Spine (Phila Pa 1976). 1994;19(9):1066–9. https://doi.org/10.1097/00007632-199405000-00013.

Radiological Assessment of the Lumbar Spine

5

Joshua Chalif, James Tanner McMahon, David Liu, and Hasan Zaidi

Introduction

Radiological imaging plays a pivotal role in the diagnosis, management, surgical planning, and outcomes assessment of lumbar spine pathologies. Given the complexity of the lumbar spine, accurate imaging is crucial for understanding the underlying anatomical and pathological conditions. Indeed, innovations in spinal surgery have often paralleled historic innovations in imaging, such as development of the X-ray, myelogram, CT scan, and MRI scan. Prior to the development of these imaging tools, spinal surgery was generally considered extremely high risk and was rarely performed. For example, the first lumbar discectomy was performed in 1934, prior to the advent of advanced imaging, and was thought to be due to a tumor [1]. The development of advanced imaging tools has greatly expanded the number of patients who undergo surgery as well as the safety of surgery itself. Conversely, the ubiquity of spinal imaging has reminded surgeons that radiological findings must be taken in the context of clinical symptoms [2]. This chapter explores the various radiological modalities available for assessing the lumbar spine and highlights their indications, techniques, and interpretation.

J. Chalif · J. T. McMahon · D. Liu · H. Zaidi (✉)
Department of Neurosurgery, Brigham and Women's Hospital, Boston, MA, USA
e-mail: jchalif@bwh.harvard.edu; jtmcmahon@bwh.harvard.edu; ddliu@mgb.org; hzaidi1@bwh.harvard.edu

Plain Radiography

Indications

Due to low cost and low radiation dose, plain radiography remains the first-line imaging modality for evaluating many lumbar spine disorders. For patients who initially present to their primary care provider or the emergency room, plain radiography is the first imaging study of choice, according to several guidelines [2]. Indications for lumbar spine X-ray include the initial evaluation of mechanical back pain, low-impact trauma, and degenerative changes. For surgeons evaluating the patient with mechanical back pain, flexion-extension and lateral bending views can be helpful to determine if there is dynamic instability which may be an indication for stabilization.

Techniques

The standard views include anteroposterior (AP) and lateral projections, which provide essential information on the overall alignment of the lumbar vertebrae, including the presence of spondylolisthesis, and normal lordosis (or lack thereof)

A. A. Baaj et al. (eds.), *Surgery of the Lumbar Spine*, https://doi.org/10.1007/978-3-032-18097-1_5

(Fig. 5.1). Oblique views are not commonly used due to presence of CT/MRI, but are still being used in transforaminal facet injections, and sometimes can be used to evaluate the integrity of the pars interarticularis [3]. Disc space narrowing and vertebral body height can also be evaluated. They help in identifying conditions such as osteophytes, disc space narrowing, and vertebral body alignment. Flexion-extension and bending films can help identify dynamic instability (due to spondylolisthesis, fracture, or ligamentous injury) by assessing changes in alignment with motion—a translation of more than 3 mm or an angular change of 10–15 degrees can indicate some degree of mechanical instability.

For flexion-extension films, the patient is typically positioned standing to maximize physiologic loading of the spine. Lateral radiographs are obtained in full forward flexion and maximal extension. The patient's pain should be well-controlled, and the patient should be encouraged to actively participate with maximal effort to avoid underestimating instability. The iliac crests and at least L1 through S1 should be visualized.

Interpretation

Radiographic interpretation focuses on evaluating vertebral alignment, detecting fractures, and assessing intervertebral disc space. Common findings include spondylolisthesis, scoliosis, and degenerative changes like osteophyte formation. Radiographs are often the first step in a comprehensive diagnostic workup and may guide the need for advanced imaging. For surgeons, they can also be a key component in evaluating instability and the subsequent need for stabilization.

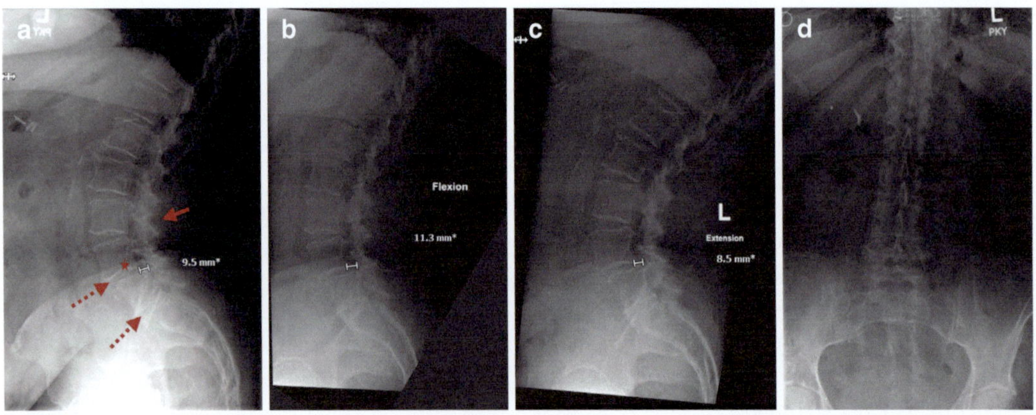

Fig. 5.1 Lumbar plain films. Depicted are four-view lumbar X-rays for the workup of degenerative lumbar spinal stenosis. Images are taken while the patient is standing. (**a**) *Lateral neutral.* Solid arrow demonstrates facet arthropathy, where bone is hypertrophied and joint lines are not clearly visible. Dashed arrows demonstrate disc space height loss at L4–5 and L5-S1. Star demonstrates grade I anterolisthesis of L4 on L5. (**b**) On flexion, the spondylolisthesis increases to 11.3 mm. (**c**) On extension, the spondylolisthesis reduces to 8.5 mm. (**d**) *Anterior-posterior.* There is no scoliosis on this view, and there is mild degeneration of both SI joints

Computed Tomography (CT)

Indications

CT imaging is highly valuable for detailed assessment of bony anatomy. It is particularly indicated in trauma cases to evaluate fractures, preoperative planning to assess pedicle morphology and bone quality, and in situations where MRI is contraindicated [4, 5].For patients with spondylolisthesis, a CT scan can help determine if there is a defect in the pars, or if there are other subtle bony defects. CT scans are also crucial for determining the quality of a fusion mass and for identifying evidence of screw pullout or pseudoarthrosis. Therefore, it is often obtained as part of an inpatient workup with trauma, as part of the preoperative planning process when it has already been decided that the patient will undergo surgery, or as part of the postoperative clinic visit.

Techniques

CT scans provide high-resolution images in axial, coronal, and sagittal planes (Fig. 5.2), taken in slice thickness ranges from 0.5 mm to 1.25 mm. Multiplanar reconstructions allow for a thorough evaluation of bony structures, which is critical in surgical planning, especially for spinal fusion procedures. Metal artifact, although greatly reduced with the introduction of new algorithms [6], can still significantly degrade image quality in patients with spinal hardware. A lumbar CT scan delivers about 4 millisieverts of ionizing radiation, which has a very small but non-zero increased lifetime cancer risk (estimated at about 1 in 4000 to 1 in 5000) [7].

Interpretation

CT imaging is the gold standard for assessing fractures, bone abnormalities, and postoperative evaluation of instrumentation. Although lumbar X-rays can demonstrate the presence of a fracture, characterizing it further often requires a CT scan to more clearly define the bony anatomy. CT is often used by surgeons to plan the insertion of pedicle screws, since it is the optimal method to evaluate the width and length of the pedicles. It provides detailed information on bone density,

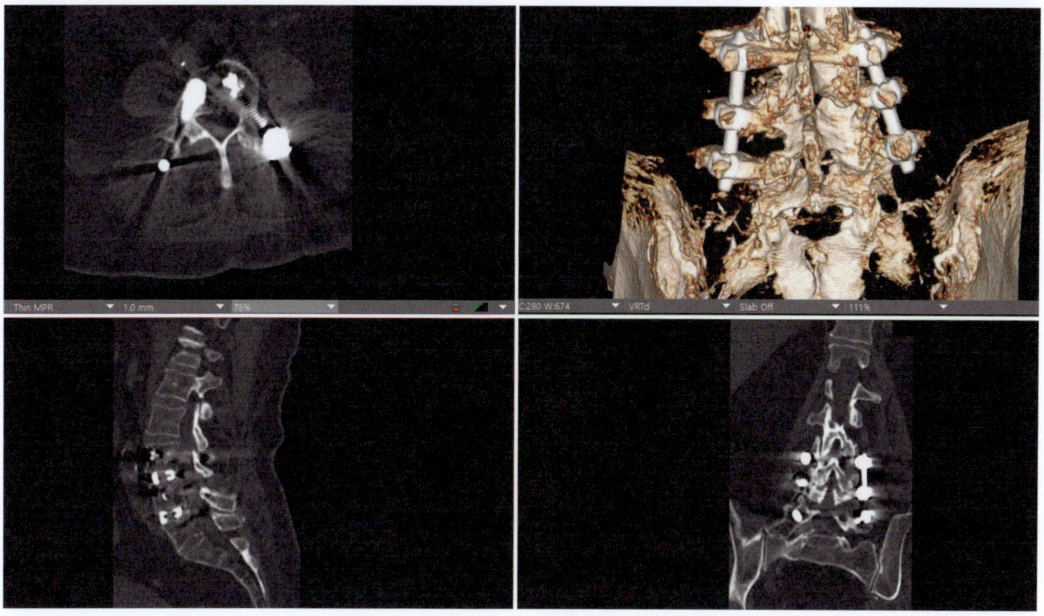

Fig. 5.2 CT of lumbar spine. A postoperative CT scan is depicted of the patient in Fig. 5.1, who underwent an L3–5 transforaminal interbody fusion with PMMA-augmented pedicle screws. Note the reduction of spondylolisthesis. CT scans can be used to evaluate integrity of postoperative hardware and alignment. The 3D reconstruction can be of utility when assessing complex anatomy

the presence of sclerotic lesions, and the integrity of the spinal canal [8]. Haloing around the screws or low Hounsfield units in the area of a fusion mass can be indicative of hardware or fusion failure. Poor bone quality may affect which spinal levels will be treated or whether the hardware needs to be augmented with adjuncts such as cement. However, it does have limited utility in assessing soft tissue structures, including nerve roots, discs, ligaments, and the spinal cord itself. Additionally, CT myelography, which involves the injection of contrast material, enhances visualization of the spinal cord and nerve roots, especially in patients who cannot undergo MRI [9].

Magnetic Resonance Imaging (MRI)

Indications

MRI is the imaging modality of choice for evaluating soft tissue structures of the lumbar spine, including intervertebral discs, spinal cord, nerve roots, and surrounding ligaments. It is particularly useful in cases of suspected disc herniation, spinal stenosis, infectious, inflammatory, or neoplastic conditions [10–12].

Techniques

A standard lumbar MRI spine protocol typically includes several sequences, in both the axial and sagittal planes; the images may also be reconstructed to be parallel to the axis of the spinal cord, which aids in visualization. T1 imaging is obtained to evaluate vertebral body marrow, anatomy, and disc desiccation. T2 imaging highlights cerebrospinal fluid and therefore is optimal for visualizing nerve root impingement, lateral recess stenosis, or foraminal narrowing. These images may be further processed into STIR or fat-suppressed sequence for highlighting edema and inflammation. Additionally, post-contrast T1 images with gadolinium are indicated in cases of suspected infection or tumor. Advanced techniques such as diffusion-weighted imaging (DWI) and MR myelography can further enhance diagnostic accuracy.

Interpretation

MRI provides detailed visualization of soft tissues, allowing for the assessment of disc degeneration, herniation, and nerve root compression. The full range of pathologies that can be evaluated and interpreted is beyond the scope of this chapter; the reader is referred to a formal neuroradiology textbook for this. Most commonly, lumbar MRIs are used to evaluate spinal stenosis which is readily identifiable on T2-weighted images, where the degree of canal narrowing can be assessed. Several grading systems for lumbar stenosis exist, such as the Lurie and Lee grading scales, which are commonly used by radiologists [13] (Fig. 5.3). These may guide—in conjunction with the clinical exam—whether the patient is a candidate for surgery. Additionally, MRI is invaluable in identifying infection, neoplasms, and other complex pathologies that may not be apparent on CT or plain radiography.

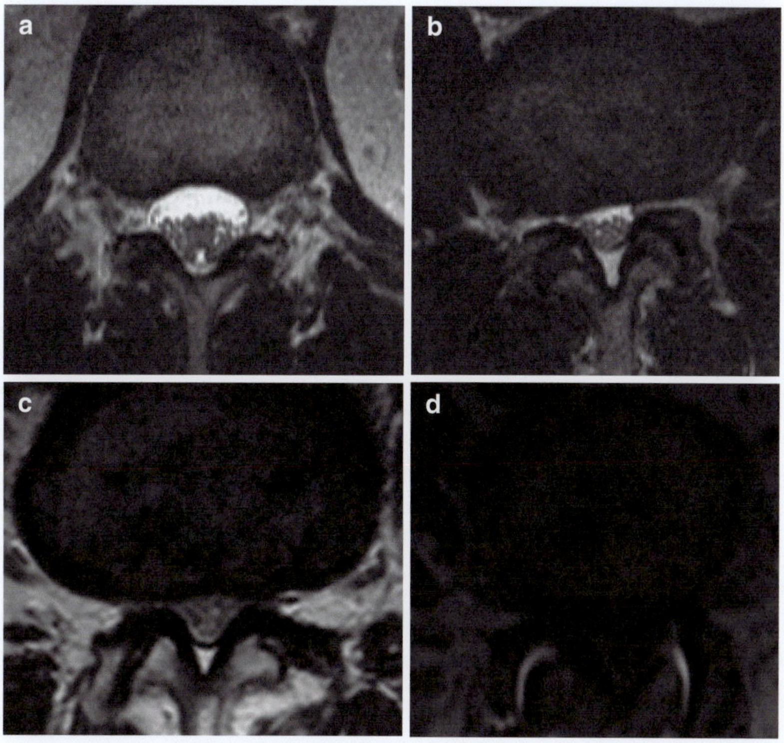

Fig. 5.3 Example of central lumbar spinal stenosis grading on MRI (Lee). Degree of stenosis is defined by degree of obliteration of anterior CSF space and degree of visualization of cauda equina nerve roots. Note that although the grades are discrete, stenosis lies upon a spectrum, so designations such as "moderate-severe" are not uncommon. (**a**) *Grade 0 (no stenosis).* Anterior CSF space is not obliterated. (**b**) *Grade 1 (mild stenosis).* Mild obliteration of the anterior CSF space, but all nerve roots are discernible. (**c**) *Grade 2 (moderate stenosis).* Moderate obliteration of the anterior CSF space, but nerve roots are discernible. (**d**) *Grade 3 (severe stenosis).* Complete obliteration of the anterior CSF space, but nerve roots are not discernible

Myelography

Indications

CT myelography is used when MRI is contraindicated or when further clarification of spinal canal pathology is needed [9]. It is particularly useful for visualizing spinal cord compression, nerve root anomalies, and postoperative scarring. A more recent indication has been to detect the presence of idiopathic CSF leaks. Therefore, it is usually only obtained in patients with more complex spinal pathology and is not part of the typical workup for lumbar spine pathology.

Techniques

This procedure involves the injection of contrast material into the subarachnoid space, followed by imaging under fluoroscopy or CT. This is done by lumbar puncture under fluoroscopic guidance, typically at the L3–4 or L4–5 level. The patient is placed in the Trendelenburg or lateral decubitus position to allow contrast to flow cranially. CT scan is performed shortly afterwards. Contrast outlines the spinal cord and nerve roots, providing detailed information on compressive lesions. The radiation dose is slightly higher than a standard lumbar CT, in the range of 6 to 10 millisieverts.

Interpretation

Myelography is effective in detecting spinal cord compression, arachnoiditis, and nerve root abnormalities. It is particularly useful in complex cases where MRI findings are inconclusive or in patients with contraindications to MRI, for example, if a patient has a spinal cord stimulator or an implantable cardiac device that is not MRI compatible.

Bone Scintigraphy

Indications

Bone scintigraphy is employed to detect areas of increased osteoblastic activity, such as in cases of metastases, infection, or stress fractures. It is particularly useful when there is a suspicion of metastatic disease or osteomyelitis. Though largely supplanted by MRI and CT in many diagnostic contexts, bone scintigraphy retains utility in specific clinical scenarios where metabolic bone activity must be assessed.

Techniques

The most commonly used technique is single-photon emission computed tomography (SPECT), which allows for the detection of increased metabolic activity in bone [14]. It involves the intravenous injection of a radiotracer, typically technetium-99 m-labeled methylene diphosphonate (Tc-99 m MDP), which is preferentially taken up by areas of increased bone metabolism. Images are typically obtained in three phases: (1) Perfusion (dynamic) phase: Immediately post-injection to assess blood flow; (2) Blood pool phase: Minutes after injection, reflects soft tissue vascularity; (3) Delayed (bone) phase: 2–4 h post-injection, reveals osseous uptake patterns.

Interpretation

Bone scintigraphy identifies areas of increased radiotracer uptake, indicating active bone formation or repair. This modality is extremely sensitive for detecting early bone changes that may not be visible on plain radiography or CT, making it valuable in the detection of occult fractures or early-stage infections which may not be readily apparent in other imaging modalities.

Ultrasound

Indications

Although ultrasound has a limited role in spinal imaging, it can be useful in specific cases, such as guiding injections or evaluating soft tissue masses adjacent to the spine [15]. It is more commonly used during injections in pain clinic or intraoperatively to visualize the spinal cord and nerve roots.

Techniques

Doppler ultrasound is sometimes used to assess vascular structures and blood flow near the spine. In the operative setting, it can be used to visualize the intrathecal contents, for example, during spinal tumor surgery.

Interpretation

Ultrasound can help in evaluating soft tissue structures, including ligaments and muscles, as well as vascular abnormalities. However, its use is generally limited due to the complex anatomy and the presence of bony structures that obstruct sound waves. It is an attractive modality of imaging since it is real-time and does not involve radiation; however, it has limited use cases and is still under active development for spinal pathologies.

Radiological Findings in Common Lumbar Spine Pathologies

Degenerative Disc Disease

Degenerative disc disease is characterized by loss of disc height, disc desiccation, and the presence of osteophytes. MRI is the preferred modality for evaluating the extent of disc degeneration and its impact on adjacent structures [16]. On MRI, disc desiccation will appear as decreased T2 signal; Modic changes may also be seen (the reader is referred to a formal neuroradiology text for full discussion of Modic changes). Osteophyte formation may also be present on radiographs and CTs as bony spurs at endplates, but is less easily visualized on MRIs.

Lumbar Spinal Stenosis

Spinal stenosis is often identified on MRI by narrowing of the spinal canal, which may be due to disc bulging, ligamentum flavum hypertrophy, or osteophyte formation. The degree of stenosis and its clinical relevance are assessed by correlating imaging findings with patient symptoms [11]. Typically, the degree of effacement of CSF signal around the thecal sac on T2 MRI is directly reflective of the degree of central stenosis. The loss of perineural fat signal surrounding the nerve root on sagittal T2 MRI is proportional to the degree of foraminal stenosis. Several grading systems exist, for which we refer the reader to other texts.

Lumbar Disc Herniation

Disc herniation is readily identifiable on MRI, where the displaced disc material can be visualized compressing adjacent nerve roots. T2-weighted images are particularly useful in showing the extent of disc herniation and its effect on the spinal canal [17]. The surgeon may see focal disc extension beyond the vertebral body margin, and if the fragment is fully separated from the parent disc (often caudally), this is called sequestered. The location of disc herniation is important for preoperative planning, as this will dictate how much bone and ligament needs to be resected in an operation.

Lumbar Deformity

Long-cassette standing lumbar films can be obtained for the workup of degenerative lumbar scoliosis. A lateral film evaluates for sagittal deformity while an anterior-posterior film evaluates for coronal deformity (Fig. 5.4). The patient is asked to stand and an X-ray spanning from the femoral shafts to the skull base is obtained. It is critical that the femoral heads be overlapping for proper interpretation. The specific theory and measurements for sagittal balance parameters such as pelvic incidence, lumbar lordosis, and sagittal vertical axis will not be addressed in this chapter.

Spondylolisthesis

Spondylolisthesis is typically evaluated using plain radiography, where the degree of vertebral slippage can be measured. This is graded with the Meyerding classification, which ranges from 1 to 5, with increasing number indicating increasing slippage. These may be due to pars interarticularis defects, which are typically best evaluated with CT. MRI or CT may be used to assess associated disc degeneration or nerve root compression [18]. Standing flexion-extension plain radiographs can also be useful in evaluating "dynamic instability" of a spondylolisthesis [19].

Infections and Neoplasms

Infections such as discitis or osteomyelitis are best evaluated with MRI with gadolinium contrast, which can show early inflammatory changes and abscess formation [20]. Neoplasms may present with bone destruction or soft tissue masses, which are well visualized on both MRI and CT [21].

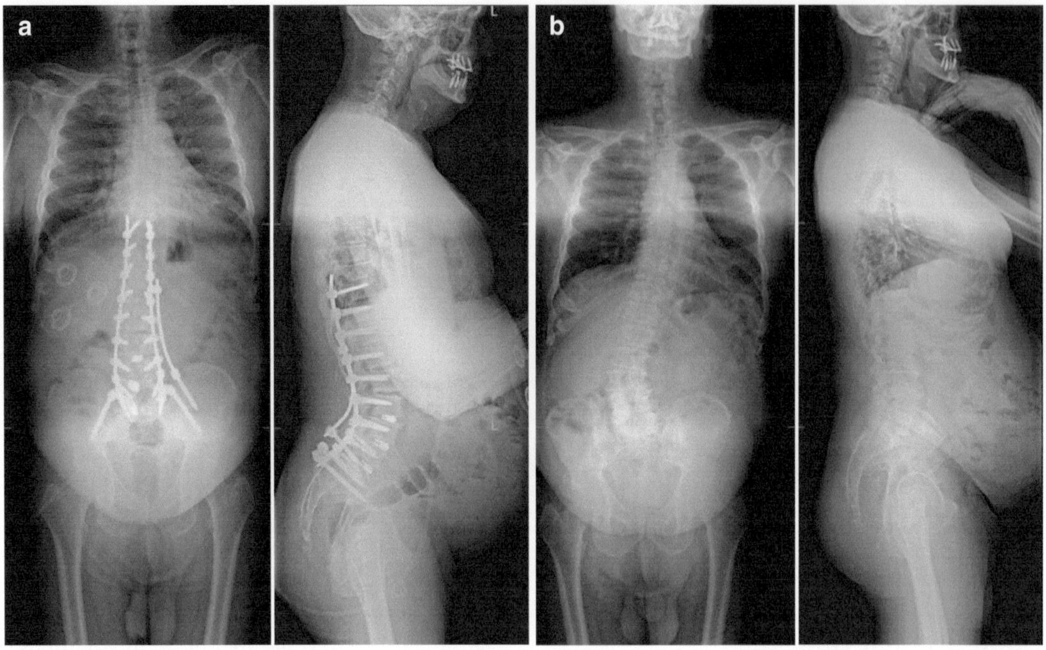

Fig. 5.4 Scoliosis standing films. Postoperative (**a**) and preoperative (**b**) standing lumbar X-rays from T10-Pelvis fusion surgery for lumbar sagittal deformity. The patient also has a thoracic deformity as well. Postoperative films demonstrate improvement in alignment and new spinal hardware

Role of Radiological Imaging in Pre- and Postoperative Assessment

Preoperative Planning

Radiological imaging is critical in preoperative planning, allowing for detailed assessment of anatomical structures and identification of potential challenges. For instance, CT scans are invaluable in planning the placement of pedicle screws, while MRI can identify soft tissue pathology that might affect surgical outcomes.

Postoperative Imaging

Postoperative imaging is essential for monitoring the placement of hardware, assessing fusion status, and identifying complications such as infection or hardware failure. CT is often used to evaluate bone fusion, while MRI can be employed to assess soft tissue healing and any recurrent pathology [22].

Emerging Technologies in Lumbar Spine Imaging

3D Imaging and Navigation

Advances in 3D imaging using augmented reality and navigation systems have revolutionized spinal surgery, allowing for more precise planning and execution of surgical procedures [23, 24]. These technologies integrate preoperative imaging with real-time surgical navigation, enhancing accuracy and reducing the risk of complications.

Artificial Intelligence (AI) and Machine Learning

AI and machine learning are increasingly being applied to radiological imaging, offering the potential for automated image analysis and predictive modeling [25]. These technologies may improve diagnostic accuracy and efficiency, particularly in identifying subtle pathologies and guiding treatment decisions.

Conclusion

Radiological assessment is a cornerstone of lumbar spine surgery, providing essential information for diagnosis, surgical planning, and postoperative monitoring. Each imaging modality offers unique strengths, and their combined use allows for a comprehensive evaluation of the lumbar spine. As technology continues to advance, emerging imaging techniques and AI applications hold promise for further enhancing the precision and effectiveness of lumbar spine surgery.

References

1. Mixter WJ, Barr JS. Rupture of the intervertebral disc with involvement of the Spinal Canal. N Engl J Med. 1934;211(5):210–5. https://doi.org/10.1056/NEJM193408022110506.
2. Jarvik JG, Deyo RA. Diagnostic evaluation of low back pain with emphasis on imaging. Ann Intern Med. 2002;137(7):586–97. https://doi.org/10.7326/0003-4819-137-7-200210010-00010.
3. Libson E, Bloom RA, Dinari G, Robin GC. Oblique lumbar spine radiographs: importance in young patients. Radiology. 1984;151(1):89–90. https://doi.org/10.1148/radiology.151.1.6701343.
4. Bernstein MP, Young MG, Baxter AB. Imaging of spine trauma. Radiol Clin North Am. 2019;57(4):767–85. https://doi.org/10.1016/j.rcl.2019.02.007.
5. Zhang Q, Zhao F, Zhang Y, Huang M, Gong X, Deng X. Automated measurement of lumbar pedicle screw parameters using deep learning algorithm on preoperative CT scans. J Bone Oncol. 2024;47:100627. https://doi.org/10.1016/j.jbo.2024.100627.
6. Kotsenas AL, Michalak GJ, DeLone DR, et al. CT metal artifact reduction in the spine: can an iterative reconstruction technique improve visualization? AJNR Am J Neuroradiol. 2015;36(11):2184–90. https://doi.org/10.3174/ajnr.A4416.
7. National Research Council Committee on Health Effects of Exposure to Low Levels of Ionizing R. Health Effects of Exposure to Low Levels of Ionizing Radiations: Time for Reassessment? National Academies Press (US). Copyright 1998 by the National Academy of Sciences. All rights reserved; 1998.
8. Ahmad A, Crawford CH 3rd, Glassman SD, Dimar JR 2nd, Gum JL, Carreon LY. Correlation between bone density measurements on CT or MRI versus DEXA scan: a systematic review. N Am Spine Soc J. 2023;14:100204. https://doi.org/10.1016/j.xnsj.2023.100204.
9. Patel DM, Weinberg BD, Hoch MJ. CT myelography: clinical indications and imaging findings. Radiographics. 2020;40(2):470–84. https://doi.org/10.1148/rg.2020190135.
10. Zhang AS, Xu A, Ansari K, et al. Lumbar disc herniation: diagnosis and management. Am J Med. 2023;136(7):645–51. https://doi.org/10.1016/j.amjmed.2023.03.024.
11. Katz JN, Zimmerman ZE, Mass H, Makhni MC. Diagnosis and Management of Lumbar Spinal Stenosis: a review. JAMA. 2022;327(17):1688–99. https://doi.org/10.1001/jama.2022.5921.
12. Mechri M, Riahi H, Sboui I, Bouaziz M, Vanhoenacker F, Ladeb M. Imaging of malignant primitive tumors of the spine. J Belg Soc Radiol. 2018;102(1):56. https://doi.org/10.5334/jbsr.1410.
13. Guen YL, Joon WL, Hee SC, Kyoung-Jin O, Heung SK. A new grading system of lumbar central canal stenosis on MRI: an easy and reliable method. Skeletal Radiol. 2011;40(8):1033–9. https://doi.org/10.1007/s00256-011-1102-x.
14. Varga M, Kantorová L, Langaufová A, et al. Role of single-photon emission computed tomography imaging in the diagnosis and treatment of chronic neck or Back pain caused by spinal degeneration: a systematic review. World Neurosurg. 2023;173:65–78. https://doi.org/10.1016/j.wneu.2023.02.058.
15. Vasudeva VS, Abd-El-Barr M, Pompeu YA, Karhade A, Groff MW, Lu Y. Use of intraoperative ultrasound during spinal surgery. Global Spine J. 2017;7(7):648–56. https://doi.org/10.1177/2192568217700100.
16. Taher F, Essig D, Lebl DR, et al. Lumbar degenerative disc disease: current and future concepts of diagnosis and management. Adv Orthop. 2012;2012:970752. https://doi.org/10.1155/2012/970752.
17. Pojskic M, Bisson E, Oertel J, Takami T, Zygourakis C, Costa F. Lumbar disc herniation: epidemiology, clinical and radiologic diagnosis WFNS spine committee recommendations. World Neurosurg X. 2024;22:100279. https://doi.org/10.1016/j.wnsx.2024.100279.
18. Vilanilam GK, Kumar S, Vattoth S. MR imaging differentiating features between lytic and degenerative lumbosacral spondylolisthesis. Neuroradiol J. 2024;37(3):276–84. https://doi.org/10.1177/19714009231177409.
19. Câmara JR, Keen JR, Asgarzadie F. Functional radiography in examination of spondylolisthesis. AJR Am J Roentgenol. 2015;204(4):W461–9. https://doi.org/10.2214/ajr.14.13139.
20. Dhodapkar MM, Patel T, Rubio DR. Imaging in spinal infections: current status and future directions.

N Am Spine Soc J. 2023;16:100275. https://doi.org/10.1016/j.xnsj.2023.100275.
21. Motamedi K, Ilaslan H, Seeger LL. Imaging of the lumbar spine neoplasms. Semin Ultrasound CT MR. 2004;25(6):474–89. https://doi.org/10.1053/j.sult.2004.09.004.
22. Choudhri TF, Mummaneni PV, Dhall SS, et al. Guideline update for the performance of fusion procedures for degenerative disease of the lumbar spine. Part 4: radiographic assessment of fusion status. J Neurosurg Spine. 2014;21(1):23–30. https://doi.org/10.3171/2014.4.Spine14267.
23. Pierzchajlo N, Stevenson TC, Huynh H, et al. Augmented reality in minimally invasive spinal surgery: a narrative review of available technology. World Neurosurg. 2023;176:35–42. https://doi.org/10.1016/j.wneu.2023.04.030.
24. Sommer F, Hussain I, Kirnaz S, et al. Safety and feasibility of augmented reality assistance in minimally invasive and open resection of benign intradural extramedullary tumors. Neurospine. 2022;19(3):501–12. https://doi.org/10.14245/ns.2244222.111.
25. Martín-Noguerol T, Oñate Miranda M, Amrhein TJ, et al. The role of artificial intelligence in the assessment of the spine and spinal cord. Eur J Radiol. 2023;161:110726. https://doi.org/10.1016/j.ejrad.2023.110726.

6 Intraoperative Neuromonitoring in Lumbar Spine Surgery

Sarah Bin Abdulqader, Muhammad Tariq Imtiaz, and Sultan Aldebeyan

Introduction

Intraoperative neurophysiology monitoring (IONM) has been established as a major and cornerstone ancillary prerequisite for many spine procedures [1]. Its utilization has led to improved neurological outcomes attributed to the immediate real-time feedback on spinal cord function [2]. This immediate and instant feedback can help the surgical team in intraoperative decision-making and guide them to reduce or reverse this damage [3]. Furthermore, it can help the surgeon guesstimate the nature of damage allowing them to complete the procedure while minimizing further injury [3, 4]. This consequently made the use of IONM a standard of care in many spine procedures and for scoliosis surgery in particular [5]. Various electrophysiological monitoring modalities have been used to monitor central and peripheral nervous system function with their unique sets of benefits, limitations, sensitivity, and specificity. These modalities include somatosensory evoked potentials (SSEPs), motor evoked potentials (MEPs), free-run or spontaneous EMG (sEMG), and triggered EMG (tEMG) [1] (Fig. 6.1).

This chapter will focus on the utility of IONM in different lumbar spine surgeries.

S. B. Abdulqader
Department of Neurosurgery, National Neuroscience Institute, King Fahad Medical City, Riyadh, Saudi Arabia

M. T. Imtiaz
Department of Neurophysiology, National Neuroscience Institute, King Fahad Medical City, Riyadh, Saudi Arabia

S. Aldebeyan (✉)
Department of Spine Surgery, National Neuroscience Institute, King Fahad Medical City, Riyadh, Saudi Arabia

A. A. Baaj et al. (eds.), *Surgery of the Lumbar Spine*, https://doi.org/10.1007/978-3-032-18097-1_6

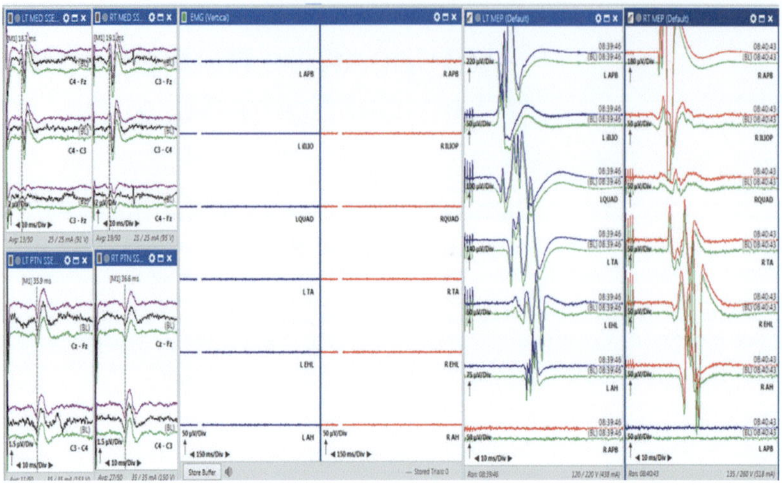

Fig. 6.1 A view of multimodality intraoperative neurophysiology monitoring data showing upper and lower SSEPs, EMGs, and left and right TcMEPs in one screen

Monitoring Modalities

Somatosensory Evoked Potentials

SSEPs were the earliest spinal cord electrophysiological monitoring modality described for the surgical correction of scoliosis in the 1970s [6]. Since then, SSEPs have remained the mainstay modality for assessing intraoperative spinal cord function during various spinal procedures. It provides monitoring of the dorsal column which mediates tactile sensation, vibration, and proprioception [1, 7]. Although it has been used widely with excellent reliability, a few drawbacks have been raised concerning the safety of using SSEPs as a standalone monitoring modality [1]. Interruptions in monitoring lead to temporal summation resulting in a delay in detecting signal changes up to 16 min [8]. However, delays have been minimized now with collaboration from anesthesia teams regarding the use of optimal anesthetic regimens and achieving data within seconds with minimal averages [1]. Still, there have been reports of false positives and false negatives using this modality [8–10]. For these reasons, the modern technique of using IONM doesn't solely rely on one modality but rather the reading of data together from all modalities before making a decision (Multi-Modality IONM) (Fig. 6.1).

For lumbar spine surgery, the posterior tibial nerve (L4, L5, S1, and S2) and the peroneal nerve (L4, L5, and S1) are usually selected for monitoring (Fig. 6.3) [1]. Stimulation of electrodes placed on the lower limbs is recorded using scalp or posterior neck coherent with the primary somatosensory cortex (using the 10/20 EEG system) [1]. A 50% reduction in amplitude and/or a 10% increase in latency (the time it takes for waves from the point of stimulation to the point of recording) are considered alarming and corrective measures should be taken [1]. Other factors that might affect the SSEPs'amplitude need to be eliminated such as hypothermia, hypotension, halogenated agents, and nitrous oxide [1].

Motor Evoked Potentials

MEPs have emerged as a viable and valuable monitoring modality in the 1980s [11]. The main advantage of MEPs is the ability and sensitivity to predict postoperative motor deficits as it primarily monitors the corticospinal tract pathway [1, 12]. Additionally, MEPs can detect ischemic insults during various spine procedures [1]. Before the use of MEPs, the only reliable method to assess corticospinal tract integrity and motor function during spine surgery was the Stagnara wake-up test [13]. This test requires waking up

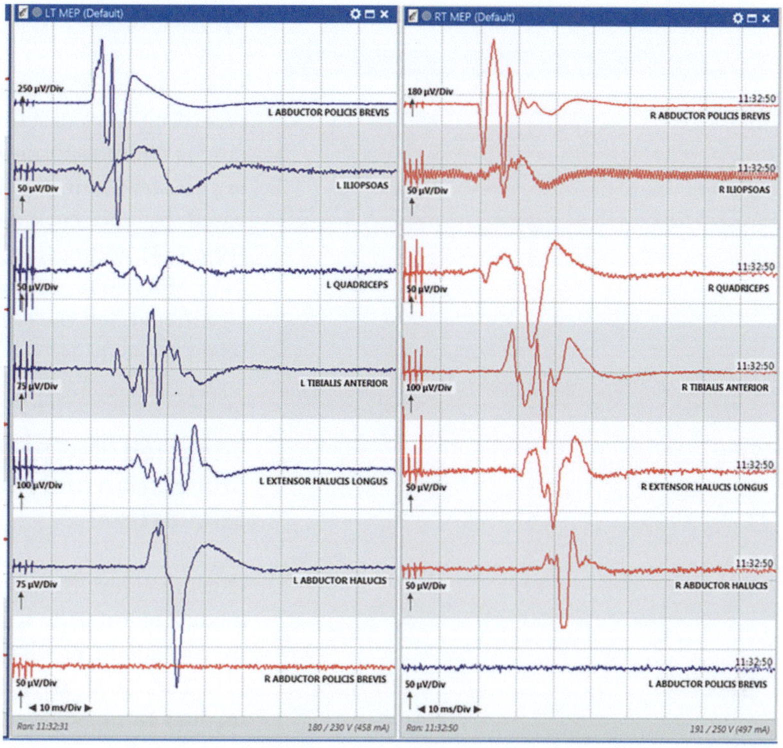

Fig. 6.2 Left and right side TcMEPs (left side body responses (CMAPs) in blue while right side body responses in red colors to identify laterality clearly). Muscles on the top are left and right upper limb (hand muscles) which serves as a control for lumbar spinal surgeries. Later responses are from lower limb muscles corresponding to several Lumbar nerve roots. Data is continuously monitored as much as possible especially during important surgical steps and compared with starting pre-incision data (baselines)

the patient during surgery and asking them to move their feet [1, 13]. Although it is useful in some cases, it is practically time-consuming and lacks accuracy.

Transcranial MEPs (TcMEPs) in spine surgery are acquired using transcranial stimulation with the placement of electrodes on the scalp coherent with the primary motor cortex (using the 10/20 EEG system) [1, 3] (Fig. 6.2). Signals can be recorded at the level of the muscle (compound muscle action potential [CMAP]), nerve (neurogenic MEPs), or spinal cord (direct corticospinal wave [D-wave] recording) [1]. Direct spinal cord stimulation can also be performed with electrodes recorded at the level of the nerves or muscles. In direct TcMEP, electrodes are placed at C3 and C4 if stimulation for both upper and lower extremities is desired and at C1 and C2 if more focal activation of the lower extremity is needed [1].

Four methods are generally employed for the interpretation of MEP recordings. (1) the all-or-nothing criterion [1, 14], (2) the amplitude criterion [1, 15], (3) the threshold criterion [1, 16], and (4) the morphology criterion [1, 17]. In the all-or-nothing criterion, a complete loss of MEP signals is considered a clinically significant event [1]. The amplitude criterion uses a decrease of 80% in amplitude in at least 1 out of 6 recorded sites as a clinically significant event [15]. The threshold criterion analyzes the increment in stimulation threshold required to maintain the compound muscle action potential [16]. The morphology criterion evaluates changes in the pattern and duration of MEP waveform morphology [1, 17]. The most common practice these days is to assess the data quickly amongst all criteria and establish an intervention relevant to surgical maneuvers.

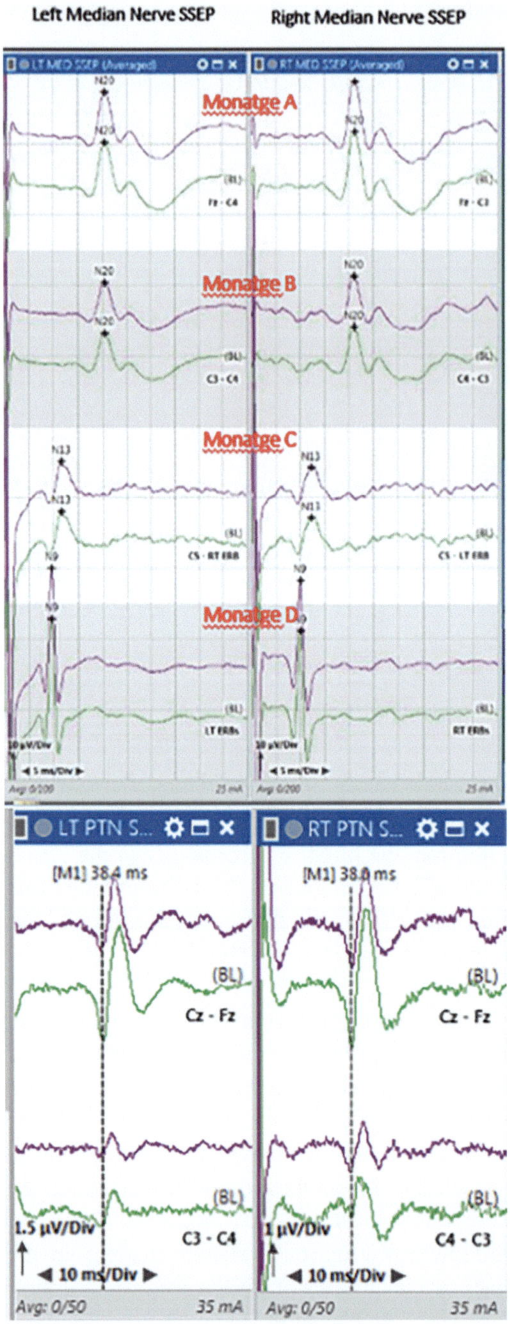

Fig. 6.3 Left and right median nerve SSEPs (top picture) with stimulation at median nerves at the wrist. Montage D recorded at Erbs point (brachial plexus) shows peripheral conduction at 9 milliseconds N9. Montage C recorded at brain stem or medulla at 13 milliseconds N13. Montages A & B are central nervous system recordings from scalp electrodes at 20 milliseconds N20 (primary sensory cortex). Bottom Picture: Scalp electrodes recordings from posterior tibial nerves stimulation at ankles (left and right sides) with latency at 38 milliseconds. Data is continuously monitored as much as possible especially during important surgical steps and compared with starting pre-incision data (baselines)

Spontaneous EMG

Spontaneous EMG (sEMG) is used where the recording of a certain nerve root is required [1, 3]. These recordings are obtained by placing electrodes in the muscle of interest innervated by the corresponding nerve root [1] (Fig. 6.4). Repetitive, continuous EMG firing or sEMG trains are considered to be clinically significant and the surgeon should be notified when present [1].

Triggered EMG (tEMG-Pedicle Screw Stimulation and Direct Nerve Stimulation)

During spine instrumentation, identifying a medial or inferior breach of the pedicle wall may result in preventable nerve root damage [1]. Therefore, triggered EMG evolved as a method to detect medial/inferior pedicle wall breaches during instrumentation [3]. This technique uses a monopolar that directly stimulates the pedicle screw at various intensities. Needles placed at the corresponding muscles will measure CMAP time-locked to the stimulation [1]. In lumbar spine surgery, a threshold acquired between 10 and 20 milliamperes indicates that no breach of the medial (drop in TcMEPs) or lateral wall (Significant sEMG activity) has occurred [1]. Generally, a threshold higher than 10 milliamperes for lumbar levels and higher than 8 milliamperes for thoracic levels are safe screws.

Moreover, tEMG has become a viable monitoring tool during cauda equina surgery [18]. During cauda equina tumor resection, tEMG can detect if the involved rootlets can be resected safely or not with a sensitivity of 37% and specificity of 97% [18]. Healthy spinal motor nerve roots can be safely stimulated with responses acquired at less than 1 milliamperes up to 2–3 milliamperes. However, higher milliamperes may suggest an inherent pathology in the nerve roots and need to be carefully assessed.

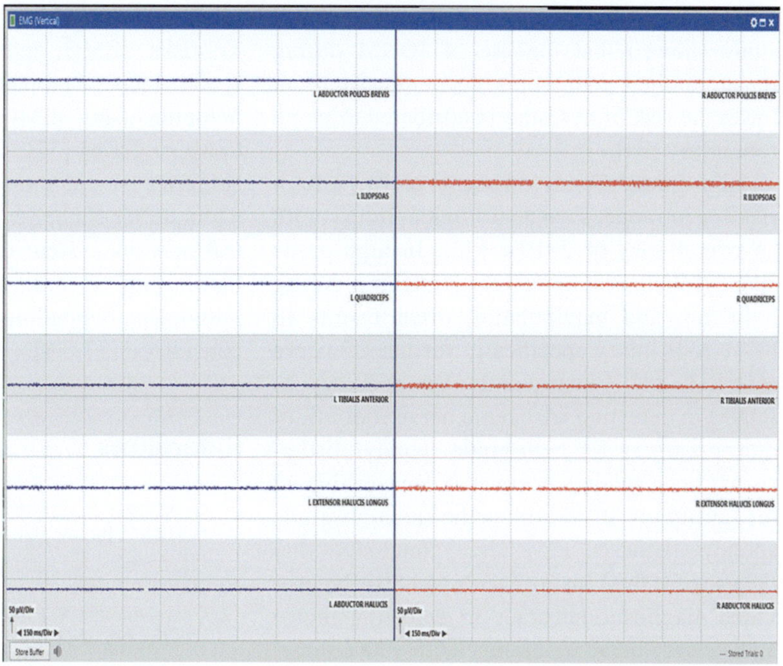

Fig. 6.4 Left and right spontaneous EMG (sEMG) from multiple lumbar root levels showing no discharges

Monitoring in Lumbar Spine Surgery

IONM plays a major role in different lumbar spine surgery procedures, including oncology surgery, degenerative spine conditions, and deformity surgery [3]. In lumbar spine oncology cases, intraoperative SSEPs and MEPs are usually monitored [19]. In addition, preoperative evoked potentials, SSEPs and MEPs can be used to complement the clinical examination and assess the extent of spinal cord dysfunction [19]. Moreover, direct waves (D-waves) have emerged lately as an adjunct to MEPs in assessing the integrity of the corticospinal tract function [20]. The main advantage of D-waves over MEPs is their predictability of long-term functional outcomes [21]. However, D-waves are not useful in lumbar spine tumors given their inability to detect signals below the thoracic 10–11 level [20, 21].

The role of IONM in degenerative spine conditions has been widely discussed lately and remains controversial [5]. Lateral interbody lumbar fusion is considered a minimally invasive technique targeted at treating various lumbar spine conditions [22]. This technique has a risk of injuring the lumbar plexus especially when done through a trans-psoas approach [22]. EMG monitoring has been routinely implemented in such cases with growing literature on the utility of other monitoring modalities such as saphenous SSEP and MEP [23–25]. Moreover, literature is evolving on the utility of IONM in degenerative spine cases specifically for revisions and instrumented fusion with high sensitivity and specificity [2, 26].

Posterior spinal fusion is a commonly performed procedure with a risk of iatrogenic paraplegia ranging between 0.6% and 3.5% [27, 28]. A recent study found that 3.3% of patients had changes in SSEPs or MEPs after posterior spinal fusion [28]. However, these signal changes were evident at the cervical and cervicothoracic levels with no significant signal alteration in the lumbar spine levels [28]. Moreover, there was no added benefit of the use of IONM during minimally invasive transforaminal lumbar interbody fusion in one study [29].

In endoscopic lumbar spine surgery, the utility of IONM has been discussed in small case series; however, no evidence supports its true efficacy in those cases [30]. However, a recent study showed that the use of IONM during transforaminal endoscopic decompression can lower the risk of dysesthesia attributed to nerve root injury [31].

High-grade spondylolisthesis carries a high risk for intraoperative neurological injury with an overall risk of 2–10% [32]. In high-grade spondylolisthesis, nerve root stretching during reduction and manipulation often results in nerve root injury specifically for the L5 nerve root [33, 34]. Consequently, the accuracy of IONM in detecting iatrogenic nerve root injury during surgery for high-grade spondylolisthesis has been studied. Lorio et al. have evaluated the utility of IONM in pediatric high-grade spondylolisthesis. [35] They concluded that the use of IONM (using MEPs and SSEPs) provided diagnostic accuracy in detecting motor and sensory nerve root injury with 100% sensitivity and 80.5–97.1% specificity [35]. However, IONM did not add significant value in reducing the risk of L5 nerve root injury in adult high-grade spondylolisthesis with a sensitivity of 20% and specificity of 100% [36]. If IONM is indicated, monitoring of peroneal and posterior tibial nerves SSEPs, sEMG, and TcMEPs using relevant muscles including anal sphincters monitoring can be useful (Table 6.1).

IONM has strong implications during spinal dysraphism, cerebral palsy-spastic diaplegia, and tethered cord surgeries [37, 38]. Similar to other lumbar spine procedures, SSEPs, TcMEPs, sEMG, and special techniques with specific sets of parameters for monitoring and mapping using tEMGs are monitored during these surgeries [37]. Given that most of these surgeries are commonly performed in children, a unique set of challenges attributed to the central nervous system maturity might affect the monitoring techniques, and individualized monitoring depending on age group should be considered [37, 38].

Table 6.1 Muscles tested

Root	Muscle	Nerve
L2-3-4	Illiacus	Lumbar plexus
L2-3-4	Rectus femoris	Femoral
L4-5 S1	Semitendinosus/ membranosus	Sciatic
L4-5	Tibilais anterior	Peroneal
L5-S1	Extensor hallucis	Peroneal
L5-S1	Extensor digitorum brevis	Peroneal
L5-S1	Gastrocnemius lateral	Tibial
S1-2	Gastrocnemius medial	Tibial
S1-2	Abductor hallucis	Tibial
S3-4-5	External anal sphincter	Pudendal
S3-4-5	External urethral sphincter	Pedendal

References

1. Gonzalez AA, Jeyanandarajan D, Hansen C, Zada G, Hsieh PC. Intraoperative neurophysiological monitoring during spine surgery: a review. Neurosurg Focus. 2009;27(4):E6.
2. Charalampidis A, Jiang F, Wilson JR, Badhiwala JH, Brodke DS, Fehlings MG. The use of intraoperative neurophysiological monitoring in spine surgery. Glob Spine J. 2020;10(1_suppl):104S–14S.
3. Fehlings MG, Brodke DS, Norvell DC, Dettori JR. The evidence for intraoperative neurophysiological monitoring in spine surgery: does it make a difference? Spine. 2010;35(9S):S37–46.
4. Pajewski TN, Arlet V, Phillips LH. Current approach on spinal cord monitoring: the point of view of the neurologist, the anesthesiologist and the spine surgeon. Eur Spine J. 2007;16:115–29.
5. Sharan A, Groff MW, DAiley AT, Ghogawala Z, Resnick DK, Watters WC, et al. Guideline update for the performance of fusion procedures for degenerative disease of the lumbar spine. Part 15: electrophysiological monitoring and lumbar fusion. J Neurosurg Spine. 2014;21(1):102–5.
6. Nash JCL, Lorig RA, Schatzinger LA, Brown RH. Spinal cord monitoring during operative treatment of the spine. Clin Orthop Relat Res (1976–2007). 1977;126:100–5.
7. Chiappa KH. Short-latency somatosensory evoked potentials: methodology. In: Evoked potentials in clinical medicine; 1990. p. 307–435.
8. Hilibrand AS, Schwartz DM, Sethuraman V, Vaccaro AR, Albert TJ. Comparison of transcranial electric motor and somatosensory evoked potential monitoring during cervical spine surgery. JBJS. 2004;86(6):1248–53.
9. Gunnarsson T, Krassioukov AV, Sarjeant R, Fehlings MG. Real-time continuous intraoperative electromyographic and somatosensory evoked potential recordings in spinal surgery: correlation of clinical and electrophysiologic findings in a pro-

spective, consecutive series of 213 cases. Spine. 2004;29(6):677–84.
10. Minahan RE, Sepkuty JP, Lesser RP, Sponseller PD, Kostuik JP. Anterior spinal cord injury with preserved neurogenic 'motor'evoked potentials. Clin Neurophysiol. 2001;112(8):1442–50.
11. Merton P, Morton H. Stimulation of the cerebral cortex in the intact human subject. Nature 1980;285(5762):227-.
12. Hsu B, Cree AK, Lagopoulos J, Cummine JL. Transcranial motor-evoked potentials combined with response recording through compound muscle action potential as the sole modality of spinal cord monitoring in spinal deformity surgery. Spine. 2008;33(10):1100–6.
13. Ben-David B, Taylor PD, Haller GS. Posterior spinal fusion complicated by posterior column injury: a case report of a false-negative wake-up test. Spine. 1987;12(6):540–3.
14. Kothbauer KF, Deletis V, Epstein FJ. Motor-evoked potential monitoring for intramedullary spinal cord tumor surgery: correlation of clinical and neurophysiological data in a series of 100 consecutive procedures. Neurosurg Focus. 1998;4(5):E3.
15. Langeloo DD, Lelivelt A, Journée HL, Slappendel R, de Kleuver M. Transcranial electrical motor-evoked potential monitoring during surgery for spinal deformity: a study of 145 patients. Spine. 2003;28(10):1043–50.
16. Calancie B, Molano MR. Alarm criteria for motor-evoked potentials: what's wrong with the "presence-or-absence" approach? Spine. 2008;33(4):406–14.
17. Quiñones-Hinojosa A, Lyon R, Zada G, Lamborn KR, Gupta N, Parsa AT, et al. Changes in transcranial motor evoked potentials during intramedullary spinal cord tumor resection correlate with postoperative motor function. Neurosurgery. 2005;56(5):982–93.
18. Lee S, Cho D-C, Rhim SC, Lee BJ, Hong SH, Koo YS, Park JH. Intraoperative monitoring for cauda equina tumors: surgical outcomes and neurophysiological data accrued over 10 years. Neurospine. 2021;18(2):281.
19. Ilhan F, Boulogne S, Morgado A, Dauleac C, André-Obadia N, Jung J. The impact of neurophysiological monitoring during Intradural spinal tumor surgery. Cancer. 2024;16(12):2192.
20. Deletis V, Sala F. Intraoperative neurophysiological monitoring of the spinal cord during spinal cord and spine surgery: a review focus on the corticospinal tracts. Clin Neurophysiol. 2008;119(2):248–64.
21. Olmsted ZT, Ryu B, Phayal G, Green R, Lo S-FL, Sciubba DM, et al. Direct wave intraoperative neuromonitoring for spinal tumor resection: a focused review. World neurosurgery: X. 2023;17:100139.
22. Cofano F, Zenga F, Mammi M, Altieri R, Marengo N, Ajello M, et al. Intraoperative neurophysiological monitoring during spinal surgery: technical review in open and minimally invasive approaches. Neurosurg Rev. 2019;42:297–307.
23. Alluri R, Mok JK, Vaishnav A, Shelby T, Sivaganesan A, Hah R, Qureshi SA. Intraoperative neuromonitoring during lateral lumbar interbody fusion. Neurospine. 2021;18(3):430.
24. Riley MR, Doan AT, Vogel RW, Aguirre AO, Pieri KS, Scheid EH. Use of motor evoked potentials during lateral lumbar interbody fusion reduces postoperative deficits. Spine J. 2018;18(10):1763–78.
25. Jain N, Alluri R, Phan K, Yanni D, Alvarez A, Guillen H, et al. Saphenous nerve somatosensory-evoked potentials monitoring during lateral interbody fusion. Global Spine Journal. 2021;11(5):722–6.
26. Sutter MA, Eggspuehler A, Grob D, Porchet F, Jeszenszky D, Dvorak J. Multimodal intraoperative monitoring (MIOM) during 409 lumbosacral surgical procedures in 409 patients. Eur Spine J. 2007;16:221–8.
27. Qiu Y, Wang S, Wang B, Yu Y, Zhu F, Zhu Z. Incidence and risk factors of neurological deficits of surgical correction for scoliosis: analysis of 1373 cases at one Chinese institution. Spine. 2008;33(5):519–26.
28. Agarwal N, Hamilton DK, Ozpinar A, Choi P, Hart R, Yaylali I. Intraoperative neurophysiologic monitoring for adult patients undergoing posterior spinal fusion. World Neurosurg. 2017;99:267–74.
29. Garces J, Berry JF, Valle-Giler EP, Sulaiman WA. Intraoperative neurophysiological monitoring for minimally invasive 1-and 2-level transforaminal lumbar interbody fusion: does it improve patient outcome? Ochsner J. 2014;14(1):57–61.
30. He S, Ren Z, Zhang X, Li J. Neurophysiologic monitoring for treatment of upper lumbar disc herniation with percutaneous endoscopic lumbar discectomy: a case report on the significance of an increase in the amplitude of motor evoked potential responses after decompression and literature review. Int J Surg Case Rep. 2020;67:271–6.
31. de Carvalho PST, Ramos MRF, da Silva Meireles AC, Peixoto A, de Carvalho P Jr, Ramírez León JF, et al. Feasibility of using intraoperative neuromonitoring in the prophylaxis of dysesthesia in transforaminal endoscopic discectomies of the lumbar spine. Brain Sci. 2020;10(8):522.
32. Rocos B, Strantzas S, Zeller R, Lewis S, Tan T, Lebel D. What is the optimal surgical method for achieving correction and avoiding neurological complications in pediatric high-grade spondylolisthesis? J Pediatr Orthop. 2021;41(3):e217–e25.
33. Yang J, Peng Z, Kong Q, Wu H, Wang Y, Li W, et al. Stretch on the L5 nerve root in high-grade spondylolisthesis reduction. J Neurosurg Spine. 2022;37(2):232–40.
34. Petraco DM, Spivak JM, Cappadona JG, Kummer FJ, Neuwirth MG. An anatomic evaluation of L5

nerve stretch in spondylolisthesis reduction. Spine. 1996;21(10):1133–8.
35. Iorio C, Koucheki R, Strantzas S, Vandenberk M, Lewis SJ, Zeller R, et al. Utility of intraoperative neurophysiological monitoring in detecting motor and sensory nerve injuries in pediatric high-grade spondylolisthesis. Spine J. 2023;23(12):1920–7.
36. Schär RT, Sutter M, Mannion AF, Eggspühler A, Jeszenszky D, Fekete TF, et al. Outcome of L5 radiculopathy after reduction and instrumented transforaminal lumbar interbody fusion of high-grade L5–S1 isthmic spondylolisthesis and the role of intraoperative neurophysiological monitoring. Eur Spine J. 2017;26:679–90.
37. Pasquali C, Tramontano V, Sala F. Intraoperative neurophysiological monitoring in tethered cord surgery. In: Neurophysiology in Neurosurgery. Elsevier; 2020. p. 365–79.
38. Sala F, Barone G, Tramontano V, Gallo P, Ghimenton C. Retained medullary cord confirmed by intraoperative neurophysiological mapping. Childs Nerv Syst. 2014;30:1287–91.

Bone Health Optimization

7

Zach Pennington, Anthony L. Mikula, and Benjamin D. Elder

Introduction

Over 250,000 lumbar fusion operations are performed annually in the United States [1, 2] with utilization rates expected to rise approximately 20% by 2040 [1]. Broadly, instrumentation is used to correct sagittal and coronal plane deformity, achieve indirect decompression (through interbody placement), and address instability. Successful fusion relies upon effective apposition of the fusion surfaces, which is itself reliant upon a strong implant-bone interface. As the US population continues to age, so does the prospective lumbar fusion population [1]. Given the known decrease in bone quality that occurs with age, there is likely to be a commensurately increasing population of patients with indications for surgical fusion but with poor underlying bone quality. It is therefore of critical importance to the practicing spine surgeon to identify methods for successful preoperative evaluation of bone integrity and strategies for preoperative bone health optimization.

Z. Pennington · A. L. Mikula · B. D. Elder (✉)
Department of Neurologic Surgery, Mayo Clinic, Rochester, MN, USA
e-mail: Pennington.Zachary@mayo.edu; mikula.anthony@mayo.edu; elder.benjamin@mayo.edu

Bone Quality and Complications Following Instrumented Spine Surgery

Osteoporosis—defined by bone density diminution resulting in an increased risk of fracture—is estimated to affect one in ten Americans ≥50 years of age [3] with a worldwide prevalence expected to exceed 300 million people by the year 2040 [4]. The World Health Organization (WHO) defines osteoporosis based on the results of dual-energy X-ray absorptiometry (DXA) [5]. Measured bone mineral densities (BMD) ≥2.5 standard deviations below the average for young, healthy, sex-matched controls are defined as osteoporosis, and t-scores between −1.0 and − 2.5 are defined as osteopenia or low BMD. Currently, the United States Preventative Task Force recommends screening for osteoporosis in all women ≥65 years old and postmenopausal women <65 years of age with elevated fracture risk as determined by the Simple Calculated Osteoporosis Risk Estimation (SCORE) tool, Osteoporosis Risk Assessment Instrument (ORAI) [6], Osteoporosis Index of Risk (OSIRIS), Fracture Risk Assessment (FRAX) tool, [7] or Osteoporosis Self-Assessment Tool (OST) [8, 9]. Similar recommendations have been made by the International Society of Clinical Densitometry (ISCD), though the latter also include men aged ≥70 as well as women <65 and men <70 with an increased risk

A. A. Baaj et al. (eds.), *Surgery of the Lumbar Spine*, https://doi.org/10.1007/978-3-032-18097-1_7

of fracture, a condition associated with bone loss, or low body weight, and anyone with a known fragility fracture, or who is being considered for pharmacologic therapy [10]. Of note, both the FRAX and ORAI scores factor in prior history of fragility fracture, which is a strong predictor of future fracture.

In vitro data has consistently demonstrated a positive association of bone density with both implant pullout strength [11, 12] and construct cycles to failure [13]. Weiser and colleagues showed that osteoporotic vertebrae experienced implant loosening after 55% fewer loading cycles as compared to normal bone and peak fatigue loads 40% lower than vertebrae with normal bone mineral density. Clinical series have also demonstrated increased mechanical complications, including proximal junctional kyphosis, instrumentation failure, and pseudarthrosis [14–16]. In patients undergoing interbody fusion, those with poor bone quality also experience higher rates of interbody cage subsidence with Oh and colleagues [17] noting an 8.5-fold higher risk of interbody subsidence in patients with osteoporotic aBMD.

Assessing Bone Quality

DXA has long been considered the gold standard for assessing underlying bone mineral density among spine surgeons [18], and it remains a recommended screening method based upon the 2018 USPTF Recommendation Statement [8]. However, DXA is suboptimal for assessments in the adult spine population, as degenerative changes are associated with false elevations in measured areal BMD (aBMD) [19]. aBMD is defined by measuring photon absorption at the two energy levels on DEXA in the region of interest (e.g., vertebral body), which is then converted to an apparent bone mineral content (BMC) based upon the known absorption of bone versus soft tissue. This BMC value measure is divided by the area of the region of interest to yield an aBMD value in grams per cm^2 [20]. A similar measure called volumetric BMD (vBMD) is defined by dividing the BMC measure by an estimate of the volume of the imaged bone, which is determined by radiographs and skeletal measures [21]. The degenerative changes that can falsely elevate aBMD are common in the aging spine and for this reason, the ISCD recommends utilizing aBMD measures obtained from the femoral neck, total hip, or distal radius, in cases of significant spinal degeneration [22]. However, such measures are merely surrogates for vertebral bone quality and operate on the presumption that bone loss in the appendicular skeleton effectively mimics bone loss in the axial skeleton. Additionally, utilization of DXA requires surgeons to obtain additional testing in the preoperative setting, which may further delay patient surgeries.

Because of these reasons, alternative methods for assessing bone quality and osteoporosis risk have been developed. The FRAX tool [7] (https://frax.shef.ac.uk/FRAX/tool.aspx) was developed with support from the WHO as a means of identifying patients at risk of fragility fracture given most patients suffering from these fractures do not have BMD-defined osteoporosis. FRAX takes into account patient age, sex, height, weight, prior fracture history, smoking status, alcohol use, and history of glucocorticoid use, secondary osteoporosis, and rheumatoid arthritis, and uses these to provide estimates of 10-year risk of hip fracture and major osteoporotic fracture. FRAX is most useful in patients with osteopenia, in which a risk of major osteoporotic fracture >20% or a risk of hip fracture >3% is diagnostic of osteoporosis. Additionally, femoral neck BMD and trabecular bone score (TBS) can be incorporated into the algorithm to further refine risk calculations.

TBS (trabecular bone score) is a form of textural analysis originally developed by Pothuaud, [23] designed to convert variations in DXA pixel density into an estimation of trabecular bone structure. It has been correlated with trabecular thickness, spacing, and number in cadaveric lumbar spine preparations [24] and shown to offer superior fracture risk stratification to BMD alone [25]. However, the correlation of TBS with microarchitectural parameters is not consistent [26] as it correlates negatively with trabecular number and positively with trabecular thickness, [24] although both trabecular number and thickness correlate positively with bone compressive strength. To this end, cadaveric testing [27] has suggested TBS may poorly model vertebral failure load, suggesting the TBS to have criterion but not construct validity. Nevertheless, Leslie and colleagues [28] demonstrated in a cohort of 33,352 women that lumbar spine TBS better predicts 10-year risk of major osteoporotic fracture compared to FRAX with aBMD.

Yet additional methods have been developed that focus on assessing axial bone quality, as these are the bones that will be instrumented and bear the stresses of the spinal instrumentation (Fig. 7.1). Two methods that have garnered attention are Hounsfield units (HU) on axial non-contrast-enhanced computed tomography and the Vertebral Bone Quality (VBQ) score on T1-weighted magnetic resonance imaging sequences. HU-based qualitative assessment of bone quality makes use of standard non-contrast CT volumes routinely acquired as part of presurgical patient evaluation. HU is a dimensionless unit of density with the HU of water set to zero, and is conventionally measured as illustrated in (Fig. 7.1A) [29–31]. HU-based measures of bone quality are based upon the principle that bone quality, [32] specifically vertebral trabecular bone density, is highly correlated with bone stiffness and yield strength [33, 34]. With cancellous bone loss, there is a commensurate decrease in photon scattering within the cancellous bone, which manifests as lower HU. HU measures on multidetector CT have been correlated with micro-CT (μCT) based measures of trabecular bone volume [35] that are in turn correlated with vertebral body compressive strength and elastic modulus [36]. This is in contrast to DXA-based BMD measures, which correlate poorly with biomechanical CT-based measures of vertebral compressive strength [31]. Based upon their recent analysis of 114 patients with both qualitative CT and biomechanical CT data, Martini et al. [31] posited HU thresholds of 106 and 122 for osteoporosis and low BMD, respectively. This is similar to the previous threshold of <118.4 identified by Schreiber et al. [37] who also noted a near-perfect linear correlation between elastic modulus and HU ($r^2 = 0.998$) in polyurethane blocks subjected to pure vertical compression.

HU has been correlated with several mechanical spine complications, including proximal junctional kyphosis following long-segment fusion for adult spinal deformity, [15, 16, 38] pathologic fracture following radiotherapy for spinal metastases, [30] intraoperative endplate violation during interbody placement, [39] and postoperative interbody subsidence [40]. Multiple thresholds for poor bone density have been suggested, with a recent review by Agaronnik and colleagues [41] suggesting a threshold of 125–150 HU for the prediction of vertebral compression fractures. Girdler and colleagues [5] recommended the use of a tiered system, wherein HU<150 predicted pseudoarthrosis and adjacent segment fracture, <135 was a surrogate for low bone density (osteopenia), <120 suggested increased risk of screw loosening or interbody subsidence, and < 110 was a surrogate for osteoporosis. However, there is no accepted HU threshold below which patients have an appreciably higher risk of postoperative complications.

VBQ (Vertebral Bone Quality) score [42] employs non-contrast enhanced T1-weighted MRI images and is based upon the principle that as bone ages, marrow is progressively replaced with fatty tissue [43] with a commensurate increase in the T1 signal intensity of the medullary bone (Fig. 7.1B). Its chief benefits are that it does not require ionizing radiation and employs imaging routinely obtained as part of the preoperative evaluation [41]. It has been correlated with DXA t-scores at the femoral neck and hip [44], and several groups have found it to be useful for the diagnosis of osteoporosis [41]. Reported thresholds for diagnosing low bone density or osteoporosis based on VBQ score are variable as is the reported diagnostic accuracy, though it is suggested that VBQ >3 may identify patients with poor underlying bone quality meriting referral to a specialist for further evaluation [41]. VBQ has similarly been correlated with mechanical spine complications, including interbody subsidence following TLIF [45] and pedicle screw loosening after multilevel interbody fusion

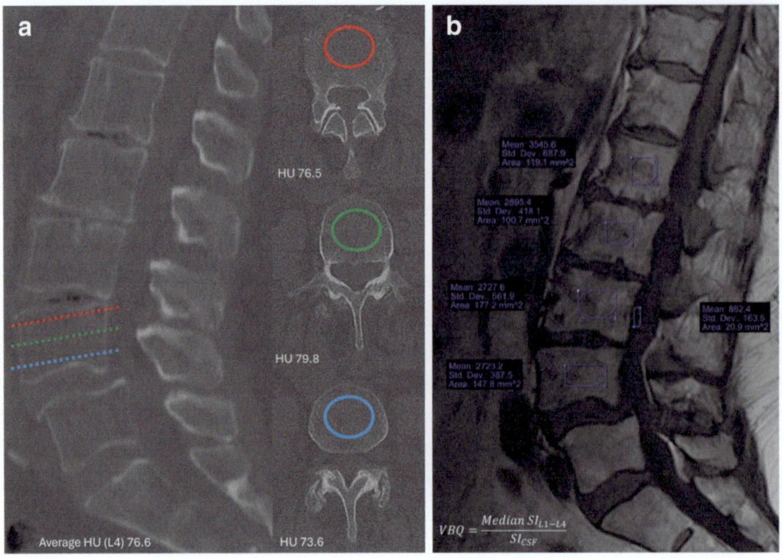

Fig. 7.1 Alternative methods for assessing underlying bone quality. (**a**) Hounsfield units measured from non-contrast enhanced computed tomography can be used to estimate bone quality and is based on the principle that with osteoporosis, there is a diminution in cancellous bone trabeculae, resulting in a decrease in the average radiopacity of the cancellous/trabecular bone. The figure shows estimation of HU for the L4 body with regions of interest (ROIs) constructed on axial slices through the superior, mid-, and inferior vertebral body; values are averaged to find the HU for the body in question. References commonly cite lumbar HU < 125–150 as a threshold meriting further evaluation for poor bone quality. (**b**) Vertebral Bone Quality (VBQ) score is based upon the principle that with osteoporosis, cancellous bone experienced progressive fatty infiltration, which is detectable as increased average signal on T1-weighted sequences. VBQ is calculated by placing ROIs on the L1–4 bodies and in the CSF space posterior to the L3 body. VBQ is given by the median value for the L1–4 vertebral body ROI average signals divided by the average signal of the CSF ROI. VBQ greater than 3 suggests poor bone quality and the need for additional workup

for degenerative disease [46] or multilevel fusion for adult spinal deformity [47]. Literature is sparser though, as are direct comparisons between HU and VBQ. Of those previously published, HU has been found to be superior for the prediction of both pathologic fracture following radiotherapy in patients with spine metastases [30] and proximal junctional kyphosis following thoracolumbar fusion for adult spinal deformity [38]. Further research is merited to investigate the relative diagnostic accuracy of these two modalities. Additionally, alternative MR-based measures, notably the endplate bone quality (EBQ) score, have been suggested as superior risk stratification tools for interbody subsidence [48, 49] though EBQ scores are notably susceptible to Modic changes [50].

A third alternative method is biomechanical computed tomography (BCT), a technique developed in the research setting that converts HU data into calibrated BMD values, which are used to construct a finite element model based upon material-property-density correlations derived from cadaveric experiments [51]. The finite element models are then subjected to loading conditions with 700 N simulated loads seen in everyday life as a "virtual stress test" to estimate bone strength and load-to-strength ratio. It has been shown to better predict lumbar vertebral fracture risk than vBMD (volumetric BMD) [52–54] and has been suggested as a cost-effective alternative to DXA for fracture risk screening, [55] that utilizes previously acquired CT volumes. To this end, it is now available as a Medicare screening benefit for osteoporosis diagnosis and can be used with most existing CT scans [56]. Recently, it has also been shown to predict risk of reoperation and subsequent vertebral fracture in patients undergoing thoracolumbar fusion, with Keaveny et al. [57] suggesting patients found to be osteoporotic on BCT had a 4.7-fold higher risk of vertebral fracture within 5 years of surgery.

Agents for Preoperative Bone Health Optimization

Agents for bone health optimization can be grossly divided into anabolic and antiresorptive therapies. For all patients being considered for lumbar fusion, our practice is to measure calcium and vitamin D_3 levels, and place patients on scheduled vitamin D_3 (2000–5000 international units daily) and calcium supplementation (1200 mg/daily) if necessary, similar to that recommended by Anderson et al. [58] This recommendation exceeds that currently recommended by the USPTF [59]; however, such guidelines were designed for the average, non-osteoporotic community-dwelling adult. Antiresorptive medications—the bisphosphonates—are the older class and include both oral (risedronate, alendronate, ibandronate) and intravenous formulation (zoledronic acid). Bisphosphonates function as pyrophosphate analogs and bind to calcium ions in the hydroxyapatite crystals of bone [60]. From there, the bisphosphonates are taken up by osteoclasts from the bone mineral surface and incorporated into new adenosine triphosphate molecules, where they prove cytotoxic and promote osteoclast apoptosis [60]. Second-generation bisphosphonates (nitrogen-containing bisphosphonates, e.g., alendronate, risedronate, zoledronic acid) use an alternative mechanism, binding to and inhibiting farnesyl pyrophosphate. This disrupts posttranslational protein modification within osteoclasts, again leading to osteoclast apoptosis [60]. These second-generation medications are 10–10,000 times more potent than first-generation bisphosphonates and consequently comprise those medications that are currently employed in the clinical setting. As a whole, bisphosphonate therapy can help to maintain underlying bone mineral density, and small clinical trials have suggested they may improve radiographic fusion rates and decrease the risk of interbody subsidence [61, 62]. More importantly, oral bisphosphonate use has been associated with reduced rates of vertebral and non-vertebral fragility fractures [63]. In the VERT-NA trial, daily risedronate was associated with a 41% cumulative decrease in new vertebral fractures and 39% decreases in new nonvertebral fractures over 3 years [64, 65]. It was also associated with significant BMD increases relative to placebo. Ibandronate similarly reduced the rate of new vertebral fractures by 62% relative to placebo and increased lumbar spine BMD (6.5%) in the BONE trial. [66] Oral bisphosphonates are taken as a daily (risedronate, alendronate), weekly (risedronate, alendronate), or monthly (ibandronate) medication, and side effects include gastrointestinal side effects, hypocalcemia, atrial fibrillation, atypical femur fractures, and osteonecrosis of the jaw [60]. However, bisphosphonate therapy does not appear to improve underlying bone quality [67] and may therefore not be suitable as a first-line agent for patients with poor underlying bone quality who require improvement in said bone quality preoperatively.

Denosumab—a monoclonal antibody designed to bind and inhibit receptor-activated nuclear factor κB ligand (RANKL-L)—is an alternative antiresorptive therapy that has seen applications in both the oncology populations and patients with osteoporosis. It is administered as a subcutaneous injection of 60 mg every six months and has been demonstrated to improve underlying bone quality on both DXA areal BMD and volumetric BMD assessed with quantitative CT [68]. In the FREEDOM trial, in which postmenopausal women 60–90 years of age were treated with 36-months of denosumab (60 mg s.c.) and daily calcium and vitamin D supplementation, spine trabecular vBMD increased 12.6% relative to baseline and 21.8% relative to patients treated with placebo. Subsequent follow-up of patients in the FREEDOM trial has demonstrated continued improvements in aBMD on DXA with a commensurate decrease in patients at high-risk for fragility fractures [69]. Denosumab therapy is limited to 6 to 10 years. Withdrawal of denosumab is associated with a significant worsening in bone mineral density (rebound phenomenon), which requires continued management with either a lower dose denosumab regimen or bisphosphonate therapy. For this reason, many surgeons disfavor denosumab for bone health optimization. Importantly, denosumab is a poor first-line agent in the spinal surgery population to improve bone density preoperatively, as it can significantly inhibit the maximal benefit of some of the anabolic treatments described below [70].

Anabolic agents can be grouped into recombinant parathyroid hormone (rPTH) analogs and anti-sclerostin therapy. PTH analogs include the 34 amino acid synthetic PTH peptide teriparatide and the 34 amino acid synthetic parathyroid hormone-related peptide analog abaloparatide. Teriparatide was FDA-approved in 2002 (generics approved late 2023) and stimulates osteoblast activity, gastrointestinal calcium absorption, and resorption of calcium in the kidneys. It is administered as a 20mcg daily subcutaneous injection and has been demonstrated to both increase aBMD and reduce the risk of fragility fractures [71]. It has been suggested to improve lumbar fusion rates [72, 73] and also to reduce rates of screw loosening relative to bisphosphonate treatment [74]. Additionally, it has been suggested to improve baseline radiographic bone quality as assessed by HU, which may be a more sensitive measure for these changes as compared to DXA. [75] However, the current FDA label recommends against use of teriparatide therapy beyond 2 years owing to the potential increased risk of osteosarcoma. Abaloparatide, FDA-approved in 2017, has a similar mechanism of action in that it stimulates osteoblast function by binding to and activating PTH1 receptors. It possesses amino acid residue substitutions designed to improve shelf stability and potentiate osteogenic effects relative to teriparatide. In the ACTIVE study [76] that compared abaloparatide, teriparatide, and placebo, daily subcutaneous injection of abaloparatide was associated with significantly lower rates of hypercalcemia relative to teriparatide and lower rates of major osteoporotic fractures. Overall fracture rates and improvements in DXA-measured aBMD were not significantly different between teriparatide and abaloparatide, though there were trends toward superior outcomes for both endpoints in the abaloparatide cohort. Investigations in the spine population are heretofore wanting, and abaloparatide therapy is similarly limited to 2 years on the FDA warning, owing to the theoretical increased risk of osteosarcoma.

The last anabolic medication in current use is the monoclonal antibody romosozumab, an anti-sclerostin humanized antibody FDA-approved in 2019, which is both anabolic and anti-resorptive. A total of 210 mg is administered in two subcutaneous injections (105 mg per 1.17 mL each) per month for up to a one-year period. Romosozumab promotes bone formation by removing sclerostin-mediated inhibition of canonical Wnt signaling in bone. In the phase III FRAME trial [77], romosozumab was shown to significantly improve DXA-measured aBMD and reduce the risk of vertebral fracture (73%) relative to placebo in ambulatory postmenopausal women with DXA-diagnosed osteoporosis. It has also been shown on quantitative CT to improve vBMD of both the vertebral body and pedicles [78]. Direct comparisons of various anabolic agents have suggested romosozumab may be superior to rPTH analogs. Genant and colleagues [79] demonstrated with quantitative CT that while improvements in cancellous bone vBMD were similar following 12-months of therapy with teriparatide or romosozumab, romosozumab therapy was associated with significantly greater gains in spine cortical vBMD (13.7 vs 5.7%; $p < 0.0001$). Romosozumab has additionally been shown to significantly improve lumbar BMD even among patients previously treated with antiresorptive or anabolic therapies [70].

For all of the anabolic agents, discontinuation is typically associated with loss of the bone mineral density gains over several months. Therefore, it is critical that patients be transitioned to maintenance therapy with an anti-resorptive agent following completion of the two-year treatment with the rPTH analogues, or one year of therapy with romosozumab. Initiation of denosumab has been recommended by some, owing to its ability to improve lumbar spine aBMD relative to treatment with bisphosphonates following completion of romosozumab therapy, while rPTH analogues are often followed with bisphosphonate maintenance therapy [80]. From a surgeon's perspective, the advantage of romosozumab and denosumab is that they are administered as infusions by medical professionals and so are commonly covered by Medicare Part B and private insurance, as compared to teriparatide and abaloparatide, which may not be covered or only partly covered on Medicare Advantage or Medicare Part D plans [5].

Examinations of the impact of abaloparatide and romosozumab in the spine surgery populations are very limited. One retrospective study from our own group [67] did evaluate improvements in spine bone quality, as measured by HU, following treatment with alendronate, teriparatide, denosumab, or romosozumab in patients undergoing outpatient treatment for osteoporosis. Significant improvements in lumbar spine HU were noted for teriparatide and romosozumab therapies, but not for antiresorptive therapies alone (alendronate and denosumab), and romosozumab demonstrated its anabolic effects on HU more quickly than teriparatide. [67] This may be explained in part by the dual anabolic and anti-resorptive effects of romosozumab compared to teriparatide which is anabolic and pro-resorptive. Additionally, prior work has shown romosozumab to have a very rapid rise in bone formation markers during the first three months of treatment [81]. However, it is unclear whether adjustments for baseline HU, age, sex, and BMI would alter the improvements seen. Nevertheless, based upon these data, our current practice is to refer patients with low baseline bone density to endocrinology specialists for initiation of anabolic therapy. This aligns with the recent recommendation of the AOSpine Knowledge Forum Deformity group [82] which recommended patients undergoing surgery for adult spinal deformity undergo treatment with ≥3 months of anabolic agents prior to surgery to reduce mechanical complications. With regard to agent selection, teriparatide has the greatest clinical data but requires daily administration and can only be used for up to 2 years [83]. It can also be associated with hypercalcemia and carries a theoretical risk of osteosarcoma. For this reason, it is contraindicated in those with bone metastases, skeletal malignancies, and metabolic bone diseases. For commercially insured patients in the United States, teriparatide has been reported to have an out-of-pocket cost of \$37/month (versus \$59/month for zoledronic acid, \$61/month for abaloparatide, \$104/month for denosumab, and \$51/month for romosozumab) [84]. Overall costs are notably higher though, varying from \$1200–\$4000/month for teriparatide, \$2700–4400/month for abaloparatide, \$1800–2200/month for denosumab (search of GoodRx at time of writing). Abaloparatide generally has the same indications/contraindications as teriparatide and is also administered subcutaneously daily but has more limited safety data. Romosozumab, the newest of the anabolic agents, is administered as a subcutaneous injection monthly, but can only be administered for 12 months due to exhaustion of therapeutic benefit beyond this timeframe. It is also associated with increased rates of injection site reactions and may be associated with increased rates of cardiovascular events, though this is an ongoing area of investigation. Yet in a recent cost-effectiveness analysis, [85] it and denosumab were both shown to be cost-effective versus bisphosphonate therapy. Both agents are also administered in the clinic setting, meaning that for Medicare patients they are covered by Part B, and so may have lower patient costs than teriparatide and abaloparatide, which may only be partially covered by prescription medication plans (e.g., Part D) [5]. For those for whom anabolic agents are contraindicated, denosumab is a good option as it only requires injections ever six months and results in greater bone improvement relative to bisphosphonates. However, it is contraindicated in those with hypocalcemia and has been associated with osteonecrosis of the jaw, atypical fractures, and discontinuation is associated with a significant increase in fracture risk. For this reason, patients discontinuing denosumab should be placed on another antiresorptive therapy (e.g., bisphosphonates) prior to discontinuation. Data from the FREEDOM trial extension has demonstrated the safety of using denosumab for up to 10 years, though routine follow-up is still recommended throughout the treatment course [86].

Conclusions

Osteoporosis is a common comorbidity within the aging population (1 in 10 Americans over age 50) and is associated with increased risk of vertebral and nonvertebral fragility fractures. Vertebral compression fractures are correlated with significant increases in both care dependency and prolonged analgesic use, [87] and are a leading cause of disability globally [88]. They are also associated with significantly increased healthcare costs, with a recent analysis noting an 82% increase in medical costs compared to age-matched controls [89]. The occurrence of a prior vertebral fragility fracture portends a four-to-five-fold increased risk of subsequent fracture in community-dwelling adults [90, 91] and a greater than six-fold increase in patients undergoing lumbar fusion [92]. Consequently, early screening for patients at high risk for osteoporosis and intervention can help to prevent future disability.

Good underlying bone quality is particularly important to successful outcomes following lumbar fusion, with bone playing a role akin to the bedrock on which buildings are constructed. Given the high prevalence of osteoporosis, it is our general practice to screen all patients considering an instrumented spinal fusion operation aged ≥50 and all patients of any age with a history of significant risk factors, such as prolonged steroid use or smoking. We additionally routinely evaluate vitamin D_3 levels in all patients. All patients undergo DXA screening as that remains the gold standard test worldwide, though we find opportunistic HU assessment on the routinely obtained non-contrast CT scan of the lumbar spine to be most useful. If patients have osteoporosis based on any assessment, namely DXA with a t-score < −2.5, FRAX major osteoporotic fracture risk >20% or hip fracture risk >3%, history of any fragility fracture, or reduced TBS score, then they are referred for bone health optimization prior to surgery. We generally use HU <110 at L1 as an additional screening test for a more spine-specific assessment for patients who should be considered for preoperative anabolic therapy, though there is currently more limited acceptance from third-party payors for this assessment tool, and CT bone strength assessments have provided further utility for these patients. The time course of preoperative treatment with anabolic therapy is variable and generally guided by the quality of the bone on the aforementioned assessments, and the magnitude of the surgery, though we have found that romosozumab seems to have the most rapid effects. Additionally, it is critical that when spine surgeons are consulted on patients with newly diagnosed fragility fractures, we identify this as diagnostic for osteoporosis regardless of the DXA t-score, and it is of paramount importance that these patients get referred for bone health optimization at the same time as any acute intervention for the fracture.

References

1. Neifert SN, Martini ML, Hanss K, Rothrock RJ, Gilligan J, Zimering J, Caridi JM, Oermann EK. Large rises in thoracolumbar fusions by 2040: a cause for concern with an increasingly elderly surgical population. World Neurosurg. 2020;144:e25–33.
2. Martin BI, Mirza SK, Spina N, Spiker WR, Lawrence B, Brodke DS. Trends in lumbar fusion procedure rates and associated hospital costs for degenerative spinal diseases in the United States, 2004 to 2015. Spine (Phila Pa 1976). 2019;44:369–76.
3. Wright NC, Looker AC, Saag KG, Curtis JR, Delzell ES, Randall S, Dawson-Hughes B. The recent prevalence of osteoporosis and low bone mass in the United States based on bone mineral density at the femoral neck or lumbar Spine. J Bone Miner Res. 2014;29:2520–6.
4. Odén A, McCloskey EV, Kanis JA, Harvey NC, Johansson H. Burden of high fracture probability worldwide: secular increases 2010–2040. Osteoporos Int. 2015;26:2243–8.
5. Girdler SJ, Lindsey MH, Sebastian AS, Nassr A. Osteoporosis evaluation and management in spine surgery. J Am Acad Orthop Surg. 2024; https://doi.org/10.5435/JAAOS-D-24-00311.
6. Sedrine WB, Chevallier T, Zegels B, Kvasz A, Micheletti M-C, Gelas B, Reginster J-Y. Development and assessment of the Osteoporosis Index of Risk

(OSIRIS) to facilitate selection of women for bone densitometry. Gynecol Endocrinol. 2002;16:245–50.
7. Kanis JA, Johansson H, Harvey NC, McCloskey EV. A brief history of FRAX. Arch Osteoporos. 2018;13:118.
8. Curry SJ, Krist AH, Owens DK, et al. Screening for osteoporosis to prevent fractures. JAMA. 2018;319:2521–31.
9. Pennington Z, Ehresman J, Lubelski D, Cottrill E, Schilling A, Ahmed AK, Feghali J, Witham TF, Sciubba DM. Assessing underlying bone quality in spine surgery patients: a narrative review of dual-energy X-ray absorptiometry (DXA) and alternatives. Spine J. 2021;21:321–31.
10. Densitometry IS for C (2023) 2023 ISCD official positions adult. Northbrook, Illinois.
11. Halvorson TL, Kelley LA, Thomas KA, Whitecloud TS, Cook SD. Effects of bone mineral density on pedicle screw fixation. Spine (Phila Pa 1976). 1994;19:2415–20.
12. Hadjipavlou AG, Nicodemus CL, Al-Hamdan FA, Simmons JW, Pope MH. Correlation of bone equivalent mineral density to pull-out resistance of triangulated pedicle screw construct. J Spinal Disord. 1997;10:12–9.
13. Weiser L, Huber G, Sellenschloh K, Viezens L, Püschel K, Morlock MM, Lehmann W. Insufficient stability of pedicle screws in osteoporotic vertebrae: biomechanical correlation of bone mineral density and pedicle screw fixation strength. Eur Spine J. 2017;26:2891–7.
14. Bjerke BT, Zarrabian M, Aleem IS, Fogelson JL, Currier BL, Freedman BA, Bydon M, Nassr A. Incidence of osteoporosis-related complications following posterior lumbar fusion. Glob Spine J. 2018;8:563–9.
15. Mikula AL, Fogelson JL, Lakomkin N, et al. Lower Hounsfield units at the upper instrumented vertebrae are significantly associated with proximal junctional kyphosis and failure near the thoracolumbar junction. Oper Neurosurg. 2021;21:270–5.
16. Mikula AL, Lakomkin N, Pennington Z, et al. Association between lower Hounsfield units and proximal junctional kyphosis and failure at the upper thoracic spine. J Neurosurg Spine. 2022;37:694–702.
17. Oh KW, Lee JH, Lee J-H, Lee D-Y, Shim HJ. The correlation between cage subsidence, bone mineral density, and clinical results in posterior lumbar interbody fusion. Clin Spine Surg. 2017;30:E683–9.
18. Berven SH, Kamper SJ, Germscheid NM, et al. An international consensus on the appropriate evaluation and treatment for adults with spinal deformity. Eur Spine J. 2018;27:585–96.
19. Liu G, Peacock M, Eilam O, Dorulla G, Braunstein E, Johnston CC. Effect of osteoarthritis in the lumbar spine and hip on bone mineral density and diagnosis of osteoporosis in elderly men and women. Osteoporos Int. 1997;7:564–9.
20. Ott SM, O'Hanlan M, Lipkin EW, Newell-Morris L. Evaluation of vertebral volumetric vs. areal bone mineral density during growth. Bone. 1997;20:553–6.
21. Katzman DK, Bachrach LK, Carter DR, Marcus R. Clinical and anthropometric correlates of bone mineral acquisition in healthy adolescent girls. J Clin Endocrinol Metab. 1991;73:1332–9.
22. Baim S, Binkley N, Bilezikian JP, Kendler DL, Hans DB, Lewiecki EM, Silverman S. Official positions of the International Society for Clinical Densitometry and Executive Summary of the 2007 ISCD Position Development Conference. J Clin Densitom. 2008;11:75–91.
23. Pothuaud L. Process of interpretation of two-dimensional densitometry images for the prediction of bone mechanical strength. In: Barillot C, Haynor DR, Hellier P, editors. Med. Image Comput. Comput. Interv—MICCAI 2004. Berlin, Heidelberg: Springer; 2004. p. 1079–80.
24. Swartz EE, Boden BP, Courson RW, Decoster LC, Horodyski MB, Norkus SA, Rehberg RS, Waninger KN. National Athletic Trainers' Association Position Statement: Acute Management of the Cervical Spine–Injured Athlete. J Athl Train. 2009;44:306–31.
25. Pothuaud L, Barthe N, Krieg M-A, Mehsen N, Carceller P, Hans D. Evaluation of the potential use of trabecular bone score to complement bone mineral density in the diagnosis of osteoporosis: a preliminary Spine BMD–matched, case-control study. J Clin Densitom. 2009;12:170–6.
26. Bousson V, Bergot C, Sutter B, Levitz P, Cortet B, Ostéoporoses SC of the G de R et d'Information sur les. Trabecular bone score (TBS): available knowledge, clinical relevance, and future prospects. Osteoporos Int. 2012;23:1489–501.
27. Maquer G, Lu Y, Dall'Ara E, Chevalier Y, Krause M, Yang L, Eastell R, Lippuner K, Zysset PK. The initial slope of the Variogram, Foundation of the Trabecular Bone Score, is not or is poorly associated with vertebral strength. J Bone Miner Res. 2016;31:341–6.
28. Leslie WD, Johansson H, Kanis JA, Lamy O, Oden A, McCloskey EV, Hans D. Lumbar spine texture enhances 10-year fracture probability assessment. Osteoporos Int. 2014;25:2271–7.
29. Mikula AL, Pennington Z, Lakomkin N, et al. Independent predictors of vertebral compression fracture following radiation for metastatic spine disease. J Neurosurg Spine. 2022;37:617–23.
30. Pennington Z, Mikula AL, Lakomkin N, et al. Comparison of Hounsfield units and vertebral bone quality score for the prediction of time to pathologic fracture in mobile spine metastases treated with radiotherapy. J Neurosurg Spine. 2023;40:19–27.
31. Martini ML, Mikula AL, Lakomkin N, et al. Opportunistic CT-based hounsfield units strongly correlate with biomechanical CT measurements in the thoracolumbar spine. Spine (Phila Pa 1976). 2024;49:1021–8.

32. Krischak GD, Augat P, Wachter NJ, Kinzl L, Claes LE. Predictive value of bone mineral density and Singh Index for the in vitro mechanical properties of cancellous bone in the femoral head. Clin Biomech. 1999;14:346–51.
33. Nazarian A, von Stechow D, Zurakowski D, Müller R, Snyder BD. Bone volume fraction explains the variation in strength and stiffness of cancellous bone affected by metastatic cancer and osteoporosis. Calcif Tissue Int. 2008;83:368–79.
34. Öhman-Mägi C, Holub O, Wu D, Hall RM, Persson C. Density and mechanical properties of vertebral trabecular bone—a review. JOR SPINE. 2021;4:e1176.
35. Issever AS, Link TM, Kentenich M, Rogalla P, Schwieger K, Huber MB, Burghardt AJ, Majumdar S, Diederichs G. Trabecular bone structure analysis in the osteoporotic Spine using a clinical in vivo setup for 64-slice MDCT imaging: comparison to μCT imaging and μFE modeling. J Bone Miner Res. 2009;24:1628–37.
36. Lang SM, Moyle DD, Berg EW, Detorie N, Gilpin AT, Pappas NJ, Reynolds JC, Tkacik M, Waldron RL. Correlation of mechanical properties of vertebral trabecular bone with equivalent mineral density as measured by computed tomography. J Bone Joint Surg Am. 1988;70:1531–8.
37. Schreiber JJ, Anderson PA, Rosas HG, Buchholz AL, Au AG. Hounsfield units for assessing bone mineral density and strength: a tool for osteoporosis management. J Bone Jt Surg. 2011;93:1057–63.
38. Pennington Z, Mikula AL, Lakomkin N, et al. Bone quality as measured by Hounsfield units more accurately predicts proximal junctional kyphosis than vertebral bone quality following long-segment thoracolumbar fusion. World Neurosurg. 2024;186:e584–92.
39. Wu H, Cheung JPY, Zhang T, Shan Z, Zhang X, Liu J, Fan S, Zhao F. The role of Hounsfield unit in intraoperative endplate violation and delayed cage subsidence with oblique lateral Interbody fusion. Glob Spine J. 2023;13:1829–39.
40. Guha D, Mushlin HM, Muthiah N, Vodovotz LL, Agarwal N, Alan N, Hamilton DK, Okonkwo DO, Kanter AS. Computed tomography Hounsfield units as a predictor of reoperation and graft subsidence after standalone and multilevel lateral lumbar Interbody fusion. World Neurosurg. 2022;161:e417–26.
41. Agaronnik ND, Giberson-Chen C, Bono CM. Using advanced imaging to measure bone density, compression fracture risk, and risk for construct failure after spine surgery. Spine J. 2024;24:1135–52.
42. Ehresman J, Schilling A, Pennington Z, et al. A novel MRI-based score assessing trabecular bone quality to predict vertebral compression fractures in patients with spinal metastasis. J Neurosurg Spine. 2020;32:499–506.
43. Yang T-L, Shen H, Liu A, Dong S-S, Zhang L, Deng F-Y, Zhao Q, Deng H-W. A road map for understanding molecular and genetic determinants of osteoporosis. Nat Rev Endocrinol. 2020;16:91–103.
44. Ehresman J, Pennington Z, Schilling A, Lubelski D, Ahmed AKK, Cottrill E, Khan M, Sciubba DM. Novel MRI-based score for assessment of bone density in operative spine patients. Spine J. 2020;20:556–62.
45. Hu Y-H, Yeh Y-C, Niu C-C, Hsieh M-K, Tsai T-T, Chen W-J, Lai P-L. Novel MRI-based vertebral bone quality score as a predictor of cage subsidence following transforaminal lumbar interbody fusion. J Neurosurg Spine. 2022;37:654–62.
46. Li W, Zhu H, Hua Z, Miao D, Wang F, Tong T, Wang L. Vertebral bone quality score as a predictor of pedicle screw loosening following surgery for degenerative lumbar disease. Spine (Phila Pa 1976). 2023;48:1635–41.
47. Kuo CC, Soliman MAR, Aguirre AO, et al. Vertebral bone quality score independently predicts proximal junctional kyphosis and/or failure after adult spinal Deformity surgery. Neurosurgery. 2023;92:945–54.
48. Jones C, Okano I, Arzani A, et al. The predictive value of a novel site-specific MRI-based bone quality assessment, endplate bone quality (EBQ), for severe cage subsidence among patients undergoing standalone lateral lumbar interbody fusion. Spine J. 2022;22:1875–83.
49. Ai Y, Zhu C, Chen Q, Huang Y, Wang J, Ding H, Deng W, Song Y, Feng G, Liu L. Comparison of predictive value for cage subsidence between MRI-based endplate bone quality and vertebral bone quality scores following transforaminal lumbar interbody fusion: a retrospective propensity-matched study. Spine J. 2024;24:1046–55.
50. Li C, Gao W, Yao X, et al. The magnetic resonance imaging-based vertebral bone quality scoring system: a novel method to evaluate endplate changes in patients with primary single-level disk herniation and Modic changes. Jt Dis Relat Surg. 2024;35:257–66.
51. Keaveny TM. Biomechanical computed tomography—noninvasive bone strength analysis using clinical computed tomography scans. Ann N Y Acad Sci. 2010;1192:57–65.
52. Faulkner KG, Cann CE, Hasegawa BH. Effect of bone distribution on vertebral strength: assessment with patient-specific nonlinear finite element analysis. Radiology. 1991;179:669–74.
53. Song F, Wei Y, Feng W, Fu R, Li Z, Gao X, Cheng X, Yang H. Biomechanical CT-computed bone strength predicts the risk of subsequent vertebral fracture. Bone. 2023;166:116601.
54. Wei Y, Feng W, Li G, Li Z, Liu Z, Cheng X, Yang H. Experimental testing and biomechanical CT analysis of Chinese cadaveric vertebrae with different modeling approaches. Med Eng Phys. 2021;93:8–16.
55. Pisu M, Kopperdahl DL, Lewis CE, Saag KG, Keaveny TM. Cost-effectiveness of osteoporosis screening using biomechanical computed tomography for patients with a previous abdominal CT. J Bone Miner Res. 2019;34:1229–39.
56. Keaveny TM, Clarke BL, Cosman F, Orwoll ES, Siris ES, Khosla S, Bouxsein ML. Biomechanical computed tomography analysis (BCT) for clini-

cal assessment of osteoporosis. Osteoporos Int. 2020;31:1025–48.
57. Keaveny TM, Adams AL, Fischer H, Brara HS, Burch S, Guppy KH, Kopperdahl DL. Increased risks of vertebral fracture and reoperation in primary spinal fusion patients who test positive for osteoporosis by biomechanical computed tomography analysis. Spine J. 2023;23:412–24.
58. Anderson PA, Kadri A, Hare KJ, Binkley N. Preoperative bone health assessment and optimization in spine surgery. Neurosurg Focus. 2020;49:E2.
59. Grossman DC, Curry SJ, Owens DK, et al. Vitamin D, calcium, or combined supplementation for the primary prevention of fractures in community-dwelling adults. JAMA. 2018;319:1592.
60. Drake MT, Clarke BL, Khosla S. Bisphosphonates: mechanism of action and role in clinical practice. Mayo Clin Proc. 2008;83:1032–45.
61. Nagahama K, Kanayama M, Togawa D, Hashimoto T, Minami A. Does alendronate disturb the healing process of posterior lumbar interbody fusion? A prospective randomized trial. J Neurosurg Spine. 2011;14:500–7.
62. Chen F, Dai Z, Kang Y, Lv G, Keller ET, Jiang Y. Effects of zoledronic acid on bone fusion in osteoporotic patients after lumbar fusion. Osteoporos Int. 2016;27:1469–76.
63. Barrionuevo P, Kapoor E, Asi N, et al. Efficacy of pharmacological therapies for the prevention of fractures in postmenopausal women: a network meta-analysis. J Clin Endocrinol Metab. 2019;104:1623–30.
64. Harris ST, Watts NB, Genant HK, et al. Effects of risedronate treatment on vertebral and nonvertebral fractures in women with postmenopausal osteoporosis: a randomized controlled trial. Vertebral Efficacy With Risedronate Therapy (VERT) Study Group. JAMA. 1999;282:1344–52.
65. Reginster J-Y, Minne HW, Sorensen OH, et al. Randomized trial of the effects of Risedronate on vertebral fractures in women with established postmenopausal osteoporosis. Osteoporos Int. 2000;11:83–91.
66. Chesnut CH, Skag A, Christiansen C, et al. Effects of oral Ibandronate administered daily or intermittently on fracture risk in postmenopausal osteoporosis. J Bone Miner Res. 2004;19:1241–9.
67. Mikula AL, Lakomkin N, Hamouda AM, et al. Change in spinal bone mineral density as estimated by Hounsfield units following osteoporosis treatment with romosozumab, teriparatide, denosumab, and alendronate: an analysis of 318 patients. J Neurosurg Spine. 2024;41:309–15.
68. McClung MR, Zanchetta JR, Høiseth A, et al. Denosumab Densitometric changes assessed by quantitative computed tomography at the Spine and hip in postmenopausal women with osteoporosis. J Clin Densitom. 2013;16:250–6.
69. Hans D, McDermott M, Huang S, Kim M, Shevroja E, McClung M. Long-term effect of denosumab on bone microarchitecture as assessed by tissue thickness–adjusted trabecular bone score in postmenopausal women with osteoporosis: results from FREEDOM and its open-label extension. Osteoporos Int. 2023;34:1075–84.
70. Ebina K, Hirao M, Tsuboi H, et al. Effects of prior osteoporosis treatment on early treatment response of romosozumab in patients with postmenopausal osteoporosis. Bone. 2020;140:115574.
71. Neer RM, Arnaud CD, Zanchetta JR, et al. Effect of parathyroid hormone (1-34) on fractures and bone mineral density in postmenopausal women with osteoporosis. N Engl J Med. 2001;344:1434–41.
72. Ohtori S, Inoue G, Orita S, et al. Teriparatide accelerates lumbar posterolateral fusion in women with postmenopausal osteoporosis. Spine (Phila Pa 1976). 2012;37:E1464–8.
73. Mohanty S, Sardar ZM, Hassan FM, Lombardi JM, Lehman RA, Lenke LG. Impact of Teriparatide on complications and patient-reported outcomes of patients undergoing long spinal fusion according to bone density. J Bone Jt Surg. 2024;106:206–17.
74. Ohtori S, Inoue G, Orita S, et al. Comparison of Teriparatide and bisphosphonate treatment to reduce pedicle screw loosening after lumbar spinal fusion surgery in postmenopausal women with osteoporosis from a bone quality perspective. Spine (Phila Pa 1976). 2013;38:E487–92.
75. Mikula AL, Puffer RC, Jeor JDS, et al. Teriparatide treatment increases Hounsfield units in the lumbar spine out of proportion to DEXA changes. J Neurosurg Spine. 2020;32:50–5.
76. Miller PD, Hattersley G, Riis BJ, et al. Effect of Abaloparatide vs placebo on new vertebral fractures in postmenopausal women with osteoporosis. JAMA. 2016;316:722.
77. Cosman F, Crittenden DB, Adachi JD, et al. Romosozumab treatment in postmenopausal women with osteoporosis. N Engl J Med. 2016;375:1532–43.
78. Ishikawa K, Tani S, Toyone T, et al. The potential effect of romosozumab on perioperative management for instrumentation surgery. JOR Spine. 2024;7:e1356.
79. Genant HK, Engelke K, Bolognese MA, et al. Effects of Romosozumab compared with Teriparatide on bone density and mass at the Spine and hip in postmenopausal women with low bone mass. J Bone Miner Res. 2017;32:181–7.
80. Kobayakawa T, Miyazaki A, Takahashi J, Nakamura Y. Verification of efficacy and safety of ibandronate or denosumab for postmenopausal osteoporosis after 12-month treatment with romosozumab as sequential therapy: the prospective VICTOR study. Bone. 2022;162:116480.
81. McClung MR, Grauer A, Boonen S, et al. Romosozumab in postmenopausal women with low bone mineral density. N Engl J Med. 2014;370:412–20.
82. Kato S, Rocos B, Yoshida G, Sardar Z, Jones KE, Oe S, Fisher C, Lewis SJ, AO Spine Knowledge Forum Deformity. AO Spine clinical practice recommendations: evaluation, implications and management of

osteoporosis in adult spinal deformity. Glob Spine J. 2025; 21925682251357200
83. Eastell R, Rosen CJ, Black DM, Cheung AM, Murad MH, Shoback D. Pharmacological management of osteoporosis in postmenopausal women: an Endocrine Society Clinical Practice Guideline. J Clin Endocrinol Metab. 2019;104:1595–622.
84. Wadhwa H, Wu JY, Lee JS, Zygourakis CC. Anabolic and antiresorptive osteoporosis treatment: trends, costs, and sequence in a commercially insured population, 2003–2021. JBMR Plus. 2023;7:e10800.
85. Luo C, Qin S-X, Wang Q-Y, Li Y-F, Qu X-L, Yue C, Hu L, Sheng Z-F, Wang X-B, Wan X-M. Cost-effectiveness analysis of five drugs for treating postmenopausal women in the United States with osteoporosis and a very high fracture risk. J Endocrinol Investig. 2022;46:367–79.
86. Bone HG, Wagman RB, Brandi ML, et al. 10 years of denosumab treatment in postmenopausal women with osteoporosis: results from the phase 3 randomised FREEDOM trial and open-label extension. Lancet Diabetes Endocrinol. 2017;5:513–23. https://doi.org/10.1016/S2213-8587(17)30138-9.
87. Honda A, Yamana H, Sasabuchi Y, et al. Mortality, analgesic use, and care requirements after vertebral compression fractures. J Bone Joint Surg. 2024;106:1453–60.
88. Dong Y, Peng R, Kang H, Song K, Guo Q, Zhao H, Zhu M, Zhang Y, Guan H, Li F. Global incidence, prevalence, and disability of vertebral fractures: a systematic analysis of the global burden of disease study 2019. Spine J. 2022;22:857–68.
89. Kim SH, Jang S-Y, Nam K, Cha Y. Analysis of long-term medical expenses in vertebral fracture patients. Clin Orthop Surg. 2023;15:989.
90. Klotzbuecher CM, Ross PD, Landsman PB, Abbott TA, Berger M. Patients with prior fractures have an increased risk of future fractures: a summary of the literature and statistical synthesis. J Bone Miner Res. 2000;15:721–39.
91. Lindsay R. Risk of new vertebral fracture in the year following a fracture. JAMA. 2001;285:320.
92. Zhao AY, Agarwal AR, Durand WM, Raad M, Seibold BT, Thakkar SC, Jain A. Prior fragility fractures are associated with higher risk of bone health-related complications within 8-years following lumbar fusion. Spine (Phila Pa 1976). 2023;49:1046–51.

8 Interventional Pain Techniques in the Lumbar Spine

Andrew Lederman

The management of lumbar spine-related pain begins with the principle that conservative measures should always be exhausted before considering more invasive options. Initial treatment typically includes physical therapy to improve strength, flexibility, and mechanics, whereas the judicious use of pain medications—with a focus on limiting opioid use whenever possible—is essential. Medications such as nonsteroidal anti-inflammatory drugs (NSAIDs), muscle relaxants, and nerve pain medications may be considered, with opioids reserved for short-term use in acute, severe pain scenarios due to the risk of dependency and adverse effects.

There are, however, critical exceptions when conservative treatments may need to be bypassed. These include (Eg. motor weakness/ foot drop) or loss of bowel or bladder control, all of which can indicate severe nerve root or spinal cord compression. Urgent intervention is also warranted in cases of infection (e.g., spinal abscesses) or cancer involving the spine. In these situations, urgent diagnosis and definitive treatment are prioritized, as the natural course of these pathologies poses a greater risk for long-term disease and impairment than a pure degenerative process, which varies broadly in its clinical presentation.

For most individuals, acute back pain resolves within approximately 6 weeks. During this period, conservative management, including physical therapy, activity modification, and over-the-counter medications, is typically effective. However, when these measures fail to reduce pain or restore function, interventional options can be utilized to diagnose the source of pain and provide pain relief.

A challenge in treating lumbar spine pain is the frequent appearance of incidental radiologic findings on imaging—such as disc degeneration, desiccation, or mild bulges—that may not correlate with the patient's symptoms, particularly in older adults. This lack of specificity in imaging makes it necessary to combine all available clinical information, including the patient's history, physical examination, and imaging studies, and to use diagnostic blocks to identify individual pain generators. An effective treatment plan often requires a combination of physical therapy, oral and topical medications, activity modifications, assistive devices, and, when appropriate, the interventional options outlined in this chapter.

A. Lederman (✉)
Department of Orthopedic Surgery, New England Baptist Hospital, Boston, MA, USA
e-mail: alederma@nebh.org

A. A. Baaj et al. (eds.), *Surgery of the Lumbar Spine*, https://doi.org/10.1007/978-3-032-18097-1_8

Treatment of Radicular Pain: Selective Nerve Root Blocks, Transforaminal Epidural Steroid Injections, and Interlaminar Epidural Steroid Injections

Radicular pain, often resulting from irritation or compression of a spinal nerve root, can lead to significant discomfort and functional impairment. Interventional procedures such as selective nerve root blocks (SNRBs), transforaminal epidural steroid injections (TFESIs), and interlaminar epidural steroid injections (ILESIs) are commonly employed to diagnose and reduce radicular pain. Each technique has distinct diagnostic and therapeutic roles.

Selective nerve root blocks (SNRBs) involve the injection of a local anesthetic, with or without corticosteroids, around a specific nerve root outside the epidural space. The primary role of SNRBs is diagnostic, aiding in the precise identification of the symptomatic nerve root by temporarily anesthetizing it. The injectate is confined to the foraminal canal and extraforaminal space, allowing accurate targeting of the nerve root with minimal spread to surrounding tissues, making this technique highly specific [1–4]. SNRBs are particularly useful when differentiating between multiple potential pain sources or when imaging findings are ambiguous. SNRBs are most appropriate when a localized diagnosis is needed or when avoiding the broader effects of steroids in the epidural space is critical [5, 6].

Transforaminal epidural steroid injections (TFESIs), on the other hand, serve both diagnostic and therapeutic purposes. TFESIs involve injecting corticosteroids and anesthetic agents into the neural foramen, allowing the medication to spread along the nerve root into the epidural space. This method provides a more localized distribution than do interlaminar epidural injections but a broader spread than do SNRBs [7–9]. TFESIs are particularly effective for treating unilateral radicular pain due to specific nerve root inflammation or compression, such as foraminal or subarticular recess stenosis. TFESIs are typically indicated for targeted therapeutic intervention when pathology is localized to a specific nerve root or in patients with prior spine surgery, where scar tissue may complicate or increase the risks associated with epidural access via the interlaminar approach [10–12].

Interlaminar epidural steroid injections (ILESIs) involve delivering corticosteroids into the epidural space via an interlaminar approach, allowing for a broader distribution of medication across the epidural space. This approach makes ILESIs suitable for diffuse pain or multiple levels of nerve root compression or irritation [13, 14]. ILESIs are indicated for bilateral or multilevel lumbar radicular pain. The wider distribution of the injectate can provide comprehensive pain relief, but it lacks the precision needed for targeting a specific nerve root, unlike TFESIs and SNRBs [15–17].

Interventional Treatments for Axial Low Back Pain

Introduction to Axial Low Back Pain

Axial low back pain, which is confined to the lumbar region without leg radiation, poses diagnostic and treatment challenges because of its complex, multifactorial nature. Unlike radicular pain, where nerve root compression can often be pinpointed as the pain source, axial low back pain often lacks a single identifiable cause [18–20]. The difficulty in identifying the specific pain generator stems from the overlap in pain pathways and the various lumbar spine structures that can contribute to the condition, including intervertebral discs, facet joints, muscles, ligaments, and nerves.

Effectively managing axial low back pain requires integrating findings from the patient's history, physical examination, and imaging studies to develop a comprehensive differential diagnosis. A thorough history provides insights into the nature and duration of the pain, aggravating and alleviating factors, and any previous treatments attempted. The physical examination helps identify pain generators through specific maneuvers, such as palpation of tender points, range of motion testing, and provocative tests. Imaging studies, including X-ray, MRI, and CT scans, are crucial for visualizing structural abnormalities that may correlate with a patient's symptoms [21–23]. Combining these elements enables clinicians to tailor their interventional approaches to address the specific underlying causes of pain [24, 25].

Myofascial Pain and Trigger Point Injections

Myofascial pain, often arising from muscle dysfunction or injury, is a common contributor to axial low back pain. Trigger points, or hyperirritable spots within muscle fascia, can cause localized and referred pain patterns. Trigger point injections (TPIs) are a common intervention for myofascial pain. Studies indicate no significant difference in pain relief outcomes when TPIs are compared with anesthetics, steroids, or saline alone, suggesting that pain relief may stem from the mechanical disruption of the trigger point rather than the pharmacologic properties of the injectate [26–28].

Newer approaches, such as peripheral nerve stimulation (PNS), have shown promise in treating myofascial pain and dysfunction by targeting the motor nerves that innervate the multifidi, which are crucial for stabilizing the lumbar spine [29, 30]. Both temporary and permanent PNS options can help improve multifid function, which is often weakened in patients with chronic low back pain. Physical examination maneuvers revealing multifidus weakness, such as prone instability tests and lumbar extension endurance tests, have been validated as indicators for these treatments [27, 31]. Imaging findings, including MR images showing fatty infiltration or atrophy of the multifidi, can also support the decision to implement PNS [32]. Temporary PNSs may be used for diagnostic purposes or when short-term improvement is desired, whereas permanent PNSs might be appropriate for chronic, refractory myofascial pain patients who show a favorable response to temporary stimulation [33, 34].

Facet Joint Pain: Intraarticular Injections and Radiofrequency Ablation

Facet joint pain, another frequent cause of axial low back pain, can be treated via intraarticular facet steroid injections or radiofrequency ablation (RFA) of the medial branches of the dorsal rami [35–37]. Intraarticular injections deliver corticosteroids directly into the facet joint to reduce inflammation and provide pain relief. This approach is best suited for patients with acute or subacute facet joint pain, where inflammation is suspected to be a significant contributor [38]. Conversely, RFA of the medial branches is a potentially longer-lasting option that disrupts pain transmission from the facet joints to the brain by delivering a current, increasing the temperature around the nerves responsible for pain signals. RFA is typically indicated for patients with chronic facet joint pain who have not responded to conservative treatments and have shown significant relief from diagnostic medial branch blocks [7, 39, 40]. While the primary intent of this procedure is to reduce pain emanating from the facet joints, given that the medial branches are also responsible for innervating the multifidi, increasing attention is being given to the risks and benefits of this procedure compared with nonablative procedures that reduce similar pain, such as peripheral nerve stimulation or regenerative injection approaches, to treating these pains.

Vertebrogenic Low Back Pain and Basivertebral Nerve Ablation

Vertebrogenic low back pain, associated with changes in the vertebral endplates known as Modic changes, represents a distinct subset of axial pain. These changes, often visible on MRI as signal alterations in the bone marrow of the vertebral endplates, suggest an inflammatory or degenerative process potentially contributing to pain [41, 42]. Basivertebral nerve ablation (BVNA) is a novel intervention that targets the basivertebral nerve, which innervates the vertebral endplates. Unlike other ablative techniques, BVNA does not typically involve a diagnostic block to confirm the pain source; instead, it relies on a patient's history of lumbar flexion-based pain and MRI findings of Modic changes to guide treatment [43, 44].

Spinal Cord Stimulation for Persistent Spinal Pain Syndrome

Spinal cord stimulation (SCS) is an established treatment option for persistent spinal pain syndrome (PSPS), a term that is now preferred over "failed back surgery syndrome" or "postlaminectomy syndrome" [45]. PSPS refers to persistent back and/or leg pain despite successful radiological decompression surgery. Once a patient has been selected, a trial procedure is performed to ensure adequate efficacy before committing to a permanent implant. The procedure involves placing electrodes in the epidural space, which, via an external battery, imparts an electrical current onto precise locations of the dorsal columns of the spinal cord to modulate pain signals before they reach the brain. When the trial procedure can significantly improve a patient's pain and function and potentially reduce the burden of pain medication needed, a permanent version with an implanted pulse generator is placed. Advancements in battery, wire, and software technology continue to evolve to enhance this option for the most refractory pain management cases. Dorsal root ganglion (DRG) stimulation, a variation of the SCS, has shown potential in treating low back pain more precisely by targeting specific nerve roots associated with the pain [46–48].

Provocative Discography and Discogenic Low Back Pain

Provocative discography is a diagnostic tool used to identify discogenic low back pain by pressurizing intervertebral discs to reproduce the patient's pain. Depending on the protocol used and the extent of spread, discography may also help diagnose vertebrogenic low back pain, although further studies are needed, as most discography research was conducted before the acceptance of vertebrogenic endplate pain and BVNA [49, 50]. Despite the historical use of various procedures to reduce discogenic pain, including intradiscal steroids, electrothermal therapy (IDET), and biacuplasty, there is still no clear evidence supporting a standard of care that effectively reduces discogenic pain or slows the degenerative process [51, 52]. Regenerative medicine approaches to improve disc-related pain outcomes show promise but are still early in developing a robust evidence base supporting their routine use.

Vertebral Augmentation for Compression Fractures

Compression fractures due to osteoporosis or oncologic disease are another source of axial low back pain that can be addressed through vertebral augmentation procedures, such as vertebroplasty or kyphoplasty [53, 54]. These procedures involve injecting bone cement into the fractured vertebral body to stabilize the fracture and alleviate pain. In cases of oncologic compression fractures, augmentation may be combined with tumor radiofrequency ablation to reduce the tumor burden and provide additional pain relief [55, 56].

Frontiers of Interventional Pain Management

The landscape of interventional pain management is rapidly evolving. Recently, regenerative approaches such as platelet-rich plasma (PRP) and bone marrow aspirate concentrate (BMAC) have been explored as alternatives to traditional treatments such as steroids or ablations. These biologic therapies offer the potential for healing and tissue regeneration rather than temporary symptom relief and potential long-term side effects of denervating structures or implanting devices. While the foundation of peer-reviewed evidence supporting these therapies continues to grow, they represent a promising frontier for managing spine-related pain with fewer long-term side effects.

At the bleeding edge of innovation are minimally invasive procedures that aim to address the biomechanical causes of back and leg pain. Techniques such as the percutaneous image-guided lumbar decompression (PILD) procedure are indicated for lumbar spinal stenosis due to hypertrophied ligamentum flavum. Patients presenting with neurogenic claudication syndrome, limiting standing and walking tolerance alongside advanced imaging demonstrating a thickened ligamentum flavum contributing to the symptomatic level of central canal stenosis, are candidates. Under fluoroscopic guidance, small amounts of thickened ligamentum flavum are removed via a cannula with the ultimate goal of reducing pressure exerted in the central canal at the targeted level [57, 58]. Additional procedures being explored include interspinous process fixation and sacroiliac joint fusion devices, which offer potential solutions for patients who are unable to undergo surgery or who wish to avoid more invasive surgical options [59, 60]. These procedures may provide pain relief and improve function, although further studies are needed to ensure both their safety and long-term efficacy as compared to current established standards of care.

Given the expanding scope and invasiveness of these interventions, refining training curricula in residency and/or fellowship is necessary.

These procedures potentially offer the benefits of smaller incisions, reduced postoperative pain, shorter hospital stays, and quicker recovery times than traditional open surgeries do.

Cancer-Related Pain in the Lumbar Spine

Patients with cancer, particularly those with spinal metastases, often experience significant pain in the lumbar spine. Metastatic disease of the lumbar vertebrae can cause both axial pain due to bone destruction and radicular pain due to nerve root compression. Management of cancer-related pain requires a multidisciplinary approach that includes both medical and interventional strategies. Interventional procedures such as vertebral augmentation (e.g., kyphoplasty) can provide stabilization of pathologic fractures and significant pain relief in patients with vertebral metastases [61, 62]. Additionally, nerve blocks, neurolysis, and intrathecal drug delivery systems can be used to manage pain in cancer patients, offering significant improvements in quality of life when medical management alone is insufficient [63–65].

Conclusion

In conclusion, interventional techniques play a critical role in the management of lumbar spine-related pain, including radicular pain, axial low back pain, and cancer-related pain. Each technique, whether it is a nerve root block, epidural injection, or a more advanced procedure like spinal cord stimulation or vertebral augmentation, must be carefully selected based on the patient's diagnosis, symptoms, and overall treatment goals. Ongoing research and advancements in technology continue to refine these procedures, offering patients more precise, effective, and minimally invasive treatment options for managing chronic pain.

References

1. Derby R, Kine G, Saal JA, Saal JS, Dleikanovitz M. Response to steroid and duration of radicular pain as predictors of surgical outcome. Spine. 1992;17(6)
2. Bogduk N. Lumbar selective nerve root blocks. Spine. 1997;22(3):445–52.
3. Windsor RE, Pinzon EG. Selective nerve root blocks in the diagnosis of radicular pain. In: Waldman SD, editor. Pain management. 2nd ed. Philadelphia: Saunders; 2011. p. 601–7.
4. Kapural L, Mekhail NA. Diagnostic selective nerve root blocks for lumbosacral radiculopathy: correlation with surgery outcome. Spine. 2003;28(24):2409–16.
5. Malmivaara A, Hakkinen U, Aro T, et al. The treatment of acute low back pain—bed rest, exercises, or ordinary activity? N Engl J Med. 1995;332(6):351–5.
6. Manchikanti L, Cash KA, Pampati V, et al. Preliminary results of a randomized, double-blind, active-controlled trial of fluoroscopic caudal epidural

injections in the management of chronic low back pain. Pain Physician. 2008;11(2):121–31.
7. Manchikanti L, Cash KA, McManus CD, et al. A randomized, double-blind, controlled trial of lumbar interlaminar epidural injections in central spinal stenosis: 2-year follow-up. Pain Physician. 2015;18(1):79–92.
8. Manchikanti L, Kaye AD, Boswell MV, Hirsch JA. A systematic review of randomized trials of interlaminar epidural injections in the management of chronic spinal pain. Pain Physician. 2016;19(2)
9. Riew KD, Yin Y, Gilula L, Lenke LG, Bridwell KH, Lauryssen C. The effect of nerve-root injections on the need for operative treatment of lumbar radicular pain. J Bone Joint Surg Am. 2000;82-A(11):1589–93.
10. Manchikanti L, Kaye AD, Falco FJE, Hirsch JA. Interventional techniques in chronic spinal pain: evidence-based practice guidelines. Pain Physician. 2013;16(2 Suppl)
11. Manchikanti L, Kaye AD, Boswell MV, Hirsch JA. A systematic review and best evidence synthesis of the effectiveness of therapeutic lumbar transforaminal epidural steroid injections. Pain Physician. 2015;18(2)
12. Manchikanti L, Pampati V, Boswell MV, Hirsch JA. Randomized trial of fluoroscopic caudal epidural injections in chronic pain of lumbar disc herniation: a two-year follow-up. Pain Physician. 2012;15(5):371–84.
13. Ackerman WE 3rd, Ahmad M. The efficacy of lumbar epidural steroid injections in patients with lumbar disc herniations. Anesth Analg. 2007;104(5):1217–22.
14. Gharibo CG, Koo J, Christiansen SE, Kerezoudis P, McClellan J. The role of interlaminar and transforaminal epidural steroid injections in managing radicular pain. Curr Phys Med Rehabil Rep. 2013;1(1):12–20.
15. Manchikanti L, Pampati V, Cash KA, et al. Results of 2-year follow-up of a randomized, double-blind, controlled trial of lumbar interlaminar epidural injections in central spinal stenosis. Pain Physician. 2016;19(4):253–66.
16. Boswell MV, Trescot AM, Datta S, et al. Interventional techniques: evidence-based practice guidelines in the management of chronic spinal pain. Pain Physician. 2007;10(1):7–111.
17. Manchikanti L, Hirsch JA, Cohen SP, et al. Assessment of the efficacy and safety of epidural injections in the management of chronic spinal pain: a systematic review. Pain Physician. 2017;20(2 Suppl)
18. Chou R, Qaseem A, Snow V, et al. Diagnosis and treatment of low back pain: a joint clinical practice guideline from the American College of Physicians and the American Pain Society. Ann Intern Med. 2007;147(7):478–91.
19. Peng B, DePalma MJ. Cervical disc degeneration and neck pain. J Bone Joint Surg Am. 2017;99(2):121–36.
20. Kuslich SD, Ulstrom CL, Michael CJ. The tissue origin of low back pain and sciatica: a report of pain responses to tissue stimulation during operations on the lumbar spine using local anesthesia. Orthop Clin North Am. 1991;22(2):181–7.
21. Modic MT, Ross JS. Lumbar degenerative disk disease. Radiology. 2007;245(1):43–61.
22. Tosteson ANA, Lurie JD, Tosteson TD, et al. Surgical vs. nonoperative treatment for lumbar disc herniation: the Spine Patient Outcomes Research Trial (SPORT) observational cohort. JAMA. 2006;296(20):2451–9.
23. Deyo RA, Weinstein JN. Low back pain. N Engl J Med. 2001;344(5):363–70.
24. McCarron RF, Wimpee MW, Hudkins PG, Laros GS. The inflammatory effect of nucleus pulposus: a possible element in the pathogenesis of low-back pain. Spine. 1987;12(8):760–4.
25. Bogduk N. Pathophysiology of lumbar radiculopathy. Neurol Clin. 2007;25(2):495–506.
26. Cummings TM, White AR. Needling therapies in the management of myofascial trigger point pain: a systematic review. Arch Phys Med Rehabil. 2001;82(7):986–92.
27. Simons DG, Travell JG, Simons LS. Myofascial pain and dysfunction: the trigger point manual, vol. 1. 2nd ed. Baltimore: Lippincott Williams & Wilkins; 1999.
28. Borg-Stein J, Simons DG. Myofascial pain. Arch Phys Med Rehabil. 2002;83(3 Suppl 1)
29. Cahana A, Deer TR, Mekhail N, et al. Spinal cord stimulation: state of the art. Pain Pract. 2006;6(4):268–75.
30. Sluka KA, Walsh DM. Transcutaneous electrical nerve stimulation: basic science mechanisms and clinical effectiveness. J Pain. 2003;4(3):109–21.
31. Jacobson E. Progressive relaxation: a physiological and clinical investigation of muscular states and their significance in psychology and medical practice. Chicago: University of Chicago Press; 1929.
32. Medlock MD, Stephens CD, Shipley CF, et al. Treatment of myofascial pain syndrome. J Manipulative Physiol Ther. 1989;12(2):115–20.
33. Melzack R, Wall PD. Pain mechanisms: a new theory. Science. 1965;150(3699):971–9.
34. Berman B, Colson J, Burman L, et al. Trigger-point injections in primary fibromyalgia. South Med J. 1994;87(10):1021–3.
35. Niemtzow RC, Baxter GD. Trigger point therapy in the treatment of myofascial pain syndrome. Arch Phys Med Rehabil. 1992;73(12):1121–3.
36. Kostopoulos D, Rizopoulos K. The manual of trigger point and myofascial therapy. Boston: SLACK Incorporated; 2001.
37. Kalichman L, Vulfsons S. Dry needling in the management of myofascial trigger points. J Am Board Fam Med. 2010;23(5):640–6.
38. Travell JG, Simons DG. Myofascial pain and dysfunction: the trigger point manual, vol. 1. 2nd ed. Baltimore: Lippincott Williams & Wilkins; 1999.
39. Fernandez-de-Las-Penas C, Dommerholt J, Gerwin RD. Myofascial trigger points: pathophysiology and evidence-informed diagnosis and management. Philadelphia: Lippincott Williams & Wilkins; 2013.

40. Cohen SP, et al. Lumbar facet joint pain: a comprehensive review of prevalence, diagnostic tools, and treatment options. Pain Physician. 2014;17(2)
41. McCormick ZL, Cushman D, Marshall B, et al. Spinal cord stimulation for chronic pain: a review of recent advances. Curr Pain Headache Rep. 2019;23(2):11.
42. Cohen SP, Raja SN. Pathogenesis, diagnosis, and treatment of lumbar zygapophysial (facet) joint pain. Anesthesiology. 2007;106(3):591–614.
43. Modic MT, Ross JS. Imaging of degenerative disc disease. Radiology. 2007;245(1):43–61.
44. Bogduk N. Cervical zygapophysial joint pain: diagnosis and management. Curr Rev Pain. 1999;3(5):353–8.
45. Manchikanti L, Cash KA, Pampati V, et al. A comparative study of lumbar interlaminar epidural injections in managing lumbar radiculopathy secondary to disc herniation. Pain Physician. 2010;13(2):143–53.
46. Manchikanti L, Pampati V, Falco FJE, Hirsch JA. A randomized, double-blind, active-control trial of fluoroscopic caudal epidural injections in managing chronic low back pain. Pain Physician. 2015;18(5):523–35.
47. Beall DP, Chambers MR, Thomas S, et al. Percutaneous lumbar decompression using an interspinous needle device. AJNR Am J Neuroradiol. 2013;34(2):435–42.
48. Chou R, Qaseem A, Snow V, et al. Diagnostic imaging for low back pain: advice for high-value health care from the American College of Physicians. Ann Intern Med. 2011;154(3):181–9.
49. Modic MT, Steinberg PM, Ross JS, et al. Degenerative disk disease: assessment of changes in vertebral body marrow with MR imaging. Radiology. 1988;166(1):193–9.
50. Barrey C, Darnis A. Current strategies for the restoration of adequate lordosis during lumbar fusion. World J Orthop. 2015;6(1):117–26.
51. Kraemer WJ, Ratamess NA. Fundamentals of resistance training: progression and exercise prescription. Med Sci Sports Exerc. 2004;36(4):674–88.
52. Peng B, Wu W, Li Z, Guo J, Wang X. Modic changes in lumbar disc disease and the therapeutic efficacy of intradiscal steroid injections. A prospective controlled study with 2-year follow-up. Eur Spine J. 2007;16(9):1434–40.
53. Fourney DR, Schomer DF, Nader R, et al. Percutaneous vertebroplasty and kyphoplasty for painful vertebral body fractures in cancer patients. J Neurosurg. 2003;98(1):21–30.
54. Berenson J, Pflugmacher R, Jarzem P, et al. Balloon kyphoplasty versus non-surgical care for vertebral compression fractures secondary to multiple myeloma: a randomized trial. Lancet Oncol. 2011;12(3):225–35.
55. Tomasian A, Wallace A, Jennings JW. Spine cryoablation: indications, techniques, and clinical outcomes for the management of spinal metastases. Semin Intervent Radiol. 2020;37(3):304–12.
56. Greenwood TJ, Wallace A, Friedman MV, et al. Combined ablation and cementoplasty for the treatment of painful malignant bone tumors. AJR Am J Roentgenol. 2019;213(1):175–83.
57. Lingreen R, Grider JS. Retrospective review of the long-term effectiveness of minimally invasive lumbar decompression (MILD) in patients with symptomatic lumbar spinal stenosis. Pain Physician. 2010;13(6):555–60.
58. Benyamin RM, Staats PS, Mi D, et al. The MILD procedure: a systematic review of the current literature. Pain Physician. 2016;19(8)
59. Patwardhan AG, Havey RM, Voronov LI, et al. Biomechanics of a minimally invasive interspinous fixation device for motion preservation: effects on kinematics and load-sharing at the implanted and adjacent levels. Spine J. 2011;11(8):790–9.
60. Bae HW, Lauryssen C, Maislin G, et al. Clinical and radiographic outcomes of interspinous process decompression with the X STOP device for lumbar spinal stenosis: two-year results of a randomized controlled trial. Spine (Phila Pa 1976). 2010;35(1):28–34.
61. Polly DW Jr, Cher DJ, Wine KD, et al. Randomized controlled trial of minimally invasive sacroiliac joint fusion using triangular titanium implants vs. non-surgical management for sacroiliac joint dysfunction: 12-month outcomes. Neurosurgery. 2015;77(5):674–91.
62. Ledonio CGT, Polly DW Jr, Swiontkowski MF. Minimally invasive versus open sacroiliac joint fusion: are they similarly safe and effective? Clin Orthop Relat Res. 2014;472(6):1831–8.
63. Duhon BS, Bitan F, Lockstadt H, et al. Triangular titanium implants for minimally invasive sacroiliac joint fusion: a prospective study. Glob Spine J. 2016;6(3):257–69.
64. Manchikanti L, Hirsch JA, Falco FJE, et al. Management of lumbar zygapophysial (facet) joint pain. World J Orthop. 2016;7(5):315–37.
65. Smith TJ, Coyne PJ, Staats PS, et al. Implantable drug delivery systems for refractory cancer pain: a guided review. Oncologist. 2005;10(1):75–83.

9 Physiotherapy for Degenerative Lumbar Spine Disease

Hana Alsobayel and Dalia Alimam

Physiotherapy, as an autonomous medical discipline, focuses on bringing the human body to its maximum functional ability in order for the individual to live independently with the best possible quality of life. Physiotherapy plays a critical role in the assessment and management of degenerative lumbar spine diseases. It utilizes a variety of tools and approaches to determine the functional status of the lumbar spine and its impact on the individual's daily living activities and quality of life. Once the functional status is determined, the physiotherapists through their clinical reasoning and the guidance of the best available evidence set up management goals based on the individual's needs and preferences. In this chapter, physiotherapy assessment and management tools and approaches for the degenerative lumbar spine diseases will be presented in light of the latest evidence and guidelines.

Physiotherapy Assessment of the Degenerative Lumbar Spine

Degenerative lumbar spine disorders are considered one of the leading causes of pain and disability globally. The physiotherapy assessment of such conditions incorporates biomechanical evaluation, functional movement assessments, and patient-reported outcome measures in light of the International Classification of Functioning, Disability, and Health (ICF) framework [1]. The physiotherapy assessment emphasizes not only impairments in body structures and function but also activity limitations and participation restrictions. Clinical Practice Guidelines (CPGs) provide further structure for the assessment, ensuring evidence-based decision-making. Guidelines, such as the National Institute for Health and Care Excellence (NICE) [2] and the American Physical Therapy Association [3], have refined best practices in physiotherapy assessment, placing greater emphasis on multidimensional evaluation approaches, red flag screening, and movement-based assessment. These guidelines also emphasize the adoption of patient-centered and value-based care to enhance management outcomes. The foundation of effective, patient-centered rehabilitation is a thorough, individualized assessment, incorporating physical, medical, and psychosocial evaluations to understand each patient's unique challenges.

Subjective Assessment

A structured subjective assessment ensures that physiotherapists collect relevant information to guide management, whether the physiotherapist

H. Alsobayel (✉) · D. Alimam
Department of Rehabilitation Sciences, College of Applied Medical Sciences, King Saud University, Riyadh, Saudi Arabia
e-mail: hsobayel@ksu.edu.sa; dalimam@ksu.edu.sa

A. A. Baaj et al. (eds.), *Surgery of the Lumbar Spine*, https://doi.org/10.1007/978-3-032-18097-1_9

was the first contact clinician or otherwise. A thorough bio-psycho-social approach to assessment that goes beyond pain intensity and mechanical symptoms is crucial. This includes evaluation of pain characteristics to distinguish between mechanical pain (exacerbated by movement or prolonged postures) and neuropathic pain (burning, tingling, or radiating symptoms). It is recommended by several guidelines using STarT Back screening tool to identify people with a high risk of developing disability and chronic pain [4].

Beyond pain assessment, physiotherapists evaluate how lumbar spine degeneration affects movement, work, daily activities, and quality of life. Two of the most commonly used Patient Reported Outcome Measures (PROM) to assess disability are Oswestry Disability Index (ODI) [5] and Roland Morris Disability Questionnaire (RMDQ) [6]. Screening mobility and balance deficits, particularly in older adults, is crucial as degenerative changes can contribute to falls and decreased independence [7].

Screening for red and yellow flags is a major aspect in subjective assessment. Clinical guidelines strongly emphasize the screening for red flags to rule out serious pathology. Screening for yellow flags is important to identify psychosocial risk factors that may contribute to persistent symptoms and may interfere with management outcomes [8]. Red flags include, for example, unexplained weight loss, night pain, progressive neurological deficits, and bladder or bowel dysfunctions, which may indicate spinal tumors, infections, or cauda equina syndrome [9]. Yellow flags refer to psychosocial barriers such as fear-avoidance behavior, catastrophizing, and work dissatisfaction, which can increase the risk of chronic disability and persistent symptoms [10]. Screening tools like Fear-Avoidance Beliefs Questionnaire (FABQ) and Tampa Scale of Kinesiophobia (TSK) are endorsed by CPGs for their predictive value in chronicity risk assessment [11].

The research on physiotherapy screening and stratification for spinal disorders presents a complex and evolving landscape. Studies consistently emphasize the importance of structured red flag screening, yet many red flags remain unreliable in practice [12].

Beyond screening for serious pathology, physiotherapists use stratification tools to tailor interventions based on patient risk profiles. Stratification tools show promise but require better integration into clinical workflows [13].

Objective Assessment

Objective assessment integrates clinical movement analysis, physical function tests, and biomechanical evaluation to establish a patient's functional abilities within the ICF framework. It is well-documented that pain and disability correlate poorly with imaging findings; therefore, functional assessment is prioritized over structural evaluation in the absence of red flags. Selecting outcome measures with adequate measurement properties is key for accurate interpretation of information gained during a clinical assessment and for measuring the effectiveness of interventions in research and clinical practice. The COnsensus-based Standards for the selection of health Measurement Instruments (COSMIN) initiative aims to facilitate selecting high-quality outcome measures through a systematic evaluation of validity, responsiveness, reliability, and measurement error of PROMs and physical measures [14].

- *Functional Movement Screening*

Movement-based assessments are important to detect mechanical dysfunctions. Tools such as the Timed Up and Go (TUG) test, Five-Repetition Sit-to-Stand (5R-STS) test, and Functional Movement Screen (FMS) are validated tools for assessing physical mobility and functional ability [15]. The strongest evidence supports 1-min stair climb and 50-foot walk tests for Degenerative lumbar spine physical function testing [16].

- *Manual and Neurological Examination*

Using segmental mobility testing, such as Passive Intervertebral Motion Testing (PIVM), is sometimes necessary to detect hypomobility or hypermobility. Neural tension tests, including the Slump Test and Straight Leg Raise (SLR), remain gold-standard assessments for detecting radiculopathy [17].

- *Biomechanical Assessment*

In some clinical settings, tools are available to assess specific structural dysfunctions, such as using Rehabilitative Ultrasound Imaging (RUSI) [18] for assessing multifidus and transversus abdominis activation, or Surface Electromyography (sEMG) to evaluate paraspinal muscle fatigue and function [19]. Research is controversial about the correlation between the core muscle activities and pain and disability among people with degenerative lumbar spine dysfunctions [20].

Clinical Decision-Making and Interdisciplinary Collaboration

Physiotherapy assessment findings are essential for interdisciplinary decision-making, particularly in determining conservative vs. surgical management. Clinical guidelines suggest that physiotherapy-based assessments should be integrated with orthopedic and pain management evaluations to tailor interventions. Physiotherapists play a key role in prehabilitation, preparing patients for spine surgery and improving postoperative recovery outcomes. Guidelines emphasize that patients undergoing lumbar spine surgery should receive preoperative physiotherapy to optimize function and strength [21].

By integrating subjective and objective assessments, red/yellow flag screening, functional movement analysis, and emerging biomechanical tools, physiotherapists can provide a comprehensive, patient-centered evaluation. Emerging trends such as artificial intelligence (AI) show promising tools to support decision-making and improve early detection of spinal dysfunctions [22]. Wearable sensors and machine learning-based gait analysis are also tools that could refine physiotherapy assessment accuracy aligning with precision rehabilitation principles [23].

Physiotherapy Intervention

Physiotherapy intervention plays a crucial role in managing non-specific lower back pain (LBP) conditions and lumbar radiculopathy (LR) caused by herniated disc and other degenerative conditions, offering conservative means of treatment [24, 25]. Physiotherapy intervention guidelines for degenerative lumbar spine conditions have evolved significantly, driven by the latest evidence-based research. Different guidelines emphasize a comprehensive assessment, focusing on individualized treatment plans that address an individual's specific goals, including therapeutic exercise, pain management techniques, mobility enhancement, strengthening of core muscles, and facilitating functional recovery [25–32].

Additionally, clinical practice guidelines (CPG) reported that physiotherapy and exercise may be effective in managing symptoms of lumbar spinal stenosis with neurogenic claudication in specific patient subgroups [33]. Different CPGs described the importance of applying a multimodal rehabilitation intervention for patients with limited walking ability and those who are overweight or obese with comorbidities. This should encompass education, lifestyle modifications, behavioral change techniques, and manual therapy (including spinal mobilization, manipulation, and massage) [34]. An individualized exercise program featuring stretches, strength training, cycling, and body weight-supported treadmill walking should also be integrated [34]. For post-surgical patients, include cognitive-behavioral therapy (CBT) in their rehabilitation plan [35, 36]. Addressing psychosocial factors has been shown to be beneficial in managing chronic LBP and improving patient outcomes [36].

As the understanding of degenerative spine issues deepens, the goal remains to empower patients through effective, evidence-backed strategies tailored to their unique needs [25]. Overall, studies emphasized the essential importance of patient education about self-management strategies, advice on returning to normal activity, and reassurance regarding their condition [36, 37].

Given the range of the treatment options, each with varying levels of effectiveness, risks, and impacts on patients' related outcomes, different approaches have been suggested that may allow the therapist and patient to choose the most suitable plan. Shared decision-making, for instance, is a process in which clinicians and patients work together to select treatments or management, based on clinical evidence and the patient's informed preferences [38, 39]. This approach is particularly relevant in the management of spine degeneration [40, 41].

Shared decision-making has shown to be related to lower pain levels due to improved acceptance, understanding of treatment goals, and adherence to treatment [42, 43]. It is fundamental in physiotherapy practice as it empowers patients to take an active role in their treatment, leading to more personalized care [42, 43]. For effective shared decision-making, physiotherapists should clearly communicate their expertise while actively listening to and incorporating individuals' preferences [43, 44]. Goal setting related to the patient's needs, values, and expectations, helps patients establish realistic and achievable outcomes, adopting motivation and adherence to treatment plans [45, 46]. By integrating patients' values and preferences into the decision-making process, physiotherapists can enhance engagement, satisfaction, and adherence to treatment plans.

Successful shared decision-making is closely linked to the therapist-patient alliance, which is fundamental for effective therapeutic outcomes [47, 48]. A strong therapeutic alliance relies on mutual trust, open communication, and collaboration [43]. Research demonstrates that pain perception is significantly influenced by contextual factors, including the therapeutic alliance between the physiotherapist and the patient [48, 49]. Such approaches not only encourage shared decision-making but also enhance the therapist-patient relationship, ultimately leading to better treatment outcomes [48].

Effective pain management techniques play a crucial role in managing degenerative spine conditions. Activity pacing, for example, is essential for preventing exacerbation of pain; it involves adjusting behaviors related to cycles of overactivity and underactivity, as well as addressing avoidance and excessive persistence [50]. It encourages patients to balance activity with rest, promoting gradual increases in physical activity without overexertion. Educating patients on acquiring activity pacing skills can enhance physical activity engagement and health outcomes for adults with chronic conditions [51]. However, conversely, when pain intensifies, they often engage in less activity and rest more.

For effective pacing, activity should be gradually increased according to planned targets rather than the level of pain. At the same time, strategies like graded exercise help patients manage their pain and build confidence in their ability to cope [52]. Graded exercise involves a structured increase in physical activity and has been shown to improve physical function and reduce pain in individuals with degenerative spine issues [53–56]. Weight management is another key factor, as maintaining a healthy weight can alleviate stress on the spine, preventing the occurrence of LBP, reducing pain intensity, and improving overall mobility [57, 58]. In conclusion, self-management strategies empower patients to take control of their pain through education and skill development, enhancing their ability to cope with chronic conditions. Together, these techniques form a wide-ranging approach to managing pain and improving quality of life for those with degenerative spine conditions [59].

It is essential for individuals with LBP conditions to understand that their individual preferences among numerous physiotherapy procedures should guide the choice of intervention. Clinicians must recognize that different treatment options may be more suitable for different individuals and play a crucial role in assisting everyone in selecting a management approach that aligns with their values and preferences. Evidence supports this approach, indicating that patient-centered care leads to better adherence to treatment and improved favorable outcomes [28].

In summary, recovery in individuals with degenerative lumbar spine conditions is promoted through a comprehensive approach that addresses both physical and psychological aspects of their health. Enhancements in strength, flexibility, and mobility contribute to pain reduction and improved functional outcomes. Addressing the psychological barriers associated with chronic pain fosters better coping mechanisms and encourages active participation in daily activities. Additionally, adopting healthier lifestyle choices supports overall well-being and can mitigate the impact of comorbidities that exacerbate pain and disability. By integrating these elements, patients can achieve significant improvements in their quality of life and reduce disability levels.

References

1. Organization WH. 2025 Release of the ICF in English, French, Spanish, Chinese, Turkish and Czech [Available from: https://www.icf-research-branch.org/.
2. guidelines N. Chronic pain (primary and secondary) in over 16s: assessment of all chronic pain and management of chronic primary pain. 2021.
3. Delitto A, George SZ, Van Dillen L, Whitman JM, Sowa G, Shekelle P, et al. Low back pain. J Orthop Sports Phys Ther. 2012;42(4):A1–57.
4. Hill JC, Dunn KM, Lewis M, Mullis R, Main CJ, Foster NE, et al. A primary care back pain screening tool: identifying patient subgroups for initial treatment. Arthritis Rheum. 2008;59(5):632–41.
5. Fairbank JC, Couper J, Davies JB, O'Brien JP. The Oswestry low back pain disability questionnaire. Physiotherapy. 1980;66(8):271–3.
6. Roland M, Morris R. A study of the natural history of back pain. Part I: development of a reliable and sensitive measure of disability in low-back pain. Spine (Phila Pa 1976). 1983;8(2):141–4.
7. Xing L, Bao Y, Wang B, Shi M, Wei Y, Huang X, et al. Falls caused by balance disorders in the elderly with multiple systems involved: pathogenic mechanisms and treatment strategies. Front Neurol. 2023;14:1128092.
8. Custers P, Van de Kelft E, Eeckhaut B, Sabbe W, Hofman A, Debuysscher A, et al. Clinical examination, diagnosis, and conservative treatment of chronic low back pain: a narrative review. Life (Basel). 2024;14(9)
9. Chhabra HS, Tamai K, Alsebayel H, AlEissa S, Alqahtani Y, Arand M, et al. SPINE20 recommendations 2023: one earth, one family, one future without spine disability. Brain Spine. 2023;3:102688.
10. Patel MS, Lee KC, Dhake RP, Longworth S, Sell P. Ability of spine specialists to identify psychosocial risk factors as obstacles to recovery in patients with low back pain-related disorders. Asian Spine J. 2021;15(2):224–33.
11. Swinkels-Meewisse EJ, Swinkels RA, Verbeek AL, Vlaeyen JW, Oostendorp RA. Psychometric properties of the Tampa scale for kinesiophobia and the fear-avoidance beliefs questionnaire in acute low back pain. Man Ther. 2003;8(1):29–36.
12. Finucane LM, Downie A, Mercer C, Greenhalgh SM, Boissonnault WG, Pool-Goudzwaard AL, et al. International framework for red flags for potential serious spinal pathologies. J Orthop Sports Phys Ther. 2020;50(7):350–72.
13. Keller F, Allet L, Meichtry A, Scascighini L, Scheermesser M, Wirz M, et al. Diagnostic and decision-making abilities of Swiss physiotherapists in a simulated direct access setting. Physiother Theory Pract. 2023;39(11):2336–51.
14. Mokkink LB, Boers M, van der Vleuten CPM, Bouter LM, Alonso J, Patrick DL, et al. COSMIN risk of bias tool to assess the quality of studies on reliability or measurement error of outcome measurement instruments: a Delphi study. BMC Med Res Methodol. 2020;20(1):293.
15. Klukowska AM, Ciobanu-Caraus O, Germans MR, Vandertop WP, Schroder ML, Staartjes VE. Measurement properties of the 5-repetition sit-to-stand test in patients with lumbar degenerative disorders: COSMIN systematic review. Spine J. 2025;25(4):696–718.
16. Kowalski KL, Mistry J, Beilin A, Goodman M, Lukacs MJ, Rushton A. Physical functioning in the lumbar spinal surgery population: a systematic review and narrative synthesis of outcome measures and measurement properties of the physical measures. PLoS One. 2024;19(8):e0307004.
17. Espinosa G, de Los Monteros FJ, Gonzalez-Medina G, Ardila EMG, Mansilla JR, Exposito JP, Ruiz PO. Use of Neurodynamic or orthopedic tension tests for the diagnosis of lumbar and lumbosacral radiculopathies: study of the diagnostic validity. Int J Environ Res Public Health. 2020;17(19)
18. Nabavi N, Mosallanezhad Z, Haghighatkhah HR, Mohseni Bandpeid MA. Reliability of rehabilitative ultrasonography to measure transverse abdominis and multifidus muscle dimensions. Iran J Radiol. 2014;11(3):e21008.
19. Suo M, Zhou L, Wang J, Huang H, Zhang J, Sun T, et al. The application of surface electromyography technology in evaluating paraspinal muscle function. Diagnostics (Basel). 2024;14(11)
20. Cooley JR, Jensen TS, Kjaer P, Jacques A, Theroux J, Hebert JJ. Spinal degeneration and lumbar multifidus muscle quality may independently affect clinical outcomes in patients conservatively managed for low back or leg pain. Sci Rep. 2024;14(1):9777.
21. Debono B, Wainwright TW, Wang MY, Sigmundsson FG, Yang MMH, Smid-Nanninga H, et al. Consensus statement for perioperative care in lum-

bar spinal fusion: enhanced recovery after surgery (ERAS(R)) society recommendations. Spine J. 2021;21(5):729–52.
22. NICE. Digital technologies for managing non-specific low back pain: early value assessment. Health Technol Assess. 2024.
23. Wei S, Wu Z. The application of wearable sensors and machine learning algorithms in rehabilitation training: a systematic review. Sensors (Basel). 2023;23(18)
24. Brodke DS, Ritter SM. Nonsurgical management of low back pain and lumbar disk degeneration. Instr Course Lect. 2005;54:279–86.
25. Wong J, Côté P, Sutton D, Randhawa K, Yu H, Varatharajan S, et al. Clinical practice guidelines for the noninvasive management of low back pain: a systematic review by the Ontario protocol for traffic injury management (OPTIMa) collaboration. Eur J Pain. 2017;21(2):201–16.
26. Meroni R, Piscitelli D, Ravasio C, Vanti C, Bertozzi L, De Vito G, et al. Evidence for managing chronic low back pain in primary care: a review of recommendations from high-quality clinical practice guidelines. Disabil Rehabil. 2019:1–15.
27. Foster NE, Anema JR, Cherkin D, Chou R, Cohen SP, Gross DP, et al. Prevention and treatment of low back pain: evidence, challenges, and promising directions. Lancet. 2018;391(10137):2368–83.
28. Stochkendahl MJ, Kjaer P, Hartvigsen J, Kongsted A, Aaboe J, Andersen M, et al. National Clinical Guidelines for non-surgical treatment of patients with recent onset low back pain or lumbar radiculopathy. Eur Spine J. 2018;27(1):60–75.
29. Chou R, Deyo R, Friedly J, Skelly A, Hashimoto R, Weimer M, et al. Nonpharmacologic therapies for low back pain: a systematic review for an American College of Physicians Clinical Practice Guideline. Ann Intern Med. 2017;166(7):493–505.
30. Buchbinder R, van Tulder M, Öberg B, Costa LM, Woolf A, Schoene M, et al. Low back pain: a call for action. Lancet. 2018;391(10137):2384–8.
31. Bernstein IA, Malik Q, Carville S, Ward S. Low back pain and sciatica: summary of NICE guidance. BMJ. 2017;356
32. National Guideline C. National Institute for health and care excellence: clinical guidelines. Low back pain and sciatica in over 16s: assessment and management. London: National Institute for Health and Care Excellence (UK) Copyright © NICE, 2016; 2016.
33. Watters WC, Baisden J, Gilbert TJ, Kreiner S, Resnick DK, Bono CM, et al. Degenerative lumbar spinal stenosis: an evidence-based clinical guideline for the diagnosis and treatment of degenerative lumbar spinal stenosis. Spine J. 2008;8(2):305–10.
34. Bussières A, Cancelliere C, Ammendolia C, Comer CM, Zoubi FA, Châtillon C-E, et al. Non-surgical interventions for lumbar spinal stenosis leading to neurogenic claudication: a clinical practice guideline. J Pain. 2021;22(9):1015–39.
35. Monticone M, Ferrante S, Teli M, Rocca B, Foti C, Lovi A, et al. Management of catastrophising and kinesiophobia improves rehabilitation after fusion for lumbar spondylolisthesis and stenosis. A randomised controlled trial. Eur Spine J. 2014;23:87–95.
36. Oliveira CB, Maher CG, Pinto RZ, Traeger AC, Lin CC, Chenot JF, et al. Clinical practice guidelines for the management of non-specific low back pain in primary care: an updated overview. Eur Spine J. 2018;27(11):2791–803.
37. Kreiner DS, Matz P, Bono CM, Cho CH, Easa JE, Ghiselli G, et al. Guideline summary review: an evidence-based clinical guideline for the diagnosis and treatment of low back pain. Spine J. 2020;20(7):998–1024.
38. Thomas H, Lambert M, Plummer C, Runnett C, Thomson R, Troy-Smith AM, et al. Shared decision-making for ICDs: a regional collaborative initiative. Br J Cardiol. 2020;27(3):23.
39. Fagundes F, de Melo do Espírito Santo C, de Luna Teixeira FM, Tonini TV, Cabral CM. Effectiveness of the addition of therapeutic alliance with minimal intervention in the treatment of patients with chronic, nonspecific low back pain and low risk of involvement of psychosocial factors: a study protocol for a randomized controlled trial (TalkBack trial). Trials. 2017;18(1):49.
40. Sam S, Sharma R, Corp N, Igwesi-Chidobe C, Babatunde OO. Shared decision making in musculoskeletal pain consultations in low- and middle-income countries: a systematic review. Int Health. 2019;12(5):455–71.
41. Ferrer RL, Gill JM. Shared decision making, contextualized. Annals Family Med. 2013:303–5.
42. Légaré F, Adekpedjou R, Stacey D, Turcotte S, Kryworuchko J, Graham ID, et al. Interventions for increasing the use of shared decision making by healthcare professionals. Cochrane Database Syst Rev. 2018;(7)
43. Grenfell J, Soundy A. People's experience of shared decision making in musculoskeletal physiotherapy: a systematic review and thematic synthesis. Behav Sci. 2022;12(1):12.
44. Hoffmann T, Bakhit M, Michaleff Z. Shared decision making and physical therapy: what, when, how, and why? Braz J Phys Ther. 2022;26(1):100382.
45. Kang E, Kim MY, Lipsey KL, Foster ER. Person-centered goal setting: a systematic review of intervention components and level of active engagement in rehabilitation goal-setting interventions. Arch Phys Med Rehabil. 2022;103(1):121–30.e3.
46. Turner-Stokes L, Rose H, Ashford S, Singer B. Patient engagement and satisfaction with goal planning: impact on outcome from rehabilitation. Int J Ther Rehabil. 2015;22(5):210.
47. Søndenå P, Dalusio-King G, Hebron C. Conceptualisation of the therapeutic alliance in physiotherapy: is it adequate? Musculoskelet Sci Pract. 2020;46:102131.

48. Sherriff B, Clark C, Killingback C, Newell D. Impact of contextual factors on patient outcomes following conservative low back pain treatment: systematic review. Chiropractic Manual Ther. 2022;30(1):20.
49. Kinney M, Seider J, Beaty AF, Coughlin K, Dyal M, Clewley D. The impact of therapeutic alliance in physical therapy for chronic musculoskeletal pain: a systematic review of the literature. Physiother Theory Pract. 2020;36(8):886–98.
50. Birkholtz M, Aylwin L, Harman RM. Activity pacing in chronic pain management: one aim, but which method? Part one: introduction and literature review. Br J Occup Ther. 2004;67(10):447–52.
51. Barakou I, Hackett KL, Finch T, Hettinga FJ. Self-regulation of effort for a better health-related quality of life: a multidimensional activity pacing model for chronic pain and fatigue management. Ann Med. 2023;55(2):2270688.
52. Ikemoto T, Miki K, Matsubara T, Wakao N. Psychological treatment strategy for chronic low back pain. Spine Surg Relat Res. 2019;3(3):199–206.
53. Leonhardt C, Kuss K, Becker A, Basler H-D, de Jong J, Flatau B, et al. Graded exposure for chronic low Back pain in older adults: a pilot study. J Geriatr Phys Ther. 2017;40(1):51–9.
54. Beissner K, Bach E, Murtaugh C, Parker SJ, Trachtenberg M, Reid MC. Implementing a cognitive-behavioral pain self-management program in home health care, part 1: program adaptation. J Geriatr Phys Ther. 2013;36(3):123–9.
55. Schemer L, Schroeder A, Ørnbøl E, Glombiewski JA. Exposure and cognitive-behavioural therapy for chronic back pain: an RCT on treatment processes. Eur J Pain. 2019;23(3):526–38.
56. López-de-Uralde-Villanueva I, Muñoz-García D, Gil-Martínez A, Pardo-Montero J, Muñoz-Plata R, Angulo-Díaz-Parreño S, et al. A systematic review and meta-analysis on the effectiveness of graded activity and graded exposure for chronic nonspecific low Back pain. Pain Med. 2016;17(1):172–88.
57. Zhang T-T, Liu Z, Liu Y-L, Zhao J-J, Liu D-W, Tian Q-B. Obesity as a risk factor for low Back pain: a meta-analysis. Clin Spine Surg. 2018;31(1):22–7.
58. Hartvigsen J, Hancock MJ, Kongsted A, Louw Q, Ferreira ML, Genevay S, et al. What low back pain is and why we need to pay attention. Lancet. 2018;391(10137):2356–67.
59. Elbers S, Wittink H, Pool J, Smeets R. The effectiveness of generic self-management interventions for patients with chronic musculoskeletal pain on physical function, self-efficacy, pain intensity and physical activity: a systematic review and meta-analysis. Eur J Pain. 2018;22(9):1577–96.

Lumbar Spine Trauma

10

Warren Roth, Jason Silvestre, James P. Lawrence, and Robert A. Ravinsky

Introduction

Traumatic injuries to the thoracolumbar spine represent a spectrum of different injury patterns that require varied treatment strategies. The lumbar spine has key roles in the bearing of weight, and transmission of significant loads from the trunk to the pelvis and lower extremities, while also being highly mobile. Furthermore, the biomechanical transition from the relatively rigid thoracic spine to the mobile lumbar region renders the thoracolumbar junction vulnerable to spinal trauma. Injuries of the thoracolumbar spine range from minor fractures treated non-operatively to high-energy fractures with significant ligamentous injuries and associated neurologic compromise. Successful management of thoracolumbar trauma requires a sound understanding of spinal biomechanics, surgical indications and techniques, and early identification and treatment of complications when they arise [3–5, 13–16].

Numerous advances in the classification and treatment of thoracolumbar injuries have been made in recent years. There are several validated thoracolumbar trauma classification systems that allow for characterization of different injury patterns, provide a framework for communication among surgical providers, allow for standardized treatment protocols, and offer opportunities for research and education. Nonsurgical and surgical treatment modalities have evolved significantly as well, focusing on the basic principles of restoration of appropriate alignment, creating structural stability, and decompression of the neural elements in order to allow for early patient mobilization and prevention of secondary complications. Modern techniques involve a broad variety of surgical approaches and include tissue-sparing or minimally invasive techniques. This chapter aims to provide a broad overview of the current approaches to managing lumbar spine trauma for the spinal clinician [3–7, 10, 16].

Epidemiology of Lumbar Trauma

Traumatic injuries to the spinal column are common, affecting over 150,000 individuals each year in North America alone, with high rates of associated morbidity and mortality [8, 16]. An epidemiological understanding of injury patterns aids the clinician in the evaluation and diagnosis of spinal injuries. Traumatic injuries to the thoracolumbar spine are found in roughly 7% of blunt trauma patients seen at Level 1 trauma centers. Motor vehicle collisions are the most com-

W. Roth · J. Silvestre · J. P. Lawrence · R. A. Ravinsky (✉)
Department of Orthopaedics and Physical Medicine, Medical University of South Carolina, Charleston, SC, USA
e-mail: rothw@musc.edu; silvesja@musc.edu; lawrejam@musc.edu; ravinsky@musc.edu

A. A. Baaj et al. (eds.), *Surgery of the Lumbar Spine*, https://doi.org/10.1007/978-3-032-18097-1_10

mon mechanism of injury and account for over a third of these injuries, with a median age of 44.5 [8, 16]. Burst fractures are the most common fracture pattern, with the majority occurring at the L1 level due to the unique biomechanics of the thoracolumbar junction [8, 16]. Falls and injuries as a result of sport are increasing secondarily to the high activity level of the older adult and the common presence of bone fragility with aging. When evaluating patients with traumatic injuries to the lumbar spine, the clinician should have a high index of suspicion for other associated injuries. Noncontiguous and concurrent spinal injuries to the cervical and thoracolumbar spine, with or without neurologic compromise, occur in roughly one-fourth of these patients. Other non-spinal injuries may be seen in association with thoracolumbar trauma as well, including intracranial, pelvic/intra-abdominal, and extremity injuries [8, 16].

Clinical Evaluation

ATLS Protocol for Polytrauma [20]

Advanced trauma life support (ATLS) remains the foundation on which care to polytraumatized patients is provided. The goal of ATLS is to address immediate threats to life first and then proceed with indicated treatments swiftly [10]. Securing the airway, ensuring ventilation and hemodynamic stability is achieved with a balanced resuscitation, following which musculoskeletal and spinal assessment are performed. Upon logrolling of the patient in the trauma bay, signs suggestive of spinal injury would include obvious swelling or subcutaneous ballotable fluid, crepitation, or bony malalignment.

Focused History and Physical Examination

Following the initial trauma evaluation, a focused history and physical examination by the surgical team should ensue. Important pieces of history include the mechanism of injury, the presence or absence of pre-existing neurological dysfunction, a relevant past medical and surgical history, medication use, alcohol or substance use, and social factors.

Physical examination should include a detailed neurological examination, assessment of the lumbar spine for evidence of soft tissue injury, and evaluation for sphincter dysfunction. If the patient presents with a clear neurological deficit, the presence or absence of the bulbocavernosus reflex indicates the presence of spinal shock, and classification of the precise spinal injury level is not yet possible until its resolution. The American Spinal Injury Association (ASIA) impairment scale allows for accurate classification based on motor and sensory impairment.

Imaging

Plain Films [3, 5–7, 10, 13–16]

Supine anteroposterior and cross-table lateral radiographs can be performed in the trauma bay. In patients who are ambulatory following their injury, standing radiographs can provide additional information, as to the segmental sagittal and coronal spinal alignment. This can be particularly helpful in compression and burst fracture patterns and can help illustrate subtle instability patterns. Findings such as transverse process fractures, spinous process widening, vertebral body height loss, and vertebral body translation guide the clinician as to the underlying mechanism and if further workup is required.

Computed Tomography (CT) [3, 5–7, 10, 13–16]

CT has largely supplanted plain radiographs and has become the standard of care in the acute radiographic evaluation of thoracolumbar spinal trauma, because of its high-quality visualization as well as the high sensitivity and specificity for bony injury. In modern trauma centers, pan-CT scan of the cranium, cervical spine, and chest/abdomen/pelvis with thoracolumbar reformats are performed routinely in patients presenting to the trauma bay. CT scan is required for accurate injury classification with regard to injury morphology and mechanism. The utility of CT is, however, limited with respect to evaluation of soft tissue injury and detailed evaluation of the posterior ligamentous complex (PLC). Indirectly, the presence of interspinous process gapping, distraction of the facet joints, or posterior element fractures provides clues to the integrity of the PLC.

Magnetic Resonance Imaging (MRI) [3, 5–7, 10, 13–16]

MRI is extremely sensitive in the assessment of the soft tissue structures and neural elements in patients with thoracolumbar trauma, as well as providing detailed information of the surrounding anatomy. It is indicated to evaluate injury to the PLC, the neural elements, as well as the presence of compressive hematomas. Furthermore, MRI assists greatly in determining fracture acuity, through the appreciation of acute bony and soft tissue edema, the presence of acute edema and hematoma, and the presence of concomitant muscular injury. The integrity of the PLC has been a topic of debate among spine trauma specialists, as MRI can frequently appreciate subtle ligamentous injury that may not always be clinically relevant.

Nuclear Medicine [3, 5–7, 10, 13–16]

With advancements and widespread availability in MRI and CT, these imaging modalities remain the gold standard for radiologic assessment in lumbar spine trauma. Modalities such as ultrasound and bone scan do not have widely accepted applications in this setting. That said, adaptations to accepted imaging modalities have demonstrated benefits, particularly with single photon emission computed tomography (SPECT). In the setting of lumbar spine trauma, MRI remains the gold standard for differentiating acuity in osteoporotic vertebral compression fractures, as well as in the diagnosis of sacral insufficiency fractures. In situations in which MRI is unavailable or contraindicated, SPECT/CT may be of diagnostic utility.

Classification Systems

TLICS [9, 11]

The thoracolumbar injury classification and severity score (TLICS) represents a valuable framework for classifying traumatic injuries of the thoracolumbar spine for the purpose of guiding treatment decisions [9, 11]. TLICS is based on three injury parameters: fracture morphology, neurologic status, and the integrity of the posterior ligamentous complex (Table 10.1).

AO Spine Classification [13, 14]

The AO Spine thoracolumbar classification system uses imaging characteristics and fracture morphology to describe various thoracolumbar injury patterns. In doing so, it provides a consistent language by which spine surgeons can com-

Table 10.1 Thoracolumbar Injury Classification and Severity Score (TLICS)

Category	Description (Points)
Injury Morphology	Compression (1) Burst (2) Translation/Rotation (3) Distraction (4)
Posterior Ligamentous Complex (PLC) Integrity	Intact (0) Suspected Injury (2) Disruption (3)
Neurologic Status	Intact (0) Nerve Root Injury (2) Complete Cord Injury (2) Incomplete Cord Injury (3) Cauda Equina Syndrome (3)
Total Points	1–3: Non-Surgical 4: Equivocal >4: Surgical

municate injury patterns for the purpose of guiding treatment decisions. In general, the progression from A to C and in assigned number are associated with progressive degrees of instability and need for surgical intervention.

Surgical Indications/Contraindications

Indications for surgery focus on neurologic status, the fracture pattern, the presence or absence of spinal stability, the presence of pain, and the success or failure of more conservative management in appropriate patients. Patients with new or progressive neurological deficits in the setting of acute neural compression necessitate either direct or indirect decompression to prevent further deterioration [1, 4, 9, 11–16].

Furthermore, the absence of structural stability (severe kyphosis, fracture with obvious PLC injury, or rotation/translation) of the thoracolumbar spine necessitates surgical stabilization. During surgical planning, post-traumatic deformities should be corrected and appropriate physiological alignment restored. This serves to facilitate early mobilization, improved pain and physiologic function, and avoids late kyphotic deformity and potential neurological deterioration. Moreover, patients who have undergone a trial of non-operative management, as may be seen with compression and stable burst fractures, may progress to requiring surgical intervention due to intractable pain with weight-bearing or progressive kyphotic deformity. Unstable injury patterns, either based on fracture pattern/mechanism alone (AO C Type) or diagnosed as a fracture with clear PLC injury on imaging (AO B1 and B2), heavily favor surgical treatment [1, 4, 9, 11–16].

There are few absolute contraindications to surgical intervention in lumbar spine trauma when it would otherwise be indicated to provide stability or relieve neural compression [1, 4, 9, 11–16]. However, patients with significant medical comorbidities or otherwise clinically unstable polytraumatized patients may be more appropriate for non-operative treatment in certain instances.

Common Injuries and Recommended Surgical Strategies

Vertebral Compression Fractures (AO type A1)

Vertebral compression fractures involve compromise of the anterior column and commonly occur in the elderly and patients with osteoporosis, though they may occur independently of these risk factors after trauma. These injuries can often be treated conservatively with pain control, bracing for comfort, and gentle mobilization [1, 2, 4, 7, 11, 12, 16]. All patients with fragility fractures, particularly after low-energy mechanisms, are at increased risk of subsequent future fracture. These should be referred to a multidisciplinary bone health clinic for assessment and medical optimization. In patients with delayed healing, and severe pain that is refractory to conservative measures, cement augmentation procedures such as vertebroplasty or kyphoplasty may be considered [1, 2, 4, 7, 11, 12, 16].

Burst Fractures (AO Type A3 and A4)

Burst fractures are common traumatic injuries to the lumbar spine, typically resulting from a large compressive force across the anterior and middle columns [1–3]. Some burst fractures can be treated conservatively, while some patients with these injuries benefit from surgery for stabilization, decompression, segmental realignment, or a combination thereof (Fig. 10.1). The decision to operate is based on fracture morphology, status of the PLC, and the neurological status, as detailed in TLICS [9, 11]. For burst fractures that require operative stabilization, the Load Sharing classification can assist in determining whether a 1-up-1-down fusion construct would afford sufficient stability, or alternatively if a 2-up-2-down construct is more appropriate [1, 2]. In the setting of neurological deficits or severe radicular pain due to bony compression of neural structures, decompression is indicated. The decision for direct decompression versus indirect

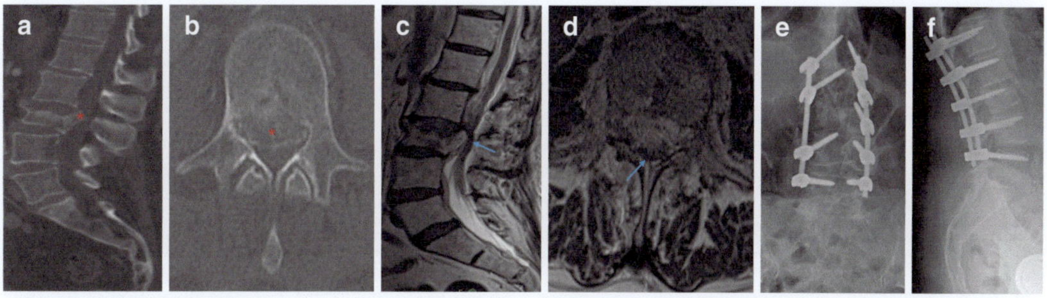

Fig. 10.1 74-year-old female involved in a motor vehicle collision with L3 burst fracture and presenting with cauda equina syndrome. Figures (**a** and **b**) demonstrate mid-sagittal and axial CT images, respectively, showing an L3 burst fracture with retropulsion of the posterior vertebral body into the spinal canal (asterisk). Figures (**c** and **d**) demonstrate mid-sagittal and axial T2-weighted MR images, respectively, illustrating severe central canal stenosis due to retropulsion of bone with compression of the thecal sac and cauda equina (arrows). Patient underwent urgent surgery for the indication of lumbar burst with cauda equina syndrome (TLICS 7). Figures (**e** and **f**) demonstrate AP and lateral post-operative radiographs, respectively, status post L1-L5 PSIF and L2-L4 decompression

decompression with ligamentotaxis is made based on imaging characteristics, the integrity of the posterior longitudinal ligament, and surgeon experience. Minimally invasive fixation with percutaneous pedicle screw instrumentation may be suitable for certain patients to allow for an internal brace effect.

Chance Fracture/Flexion Distraction (AO Type B1)

Flexion-distraction injuries occur when the vertebral column experiences a distracting force across the posterior elements, and a simultaneous compressive force across the anterior column. These injuries are commonly seen in association with seatbelts in motor vehicle collisions [14–16]. As such, these patients have a high rate of concomitant injury to abdominal viscera [14–16]. Chance fractures are a sub-category of flexion-distraction injuries, and may involve a purely osseous injury at a single level, where the fracture splits the spinous process, followed by the pedicles, and finally the vertebral body. As such, chance fractures heal well if they are reduced and there is appropriate bone-on-bone contact. In the setting of flexion-distraction injuries with injury to the PLC, surgery is indicated to restore structural stability and involves a typical instrumented fusion above and below the injury level (Fig. 10.2) [1, 2, 4, 7, 11, 12, 16].

Fracture-Dislocation (AO C Type)

Fracture-dislocation injuries in the lumbar spine result from high-energy trauma and almost invariably require surgical stabilization due to significant instability. A posterior approach is typically used, as it allows the surgeon to perform open reduction, direct decompression as needed, and instrumented stabilization and fusion of the spine. In some instances, anterior approaches may be employed as well, the benefits of this being load-sharing through the anterior column, additional surface area for fusion, improved segmental realignment, and potentially decompression. Newer methods of limited open decompression and the employment of percutaneous reduction and instrumentation techniques may offer potential advantages as well [1, 2, 4, 7, 11, 12, 16]

Fractures of the Ankylosed Spine (AS/DISH)

Special considerations are warranted in fractures of ankylosed spines, such as in ankylosing spondylitis (AS) and diffuse idiopathic skeletal

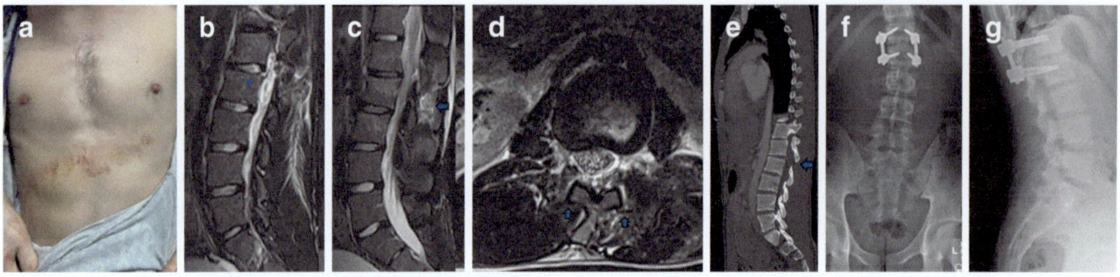

Fig. 10.2 18-year-old male involved in high-speed motor vehicle collision. Patient was restrained driver, presented to hospital with flexion distraction injury at L1–2 level. Figure (**a**) demonstrates abdominal ecchymoses with "seatbelt sign". Figures (**b** and **c**) show sagittal inverse recovery sequence images demonstrating L1–2 level injury involving the annulus of the disc (asterisk) and posterior ligamentous complex (arrow). Figure (**d**) demonstrates axial images at L1–2 with disruption of the facet capsules (arrows). Figure (**e**) shows a parasagittal CT image with L1–2 facet diastases/disruption (arrow). Imaging features were consistent with unstable flexion distraction injury (TLICS 7), and the patient was taken to the operating room for L1–2 open reduction and PSIF. Figures (**f** and **g**) are upright post-operative films

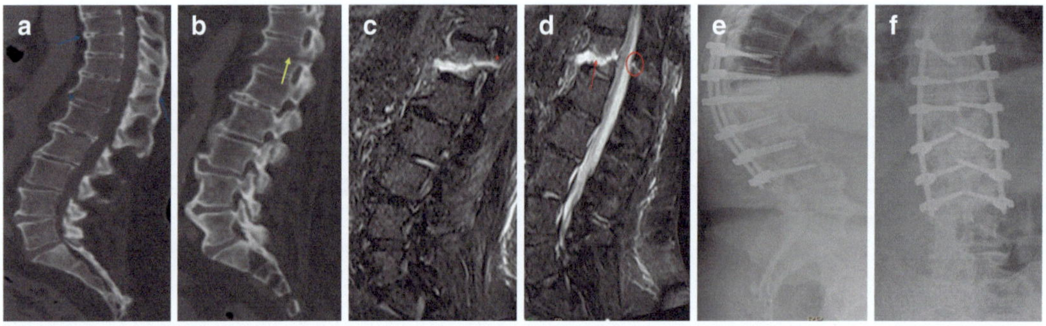

Fig. 10.3 71-year-old male with unstable 3-column injury at T12-L1 after a ground-level fall in the setting of an ankylosed spinal column. Figure (**a**) shows a mid-sagittal CT scan demonstrating a fracture through the T12 vertebral body with distraction of the fracture anteriorly (blue asterisk) and extensive ankylosis (blue arrows) consistent with ankylosing spondylitis. Figure (**b**) is a parasagittal CT image showing extension of the T12 fracture through all 3 columns (yellow arrow). Figures (**c** and **d**) show sagittal STIR MR images with injury involvement of the T12 pedicle (red asterisk), T12 vertebral body (red arrow), and extending into the posterior elements across an ossified ligamentum flavum (red circle). Figures (**e** and **f**) show AP and lateral post-operative radiographs, respectively, following T10-L3 PSIF

hyperostosis (DISH). Both conditions render patients more susceptible to fracture, even after low-energy mechanisms. Characteristically, fractures associated with AS and DISH are both extremely unstable, have a high propensity for hematoma formation, and are at high risk for radiographic underappreciation and late neurologic decline in the absence of treatment. Advanced imaging such as CT or MRI is required to identify injuries in these groups as findings may otherwise be subtle. 3-column fractures in the ankylosed spine nearly always necessitate surgical stabilization and possibly direct decompression (Fig. 10.3) [17, 18]. Fusion constructs in these patients typically involve instrumentation two or three levels above and below the injury.

Complications/Complication Management

Wound Complications [4, 8, 19]

Lumbar traumatic injuries treated surgically may be at a higher risk for post-operative spinal infections. Wound complications range from superficial dehiscence with or without associated superficial infection/hematoma to deeper fascial dehiscence and infection. The occurrence of a traumatic Morel-Lavalée lesion in association with spinal trauma, in which there is an internal degloving injury separating the fascia from the subcutaneous tissue, may be a harbinger of post-operative infection [19]. More superficial or benign post-operative wound infections can be treated with local wound care, oral antibiotics, and healing by secondary intention. Laboratory studies are useful in the identification of infection, in particular the identification of an elevated white blood cell count (WBC), erythrocyte sedimentation rate (ESR), and C-reactive protein (CRP). The CRP is considered the most sensitive indicator of infection and can also be used serially to evaluate the resolution of the infection over time. MRI can be used to assist in detection of novel or post-operative infection and, with contrast, identify the presence of discitis or epidural abscess formation. Patients with a confirmed deep infection typically require formal irrigation and debridement and often prolonged intravenous antibiotic therapy. Post-operative hematoma can often be allowed to resorb over time unless it is causing neurologic compromise or has become infected.

Loss of Fixation [4, 8, 15, 16]

Patients with poor bone quality and/or shorter constructs are at higher risk for loss of fixation. Rates are highly variable, ranging from 5% to 20% in most studies depending on factors such as patient comorbidities, surgical techniques, and biomechanical demands on the construct. When junctional failure occurs at the proximal aspect of the construct, revision is indicated to restore stability and prevent kyphotic collapse. This may be done through a combination of cement augmentation, supplemental points of fixation, or posterior tension band application. Anterior column support may be also be beneficial in some instances to relieve stress on posterior spinal instrumentation and allow for load sharing.

Durotomy [1, 2, 4, 8, 11, 12, 15, 16]

Reported rates of dural tear during a posterior-based decompressive operation range from 1% to 10%. When small and accessible, these can be repaired with direct suture closure intra-operatively. Large dural tears that are deemed irreparable are typically treated with a dural matrix substitute and often a drain for controlled CSF diversion. While dural tears may slow initiation of post-operative rehabilitation due to a 24–48-hour period of bedrest precautions, overall outcomes appear not to be significantly affected. The presence of a thoracolumbar burst fracture with a simultaneous laminar fracture is an increased risk of fracture for durotomy because of the traumatic injury.

Neurological Injury [4, 8, 15, 16]

Neurologic injury is a rare but serious complication of any spinal surgical intervention. It can occur intra-operatively due to aberrant screw placement, inadvertent injury during decompression, or infrequently from a post-operative hematoma formation. A thorough pre-operative neurologic assessment and documentation are necessary to accurately assess possible changes in function. Although the data are sparse, many surgeons opt for the use of neuromonitoring, which provides real-time information on neurologic status and allows for intra-operative interventions should possible neurologic injury be detected. Stepwise interventions include ensuring accuracy of the neuromonitoring, raising the mean arterial pressure, reversing intra-operative correction, and at a last resort performing the Stagnara wake-up test.

Pseudarthrosis [1–3, 9, 11, 14–16, 21]

Pseudoarthrosis rates in the literature range from 5% to 20%. Asymptomatic pseudoarthrosis may be managed conservatively with radiographic surveillance. Patients with refractory pain, or with evidence of instability in the setting of pseudoarthrosis, are indicated for revision fusion. A variety of strategies for revision of pseudarthrosis exist. These include increasing construct stability through larger/stronger anchors, additional levels of instrumentation, load-sharing with use of interbodies for anterior column support, and improved local biology with use of autologous iliac crest graft or osteobiologic agents.

Adjacent Segment Degeneration [4, 8, 15, 16, 21]

Long segment fusion alters the biomechanics of the spine by creating longer lever arms, imparting additional strain on the levels adjacent to the construct, and accelerating the degenerative process at these levels. The cumulative incidence increases in the years after surgery. Various studies demonstrate a range of 5–25% at 10 years after surgery in patients who underwent lumbar fusion [21]. Radiographs may demonstrate ASD in a significant number of patients, but only a small subset of patients are symptomatic and require further intervention.

Outcomes

Clinical and surgical outcomes following trauma to the lumbar spine are variable and dependent on the severity of the initial injury, comorbid medical conditions, and subsequent treatment. In general, both operative and non-operative management can be successful. In a systematic review, patients with burst fractures treated non-operatively or with posterior instrumentation were pain-free at final follow-up at rates of 26% and 45%, respectively [24]. That said, other studies demonstrate that the majority of patients treated either operatively or non-operatively do not have pain 2–7 years after injury, and 83% return to work full-time [22]. The majority of patients without neurologic injury can typically resume high-impact exercise at 1 year out from surgery [22]. Other studies demonstrate similar patient-reported outcome measures between operative and non-operative treatment, with neurologic impairment being a predictor of worse outcomes, and improved neurologic recovery with operative intervention [23]. As demonstrated above, the clinical and surgical outcomes of lumbar spine trauma vary significantly based on factors such as the nature of the injury (e.g., fracture type, neurological involvement), the timing and method of treatment, and patient-specific variables like age, comorbidities, and bone health. It is critical to take an individualized yet evidence-based approach to provide patients the best possible outcome.

Bibliography

1. Aligizakis A, Katonis P, Stergiopoulos K, Galanakis I, Karabekios S, Hadjipavlou A. Functional outcome of burst fractures of the thoracolumbar spine managed non-operatively, with early ambulation, evaluated using the load sharing classification. Acta Orthop Belg. 2002;68(3):279–87.
2. Avanzi O, Landim E, Meves R, Caffaro MF, Luyten FDAA, Faria AA. Thoracolumbar burst fracture: load sharing classification and posterior instrumentation failure. Revista Brasileira de Ortopedia (English Edition). 2010;45(3):236–40.
3. Diaz JJ Jr, Cullinane DC, Altman DT, Bokhari F, Cheng JS, Como J, et al. Practice management guidelines for the screening of thoracolumbar spine fracture. J Trauma. 2007;63(3):709–18.
4. Ghobrial GM, Maulucci CM, Maltenfort M, Dalyai RT, Vaccaro AR, Fehlings MG, et al. Operative and nonoperative adverse events in the management of traumatic fractures of the thoracolumbar spine: a systematic review. Neurosurg Focus. 2014;37(1):E8.
5. Gray L, Vandemark R, Hays M. Thoracic and lumbar spine trauma. Semin Ultrasound CT MRI. 2001;22(2):125–34. WB Saunders.
6. Hirsch BP, Sossamon J, Khan MA, Reitman C, Lawrence JP, Glaser J, et al. Applications of SPECT/CT in the evaluation of spinal pathology: a review. Int J Spine Surg. 2024;18(1):9–23.
7. Jun DS, An BK, Yu CH, Hwang KH, Paik JW. Practical use of bone scan in patients with an osteoporotic vertebral compression fracture. J Korean Med Sci. 2015;30(2):194–8.

8. Katsuura Y, Osborn JM, Cason GW. The epidemiology of thoracolumbar trauma: a meta-analysis. J Orthop. 2016;13(4):383–8.
9. Kepler CK, Vaccaro AR, Koerner JD, Dvorak MF, Kandziora F, Rajasekaran S, Aarabi B, Vialle LR, Fehlings MG, Schroeder GD, Reinhold M, Schnake KJ, Bellabarba C, Oner FC. Reliability analysis of the AOSpine thoracolumbar spine injury classification system by a worldwide group of naive spinal surgeons. Eur Spine J. 2015;25:1082.
10. Kool DR, Blickman JG. Advanced trauma life support®. ABCDE from a radiological point of view. Emerg Radiol. 2007;14:135–41.
11. Lee JY, Vaccaro AR, Lim MR, Öner FC, Hulbert RJ, Hedlund R, et al. Thoracolumbar injury classification and severity score: a new paradigm for the treatment of thoracolumbar spine trauma. J Orthop Sci. 2005;10:671–5.
12. Parker JW, Lane JR, Karaikovic EE, Gaines RW. Successful short- segment instrumentation and fusion for thoracolumbar spine fractures: a consecutive 4½-year series. Spine. 2000;25(9):1157–70.
13. Vaccaro A, Kandziora F, Fehlings M, Shanmughanathan R. Thoracic and lumbar trauma. AO Surgery Reference. n.d.. https://surgeryreference.aofoundation.org/spine/trauma/thoracolumbar.
14. Vaccaro AR, Oner C, Kepler CK, Dvorak M, Schnake K, Bellabarba C, Reinhold M, Aarabi B, Kandziora F, Chapman J, Shanmuganathan R, Fehlings M, Vialle L, AOSpine Knowledge Forum Trauma. AOSpine thoracolumbar spine injury classification system: fracture description, neurological status, and key modifiers. Spine (Phila Pa 1976). 2013;38(23):2028–37.
15. Waddell WH, Gupta R, Stephens BF. Thoracolumbar spine trauma. Orthop Clin North Am. 2021;52(4):481–9.
16. Wood KB, Li W, Lebl DS, Ploumis A. Management of thoracolumbar spine fractures. Spine J. 2014;14(1):145–64.
17. Harlianto NI, Ezzafzafi S, Foppen W, Kuperus JS, van der Horst-Bruinsma IE, de Jong PA, Verlaan JJ. The prevalence of vertebral fractures in diffuse idiopathic skeletal hyperostosis and ankylosing spondylitis: a systematic review and meta-analysis. N Am Spine Soc J. 2024;17:100312. https://doi.org/10.1016/j.xnsj.2024.100312.
18. Cabrera A, Bouterse A, Nelson M, Dietrich C, Razzouk J, Oyoyo U, Bono CM, Danisa O. Prediction of in-hospital mortality following vertebral fracture fixation in patients with ankylosing spondylitis or diffuse idiopathic skeletal hyperostosis: machine learning analysis. Int J Spine Surg. 2024;18(1):62–8. https://doi.org/10.14444/8567.
19. Mulcahy MJ, Ball JR. The Morel-Lavallée lesion in thoracolumbar spine trauma-two index cases. J Spine Surg (Hong Kong). 2018;4(3):654–7. https://doi.org/10.21037/jss.2018.06.20.
20. American College of Surgeons. About advanced trauma life support. ACS. n.d.. https://www.facs.org/quality-programs/trauma/education/advanced-trauma-life-support/about/.
21. Radcliff KE, Kepler CK, Jakoi A, Sidhu GS, Rihn J, Vaccaro AR, Albert TJ, Hilibrand AS. Adjacent segment disease in the lumbar spine following different treatment interventions. The Spine J. 2013;13(10):1339–49. https://doi.org/10.1016/j.spinee.2013.03.020.
22. Marek AP, Morancy JD, Chipman JG, Nygaard RM, Roach RM, Loor MM. Long-term functional outcomes after traumatic thoracic and lumbar spine fractures. Am Surg. 2018;84(1):20–7.
23. Stadhouder A, Buskens E, de Klerk LW, Verhaar JA, Dhert WA, Verbout AJ, Vaccaro R, Oner FC. Traumatic thoracic and lumbar spinal fractures: operative or nonoperative treatment: comparison of two treatment strategies by means of surgeon equipoise. Spine. 2008;33(9):1006–17. https://doi.org/10.1097/BRS.0b013e31816c8b32.
24. Schouten R, Lewkonia P, Noonan VK, Dvorak MF, Fisher CG. Expectations of recovery and functional outcomes following thoracolumbar trauma: an evidence-based medicine process to determine what surgeons should be telling their patients. J Neurosurg Spine. 2015;22(1):101–11. https://doi.org/10.3171/2014.9.SPINE13849.

Sacral Trauma

11

Kyle J. Holmberg, Michael T. Quinet, and John C. France

Introduction

Sacral fractures are often discussed as a component of pelvic ring fractures and are thus under the purview of the Orthopedic traumatologist. This is certainly true of the anteroposterior and lateral compression type fractures; thus, those variants will not be discussed in this chapter. The vertical shear type fracture also has traditionally been cared for by the traumatologist but in recent years the use of spinopelvic fixation has taken on a greater role and will be included here. Otherwise, our focus will be on the transverse and sacral-U or sacral-H patterns. The latter can be managed by a combination of trauma and spine surgeons.

There are two populations of patients typically affected by sacral fractures: first are the high-energy fractures seen in trauma patients and second are the low-energy, insufficiency fractures that tend to occur in the elderly with poor bone quality. These two groups are treated differently, and those differences will be highlighted in this chapter. In addition to these two groups, decision-making for treatment and treatment techniques are dictated by: the amount of fracture displacement or angulation (especially kyphosis), the presence of neurological injury, the need for mobilization, and the status of the soft tissue envelope.

Anatomy and Biomechanics

The sacrum is made up of five vertebral bones at the lowest functional portion of the spinal column and forms the only connection between the spinal column and pelvis. The sacrum functions to protect the caudal nerve roots and serves to provide stability and motion segments for the lower spine and pelvis. Motion occurs through the L5/S1 disc, the bilateral facet joints, and the articulation between the sacrum and iliac bones [1]. The upper sacral vertebrae (S1/S2) are similar in size and shape to the lumbar vertebrae, although several anatomic variants exist as in sacral dysmorphism, whereas the lower three segments are smaller in size and do not contribute significantly to spinopelvic stability [2]. The S1 vertebral body represents the largest portion of the sacrum and possesses the greatest proportion of cancellous bone. The bilateral sacral ala which forms the lateral-most portions of the sacrum have relatively less cancellous bone predisposing this area to insufficiency fractures in patients with poor bone quality [3]. Anatomic variability, bone quality, and density all play a role in treatment considerations when treating patients with sacral fractures.

K. J. Holmberg (✉) · M. T. Quinet · J. C. France
West Virginia University Department of Orthopaedic Surgery, Morgantown, WV, USA
e-mail: jfrance@hsc.wvu.edu

A. A. Baaj et al. (eds.), *Surgery of the Lumbar Spine*, https://doi.org/10.1007/978-3-032-18097-1_11

Classification

Historically, there have been many classifications used to describe sacral fractures. While many of them provide helpful information in describing sacral trauma, for our purposes we will focus on those we find most helpful in describing injury patterns and guiding treatment. The Denis classification in 1988 was the first widely adopted and continues to have utility today. It was based on a study which included 236 patients with sacral fracture and divided the sacrum into 3 zones: zone 1 lateral to the neuroforamen, zone 2 through the neuroforamen, and zone 3 through the central canal [4]. As one moves from zone 1 to 3 the risk of neurological injury increases. The incidence of neurological injury for zone 1 was 5.9% and was usually an L5 root entrapped in the fracture as it transverses over the anterior brim of the sacral ala. The incidence for zone 2 was reported as 28.4% as was usually injury of nerve roots as they pass through the corresponding foramen or the L5 root as it exits the L5-S1 foramen and moves out past the transverse process.

Finally, the incidence for zone 3 fractures was 56.7% with the injury occurring within the spinal canal and frequently creating bladder and/or bowel dysfunction [5]. It was recognized that the zone 3 fractures could take on various patterns including pure transverse fractures and those that include either unilateral or bilateral vertical fracture lines such as those of the sacral-U and sacral-H variety. Gibbons et al. looked specifically at the neurological injury associated with fractures within the Denis classification and categorized the neurological injuries into groups as follows: (1) No neurological injury, (2) Sensory paresthesia or dysesthesia only, (3) Motor deficit included without bladder/bowel dysfunction, and (4) those with bladder and/or bowel dysfunction [5]. These neurological injuries often act as drivers toward surgical intervention and are dependent of the level of transverse sacral component with fractures below S4 rarely sustaining neurological injury.

Pure transverse fractures are relatively uncommon, and most transverse fractures have vertical components and are thus considered "U", "H", "Y", or lambda patterns. The pure transverse fractures are below S2 and thus have no significant effect on pelvic ring stability nor lower extremity motor function but can result in bladder bowel dysfunction if occurring between S2 and S4 [6]. Roy Camille et al. devised a classification of transverse fractures that was based on the displacement pattern. Type 1 was a pure flexion or angulation only, type 2 was angulation with posterior displacement of the cephalad sacrum on the caudal end, and type 3 was anterior displacement of the cephalad segment on the caudal section generally without angulation but can have shortening to the sacrum [7]. For the vertical sacral fractures typical of the vertical shear pelvic ring fracture there can be impact on the spinal column and Isler et al. subclassified these injuries based on the fracture line relative to the L5-S1 facet. Type 1 exited lateral to the facet and did not affect spinal stability even though it is common to see an associated L5 transverse process fracture. Type 2 goes through and disrupts the facet potentially creating a spinal instability issue. Type 3 exits medial to the facet and can create difficulties with closed reduction. All 3 of these patterns tend to be part of a more global pelvic ring fracture [8]. The role of the spine surgeon is often to add spinopelvic fixation to supplement the reduction and stability achieved by the trauma surgeons.

The most recent effort at classification is the AO classification (See Fig. 11.1). Like other AO spine trauma classifications, it includes the pattern of fracture with corresponding instability, the neurological injury, and associated injuries that might influence treatment decisions. It should be used in conjunction with the AO pelvic trauma classification as there is great overlap. Type A are transverse fractures below the sacroiliac joint and as a result don't affect pelvic ring stability. These can be simple coccygeal fractures, nondisplaced or significantly displaced fractures. Type B are vertical patterns that disrupt the pelvic ring but does not create spinopelvic instability. Type C fractures are those that affect the spinopelvic relationship and can cause spino-

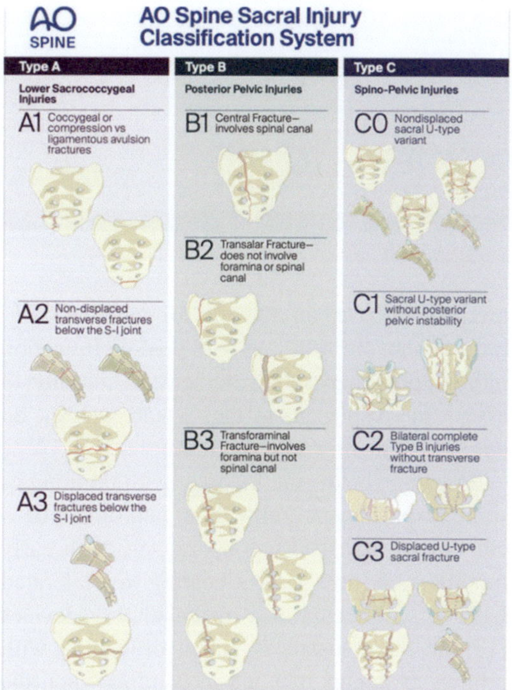

Fig. 11.1 Acknowledgement of AO Spine and the Knowledge Forums' work "The AO Spine Injury Classification Systems were developed and funded by AO Spine through the AO Spine Knowledge Forum Trauma, a focused group of international spine trauma experts. AO Spine is a clinical division of the AO Foundation, which is an independent medically guided not-for-profit organization. Study support was provided directly through AO Network Clinical Research and AO ITC, Clinical Evidence." Link: https://www.aofoundation.org/spine/clinical-library-and-tools/aospine-classification-systems

pelvic instability but do not disrupt the pelvic ring. Each group is subdivided per the illustration. The neurological component is NX unexaminable, N0 no deficit, N1 transient deficit, N2 root injury, or N3 cauda equina injury (complete or incomplete). There are 4 modifiers: M1 soft tissue injury such as open fracture or internal degloving (Morel-Lavalle), M2 metabolic bone disease such as in sacral insufficiency fractures in osteoporotic patients, M3 the inclusion of an anterior pelvic ring or acetabular injury, and M4 sacroiliac joint injury [9–14].

Finally, one must remember to consider the classifications considering the energy imparted upon the sacrum and divided the injuries into high-energy trauma that can occur despite good bone quality and those of low energy that only occur when the bone quality is significantly impaired.

Examination and Imaging

The initial evaluation of sacral fractures should include the basic ATLS assessment as the high-energy patient frequently has associated injuries. Consultation with other surgical specialists must be considered in the polytraumatized patient to determine which injuries should be addressed first based on severity and the patient's need for resuscitation. The low-energy patients require an assessment of risk factors for osteoporosis, their preinjury ambulatory status, and a thorough evaluation of comorbidities and potential medications that can affect treatment. A careful history and physical examination should be obtained with attention to neurologic function in the case of high-energy injuries. The soft tissue envelope should be thoroughly examined for open wounds; this includes the potential for rectal or vaginal injury. More frequently, the soft tissue injury is an internal degloving (Morel-Lavelle) injury and these can lead to skin necrosis or secondary infection and pose wound healing complications if surgical treatment is considered.

High-energy injury patients undergoing an ATLS assessment at trauma centers frequently undergo CT scans of the chest, abdomen, and pelvis as part of their initial imaging workup. CT scans have a sensitivity of approximately 94% in identifying sacral fractures which can be helpful in early diagnosis and treatment of these injuries. Dedicated 3D reconstruction images of the spine and pelvis can improve visualization of bony detail of the fracture characteristics which can aid in pre-operative planning or help guide treatment. In the low-energy injury patient often presenting in the ambulatory setting with complaints of low back or pelvic pain, dedicated CT scans are not always available for review. There can be an inciting event such as fall from standing but often there is no known inciting event, in this case the initial imaging study is often pelvic or lumbar spine radiographs obtained in the office.

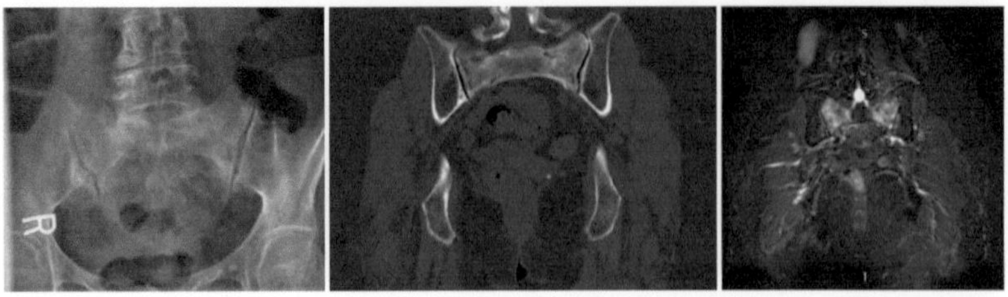

Fig. 11.2 Radiograph, CT, and MRI demonstrating a bilateral sacral insufficiency fracture in a 63-year-old female who presented with low back pain after a low-energy injury

Sacral insufficiency fractures can be challenging to identify on plain radiographs due to patient positioning and body habitus. When radiographs are indeterminant and there is a high index of suspicion for a sacral insufficiency fracture, advanced imaging may be considered. In a study of 77 patients magnetic resonance imaging (MRI) has a sensitivity of 100% in identifying sacral insufficiency fractures, compared to 94.2% in CT scans, and 28.5% on plain radiographs which included anteroposterior and lateral views of the pelvis [15]. Therefore, MRI or CT may be valuable tools in the ambulatory setting for diagnosing these injuries, with MRI being the preferred diagnostic imaging for the identification of sacral insufficiency fractures and CT being a secondary study to characterize the bony pattern. MRI excels in identifying signal change indicative of subtle edema in the bone which results from sacral insufficiency fractures (See Fig. 11.2). These patients often present with an MRI scan already obtained due to the complaint being "low back pain" [16].

Nonoperative Treatment

The goals for non-surgical treatment of sacral trauma emphasize multimodal pain control and early mobilization with or without the use of ambulatory aids. In patients who fail to mobilize, preventing medical comorbid conditions that result from prolonged immobilization such as thromboembolic events, pulmonary decline, decubiti, and ileus due to pain or narcotic use are paramount. Non-operative treatment is typically reserved only for non- or minimally displaced fractures in the *high-energy* patient population and consists of mobilization with weight-bearing precautions based on concerns for potential instability. These are followed with post-mobilization radiographs, then serial radiographs initially to assess for displacement that would warrant an upgrade of treatment to surgical.

Fractures below the S2 body with minimal or some displacement, but without neurologic deficit, can be managed non-operatively with early mobilization and weight-bearing as tolerated with or without the use of ambulatory devices [17]. In these instances, sacral offloading with pillows or donuts may aid in comfort when the patient is recumbent. Whereas most *sacral insufficiency* fractures are amenable to non-operative management as long as the patient is able to maintain their preinjury ambulation status. Serial radiographs and close clinical follow-up should be obtained to monitor for instability or deformity that may develop as a sequela of non-operative management.

Operative Treatment

Operative treatment of *high-energy* sacral fractures is indicated in open fractures, displaced or unstable vertical shear pelvic fractures, cases of spinopelvic instability such as the sacral U or H type fracture, and in cases of neurologic deficit [18]. For *insufficiency fractures* initial operative fixation is reserved for those patients that will mobilize despite significant efforts, kyphotic deformity effecting spinopelvic alignment, and those with bladder/bowel dysfunction [19]. The goals of early surgical treatment are to address neurologic compression, stabilize the spine and/or pelvis, and restore alignment. Delayed surgical treatment may be indicated in the cases of progressive deformity, typically in kyphosis, which alter the pelvic incidence and thus spinopelvic alignment. This would be true of either high-energy or insufficiency fractures that were initially treated nonoperatively. In cases of soft tissue compromise, such as in open fractures, or Morel-LaValle lesions, or skin breakdown resulting from fracture displacement open debridement may be indicated.

Surgical Technique

If the sacral fracture is displaced there are a variety of techniques which can be utilized to achieve reduction and fixation including transiliac-transsacral fixation of the sacrum, lumbopelvic fixation, or both depending on the injury pattern [20]. Because the soft tissue envelope is often compromised an effort should be made to minimize open incisions. To achieve a closed reduction of the sacrum the patient may be positioned prone with the hips extended using bumps or blankets in order to counteract the kyphotic deformity of the sacral fracture [18] (See Fig. 11.3). If available a bed that breaks into extension such as the Proaxis table may be used. Schanz pins can be placed into the iliac wings and used to lever the pelvis with the caudal sacral component further into extension to match the cephalad alignment. In some instances, traction may be required to dis-impact the sacral vertebrae and can be applied with bilateral distal femoral traction pins. Intraoperative fluoroscopy can aid in assessing fracture reduction. If the fracture is unable to be reduced in a closed fashion, then open techniques involve a short midline incision with exposure of the sacral lamina and posterior elements. A laminectomy can be performed then a cobb, bone hook, or other tools can be inserted past the sacral root into the vertebral fracture and exert more direct leverage to aid reduction.

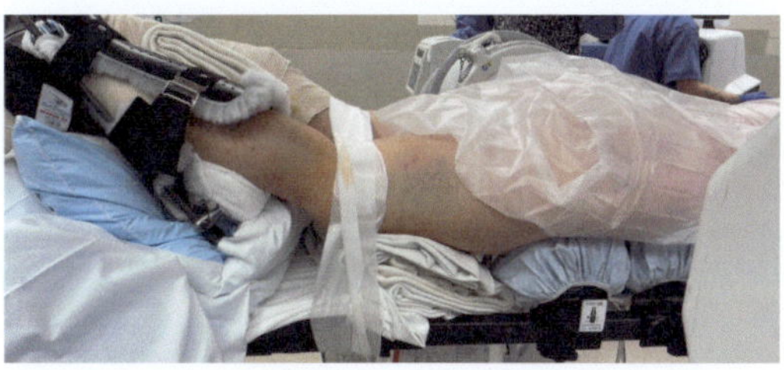

Fig. 11.3 A patient with a displaced sacral U-type fracture positioned prone with blankets under the thighs to hyperextend the hips thus aiding in fracture reduction

Lumbopelvic *fixation* is often the treatment of choice for sacral U or H-type fractures and is useful in vertical shear fracture neutralization. Lumbopelvic fixation involves placing pedicle screws at L5, and/or L4 with bilateral iliac bolts or screw constructs [21]. This allows for immediate stability of the lumbopelvic junction and thus can allow early weight bearing and mobilization. Lumbopelvic fixation can be performed in conjunction with a fusion if indicated, or as a means of internal fixation which can be removed later after the fracture is healed. This can be performed in conjunction with transiliac-transsacral fixation to complete triangular fixation either completely in the prone position or in a staged fashion, positioning the patient supine for the transiliac-transsacral fixation and then prone for the lumbopelvic fixation if the fracture is associated with anterior pelvic ring fractures requiring fixation [22]. If no transiliac-transsacral screw is required, the S1 can be utilized for the spinopelvic fixation (otherwise the corridor through S1 may be obstructed) [23]. Our preference is to place percutaneous guide pins for all the screws then place the transiliac-transsacral screw to provide the best visualization of landmarks followed by the spinopelvic screws and rods.

If decompression is warranted due to bladder/bowel dysfunction, the laminectomy is used for this purpose. Also this allows access to the anterior aspect of the sacrum and fracture fragments then using a tamp or angled instrument on the apex of the kyphosis it can be impacted forward to remove the pressure exerted on the nerves [24] (See Fig. 11.4). This can also be utilized to hold the fracture reduced while internal fixation is applied. If the sagittal alignment and anterior-posterior displacement are anatomically aligned then satisfactory decompression may indirectly be accomplished without laminectomy.

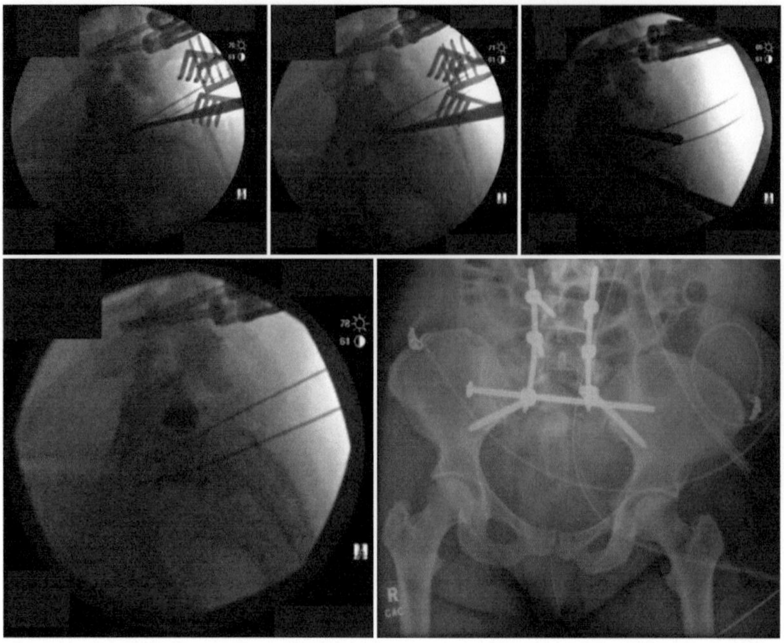

Fig. 11.4 Open reduction and internal fixation of the sacrum with lumbo-pelvic fixation for a displaced sacral U-type fracture. A laminectomy was performed, and working through the fracture site, an instrument was used to reduce the displaced sacral fracture. Once the reduction was achieved, the fracture was fixed using a trans-iliac-trans sacral screw via the S1 corridor

Summary

Sacral fractures present a challenging problem for the orthopedic and spine surgeon. In the case of insufficiency fractures, low back pain is ubiquitous in this same patient population and presents with a wide differential diagnosis. Thus, a high index of suspicion should be maintained when treating patients who are at risk for insufficiency fractures and presenting with low back pain. Advanced imaging such as MRI should be utilized when indicated due to its high sensitivity for identifying subtle edema which may be present in sacral insufficiency fractures.

While the high-energy trauma patient presenting to a trauma center often undergoes advanced imaging as part of their initial workup, these radiographic studies should be scrutinized so as not to miss a potentially devastating injury. They are often multiply injured and must be treated in the context of the overall injury burden and prioritized accordingly.

References

1. Williams PL, Warwick R, Dyson M, et al., editors. Gray's anatomy. New York: Churchill Livingstone; 1989.
2. Williams P, Warwick R, Dyson M, et al. Gray's anatomy. 37th ed. Edinburgh: Churchill Livingstone; 1989.
3. Morris H. In: Lond MB, editor. Human anatomy. Philadelphia: P. Blakiston's Son & Co; 1989.
4. Denis F. Sacral fractures. An important problem—a retrospective analysis of 236 cases. Clin Orthop. 1988;227:67–81.
5. Gibbons KJ, Soloniuk DS, Razack N. Neurological injury and patterns of sacral fractures. J Neurosurg. 1990;72:889–93.
6. Fountain SS, Hamilton RD, Jameson RM. Transverse fractures of the sacrum: a report of six cases. J Bone Joint Surg Am. 1977;59:486–9.
7. Roy-Camille R, Saillant G, Gogna G, Mazel C. Transverse fracture of the upper sacrum: suicidal jumper's fracture. Spine. 1985;10:838–45.
8. Isler B. Lumbosacral lesions associated with pelvic ring injuries. J Orthop Trauma. 1990;4:1–6.
9. Vaccaro AR, Schroeder GD, Divi SN, et al. Description and reliability of the AOSpine sacral

classification system. J Bone Joint Surg Am. 2020;102(16):1454–63. https://doi.org/10.2106/JBJS.19.01153.
10. Vaccaro AR, Schroeder GD, Divi SN, Kepler CK, Kleweno CP, Krieg JC, Wilson JR, Holstein JH, Kurd MF, Firoozabadi R, Vialle LR, Oner FC, Kandziora F, Chapman JR, Schnake KJ, Benneker LM, Dvorak MF, Rajasekaran S, Vialle EN, Joaquim AF, El-Sharkawi MM, Dhakal GR, Popescu EC, Kanna RM, Muijs SPJ, Tee JW, Bellabarba C. Description and reliability of the AOSpine sacral classification system. JBJS. 102(16):2020.
11. Schroeder GD, Karamian BA, Canseco JA, Vialle LR, Kandziora F, Benneker LM, Rajasekaran S, Holstein JH, Schnake KJ, Kurd MF, Dvorak MF, Vialle EN, Joaquim AF, Kanna RM, Fehlings M, Wilson JR, Chapman JR, Krieg JC, Kleweno CP, Firoozabadi R, Öner FC, Kepler CK, Vaccaro AR. Validation of the AO spine sacral classification system: reliability among surgeons worldwide. J Orthop Trauma. 2021;35(12):e496–501. https://doi.org/10.1097/BOT.0000000000002110. PMID: 34387567; PMCID: PMC8788941.
12. Karamian BA, Schroeder GD, Lambrechts MJ, Canseco JA, Vialle EN, Kandziora F, Benneker LM, Shanmuganathan R, Öner FC, Schnake KJ, Kepler CK, Vaccaro AR, AO Spine Sacral Classification Group Members. Validation of the hierarchical nature of the AO spine sacral classification and the development of the sacral AO spine injury score. Clin Spine Surg. 2023;36(6):E239–46. https://doi.org/10.1097/BSD.0000000000001437. Epub 2023 Mar 3.PMID: 36864585; PMCID: PMC10284127.
13. Karamian BA, Schroeder GD, Lambrechts MJ, Canseco JA, AO Spine Sacral Classification Group Members, Vialle EN, Rajasekaran S, Benneker LM, Dvorak MR, Kandziora F, Oner C, Schnake K, Kepler CK, Vaccaro AR. The influence of regional differences on the reliability of the AO spine sacral injury classification system. Glob Spine J. 2023;13(7):2025–32. https://doi.org/10.1177/21925682211068419. Epub 2022 Jan 8. PMID: 35000410; PMCID: PMC10556908.
14. Lee Y, Lambrechts M, Narayanan R, Bransford R, Benneker L, Schnake K, Öner C, Canseco JA, Kepler CK, Schroeder GD, Vaccaro AR, AO Spine Sacral Classification Group Members. The surgical algorithm for the AO spine sacral injury classification system. Spine (Phila Pa 1976). 2024;49(3):165–73. https://doi.org/10.1097/BRS.0000000000004876. Epub 2023 Nov 16. PMID: 37970681.
15. Yamauchi T, Sharma S, Chandra S, et al. Superiority of MRI for evaluation of sacral insufficiency fracture. J Clin Med. 2022;11(17) https://doi.org/10.3390/jcm11174968.
16. Graul I, Vogt S, Strube P, Holzl A. Significance of lumbar MRI in diagnosis of sacral insufficiency fracture. Glob Spine J. 2021;11(8):1197–201. https://doi.org/10.1177/2192568220941821.
17. Shin CP, Mascarenhas LD, Holderread BM, Awad M, Botros D, Avramis I, Syed I, Rizkalla JM. Treatment for sacral insufficiency fractures: a systematic review. J Orthop. 2022;34:116–22. https://doi.org/10.1016/j.jor.2022.08.021. PMID: 36060729; PMCID: PMC9433979.
18. Kellam JF, McMurtry RY, Paley D, Tile M. The unstable pelvic fracture: operative treatment. Orthop Clin North Am. 1987;18:25–41.
19. Jacquot JM, Finiels H, Fardjad S, et al. Neurological complications in insufficiency fractures of the sacrum: three case reports. Rev Rhum Engl Ed. 1999;66:109–13.
20. Routt ML Jr, Simonian PT. Closed reduction and percutaneous skeletal fixation of sacral fractures. Clin Orthop. 1996;329:121–8.
21. Gotis-Graham I, McGuigan L, Diamond T, et al. Sacral insufficiency fractures in the elderly. J Bone Joint Surg Br. 1994;76:882–6.
22. Bellabarba C, Bransford RJ. Spinopelvic fixation. In: Vialle LR, Bellabarba C, Kandziora F, editors. AOSpine Masters Series. Vol 6: Thoracolumbar spine trauma. New York: Thieme; 2016. p. 152–83.
23. Routt MLC, Simonian PT, Swiontkowski MF. Stabilization of pelvic ring disruptions. Orthop Clin North Am. 1997;28:369–88.
24. Schildhauer TA, Bellabarba C, Nork SE, et al. Decompression and lumbopelvic fixation for sacral fracture-dislocations with spino-pelvic dissociation. J Orthop Trauma. 2006;20:447–57.

Lumbar Disc Herniations

12

Michael Prim

Introduction

One of the most common pathologies encountered by spine surgeons is lumbar disc herniation. The North American Spine Society defines lumbar disc herniation as "a localized displacement of disc material beyond the normal margins of the intervertebral disc space resulting in pain, weakness, or numbness in a myotomal or dermatomal distribution" [1]. It is estimated that up to 5.5% of the world's population has symptomatic disc herniations which accounts for approximately 400 million people [1]. Additionally, the prevalence appears to be increasing as the Medicare population continues to grow [2]. Given the widespread prevalence of this condition, it is crucial for spine surgeons to have a comprehensive understanding of lumbar disc herniations. In this chapter, we cover anatomy and pathophysiology, clinical presentations, diagnostic evaluations, management strategies, and prognosis (Fig. 12.1).

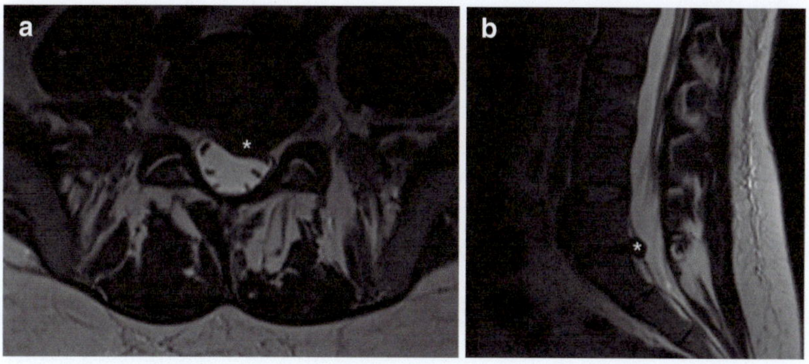

Fig. 12.1 (**a**) Axial T2-weighted MRI of focal lumbar disc herniation (white star), demonstrating compression of descending nerve roots. (**b**) Sagittal imaging of the same MRI showing the herniation outside the normal bounds of the vertebral bodies and displacement of the thecal sac and its contents

M. Prim (✉)
Department of Neurosurgery, Banner University Medical Center, University of Arizona College of Medicine, Phoenix, AZ, USA
e-mail: michael.prim@bannerhealth.com

A. A. Baaj et al. (eds.), *Surgery of the Lumbar Spine*, https://doi.org/10.1007/978-3-032-18097-1_12

Anatomy

The anatomy of the lumbar vertebrae and intervertebral discs provides the appropriate structure to carry large compressive forces while maintaining significant motion. The lumbar spine is composed of five large vertebrae, with wide bodies, whose primary function is to carry the compressive load of the body. They share this responsibility with the intervertebral disc (IVD), which also helps provide motion between lumbar segments. The IVD is composed of an inner gelatinous layer, the nucleus pulposus (NP), which is rich in proteoglycans, and an outer strength layer, the annulus fibrosus (AF), which is rich in collagen. The NP contains 70–90% water. This, combined with proteoglycans, provides hydraulic pressure to resist compression and maintains the proper spatial relationship between the facet joints [3]. The AF is a fibrous ring composed of highly organized lamellae, or concentric layers. There are approximately 15–25 lamellae per disc, and they are formed by strong, oblique collagen fibers. These fibers run about 30° relative to each vertebra it connects, and adjacent lamellae run in opposite directions. This arrangement limits rotational and bending forces between adjacent vertebrae. Of note, the lamellae are thinner in the posterior aspect of the annulus fibrosus [3].

There are other anatomical structures to consider when discussing the anatomy of an IVD. It is an avascular structure with only small arterioles supplying the most peripheral aspects of the AF. The central portion of the AF and the NP relies on the cartilaginous endplates (CEP) of the adjacent vertebral bodies to help maintain nourishment, deliver oxygen, and remove waste material [3]. The CEP is a collection of thin layers of hyaline cartilage. This binds to the underlying vertebral bodies and is a mechanical barrier between the bony surface and the IVD. Alterations or degenerative changes in the CEP can have significant effects on the IVD and lead to desiccation of the NP and central portion of the AF since they are farthest from a blood supply [3].

Pathophysiology

Many things can lead to lumbar disc degeneration and, ultimately, herniation. Some of the main risk factors that have been identified for lumbar disc herniation are repeated mechanical load/stress, traumatic injury, low nutrition supply, genetics, smoking, and obesity [3]. Patients who experience repeated mechanical stress, such as those in physically demanding jobs (e.g., construction workers, delivery personnel, assembly line workers, and even surgeons), have a higher incidence of lumbar disc herniations compared to the general population [4–6]. Additionally, the lumbar spine is a region of significant mobility and, therefore, is at risk for injury during traumatic events [7]. Traumatic disc herniations can be caused by motor vehicle accidents, falls, blunt abdominal/back injuries, or be associated with traumatic fractures of the motion segment involved [8]. These can also happen at times of significant or repeated axial loading such as weightlifting, moving furniture, jogging, or horseback riding, etc.

Other environmental factors that play a role are diabetes and smoking. Chronically elevated glucose levels lead to glycosylation of proteins, including glycans and collagen. This leads to dehydration of the NP and softening of the AF fibers, ultimately rendering the intervertebral disc inadequate [4]. A similar process happens with smoking. One study was able to demonstrate that mice exposed to smoke inhalation had decreased synthesis of proteoglycans. This, combined with the vasoconstrictive effects of smoking, in an area of low blood flow, makes it easy to conclude that smoking leads to increased risk of lumbar disc herniation [9]. Huang et al. performed a meta-analysis in 2015 and found that smokers have an overall Relative Risk of lumbar disc herniation at 1.27 (95% CI, 1.15–1.40).

Interestingly, despite the data suggesting the significant role of environmental factors, genetics likely play a key role as well. The Twin Spine Study by Battié et al. was a multicenter, multinational study aimed at further describing the pathogenesis of lumbar disc degeneration. This study was performed by interviewing and examining, including MRIs, 300 pairs of twins (147 monozygotic pairs and 153 dizygotic pairs). The twins were recruited from the Finnish Twin Cohort and were found to be representative of the general Finnish population. They concluded that disc degeneration was largely determined to be genetically influenced with environmental factors having modest effects [10].

Clinical Presentation

The way patients present with lumbar disc herniations can be varied. As with most spine pathologies, history and physical is key to establishing a correct diagnosis. It is more common in males by a factor of 2:1, and greater than 95% of disc herniations occur at L4/5 or L5/S1 [6]. The classic presentation of a lumbar disc herniation includes pain and numbness in the distribution of the affected nerve root as seen on imaging. Pain can be described as sharp or electric as well as dull or achy [7]. Both the exiting nerve root and/or the traversing nerve root can be compressed by a focal disc herniation. A broad or central disc herniation can cause compression of the entire thecal sac. This can lead to bilateral lower extremity complaints like previously mentioned such as pain, numbness, or tingling, or complaints of neurogenic claudication, which is typically described as a heavy sensation in both lower extremities after walking after a certain distance. It is important to distinguish neurogenic claudication from vascular claudication in patients with peripheral vascular disease. Severe acute compression of the thecal sac below L2 can lead to cauda equina syndrome (Fig. 12.2). Cauda equina is a spinal emergency. It is characterized by lower extremity weakness, unilateral or bilateral, saddle anesthesia, and urinary retention/incontinence. Patients who present with cauda equina require urgent decompression [7].

There are several things to evaluate on the physical examination. The patient may have decreased sensation or proprioception in unilateral or bilateral lower extremities. They could also have weakness with the appropriate myotome. Reflexes can be diminished as well. Specific maneuvers such as a straight leg raise can help localize the site of symptomatic compression. In fact, Petersen et al. performed a systematic review and were able to recommend a straight leg raise test in combination with the Hancock rule (3 positive findings out of the following: dermatomal pain in an appropriate distribution, a corresponding sensory deficit, motor weakness, and decreased reflexes) serve as excellent screening tools for lumbar disc herniation [11].

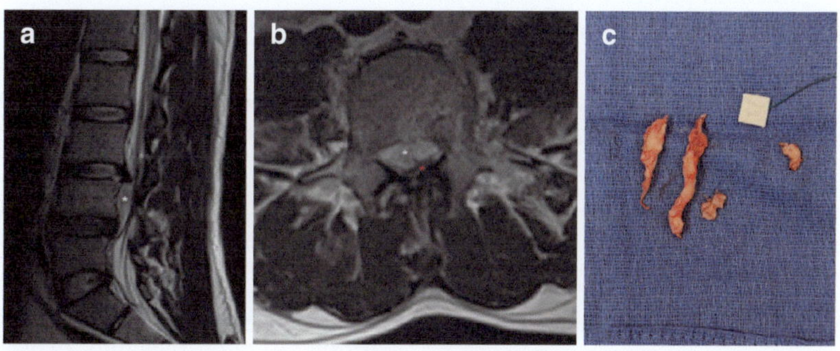

Fig. 12.2 (**a**) Sagittal T2-weighted MRI of a 37-year-old male after an auto vs pedestrian accident, which demonstrates a large traumatic disc herniation (white star). (**b**) Axial imaging demonstrating significant compression of the thecal sac (red star). The patient initially presented neurologically intact, but he had a rapid decline in his lower extremity motor exam and was taken for emergent intervention due to acute cauda equina syndrome. (**c**) Intraoperative photo of resected disc fragments

Diagnostic Evaluation

In addition to history and physical examination, multiple diagnostic studies can be obtained to make the diagnosis of a lumbar disc herniation. X-rays can demonstrate disc height loss, which may aid findings on history and physical but are not adequate for a diagnosis alone. In patients where lumbar disc herniation is suspected, an MRI is recommended as the most appropriate noninvasive test [1, 6, 12]. If an MRI cannot be obtained due to an implanted device or patient intolerance, a CT myelogram serves as a good secondary option [1]. A routine non-contrast CT scan can also be obtained, but they are not as sensitive as the previously mentioned modalities [6]. In addition to imaging, electrodiagnostic (EMG/NCS) studies can be obtained. They are typically not necessary but can be used to help find symptomatic levels in patients with multilevel disease or in patients with ambiguous symptoms [13].

This is a good time to remember to always consider other pathologies. The differential diagnosis for lumbar radiculopathy is large and includes many different categories. Other degenerative processes such as facet hypertrophy or spondylolisthesis can mimic lumbar disc herniations. Nerve root compression can be caused by oncologic processes such as schwannomas, myxopapillary ependymomas, neurofibromas, meningiomas, or even primary bone tumors such as chordomas. Infectious processes are common as well in the lumbar spine and could lead to an epidural abscess or significant destruction of the bony anatomy causing nerve root compression. One should also consider vascular (dural AV fistula), trauma (facet fracture), and even metabolic causes such as epidural lipomatosis.

Non-operative Treatment

Conservative/non-operative treatment of lumbar disc herniations is the first-line therapy. It is estimated that up to 90% of people with lumbar disc herniation will experience symptom resolution without surgical intervention [12, 13]. Nonsurgical options include pharmacotherapy, physical therapy/lumbar manipulation, and injection therapy. Pharmacotherapy should start with acetaminophen or nonsteroidal anti-inflammatory drugs (NSAIDS) as both have shown to be effective in treating low back pain caused by lumbar disc herniation without having to elevate to narcotic pain medication [12]. Other medications include gabapentin or pregabalin but their effectiveness in treating neuropathic pain from lumbar disc herniation is unknown [1]. Physical therapy/lumbar manipulation is also frequently recommended prior to surgical intervention. Some recent studies have found that back extension exercises, spinal decompression therapy, and core stabilization exercises have helped resolve patient's symptoms [12]. There are also reports that chiropractic manipulation can help alleviate back and leg pain as well [13]. However, it is unclear if resolution of symptoms is due to physical therapy/manipulation or the natural history of lumbar disc herniation resolving on its own with time [13].

If first-line pharmacotherapy and physical therapy fail, epidural steroid injections (ESIs) are often recommended prior to proceeding to surgery. Corticosteroids are powerful anti-inflammatory agents that work through multiple mechanisms including suppression of pro-inflammatory cytokines [14]. ESIs are likely to provide short-term relief, but their long-term benefits remain debatable [1, 13, 14]. Interestingly, despite their widespread use and recommendation, epidural application of corticosteroids is not approved by the US Food and Drug Administration (FDA) [14]. This makes the use of ESIs "off-label". ESIs are typically very well tolerated with a low risk profile with a complication rate <1%. Most complications are minor, such as headaches, cerebrospinal fluid leaks due to dural puncture, or vasovagal reactions. Unfortunately, there can also be severe complications such as meningitis or neurological deficit/paraplegia due to direct injury to a nerve root [14].

Surgery

If conservative measures fail to adequately relieve the patient's symptoms, surgery is an excellent option for this patient population. Surgery has been shown to decrease radicular leg pain faster when compared to conservative measures alone [12, 13]. In the absence of neurological deficits, conservative treatment should be trialed for at least 6 weeks. However, it has been shown that surgery performed prior to 6 months after onset of symptoms has led to improved symptom relief [12, 14]. Unfortunately, the long-term benefits of early surgery are less clear as similar outcomes are reported at long-term follow-up [13, 14]. This makes determining the optimal timing for surgery challenging, as the surgeon should trial conservative measures to assess symptom improvement, while being prepared to intervene within a limited window if symptoms persist. If patients are suffering from cauda equina or foot drop, a more appropriate timeline should be implemented with surgery performed on an emergent or urgent basis, respectively [12–14].

There are several surgical approaches that can be performed for the treatment of lumbar disc herniation. A traditional open microdiscectomy is considered to be the gold standard [14]. Minimally invasive (MIS) techniques, such as the use of tubular retractors or endoscopic microdiscectomy, are becoming more popular and demonstrate similar success rates compared to the gold standard in terms of symptom relief, with the added benefits of MIS, such as less soft tissue dissection, shorter hospital stays, and decreased infection rate [13].

Patients with isolated leg pain in the setting of a single lumbar disc herniation do not routinely need a fusion procedure performed in conjunction with the discectomy. The inclusion of performing a fusion may be considered if the patient is also suffering from mechanical axial back pain, severe multilevel degenerative changes, or radiographic instability [12].

Prognosis/Long-Term Outcomes

There are many variables that help predict the long-term outcomes after a lumbar microdiscectomy. As stated earlier, short-term outcomes are favorable after surgery, but long-term outcomes are less clear. Favorable long-term outcomes are associated with younger age, shorter duration of symptoms, lack of back pain, as well as less compression on imaging [1, 14]. On the other hand, factors that are associated with worse long-term outcomes are increased age, smoking status, symptoms present for >6–8 months, high body mass index, signs of preoperative psychological distress, such as somatization and/or depression, and a significant degree of neural compression on imaging [1, 15–17].

Patients with preoperative motor deficits are likely to regain function over time if their symptoms have not been present for an extended period before surgery. One study demonstrated that even severe muscle weakness prior to surgery was completely or nearly completely resolved if surgery was performed within 8 weeks of symptom onset and the muscles were innervated by the L2–5 nerve roots. Of note, patients who suffered severe L5-S1 compression demonstrated poor recovery, if any [18].

Lumbar disc herniation surgery has a reoperation rate of 3–18% [13, 15, 19]. The majority of patients who have undergone reoperation suffer from recurrent disc herniations [15, 16]. Having a prior lumbar discectomy is also a risk factor for requiring lumbar fusion. Patients with a diagnosis of lumbar radiculopathy who undergo a microdiscectomy are around 3 times more likely to have a lumbar fusion performed [14]. This may result from iatrogenic instability caused during the initial procedure or from patient factors leading to further degeneration. Also, about one-quarter of patients who undergo a microdiscectomy will have chronic back or leg pain [1, 14].

Conclusion

Lumbar disc herniation is a prevalent and impactful condition that requires a nuanced understanding of anatomy, pathophysiology, and clinical management for effective treatment. While conservative therapies often lead to symptom resolution, surgical intervention remains a vital option for patients with persistent or severe symptoms. Ultimately, an individualized approach that considers patient-specific factors and current evidence will yield the best outcomes. As the field advances, ongoing research and refinement of techniques will continue to enhance the care of patients with lumbar disc herniations.

References

1. Kreiner DS, Hwang SW, Easa JE, Resnick DK, Baisden JL, Bess S, et al. An evidence-based clinical guideline for the diagnosis and treatment of lumbar disc herniation with radiculopathy. Spine J. 2014;14(1):180–91.
2. Tosteson ANA, Skinner JS, Tosteson TD, Lurie JD, Andersson G, Berven S, et al. The cost effectiveness of surgical versus non-operative treatment for lumbar disc herniation over two years: evidence from the Spine Patient Outcomes Research Trial (SPORT). Spine. 2008;33(19):2108–15.
3. Mohd Isa IL, Teoh SL, Mohd Nor NH, Mokhtar SA. Discogenic low Back pain: anatomy, pathophysiology and treatments of intervertebral disc degeneration. Int J Mol Sci. 2022;24(1):208.
4. Li S, Du J, Huang Y, Gao S, Zhao Z, Chang Z, et al. From hyperglycemia to intervertebral disc damage: exploring diabetic-induced disc degeneration. Front Immunol. 2024;15:1355503.
5. Lavé A, Gondar R, Demetriades AK, Meling TR. Ergonomics and musculoskeletal disorders in neurosurgery: a systematic review. Acta Neurochir. 2020;162(9):2213–20.
6. Pojskic M, Bisson E, Oertel J, Takami T, Zygourakis C, Costa F. Lumbar disc herniation: epidemiology, clinical and radiologic diagnosis WFNS spine committee recommendations. World Neurosurg X. 2024;22:100279.
7. Baaj AA, Mummaneni PV, Uribe JS, Vaccaro AR, Greenberg MS. Handbook of spine surgery. 2nd ed. New York/Stuttgart/Delhi/Rio de Janeiro: Thieme; 2016. p. 1.
8. Li J, Gössel L, Kunze B, Kessler O, Alharbi Y, Gärtner O, et al. Traumatic lumbar disc herniation: a systemic case review and meta-analysis. Brain Spine. 2023;3:102350.
9. Huang W, Qian Y, Zheng K, Yu L, Yu X. Is smoking a risk factor for lumbar disc herniation? Eur Spine J. 2016;25(1):168–76.
10. Battié MC, Videman T, Kaprio J, Gibbons LE, Gill K, Manninen H, et al. The twin spine study: contributions to a changing view of disc degeneration. Spine J. 2009;9(1):47–59.
11. Petersen T, Laslett M, Juhl C. Clinical classification in low back pain: best-evidence diagnostic rules based on systematic reviews. BMC Musculoskelet Disord. 2017;18:188.
12. Penchev P, Ilyov IG, Todorov T, Petrov PP, Traykov P. Comprehensive analysis of treatment approaches for lumbar disc herniation: a systematic review. Cureus. 2024;16(8):e67899.
13. Deyo RA, Mirza SK. Herniated lumbar intervertebral disk. N Engl J Med. 2016;374(18):1763–72.
14. Beall DP, Kim KD, Macadaeg K, Donboli K, Chauhan K, Sowlay M, et al. Treatment gaps and emerging therapies in lumbar disc herniation. Pain Physician. 2024;27(7):401–13.
15. Ilyas H, Savage J. Lumbar disk herniation and SPORT: a review of the literature. Clin Spine Surg. 2018;31(9):366–72.
16. Desai A, Bekelis K, Ball PA, Lurie J, Mirza SK, Tosteson TD, et al. Spine patient outcomes research trial: do outcomes vary across centers for surgery for lumbar disc herniation? Neurosurgery. 2012;71(4):833–43.
17. Righesso O, Falavigna A, Avanzi O. Correlation between persistent neurological impairment and clinical outcome after microdiscectomy for treatment of lumbar disc herniation. Neurosurgery. 2012;70(2):390–7.
18. Postacchini F, Giannicola G, Cinotti G. Recovery of motor deficits after microdiscectomy for lumbar disc herniation. J Bone Joint Surg Br. 2002;84(7):1040–5.
19. Yang A, Goldschlager T, Daly CD, Castle-Kirszbaum M, Rogers MA. Does physical activity improve patient outcomes following lumbar microdiscectomy? Neurosurgery. 2023;69(Supplement_1):109–9.

Lumbar Spinal Stenosis

13

Stefan Motov, Felix C. Stengel,
and Martin N. Stienen

Background, Classification, and Clinical Presentation

Lumbar spinal stenosis (LSS) is a degenerative disease that primarily affects individuals over 60 years of age. It is defined as spinal canal narrowing due to degenerative changes in the intervertebral discs, surrounding soft tissues, and bone structures. This narrowing can lead to compression of neural and vascular structures, leading to ischemic symptoms of the radicular nerve roots [1, 2]. LSS can be classified according to the localization (central stenosis, recess stenosis, neuroforaminal stenosis) and according to imaging-based severity [1, 3–5]. The imaging characteristics of LSS, however, do not necessarily correlate with the severity of an individual patient's clinical symptoms. Typically, patients present with positional pain in the lower back or radiating into the legs when up and walking, which may be accompanied by feelings of heaviness, sensory disturbances, and/or muscle weakness. The so-called "neurogenic claudication" often improves with lumbar flexion, which increases the cross-sectional area of the spinal canal, which is why patients lean forward or sit down when symptoms worsen. The natural course of LSS varies; symptoms may remain stable for many years but typically show a slow progression, which eventually requires treatment [6].

Conservative Treatment Options

Conservative treatment is the first choice for many patients with LSS. The aim of each treatment is to improve function by increasing mobility and walking distance, reducing pain and disability, and thus improving health-related quality of life.

Physiotherapy

Physiotherapy plays an important role in LSS management. Key components include range-of-motion with flexion exercises, strengthening exercises to increase back and trunk stability, as well as aqua aerobics and manual therapy. Although various studies have shown some effectiveness of these measures, the overall level of evidence to support their application is classified as low [7].

S. Motov · F. C. Stengel · M. N. Stienen (✉)
H-OCH Health Ostschweiz, Interdisciplinary Spine Center & Department of Neurosurgery, Kantonsspital St.Gallen & School of Medicine, University of St. Gallen, St. Gallen, Switzerland
e-mail: felix.stengel@stengel-nuernberg.de

A. A. Baaj et al. (eds.), *Surgery of the Lumbar Spine*, https://doi.org/10.1007/978-3-032-18097-1_13

Pharmacological Treatment

Pharmacological measures, based on the staged regimen proposed by the World Health Organization, can help to treat pain and inflammation associated with LSS. These include paracetamol, NSAIDs, gabapentin, muscle relaxants, and—for acute pain exacerbation—short-term use of opioids [8].

Epidural Steroid Injections

Epidural steroid injections (ESI) serve both diagnostic and therapeutic purposes in LSS management. They can help differentiate facetogenic back pain from back pain associated with neurogenic claudication [9]. For LSS, interlaminar ESI (at the level of stenosis or adjacent segment) and sacral epidural blocks (for LSS at the L4/5 and L5/S1 levels) are most often performed. Clinically meaningful pain relief can be expected in about 60–70% of LSS patients in the short term [9], and patients with at least 50% pain reduction to the local anesthetic in the "diagnostic window" have a three-fold higher chance for a favorable 1-month response to ESI [10]. When determining the indication for ESI, it must be considered that the risk for an incidental durotomy may be higher if surgical decompression is performed within 3 months following an ESI [11]. The risk for surgical site infections does not seem to be much higher when an ESI is performed within 1 to 3 months prior to lumbar decompression [12, 13].

Effectiveness of Conservative Versus Surgical Treatment

Several studies have compared the outcomes of conservative and surgical treatment for LSS [14–17]. These studies generally show greater improvement in the surgical groups compared to non-surgical groups, particularly in long-term follow-ups. The SPORT trial was among the first randomized controlled studies, unfortunately somewhat limited by high levels of loss to follow-up, crossover, and nonadherence, which decreased the power and value of the intention-to-treat analysis. In the as-treated analysis, however, a greater improvement on the Short Form-36 (SF-36) bodily pain (BP), physical function (PF), and Oswestry Disability Index (ODI) metrics were reported for the surgical group compared with the non-surgical group at 2 years of follow-up, [18, 19] which persisted as positive effect at 4 and 8 years [18, 20]. Although the long-term effectiveness of conservative measures may be limited, they can help delay or avoid surgery in some LSS patients. Recent data shows that lumbar decompression without instrumentation leads to favorable results even in patients with predominant back pain [21], hence lumbar decompression may also be considered in patients presenting with symptoms beyond the radiating lower extremity pain. The choice of treatment should be individualized based on the clinical picture (symptom severity, quality of life), concomitant diseases (life expectancy), and patient preferences. Regular reassessment is helpful to evaluate treatment efficacy and consider alternative options when conservative measures fail to provide adequate relief.

Indication for Lumbar Decompression

Laminectomy—a midline approach with resection of the spinous process and bilateral parts of the lamina and joints, preserving the pars interarticularis—was historically the first approach to address LSS. Although generally perceived as a minimally invasive surgical (MIS) procedure and still frequently applied today, a classic laminectomy, including resection of the posterior tension band, increases the chance of instability [22] and the odds of requiring additional fusion [23]. With emerging knowledge about potential long-term effects, less destabilizing alternative decompression techniques have been developed, including but not limited to unilateral laminotomy with "over-the-top" decompression, bilateral laminotomy, or the spinous process splitting technique [24, 25]. Residents and fellows can safely perform those techniques in training without increasing complication rates and jeopardizing outcomes [26]. A recent multi-center randomized trial found no differences in the effectiveness of these three open techniques regarding complication rates and clinical outcomes [27]. Moreover, the radiological analysis revealed similar degrees of dural expansion for all three types of lumbar decompression [28]. A recent review and recommendation statement of the World Federation of Neurosurgical Societies Spine Committee indicated that lumbar decompression is the treatment of choice for symptomatic LSS. However, the best surgical technique is still under debate due to the low level of evidence [29].

There has been uncertainty about whether patients with LSS and concomitant degenerative grade-1 spondylolisthesis require fusion in addition to decompression [30]. Two recent trials now demonstrated that decompression without fusion is adequate for most of these patients without evident instability or foraminal stenosis [31, 32]. Hence, lumbar decompression without fusion can be considered the primary treatment option for most surgical candidates with LSS and a mild slip [2], as decompression with fusion was associated with higher risks for complications, longer hospital stays, and higher costs. Post-hoc analyses, focusing particularly on the sagittal balance parameters, revealed that patients with a higher pelvic incidence (PI)–lumbar lordosis (LL) mismatch experienced superior results with fusion regarding health-related quality of life and reoperation rate at 2 years postoperatively. In contrast, the addition of fusion for LSS patients with low-grade spondylolisthesis and spinopelvic harmony (low PI-LL mismatch) resulted in worse quality-of-life outcomes and higher reoperation rates [33]. It is important to note that patients suitable for lumbar decompression without fusion should not be symptomatic from foraminal stenosis and not show evident signs of segmental instability (e.g., mechanical back pain, facet joint effusion, progressive spondylolisthesis of >3 mm), as this is associated with a higher proportion of patients with insufficient improvement after decompression and higher reoperation rates [34].

Techniques for Lumbar Decompression

In the following, we will focus on two MIS techniques that have shown promising results in comparative studies and are increasingly used for LSS decompression. First, the application of tubes to use a unilateral approach in order to bilaterally decompress enables a more muscle-sparing technique with less blood loss, less approach-related back pain, and enhanced recovery with a shorter length of stay compared to open decompression. Especially in the early post-operative phase of <3 months, tubular decompression has demonstrated superior clinical outcomes [8], which justifies the broader use of tubular microscopic approaches for spinal canal decompression. However, there are no randomized controlled trials comparing complication rates and outcomes of open vs. tubular decompression in LSS, and comparative trials for sciatica resulting from a herniated lumbar disc failed to demonstrate the superiority of the tubular technique [35]. It should be noted that outcome and patient satisfaction are directly correlated with a sufficient degree of decompression. Compared to open decompression, where visualization of the complete interlaminar window during the procedure is possible, the use of the tubular retractor results in a dot-shaped, partial exposure of the pathology. Bearing this in mind, a more active surgical technique is required, repositioning the tube multiple times to decompress the whole segment sufficiently.

Second, unilateral biportal endoscopy (UBE) has demonstrated benefits in terms of less blood loss, complications, and shorter length of stay, as well as better clinical outcomes, compared to open microscopic decompression in a recent meta-analysis [36]. Pooled analyses reveal that incidental durotomy (4.5%), transient motor deficit (2.6%), insufficient decompression (2.0%), and symptomatic epidural hematoma (1.1%) constitute the most common complications and are within the range of microsurgical procedures [37]. The potentially greatest advantage of UBE over microsurgical techniques is that surgical site infections are literally non-existing (0% in large meta-analyses [36]), owing to the small skin incisions and the use of continuous irrigation, which washes out pathogens during the whole procedure. UBE is a versatile technique applicable to a multitude of lumbar pathologies that require decompression, and extension of the approach toward minimally invasive lumbar interbody fusion is possible [37, 38]. The advantages of biportal over monoportal endoscopic techniques for LSS include shorter surgical time as the use of the drill is more efficacious, improved visualization of the complete spinal canal as the instrument does not block the view, and a tendency toward lower disability outcomes [39]. As true for all MIS techniques, UBE also has a learning curve, which seems to be shorter than for monoportal endoscopic techniques, but still needs to be overcome until stable results can be achieved [40].

Microtubular Decompression

Case Presentation

An 85-year-old female presented with numeric rating scale (NRS) 6/10 lumbar pain and NRS 9/10 right-sided L5 radicular pain for 6 months without significant improvement under oral analgesics and physiotherapy. Magnetic resonance imaging (MRI) and X-ray studies revealed a combination of L4/5 LSS and a stable, degenerative spondylolisthesis Meyerding grade-I (Fig. 13.1a–c). An ESI at the L4/5 level provided symptomatic relief for only a few weeks. Due to persistent symptoms, the patient was advised for microscopic tubular right-sided unilateral laminotomy with "over-the-top" decompression.

Technique Description

After identifying the interlaminar window under ap/lateral fluoroscopy (Fig. 13.1d, e) we recommend planning a skin incision of approximately 1.5–2 cm, about 1–2 cm lateral to the midline, depending on the intended lumbar level and patient-specific anatomy. The thoracolumbar fascia is opened with a bovy, a directional guide is inserted until bony contact is established, and with circular movements, the bony structures-spinolaminar junction/caudal lamina border of upper lamina/medial facet joint border are palpated. Sequential tube insertion in a 5–10° angle, respective to the midline, and muscle dilation is performed. A tubular retractor of 1.8–2.2 cm, depending on the pathology and surgeon's level of experience, is inserted over the dilators and attached to the OR table with a holding arm (Figs. 13.1f, g and 13.2a, b).

A pedicle probe or dissector is placed in the interlaminar window for fluoroscopic verification of the spinal level. The final piece of muscle is detached with a bovy, and the bony structures are exposed under microscopic view (Fig. 13.2c). Bony decompression is performed with a 4 mm Diamant or oval burr starting at the medial inferior border of the upper lamina. Drilling begins at the base of the spinous process and rotates up and laterally at the caudal border of the upper lamina with preservation of the ipsilateral pars interarticularis of the medial facet joint (Fig. 13.2d). Drilling and (counter-)clockwise removal of the cranial border of the lower lamina is performed. After ipsilateral ligamentum flavum exposure and mobilization with a ball-tip, circumferential resection with a Kerrison rongeur follows. The tube is tilted 20–25° to the contralateral side, and the OR table is rotated 5–10° away from the surgeon to facilitate drilling of the contralateral lamina with preservation of the contralateral ligamentum flavum. The contralateral ligament is mobilized with a ball tip and resected with a Kerrison rongeur. Bilateral palpation of the pedicles and the nerve roots in the recess secures the

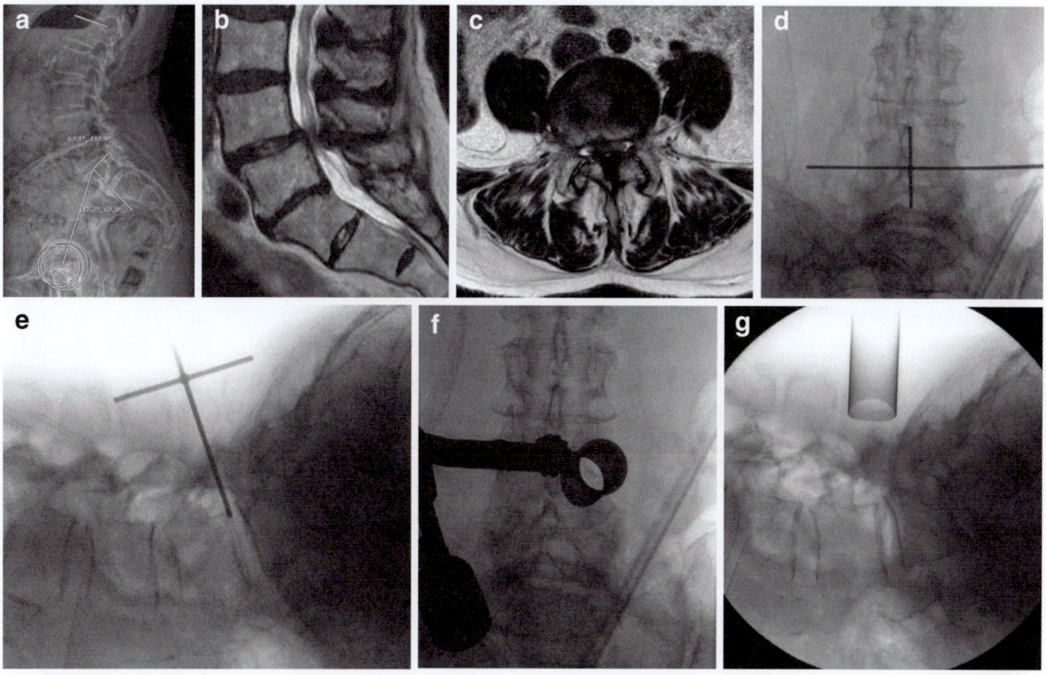

Fig. 13.1 Preoperative standing X-ray (**a**) and T2-weighted MRI studies in sagittal (**b**) and axial views (**c**) focusing on lumbar spine with L4/5 and L5/S1 disc degeneration and L4/5 LSS and grade-I spondylolisthesis, PI-LL mismatch 0°. (**d, e**) Identifying the interlaminar window and planning the skin incision. (**f, g**) Intraoperative fluoroscopy after insertion of the tubular retractor shows its relationship to the midline and interlaminar window

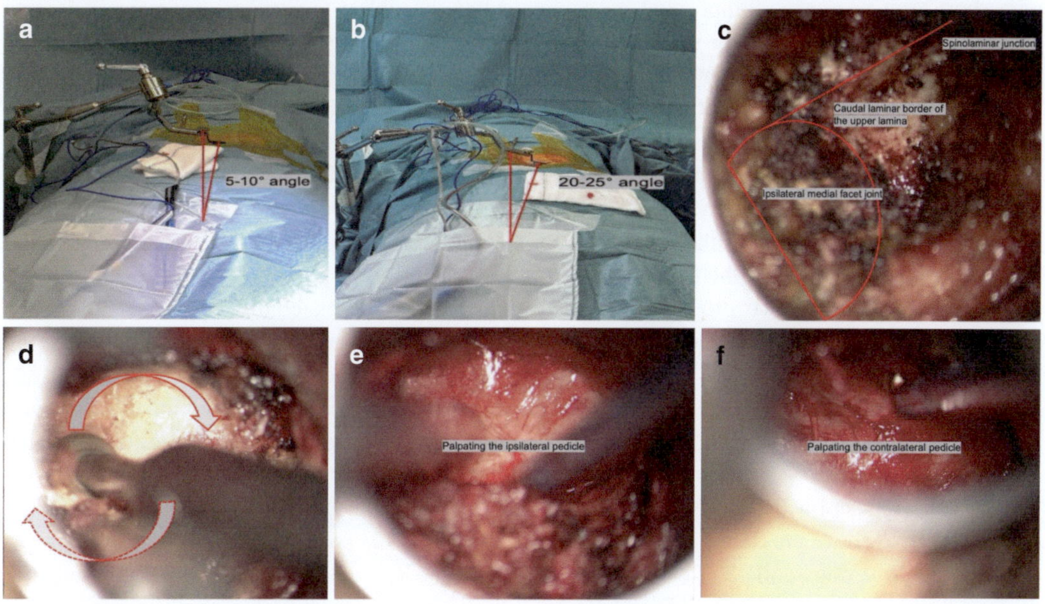

Fig. 13.2 Tube insertion and fixation on the OR table for ipsilateral decompression (**a**) in approximately 5–10° angle to the midline, centered on the interlaminar window. For the contralateral decompression (**b**), 20–25° tilt of the tube to the midline is performed. (**c**) Exposure of the anatomical structures, as visualized through the tubular retractor. (**d**) Bony anatomical structures are removed through clockwise ipsilateral drilling maneuver with ultimately exposure of the ligamentum flavum and preservation of the facet joint. Here, a right-sided approach is taken; for left-sided approaches the decompression is performed in a counterclockwise fashion. Verification of decompression sufficiency by palpating the ipsilateral (**e**) and contralateral pedicles (**f**)

satisfactory extent of the decompression (Fig. 13.2e, f). The defect is filled with saline, and the tube is finally removed via clockwise rotation, while muscle bleeders are coagulated. Fascia and subcutaneous tissue are closed with single sutures.

Case Resolution

The patient experienced an uneventful postoperative course and was discharged on the second postoperative day with mild residual low back pain (NRS 1/10) and no residual radicular pain. At the 6-week postoperative follow-up visit, the patient was symptom-free without any pain medication.

Unilateral, Biportal Endoscopic (UBE) Decompression

Case Presentation

A 77-year-old male patient presented with a history of neurogenic claudication and several ESIs with short-term response, complicated by acute onset of a sharp, radicular pain radiating to the right L5 dermatome (NRS 4/10 lumbar pain, NRS 8/10 radicular leg pain; ODI 46/100%) with new-onset foot drop for 7 days. The patient could not tolerate the pain and used heat applications on his back, in addition to high doses of analgesics, resulting in skin burns. Due to the immobilizing pain and neurological deficit, the patient was recommended surgery, and we offered right-sided UBE with decompression and sequestrectomy.

Technique Description

The patient is positioned prone, and particular care is taken to relieve pressure to the abdominal cavity to avoid venous collateral circulation via the spinal epidural space. Using AP and lateral fluoroscopy, the OR table is rotated and tilted until the spinous processes are centered between both pedicles and the target disc space is strictly vertical. For a left-sided approach, two 7-8 mm skin incisions are planned on the ipsilateral pedicle line, each about 1 cm above and below the center of the disc space. For a right-sided approach by a right-handed surgeon, both incisions are planned a few millimeters more caudally.

After the incision of the left (endoscopic) portal, serial blunt dilation to the caudal aspect of the cranial lamina (here: L4) is performed. The right (working) portal is prepared, using the muscle detacher to dock onto the cranial aspect of the inferior lamina (here: L5) and create a cavity around the interlaminar window. With the dilators and the muscle detacher in situ, we perform one-time fluoroscopic control to verify the right level (Fig. 13.2c), before bringing in and installing the endoscope tower.

The bony anatomy of the cranial and caudal laminae with a base of the spinous process, as well as the medial aspect of the facet joint, is exposed using a strong 90° radiofrequency (RF) probe. A 4 mm Diamant drill is used to remove the caudal aspect of the cranial lamina until the insertion point of the yellow ligament is reached; this ensures sufficient decompression as the cranial extension of the stenosis typically ends just caudal to this landmark (compare Fig. 13.3a). After detaching the yellow ligament, it is first removed in a cranio-caudal, then in a mediolateral direction, either in piece-meal or *en-block* fashion. The ipsilateral lateral recess is decompressed, taking the medial third of the facet joint (both inferior and superior articulating processes) until the caudal pedicle is controlled (Fig. 13.3e). The traversing nerve root can be mobilized and medialized to inspect the disc space and remove protruded or herniated disc fragments, as needed (Fig. 13.3f). After ipsilateral decompression, the base of the spinous process can be drilled off, together with the medial aspect of the contralateral facet joint, again staying outside of and keeping the yellow ligament as protection layer for the dura intact as long as possible. After blunt dissection of potential adhesions between the dura and the yellow ligament, the contralateral recess is decompressed until the pedicle, disc space, and foramen on the opposite side are controlled (Fig. 13.3g). For the work on the contralateral side and final inspection, the 0° optic can be exchanged to a 30° endoscope, which may offer superior visualization.

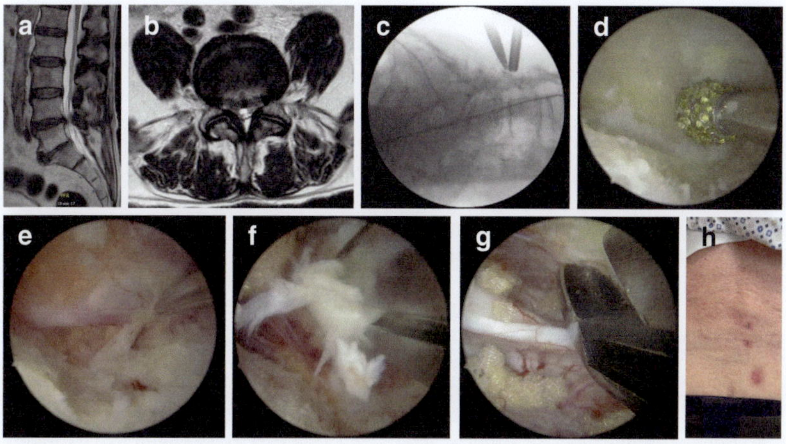

Fig. 13.3 MRI studies in sagittal (**a**) and axial view (**b**) demonstrate facet joint hypertrophy and resulting bilateral recess stenosis at L4/5, with subsequent compression of both L5 nerves. On the right side, there is suspicion of an acute lumbar disc herniation on the level of the disc space. (**c**) Intraoperative fluoroscopy is used to confirm the right level after the approach and before insertion of the endoscope. (**d**) After preparing the bony anatomy with a RF probe, a 4 mm Diamant drill is used to shave off the caudal aspect of the cranial lamina, the medial third of the ipsilateral joint, as well as the cranial aspect of the caudal lamina, keeping the yellow ligament as a protection layer for the dura. (**e**) View on the dura and traversing L5 nerve root, palpating the ipsilateral L5 pedicle with a Penfield dissector and releasing epidural adhesions. (**f**) The protruded disc material is removed with a pituitary rongeur after slight retraction of the L5 nerve and opening of the posterior longitudinal ligament with a semi-sharp knife (Indian knife). (**g**) After ipsilateral decompression, the over-the-top decompression is performed with the drill and punches. Note how the dura is folded and pushed downward by the irrigation pressure, facilitating access to the contralateral recess. (**h**) View of the patient's skin incisions at the 6-week follow-up. Note the residual stains from the self-inflicted skin burns

Case Resolution

The patient experienced an uneventful postoperative course and was seen back 6 weeks postoperative, where he reported no residual radicular leg pain (NRS 0/10) and mild low back pain (NRS 2/10); his ODI at this time was 17.8%. Figure 13.3h depicts his back at the follow-up, with well-healed incisions of the UBE procedure and residual stains from his self-inflicted skin burns.

References

1. Lee GY, et al. A new grading system of lumbar central canal stenosis on MRI: an easy and reliable method. Skeletal Radiol. 2011;40(8):1033–9.
2. Katz JN, et al. Diagnosis and Management of Lumbar Spinal Stenosis: a review. JAMA. 2022;327(17):1688–99.
3. Lurie JD, et al. Reliability of readings of magnetic resonance imaging features of lumbar spinal stenosis. Spine (Phila Pa 1976). 2008;33(14):1605–10.
4. Schizas C, et al. Qualitative grading of severity of lumbar spinal stenosis based on the morphology of the dural sac on magnetic resonance images. Spine (Phila Pa 1976). 2010;35(21):1919–24.
5. Miskin N, et al. Standardized classification of lumbar spine degeneration on magnetic resonance imaging reduces intra- and inter-subspecialty variability. Curr Probl Diagn Radiol. 2022;51(4):491–6.
6. Issack PS, et al. Degenerative lumbar spinal stenosis: evaluation and management. J Am Acad Orthop Surg. 2012;20(8):527–35.
7. Temporiti F, et al. Efficacy and characteristics of physiotherapy interventions in patients with lumbar spinal stenosis: a systematic review. Eur Spine J. 2022;31(6):1370–90.
8. Lee GW, et al. Clinical and radiological outcomes following microscopic decompression utilizing tubular retractor or conventional microscopic decompression in lumbar spinal stenosis with a minimum of 10-year follow-up. Eur J Orthop Surg Traumatol. 2014;24(Suppl 1):S145–51.
9. Brandle K, et al. Ten-day response to CT-guided spinal infiltration therapy in more than a thousand patients. J Neurol Surg A Cent Eur Neurosurg. 2016;77(3):181–94.
10. Joswig H, et al. The value of short-term pain relief in predicting the one-month outcome of lumbar

Transforaminal epidural steroid injections. World Neurosurg. 2016;96:323–33.
11. Shakya A, et al. Preoperative lumbar epidural steroid injection increases the risk of a Dural tear during minimally invasive lumbar discectomy. Int J Spine Surg. 2022;16(3):505–11.
12. Lee Y, et al. Preoperative epidural steroid injections do not increase the risk of postoperative infection in patients undergoing lumbar decompression or fusion: a systematic review and meta-analysis. Eur Spine J. 2022;31(12):3251–61.
13. Hooten WM, et al. Preoperative epidural steroid injections and postoperative infections after lumbar or cervical spine surgery: a systematic review and meta-analysis. Mayo Clin Proc Innov Qual Outcomes. 2023;7(5):349–65.
14. Atlas SJ, et al. Long-term outcomes of surgical and nonsurgical management of lumbar spinal stenosis: 8 to 10 year results from the Maine lumbar spine study. Spine (Phila Pa 1976). 2005;30(8):936–43.
15. Atlas SJ, et al. The Maine Lumbar Spine Study, Part II. 1-year outcomes of surgical and nonsurgical management of sciatica. Spine (Phila Pa 1976). 1996;21(15):1777–86.
16. Malmivaara A, et al. Surgical or nonoperative treatment for lumbar spinal stenosis? A randomized controlled trial. Spine (Phila Pa 1976). 2007;32(1):1–8.
17. Delitto A, et al. Surgery versus nonsurgical treatment of lumbar spinal stenosis: a randomized trial. Ann Intern Med. 2015;162(7):465–73.
18. Weinstein JN, et al. Surgical versus nonoperative treatment for lumbar spinal stenosis four-year results of the spine patient outcomes research trial. Spine (Phila Pa 1976). 2010;35(14):1329–38.
19. Weinstein JN, et al. Surgical versus nonsurgical therapy for lumbar spinal stenosis. N Engl J Med. 2008;358(8):794–810.
20. Lurie JD, et al. Long-term outcomes of lumbar spinal stenosis: eight-year results of the spine patient outcomes research trial (SPORT). Spine (Phila Pa 1976). 2015;40(2):63–76.
21. Stienen MN, et al. Short- and long-term outcome of microscopic lumbar spine surgery in patients with predominant Back or predominant leg pain. World Neurosurg. 2016;93:458–465 e1.
22. Lener S, et al. The effect of various options for decompression of degenerated lumbar spine motion segments on the range of motion: a biomechanical in vitro study. Eur Spine J. 2023;32(4):1358–66.
23. Overdevest GM, et al. Effectiveness of posterior decompression techniques compared with conventional laminectomy for lumbar stenosis. Cochrane Database Syst Rev. 2015;3:CD010036.
24. Voglis S, et al. Spinous-process-splitting versus conventional decompression for lumbar spinal stenosis: comparative study with respect to short-term postoperative pain and analgesics use. World Neurosurg. 2022;160:e80–7.
25. Thome C, et al. Outcome after less-invasive decompression of lumbar spinal stenosis: a randomized comparison of unilateral laminotomy, bilateral laminotomy, and laminectomy. J Neurosurg Spine. 2005;3(2):129–41.
26. Joswig H, et al. Microscopic lumbar spinal stenosis decompression: is surgical education safe? Acta Neurochir. 2016;158(2):357–66.
27. Hermansen E, et al. Comparison of 3 different minimally invasive surgical techniques for lumbar spinal stenosis: a randomized clinical trial. JAMA Netw Open. 2022;5(3):e224291.
28. Hermansen E, et al. Comparable increases in dural sac area after three different posterior decompression techniques for lumbar spinal stenosis: radiological results from a randomized controlled trial in the NORDSTEN study. Eur Spine J. 2020;29(9):2254–61.
29. Costa F, et al. Decompressive surgery for lumbar spinal stenosis: WFNS spine committee recommendations. World Neurosurg X. 2020;7:100076.
30. Haider G, et al. Progression to fusion after lumbar laminectomy for degenerative lumbar spondylolisthesis: rate and risk-factors. A national database study. Clin Neurol Neurosurg. 2023;233:107919.
31. Forsth P, et al. A randomized, controlled trial of fusion surgery for lumbar spinal stenosis. N Engl J Med. 2016;374(15):1413–23.
32. Ghogawala Z, et al. Laminectomy plus fusion versus laminectomy alone for lumbar spondylolisthesis. N Engl J Med. 2016;374(15):1424–34.
33. Mohanty S, et al. Should patients with lumbar stenosis and grade I spondylolisthesis be treated differently based on spinopelvic alignment? A retrospective, two-year, propensity matched, comparison of patient-reported outcome measures and clinical outcomes from multiple sites within a single health system. Spine J. 2023;23(1):92–104.
34. Aaen J, et al. Is the presence of foraminal stenosis associated with outcome in lumbar spinal stenosis patients treated with posterior microsurgical decompression. Acta Neurochir. 2023;165(8):2121–9.
35. Arts MP, et al. Tubular diskectomy vs conventional microdiskectomy for sciatica: a randomized controlled trial. JAMA. 2009;302(2):149–58.
36. Wang YP, et al. Efficacy and safety of unilateral biportal endoscopy compared with microscopic decompression in the treatment of lumbar spinal stenosis: a systematic review and updated meta-analysis. Exp Ther Med. 2023;26(1):309.
37. Chen Z, et al. Complications of unilateral Biportal endoscopic spinal surgery for lumbar spinal stenosis: a meta-analysis and systematic review. World Neurosurg. 2023;170:e371–9.
38. Pao JL, et al. Unilateral biportal endoscopic decompression for degenerative lumbar canal stenosis. J Spine Surg. 2020;6(2):438–46.
39. He Y, et al. Unilateral biportal endoscopic versus uniportal full-endoscopic for lumbar degenerative disease: A meta-analysis. J Orthop Sci. 2024;29(1):49–58.
40. Chen L, et al. The learning curve of unilateral Biportal endoscopic (UBE) spinal surgery by CUSUM analysis. Front Surg. 2022;9:873691.

Intradural Lumbar Spinal Tumors

14

Victor M. Lu and Allan D. Levi

Introduction

The lumbar spine portends to specific types of intradural tumors due to its specific anatomy compared to other regions of the spine. The normal adult spinal cord containing primary glial cells (astrocytic and ependymal) typically terminates by the level of the second lumbar vertebral body spine as the conus medullaris. The collection of exiting lumbar nerve roots at this point is known as the cauda equina. The filum terminale is a fibrous continuation of the pia mater containing ependymal cells that travels from the conus medullaris, through the dural layer of the caudal end of the thecal sac to ultimately attach to the coccyx. The thecal sac consists of dura mater containing meningeal cells, and houses all these elements inside it and therefore defines the intradural space.

Given the vast range of cells located within the lumbar spine, there is a corresponding vast range of possible intradural tumors that can arise. The focus of this chapter is to first review the intradural tumors that are common, uncommon, and rare in the lumbar spine, and then describe the surgical considerations specific to these tumors of this location.

V. M. Lu · A. D. Levi (✉)
Department of Neurological Surgery, University of Miami Miller School of Medicine, Miami, FL, USA
e-mail: vml43@med.miami.edu; alevi@med.miami.edu

Common Tumors

Ependymoma and Myxopapillary Ependymoma

The majority of spinal cord gliomas are ependymomas. Although intramedullary lesions are less common in the lumbar spinal cord than in other areas of the spine (Fig. 14.1a), the variant type myxopapillary ependymoma is indeed most common along the cauda equina and filum terminale [1]. In general, these lesions arise from the central ependymal lining, and therefore symmetric cord expansion is very common [2]. They typically are sporadic except in the setting of neurofibromatosis type 2 (NF2). The majority of these lesions are considered low-grade gliomas that are World Health Organization (WHO) Grades 1 and 2.

Myxopapillary ependymomas (Fig. 14.1b) are a specific variant of ependymoma that occurs predominantly in the filum terminale and conus medullaris, and constitute up to 15% of spinal ependymoma, and more than 90% of tumors in lower lumbar spine [3]. They are believed to originate from the ependymal glia of the filum terminale itself, and frequently span multiple vertebral levels. This ependymomal variant is now considered WHO Grade 2 (an upgrade from the previous classification iterations under which they were considered Grade 1) to better reflect the tendency of these tumors to recur [4].

A. A. Baaj et al. (eds.), *Surgery of the Lumbar Spine*, https://doi.org/10.1007/978-3-032-18097-1_14

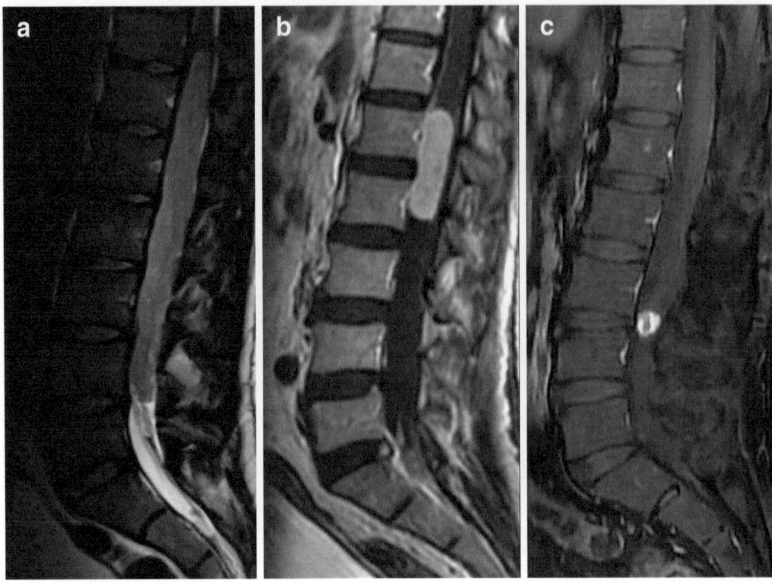

Fig. 14.1 Illustrative sagittal MRI images of common intradural lumbar spine tumors. (**a**) ependymoma on T2 sequence, (**b**) myxopapillary ependymoma on T1 sequence with contrast, and C. schwannoma on T1 sequence with contrast

Magnetic resonance imaging (MRI) of ependymomas and myxopapillary ependymomas usually reveals a well-circumscribed lesion, with iso- to hypointense T1 signal and iso- to hyperintense T2 signal throughout [5]. Contrast enhancement throughout the lesion is common. Ependymomas are known to present with intratumoral hemorrhage leading to hemosiderin deposition along the borders of the tumor (called the "cap sign"), as well as with syringomyelia and other cystic components [6]. Prognosis of spinal ependymomas in general is very promising following complete resection, with 5-year survival estimated to be approximately 85% across all variants [5]. Specific to myxopapillary ependymoma, prognosis is even better on average with an expected overall survival of greater than 98% at 5 years following complete resection [7].

Schwannoma

Nerve sheath tumors make up a large majority of intradural extramedullary tumors within the lumbar spine. Most of these tumors that are solitary and sporadic are schwannomas (Fig. 14.1c), and benign in nature [8]. Schwannomas are the second most common tumor found in the lumbar spine following ependymomas. They arise as a proliferation of Schwann cells within a nerve and as encapsulated tumors, occur adjacent to and can displace the involved nerve root itself. They usually occur in isolation, with the common exceptions of NF2 and familial schwannomatosis in which multiple lesions can occur throughout the body. These tumors rarely undergo malignant transformation and are often considered low-grade at diagnosis.

On MRI, these lesions typically show iso- and hypo-intense signal relative to the spinal cord on T1 sequence, hyperintense signal on T2 signal, and contrast enhancement. Signal heterogeneity is common, with increased T2 signal within the lesion signaling a cystic component, and decreased T2 signal corresponding to either intratumoral hemorrhage, dense cellularity as well as deposition of collagen [9]. In the cases of sporadic isolated schwannoma, gross total resection of the lesion is typically curative (Fig. 14.2). However, in syndromic cases, there is a high likelihood of new lesions arising.

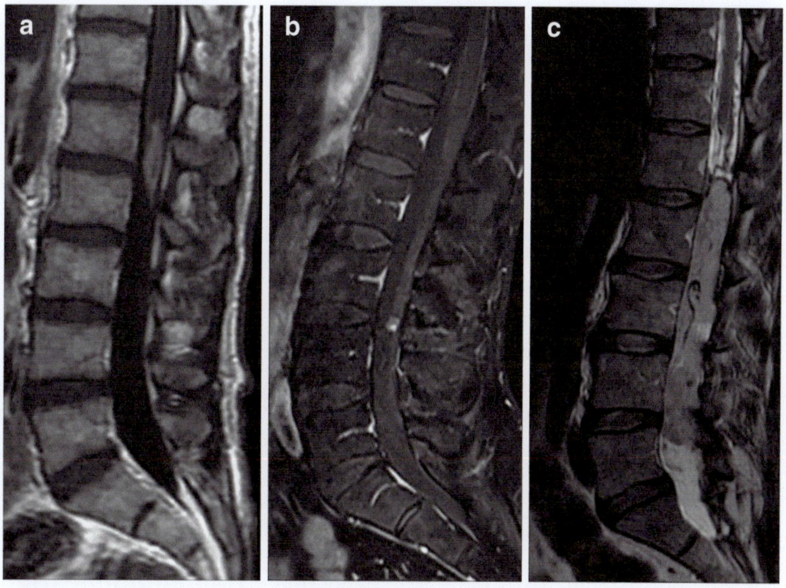

Fig. 14.2 Illustrative sagittal MRI images of uncommon intradural lumbar spine tumors. (**a**) astrocytoma on T1 sequence with contrast, (**b**) neurofibroma on T1 sequence with contrast, and C. paraganglioma on T2 sequence

Uncommon Tumors

Astrocytoma

Although astrocytomas are the second most common intramedullary spinal tumor across all regions, they do not commonly occur in the lumbar spinal cord (Fig. 14.2a) [10]. But when they do, they arise from the spinal cord parenchyma themselves, they are typically eccentric in the axial plane and rarely present with intratumoral hemorrhage [2].

Typical MRI will reveal a T1-hypointense and T2-hyperintense lesion that is diffuse with poorly defined borders. Contrast enhancement is commonly patchy or absent, with up to a third of lesions not demonstrating any enhancement at all [11]. Intratumoral cystic components and syringomyelia are common on imaging, more so than in ependymomas. Astrocytomas can occur across all WHO Grades, but less than half are expected to be high-grade. Given these tumors are highly infiltrative of spinal cord parenchyma, true complete resection is difficult to determine, and as such, prognosis is highly dependent on grade as well as radiographic extent of resection—5-year overall survival for low-grade versus high-grade lesions is approximately 95% versus 20% respectively [12, 13].

Neurofibroma and Malignant Nerve Sheath Tumors

The other type of nerve sheath tumor common to the intradural lumbar spine is neurofibroma. In contrast to schwannomas that are made up of solely Schwann cells, neurofibromas (Fig. 14.2b) are made up of multiple cellular elements, primarily perineural and Schwann cells, as well as fibroblasts and mucopolysaccharide matrix [14]. These tumors normally engulf the entire parent nerve root, and in contrast to schwannomas, typically occur in multiple locations at presentation and are associated commonly with neurofibromatosis type 1 (NF1).

On imaging, these tumors are much more homogenous on MRI compared to schwannomas, with more uniform signal intensity. These tumors can enhance with contrast, and have been known to display a "target sign" on T2 imaging—a lesional pattern of the lesion with greater peripheral intensity compared to the center of the lesion corresponding to high and low water-content [15]. Prognosis is very good with respect to overall survival given the benign nature of these tumors. However, 5–10% of these tumors are expected to undergo malignant transformation over a lifetime, more commonly in NF1 patients, which drastically shifts the prognosis [16].

The least common nerve sheath tumor of the lumbar spine are malignant nerve sheath tumors. Although these lesions mostly arise from peripheral nerves, they can have intradural involvement in the lumbar spine. Their occurrence can be secondary to malignant transformation of neurofibromas in the NF1 patients, be sporadic in nature deriving as sarcomatous lesions of the connective tissue surrounding nervous tissue, as well as be radiation-induced. Prognosis is poor, with average overall survival from diagnosis of approximately 6 years, [17] and this is despite surgical and chemoradiation treatment.

Paraganglioma

Paragangliomas (Fig. 14.2c) are neuroendocrine tumors that uncommonly occur in the spine, but when they do, they favor the cauda equina and filum terminale in the lumbar spine [18]. Their origins are believed to be from neural crest cells, neuroectodermally derived paraganglionic cells, within the lumbar sympathetic chain and are considered WHO Grade 1 lesions [19].

On imaging, these tumors are well defined within the thecal sac, and typically are isointense on T1, iso- to hyper-intense on T2 MRI sequences, and intense contrast enhancement is also universal across all tumors. These tumors are often vascular in nature, and the presence of serpentine flow voids on the surface of the tumor on preoperative imaging can be one early indication of this. Complete surgical resection is typically curative of this tumor, with recurrence rates estimated to be less than 5% of all cases [20]. However, given that these tumors are highly vascular in nature, piecemeal resection has a considerable bleed risk when compared to en-bloc resection [21].

Rare Tumors

Metastatic Disease

Metastases from primary tumors can occur within the lumbar spinal cord, as well as about the cauda equina and filum terminale which are termed "drop metastases" (Fig. 14.3a). Most of these metastases to the spinal cord are solitary whereas multiple lesions can be seen among the cauda equina and filum terminale when they present. More than half of these lesions are associated with primary lung cancer, followed by breast cancer, lymphoma, and melanoma [22]. These lesions can appear on MRI with T1-hypointense (similar to syrinx) and T2-hyperintense (secondary to associated edema) signal, and usually a disproportionate degree of contrast enhancement relative to actual size of lesion [23]. Prognosis is highly variable and dependent on primary cancer.

Hemangioblastoma

Although hemangioblastomas (Fig. 14.3b) represent the third most common spinal intramedullary spinal cord tumor, they are rare in the lumbar spine. Most of these tumors occur in isolation and except in the setting of von Hippel-Lindau syndrome where multiple lesions within the central nervous system can be seen [24]. Hemangioblastomas are vascular lesions that are classified as WHO Grade 1 tumors in the latest classification, and malignant transformation does not usually occur. Their cellular origin remains unclear, however it is believed they result from dysregulation of endothelial cells, pericytes, and stromal cells within the spinal cord parenchyma [25].

On imaging, these lesions can be cystic and are typically well-circumscribed. They are usually iso- to hyper-intense on both T1- and T2-sequences, and enhance vividly with contrast [26]. Similar to their cerebellar counterpart, spinal hemangioblastomas can also have a cystic appearance with an accompanying mural nodule. An associated syrinx is common in at least half of these tumors, and occasionally, the tumor may also demonstrate an exophytic component projecting out dorsally from the spinal cord [27]. Prognosis for these benign lesions following surgical resection is excellent, with 10-year overall survival above 90% [28].

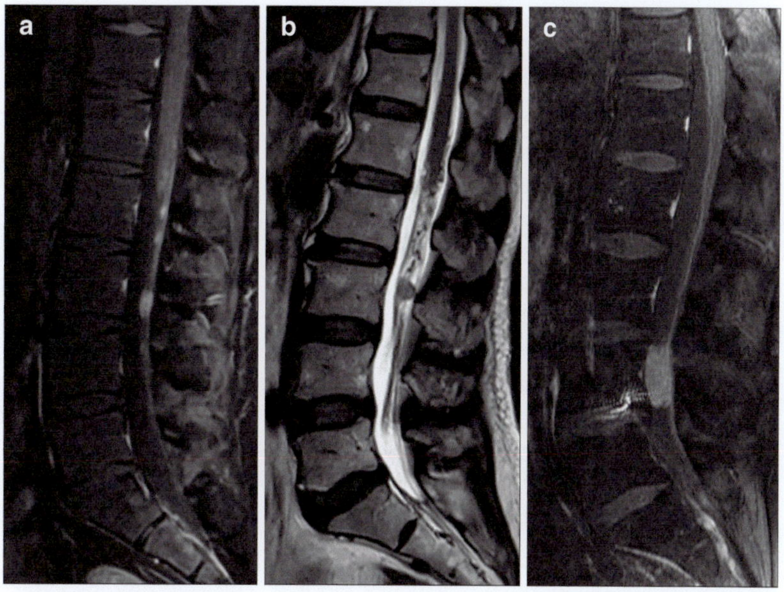

Fig. 14.3 Illustrative sagittal MRI images of rare intradural lumbar spine tumors. (**a**) metastatic disease on T1 sequence with contrast, (**b**) hemangioblastoma on T2 sequence, and (**c**) meningioma on T1 sequence with contrast

Meningioma

Meningiomas (Fig. 14.3c) have been very rarely reported in the lumbar spine [29]. They arise from the arachnoid cap cells of the arachnoid mater within the dura, and hence can occur anywhere along the thecal sac. These spinal lesions are usually slow-growing and can erode into or remodel adjacent bony elements and compress neural elements over time. On imaging, the typical dural tail seen intracranially can be seen in the lumbar spine, as well as isointense signal relative to spinal cord on T1- and T2-images and enhance strongly with contrast using MRI. These tumors show increased areas of cellularity or vascularity and calcified psammoma bodies. Prognosis is excellent following surgical treatment given the low-grade nature of the majority of these lesions [30].

Surgical Considerations

Electrophysiology

It is expected surgical practice to use electrophysiology monitoring during surgical resection of any intradural lesion in the lumbar spine. Standard preoperative preparation includes evaluating motor evoked potentials (MEPs) and somatosensory evoked potentials (SSEPs) which respectively monitor the dorsal and ventral tracts within the cord during surgery. For tumors about the filum terminale and cauda equina, it is recommended that more complex multimodal monitoring techniques be used to provide associations with functional nerve roots as well as associated with the lower lumbar spine. Free-run electromyography (EMG) monitors nerve roots in real-time that allows the surgeon to anticipate possible nerve injury. Evoked EMG is particularly useful in those tumors that encase nerve roots and the surgeon has to decide on nerve root sacrifice to improve resection. In addition to standard lower extremity lead placement, it is critically important to place leads in the external anal sphincter—so one can preserve functional rootlets innervating muscles that ultimately control bowel and bladder function.

Standard Open Technique

Posterior open approaches through the midline are generally favored in the lumbar spine to approach intradural lesions. The concern for retraction injury to the spinal cord and thecal sac at this part of the spine is less than other regions of the spine. In brief, following standard anesthesia, a classic midline subperiosteal dissection localized to the lesion can be performed after which standard laminectomy (or laminoplasty) can be performed to reveal thecal sac. There are situations where if the lesion is eccentric to one side, a surgeon may be able to visualize the entire lesion via a hemilaminectomy exposure only. Dural opening is generally performed in the midline; however, locations eccentric to one side may be reached with a paramedian incision. Dural edges should be everted and tacked to adjacent paraspinal muscle to maximize visualization within the thecal sac as well as prevent blood pooling in the operative field.

Once tumor resection has been complete, any residual subarachnoid blood is irrigated out and meticulous hemostasis is achieved. Only then is the dura re-approximated in a watertight fashion confirmed with Valsalva maneuver. In cases where watertight closure cannot be achieved, we utilize both muscle patches and dural sealants to assist in closure. Subsequent multilayer closure is used to further reduce any concerns of postoperative cerebrospinal fluid (CSF) leak, starting with the paraspinal musculature to deep and then superficial fascia, finally finishing with skin. We place a subfascial drain to self-suction for the first 6 h after surgery and then revert to gravity suction. We keep the head of bed flat as to not aggravate any increased CSF pressures at the surgical site, and allow the patient to begin to mobilize 24 h after surgery.

Minimally Invasive Approaches

Other, less invasive approaches such as mini-open and tubular approaches have also been used in treating intradural pathologies of the spine. The argument for these minimally invasive surgery (MIS) approaches is that compared to more traditional open approaches, MIS can reduce soft-tissue disruption, limit facet injury, and preserve spinal stability better without compromising surgical resection intradurally in the spine [31]. Spinal endoscopy has also emerged as an arm of the MIS armamentarium—it provides improved visualization of ventral pathologies within the thecal sac providing surgeons with a posterior option to approach these tumors that would otherwise require an anterior or lateral approach. Further, complete tumor resection is possible for intradural lumbar tumors by means of an endoscopic approach only; however, there is a reasonably steep learning curve to be able to achieve this [32].

Microscopic Technique

After the tumor has been localized to the correct level at the dura of the spinal cord using adjuncts such as ultrasound, the microscope should be brought into the field. The operative microscope allows the surgeon to obtain an optimal view of the thecal sac and its content. This then enables precise dissection and delineation of tumor tissue from normal neural elements under optimized illumination. Specific to intradural lesions, microforceps and microdissectors should be used to distinguish and separate dural and arachnoid membranes [33]. Stay sutures can be used to assist in defining the tumor, and any vessels anastomosing with the tumor can be coagulated with bipolar cautery before sectioning. This allows the tumor to begin to be mobilized, and protection between normal neural parenchyma from the tumor can be achieved with cottonoid patties.

For lesions where en-bloc resection is possible or indicated (e.g., highly vascular tumors), surface coagulation can often shrink the tumor in size to allow it to be resected easier. However, for those large tumors, piecemeal resection beginning with debulking can sometimes be the only option. Debulking can occur with sharp dissection, or with an ultrasonic aspirator which is more protective against neural tissue injury. The walls of the tumor fall into the operating view as one operates in a circumferential manner, where the planes within the normal spinal parenchyma can be protected by cottonoids as the tumor reveals itself. In the case of tumors with poorly defined margins or those without margins, surgical judgment should be used to dictate the extent of resection, and can be guided using adjuncts such as ultrasound, neuronavigation, and fluorescence.

Surgery at the Lumbar Spinal Cord

Most tumors in the lumbar spinal cord are positioned in dorsal and dorsolateral locations in the thecal sac given the most common of these tumors originate from the dorsal nerve roots [34]. However, more lateral lesions can require facetectomy from this approach to be reached, which would then require consideration for simultaneous instrumentation and fusion to limit instability. For purely ventral lesions, consideration must be given to anterior approaches via a corpectomy.

Extramedullary lesions can then be isolated along the thecal sac and surgically targeted using a combination of dissection and cauterization. For intramedullary lesions, the spinal cord can be entered through one of the known safe entry zones—these include a median approach by a midline myelotomy, a paramedian approach by a posterolateral myelotomy at the dorsal root entry zone within the posterolateral sulcus, as well as a lateral approach at the level of the dentate ligament [35]. For tumors involving nerve roots, dorsal nerve roots can be resected with impunity. However, preservation of uninvolved ventral nerve roots is critical, especially in the lumbar spine. To identify functional structures, it is critical to use evoked EMG to stimulate ventral motor roots and identify nerves with preserved motor function.

For nerve sheath tumors, schwannomas and neurofibromas, a good understanding of fascicular anatomy is required. Individual fascicles can be separated from these tumors, facilitating en bloc resection of smaller tumors, whereas larger tumors typically require debulking. While the involved nerve root in schwannomas is typically nonfunctional, fascicle preservation should still be the goal, along with any functional rootlets (Fig. 14.4). This is in contrast to neurofibromas where the nerve root from which they origin is typically indistinguishable from the lesion. In these situations, tumor debulking and preservation of the anterior rootlets found to be functional is paramount. Those nerve roots confirmed to be nonfunctional on intraoperative stimulation can be sacrificed.

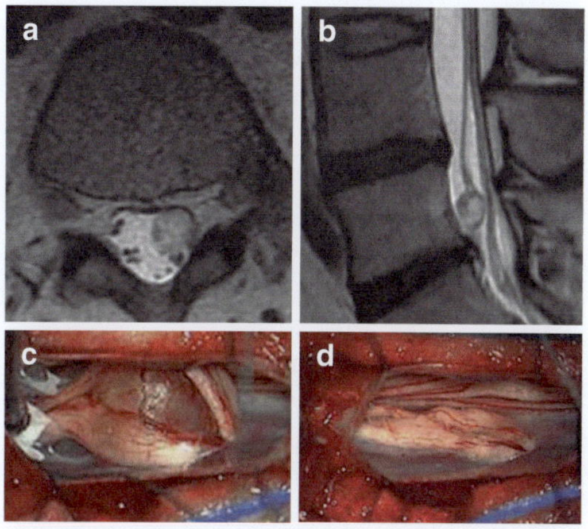

Fig. 14.4 Operative example of lumbar schwannoma seen on (**a**) axial T2 MRI and (**b**) sagittal T2 MRI. The thecal sac is opened (**c**) to reveal tumor, which is removed in its entirety after preserving surrounding fascicles to leave (**d**) the surrounding lumbar spine elements intact

Surgery at the Filum Terminale

It is recommended that lesion at the filum terminale be resected en bloc to improve recurrence and survival outcomes—for piecemeal resection increases risk of cerebrospinal fluid seeding and dissemination through the central nervous system [36]. The majority of these tumors in this area can be fully visualized from a posterior approach, using the standard techniques as described earlier—subperiosteal dissection, laminectomy,and dural opening. When tumors are less defined and/or highly vascularized (e.g., paragangliomas), close inspection after dural opening is often needed to define the relationship between the tumor and the filum, nerve roots, conus, and cauda equina. The filum should be identified using stimulation (0.5–1 mA) after which it can be coagulated with bipolar cautery and sectioned to allow for the lesion to be removed from the thecal sac [33]. When en bloc resection is not possible, subtotal resection should be a consideration to prevent neurologic deficit. Reasons this can happen about the filum terminale include intimate involvement of nerve roots and traction around other neural elements.

Conclusions

The lumbar spine is anatomically unique region of the spine as it involves both spinal cord and filum terminale. As a result, there is a wide range of intradural tumors that can occur in this region with a wide range of prognoses. Surgical considerations for these lesions include the use of electrophysiology, standard open approaches, emerging minimally invasive approaches, microscopic techniques, and specific surgical nuances based on the anatomical relation between the tumor and the spinal cord or filum terminale. Understanding these principles and techniques of treating these intradural lumbar spinal tumors will maximize outcomes.

Sources of Funding None.

References

1. Epstein FJ, Farmer JP, Freed D. Adult intramedullary spinal cord ependymomas: the result of surgery in 38 patients. J Neurosurg. 1993;79(2):204–9. https://doi.org/10.3171/jns.1993.79.2.0204.
2. Lu VM, Niazi TN. Pediatric spinal cord diseases. Pediatr Rev. 2021;42(9):486–99. https://doi.org/10.1542/pir.2020-000661.
3. Wald JT. Imaging of spine neoplasm. Radiol Clin North Am. 2012;50(4):749–76. https://doi.org/10.1016/j.rcl.2012.04.002.
4. Louis DN, Perry A, Wesseling P, Brat DJ, Cree IA, Figarella-Branger D, et al. The 2021 WHO classification of tumors of the central nervous system: a summary. Neuro-Oncology. 2021;23(8):1231–51. https://doi.org/10.1093/neuonc/noab106.
5. Smith AB, Soderlund KA, Rushing EJ, Smirniotopolous JG. Radiologic-pathologic correlation of pediatric and adolescent spinal neoplasms: part 1, intramedullary spinal neoplasms. Am J Roentgenol. 2012;198(1):34–43. https://doi.org/10.2214/AJR.10.7311.
6. Huisman TA. Pediatric tumors of the spine. Cancer Imaging. 2009;9(Special issue A):S45–8. https://doi.org/10.1102/1470-7330.2009.9012.
7. Sonneland PR, Scheithauer BW, Onofrio BM. Myxopapillary ependymoma. A clinicopathologic and immunocytochemical study of 77 cases. Cancer. 1985;56(4):883–93. https://doi.org/10.1002/1097-0142(19850815)56:4<883::aid-cncr2820560431>3.0.co;2-6.
8. Halliday AL, Sobel RA, Martuza RL. Benign spinal nerve sheath tumors: their occurrence sporadically and in neurofibromatosis types 1 and 2. J Neurosurg. 1991;74(2):248–53. https://doi.org/10.3171/jns.1991.74.2.0248.
9. Friedman DP, Tartaglino LM, Flanders AE. Intradural schwannomas of the spine: MR findings with emphasis on contrast-enhancement characteristics. AJR Am J Roentgenol. 1992;158(6):1347–50. https://doi.org/10.2214/ajr.158.6.1590138.
10. Fischer G, Brotchi J, Baleriaux D. Intramedullary spinal cord tumors. Thieme; 1996.
11. Seo HS, Kim JH, Lee DH, Lee YH, Suh SI, Kim SY, et al. Nonenhancing intramedullary astrocytomas and other MR imaging features: a retrospective study and systematic review. AJNR Am J Neuroradiol. 2010;31(3):498–503. https://doi.org/10.3174/ajnr.A1864.
12. Seki T, Hida K, Yano S, Aoyama T, Koyanagi I, Houkin K. Surgical outcomes of high-grade spinal cord gliomas. Asian Spine J. 2015;9(6):935–41. https://doi.org/10.4184/asj.2015.9.6.935.
13. Diaz-Aguilar D, ReFaey K, Clifton W, Durcanova B, Chen SG, Deen HG, et al. Prognostic factors and survival in low grade gliomas of the spinal cord: a population-based analysis from 2006 to 2012. J Clin Neurosci. 2019;61:14–21. https://doi.org/10.1016/j.jocn.2018.11.025.
14. Gouliamos AD, Kontogiannis DS, Androulidakis J, Kalovidouris AE, Vlahos LJ, Papavasiliou CG. Spinal neurilemmomas and neurofibromas: central dot sign in postgadolinium MRI. J Comput Assist Tomogr. 1993;17(3):446–8. https://doi.org/10.1097/00004728-199305000-00021.
15. Banks KP. The target sign: extremity. Radiology. 2005;234(3):899–900. https://doi.org/10.1148/radiol.2343030946.
16. Ducatman BS, Scheithauer BW, Piepgras DG, Reiman HM, Ilstrup DM. Malignant peripheral nerve sheath tumors. A clinicopathologic study of 120 cases. Cancer. 1986;57(10):2006–21.
17. Martin E, Coert JH, Flucke UE, Slooff WM, Ho VKY, van der Graaf WT, et al. A nationwide cohort study on treatment and survival in patients with malignant peripheral nerve sheath tumours. Eur J Cancer. 2020;124:77–87. https://doi.org/10.1016/j.ejca.2019.10.014.
18. Sevin IE, Dağ OD, Kahraman A, Sucu HK. A case of rare lumbar intradural tumor: paraganglioma. J Surg Case Rep. 2024;2024(2):rjae054. https://doi.org/10.1093/jscr/rjae054.
19. Wester DJ, Falcone S, Green BA, Camp A, Quencer RM. Paraganglioma of the filum: MR appearance. J Comput Assist Tomogr. 1993;17(6):967–9.

20. Gelabert-González M. Paragangliomas of the lumbar region. Report of two cases and review of the literature. J Neurosurg Spine. 2005;2(3):354–65. https://doi.org/10.3171/spi.2005.2.3.0354.
21. Corinaldesi R, Novegno F, Giovenali P, Lunardi T, Floris R, Lunardi P. Paraganglioma of the cauda equina region. Spine J. 2015;15(3):e1–8. https://doi.org/10.1016/j.spinee.2014.10.021.
22. Findlay JM, Bernstein M, Vanderlinden RG, Resch L. Microsurgical resection of solitary intramedullary spinal cord metastases. Neurosurgery. 1987;21(6):911–5. https://doi.org/10.1227/00006123-198712000-00022.
23. Sze G, Krol G, Zimmerman RD, Deck MD. Intramedullary disease of the spine: diagnosis using gadolinium-DTPA-enhanced MR imaging. AJR Am J Roentgenol. 1988;151(6):1193–204. https://doi.org/10.2214/ajr.151.6.1193.
24. Browne TR, Adams RD, Roberson GH. Hemangioblastoma of the spinal cord. Review and report of five cases. Arch Neurol. 1976;33(6):435–41. https://doi.org/10.1001/archneur.1976.00500060041009.
25. Kaelin WG. von Hippel–Lindau-associated malignancies: mechanisms and therapeutic opportunities. Drug Discovery Today Dis Mech. 2005;2(2):225–31. https://doi.org/10.1016/j.ddmec.2005.04.003.
26. Baker KB, Moran CJ, Wippold FJ 2nd, Smirniotopoulos JG, Rodriguez FJ, Meyers SP, et al. MR imaging of spinal hemangioblastoma. AJR Am J Roentgenol. 2000;174(2):377–82. https://doi.org/10.2214/ajr.174.2.1740377.
27. Corr P, Dicker T, Wright M. Exophytic intramedullary hemangioblastoma presenting as an extramedullary mass on myelography. AJNR Am J Neuroradiol. 1995;16(4 Suppl):883–4.
28. Westwick HJ, Giguère JF, Shamji MF. Incidence and prognosis of spinal Hemangioblastoma: a surveillance epidemiology and end results study. Neuroepidemiology. 2016;46(1):14–23. https://doi.org/10.1159/000441147.
29. Roux FX, Nataf F, Pinaudeau M, Borne G, Devaux B, Meder JF. Intraspinal meningiomas: review of 54 cases with discussion of poor prognosis factors and modern therapeutic management. Surg Neurol. 1996;46(5):458–63; discussion 63–4. https://doi.org/10.1016/s0090-3019(96)00199-1.
30. Hohenberger C, Hau P, Schebesch K-M, Kölbl O, Riemenschneider MJ, Pohl F, et al. Spinal meningiomas. Neuro-oncol Adv. 2023;5(Supplement_1):i112–i21. https://doi.org/10.1093/noajnl/vdad013.
31. Mende KC, Krätzig T, Mohme M, Westphal M, Eicker SO. Keyhole approaches to intradural pathologies. Neurosurg Focus. 2017;43(2):E5. https://doi.org/10.3171/2017.5.Focus17198.
32. Parihar VS, Yadav N, Yadav YR, Ratre S, Bajaj J, Kher Y. Endoscopic management of spinal intradural extramedullary tumors. J Neurol Surg A Cent Eur Neurosurg. 2017;78(3):219–26. https://doi.org/10.1055/s-0036-1594014.
33. Moriwaki T, Iwatsuki K, Ohnishi Y, Ninomiya K, Yoshimine T. Extramedullary conus Ependymoma involving a lumbar nerve root with filum Terminale attachment. Clin Med Insights Case Rep. 2015;8:101–4. https://doi.org/10.4137/CCRep.S24719.
34. Moses ZB, Barzilai O, O'Toole JE. Benign Intradural and Paraspinal nerve sheath tumors: advanced surgical techniques. Neurosurg Clin N Am. 2020;31(2):221–9. https://doi.org/10.1016/j.nec.2019.11.002.
35. Ottenhausen M, Ntoulias G, Bodhinayake I, Ruppert F-H, Schreiber S, Förschler A, et al. Intradural spinal tumors in adults—update on management and outcome. Neurosurg Rev. 2019;42 https://doi.org/10.1007/s10143-018-0957-x.
36. Bagley CA, Wilson S, Kothbauer KF, Bookland MJ, Epstein F, Jallo GI. Long term outcomes following surgical resection of myxopapillary ependymomas. Neurosurg Rev. 2009;32(3):321–34; discussion 34. https://doi.org/10.1007/s10143-009-0190-8.

Metastatic Disease to the Lumbar Spine

15

Puya Alikhani, Carballo-Cuello Cesar, Kumar Jay, and Soto-Rubio Diego

Introduction

Every year, 1.7 million people are diagnosed with cancer in the United States, of which up to 20–40% are expected to develop metastases to the spine [1]. The number of patients is expected to increase thanks to better therapeutic modalities and early detection. These advancements have led to a higher prevalence of patients diagnosed with metastatic disease, including those with spinal metastases [2, 3].

A metastatic lesion is defined as the dissemination of neoplastic cells from a primary site to an alternate location. These cells possess the ability to implant and proliferate at distant or adjacent locations [4]. Bone metastases are observed in 30% to 70% of cancer patients, with spinal involvement reported in up to 40% of this demographic. The lumbar spine accounts for approximately 20% of all spinal metastases, whereas the thoracic spine is recognized as the most affected segment [3].

P. Alikhani (✉) · C.-C. Cesar · K. Jay · S.-R. Diego
Department of Neurosurgery and Brain Repair, University of South Florida, Morsani College of Medicine, Tampa, FL, USA
e-mail: palikhan@usf.edu; cesarcarballo@usf.edu; jayk1@usf.edu; diegosotorubio@usf.edu

Pathophysiology

Direct invasion into the vertebral body can serve as the initial site of spread and may also enable tumor cells to metastasize to other distant osseous structures [5]. However, many hypotheses regarding tumor dispersion exist. The most accepted theory consists of a "seed and soil" hypothesis, where tumor cells proliferate in distant environments, providing enough resources to support their growth [6]. Spreading routes include not only direct invasion but also lymphatic, intraspinal, and hematologic routes. The Batson's vertebral plexus plays an important role in these mechanisms [7]. This valveless venous plexus provides a path for tumors invading abdominal structures to spread to axial structures, including the vertebral bodies. The ability of the primary tumor to escape immunological control is another factor that plays a role.

Prostate, lung, and breast cancer are the most common types of cancer invading the lumbar spine, followed by ovarian, multiple myeloma, and hematologic tumors [8]. Some exhibit a propensity to localize at specific vertebral levels; however, no standardized imaging follow-up protocol has been established based on the pathological characteristics or the anticipated site of dissemination within the lumbar segments [9].

A. A. Baaj et al. (eds.), *Surgery of the Lumbar Spine*, https://doi.org/10.1007/978-3-032-18097-1_15

Localization

Metastases to the lumbar spine, similar to those affecting the thoracic or cervical levels, can also be classified by location relative to the dura mater and their impact on the spinal cord. The dura acts as a robust anatomical barrier rarely breached by tumors. Most spinal metastases are extradural and compressive, although up to 6% of cases may involve intradural metastases. Lung and breast cancers are the most common causes of this type of spread, with renal cell carcinoma also reported in rare instances [10–12].

Compared with the thoracic spine, the lumbar spine poses unique challenges for decompression and stabilization because of its larger vertebrae, greater mobility, and increased loads, which raises the risk of neurologic deficits due to its nonexpendable lumbar nerve roots. Additionally, the retroperitoneal extension of lumbar malignancies is another distinct feature of metastases in this region, although its impact on surgical outcomes remains unclear [3]. Bone mineral density also plays a role in injury risk [13]. The higher mechanical stress carried by the lumbar spine often means that pathological fractures are among the first presenting symptoms, and studies suggest that tumor shape, location, and infiltration patterns also contribute to their development [14].

Scoring Systems

During a spine-invading oncological illness, patients and their care providers are often confronted with multiple treatment modalities. Decision-making is mainly influenced by disease progression and life expectancy [15]. Different therapeutic modalities have proven effective in improving symptoms and neurological conditions. However, there is still no definite consensus regarding the ideal treatment. For this reason, multiple criteria have been described to calculate scores that can objectively provide guidance.

The treatment of metastatic spine tumors is based on the premise that interventions are palliative and offered to reduce pain, improve or maintain neurological function, restore mechanical stability, and achieve local tumor control. A framework that incorporates neurologic, oncologic, mechanical stability, and systemic disease considerations (NOMS) is used to help delineate the best treatment for the patient (Fig. 15.1) [16]. The NOMS framework is a treatment paradigm that considers four key elements in a patient's clinical status to perform the optimal treatment modality [17].

The neurologic component considers the patient's degree of epidural spinal cord compression (ESCC) and its clinical manifestations, including myelopathy or functional radiculopathy. More recently, a new ESCC scale, consisting of a 6-point MRI grading system that divides ESCC according to T2-weighted axial views, was developed [18].

The oncologic component considers tumor responsiveness to conventional-dose radiation therapy (cEBRT) as either radiosensitive or radioresistant. The combination of a radioresistant tumor with ESCC has historically led patients to be offered surgery as the initial therapeutic intervention as opposed to radiation. Thus, radiosensitive tumors benefit from cEBRT alone, which leads to tumor apoptosis and immediate cord decompression [19]. Recent advances in the field have led to the development of image-guided radiation therapy (IGRT), which is a method of radiation treatment that provides conformal radiation doses with high spatial precision. This allows for the delivery of high doses of radiation to the desired treatment regions while minimizing the radiation dose to critical adjacent structures. Recent advancements in stereotactic radiosurgery (SRS) have allowed greater flexibility in the treatment of metastatic spine tumors, particularly those resistant to cEBRT, which are now considered sensitive and responsive to SRS [20]. Radiosensitive tumors such as myeloma, lymphoma, seminoma, breast, prostate, and ovarian tumors typically achieve durable local control with cEBRT. Renal, thyroid, colon, hepatocellular, sarcoma, non-small cell lung cancer, and melanoma tend to be radioresistant, and for these patients, SRS delivered by IGRT has been shown to achieve durable tumor control with low rates of toxicity [21–24].

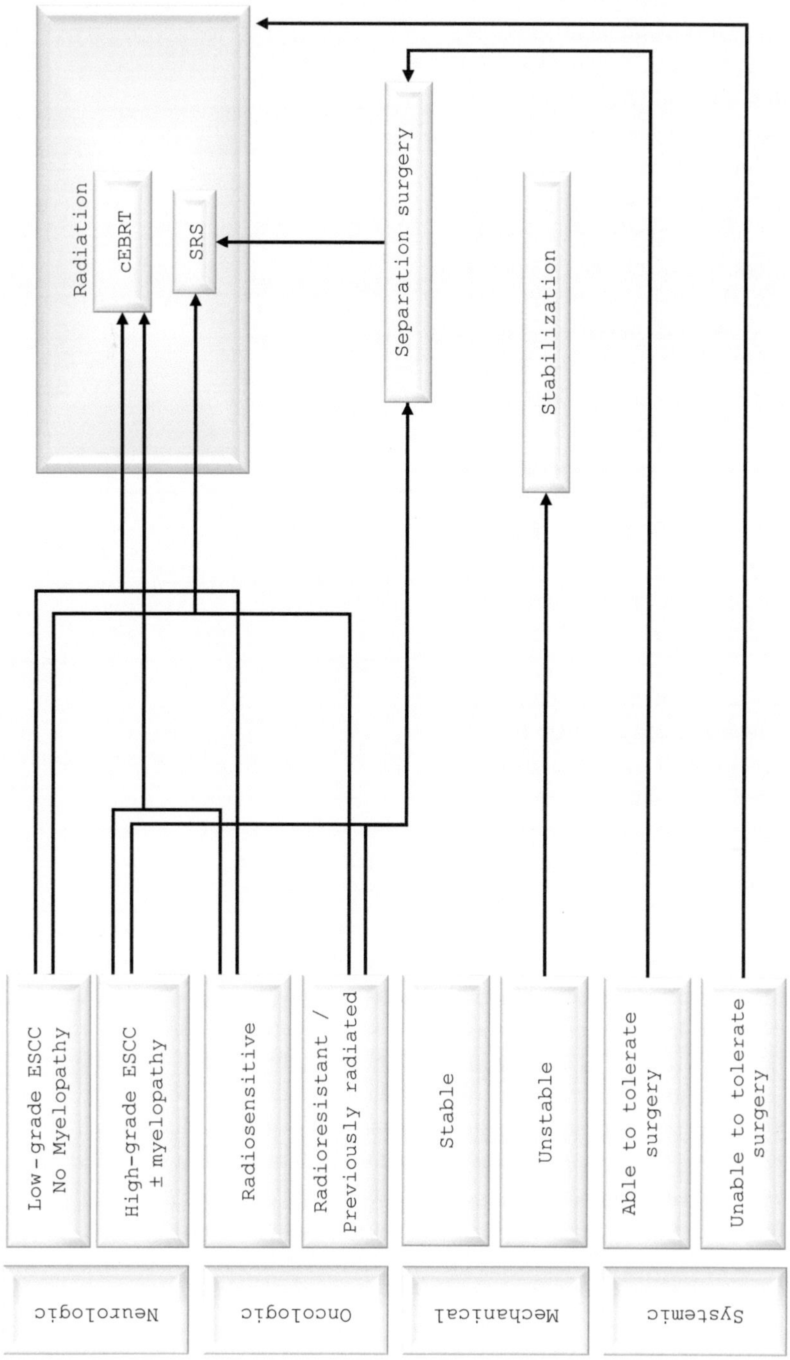

Fig. 15.1 Neurologic, oncologic, mechanical, and systemic (NOMS) decision framework. cEBRT: conventional external beam radiation therapy; ESCC: epidural spinal cord compression; SRS: stereotactic radiosurgery. (Adapted from Laufer, 2013, used with permission, ©2013)

The mechanical assessment evaluates the stability of the spine at the level of the disease, indicating the need for surgical stabilization. The Spine Oncology Study Group (SOSG) defines spinal instability as a "loss of spinal integrity as a result of a neoplastic process that is associated with movement-related pain, deformity, and/or neural compromise under physiologic loads [25]. Under this definition, the SOSG developed a scoring system, the Spinal Instability Neoplastic Score (SINS), to assess mechanical stability (Table 15.1) [25]. The score considers six parameters: location, pain, alignment, osteolysis, vertebral body collapse, and/or posterior element involvement. High SINS scores (13–18) suggest the need for surgical stabilization, whereas low SINS scores (0–6) are considered stable. Scores ranging from 7 to 12 are considered intermediate, and the need for surgical treatment is surgeon-dependent [26]. Patients with unstable fractures usually demonstrate severe movement-related pain and present with mechanical radiculopathy upon axial loading due to narrowing of the neural foramen.

Systemic component analyses are performed if the patient can physiologically tolerate the systemic disease and its medical comorbidities. This aims at survival prediction and whether surgery will be an acceptable risk owing to the patient's medical complications. A multidisciplinary team approach, including oncology, radiation oncology, and spine surgery, should be considered to determine the systemic disease of each patient, and tumor board discussions should be held.

Recently, the New England Spinal Metastasis Score (NESMS) has been described as a simple, informative scoring scheme that could be applied to both operative and nonoperative patients due to its ability to predict mortality at 3 months and 1 year and ambulatory function at 3 and 6 months [15].

Table 15.1 Radiographic features according to the Spinal Instability in Neoplasia (SINS) score

Component	Score
Location	
Junctional (O-C2; C7-T2; T11-L1; L5-S1)	3
Mobile spine (C3-6; L2-4)	2
Semirigid (T3-10)	1
Rigid (S2-S5)	0
Mechanical pain	
Yes	3
No	1
Pain free lesion	0
Bone lesion	
Lytic	2
Mixed (lytic/blastic)	1
Blastic	0
Radiographic spinal alignment	
Subluxation/translation present	4
Deformity (kyphosis/scoliosis)	2
Normal	0
Vertebral body collapse	
>50% collapse	3
<50% collapse	2
No collapse with >50% body involved	1
None of the above	0
Posterolateral involvement	
Bilateral	3
Unilateral	1
None of the above	0

Adapted from Fisher, 2010, used with permission, ©2010

Treatment

The goal of surgical treatment for spinal metastatic disease with lumbar compromise is to stabilize a spine with signs of mechanical instability, preserve neurologic function, remove epidural disease to allow stereotactic radiosurgery (SBRT) treatment, establish a histological diagnosis when needed, and provide local control when radiotherapy cannot be safely delivered [27]. This goal is to optimally obtain symptom palliation, which may lead to improved quality of life (QOL) [28].

Surgical Modalities

Historically, spinal metastasis had been treated by posterior decompression alone, resulting in poor clinical outcomes and increasing the need for treatment with a lower complication rate [28]. Direct decompressive surgery plus postoperative radiotherapy quickly became an alternative, offering superior results to radiotherapy alone for patients with spinal cord compression.

Excisional Surgery

En bloc spondylectomy, whose purpose is to remove the entirety or most of the tumor, achieve local control of the disease, and minimize tumor seeding in the surgical bed, is often followed by surgical instrumentation. Depending on the approach, this arthrodesis can be performed posteriorly, anteriorly, or through a combined approach [30]. Despite its apparent benefits, this surgical technique is restricted in the lumbar spine due to limited visualization of the ventral structures, which increases the risk of vascular injuries, given the attachment of the psoas and iliacus muscles [27].

More extensive surgical procedures have been shown to produce neurological improvement rates of up to 42%, which are higher than the rates offered by radiotherapy alone. This neurological improvement tends to be greater with more extensive decompressions; however, surgical morbidity is also strongly positively correlated, ranging from 21% to 26% in more aggressive decompressions [27].

Achieving bony union is also crucial for maintaining long-term spinal stability after reconstruction. The literature supports using anterior reconstruction with either a prefabricated prosthetic or polymethyl methacrylate (PMMA) bone cement. Evidence also supports using an anterior construct reinforced with bilateral posterior instrumentation when performing three-column reconstruction [29]. The use of bone grafts also faces a challenging environment in the context of metastatic spine disease, as it is well-documented that local irradiation and chemotherapeutic agents prevent bone remodeling and fusion [29].

Separation Surgery

This term describes the procedure, which includes circumferential resection of the epidural tumor from the thecal sac to effectively decompress it and provide an adequate margin of 2–3 mm for adjuvant radiation. Surgical goals have now been modified to maintain stability and neural function and achieve decompression of neural elements, allowing safe and effective delivery of radiosurgery to achieve local tumor control.

Separation surgery is mostly used in patients with radioresistant tumors, followed by stereotactic radiosurgery (SRS), for which the recurrence rate at 1 year is as low as 16.4%, which has increased its popularity.

Palliative Surgery

Surgical decision-making in patients with survival expectancy between 3 and 6 months is perhaps the most complex. Surgical treatment for this subset of patients should be aimed at effectively reducing pain while lowering rates of complications [30]. Within this philosophy, non-fusion surgery, without reconstruction, may be considered as a preferable choice when opting for a surgical procedure. Aimed at lowering spinal cord compression and reduction of pain [31].

Cement Augmentation

Cement augmentation, also considered a palliative measure, is the least invasive surgical treatment available for patients with lumbar metastasis. Two surgical techniques coexist: vertebroplasty and kyphoplasty. Both aim to reduce pain and, in the case of kyphoplasty, reconstruct vertebral height.

Although minimally invasive, cement augmentation has its own risk profile, which can lead to additional surgery. Different elements of the procedure have been investigated, revealing that the wall integrity of the vertebral body, the competency of the posterior tension band, and the location of the kyphoplasty at the junctional spinal level serve as risk factors leading to surgical complications [32].

The use of cement augmentation via percutaneous fenestrated pedicle screws for stability is a recent trend and has been shown to be effective as a method to increase the durability of spine surgery in cancer patients [33].

Minimally Invasive Surgery

Minimally invasive stabilization and decompression is increasingly recommended for patients with metastatic spinal disease, due to shorter postoperative recovery times and decreased morbidity. The use of tubular approaches to minimize tissue retraction may be an option when offering decompression or resection [27].

Conservative Treatment

Lumbar metastatic disease is generally painful and incapacitating. In patients in whom surgical intervention is not indicated, conservative measures are taken to improve the patient's QOL. Non-surgical interventions are used as coadjutants to the primary oncological treatment. Often provided treatments include pain management, anti-inflammatory drugs, and bisphosphonates in some instances.

Radiotherapy is an additional option for symptom control in non-operative patients. Although it is generally not recommended in the acute setting, it may also be considered postoperatively for selected patients [34].

References

1. National Cancer Institute. Cancer trends progress report [Internet]. https://progressreport.cancer.gov. 2024 [cited 2024 Oct 29]. Available from: https://progressreport.cancer.gov.
2. Rose PS, Buchowski JM. Metastatic disease in the thoracic and lumbar spine: evaluation and management. JAAOS – J Am Acad Orthop Surg. 2011;19. Available from: https://journals.lww.com/jaaos/fulltext/2011/01000/metastatic_disease_in_the_thoracic_and_lumbar.5.aspx.
3. Holman PJ, Suki D, McCutcheon I, Wolinsky J-P, Rhines LD, Gokaslan ZL. Surgical management of metastatic disease of the lumbar spine: experience with 139 patients. J Neurosurg Spine. 2005;2:550–63. Available from: https://thejns.org/spine/view/journals/j-neurosurg-spine/2/5/article-p550.xml.
4. Maccauro G, Spinelli MS, Mauro S, Perisano C, Graci C, Rosa MA. Physiopathology of spine metastasis. Int J Surg Oncol. 2011;2011:1–8.
5. Liao TY, Liaw CC, Tsui KH, Juan YH. Invasion of adjacent lumbar vertebral body from renal pelvis carcinoma: associated with bone metastasis but easily overlooked on initial CT scan. In Vivo (Brooklyn). 2019;33:939–43.
6. Langley RR, Fidler IJ. The seed and soil hypothesis revisited-the role of tumor-stroma interactions in metastasis to different organs. Int J Cancer. 2011;128:2527–35.
7. Carpenter K, Decater T, Iwanaga J, Maulucci CM, Bui CJ, Dumont AS, et al. Revisiting the vertebral venous plexus–a comprehensive review of the literature. World Neurosurg. 2021;145:381–95. Available from: https://www.sciencedirect.com/science/article/pii/S1878875020321963.
8. Jayarangaiah A, Kemp AK, Theetha Kariyanna P. Bone metastasis. Treasure Island (FL): StatPearls Publishing. 2024. [cited 2024 Oct 29]; Available from: https://www.ncbi.nlm.nih.gov/books/NBK507911/.
9. Amelot A, Terrier LM, Cristini J, LeNail LR, Buffenoir K, Pascal-Moussellard H, et al. Approaching spinal metastases spread profile. Surg Oncol. 2019;31:61–6.
10. Jacobs WB, Perrin RG. Evaluation and treatment of spinal metastases: an overview. Neurosurgical Focus FOC. 2001;11:1–11. Available from: https://thejns.org/focus/view/journals/neurosurg-focus/11/6/foc.2001.11.6.11.xml.
11. Alfieri A, Mazzoleni G, Schwarz A, Campello M, Broger M, Vitale M, et al. Renal cell carcinoma and Intradural spinal metastasis with cauda Equina infiltration: case report. Spine (Phila Pa 1976). 2005;30. Available from: https://journals.lww.com/spinejournal/fulltext/2005/01010/renal_cell_carcinoma_and_intradural_spinal.26.aspx.
12. Cansever T, Kabatas S, Civelek E, Yilmaz C, Caner H. Spinal metastasis of occult lung carcinoma causing cauda equine syndrome with lumbar spinal stenosis. Turk Neurosurg. 2011;21:408–12.
13. Salvatore G, Berton A, Giambini H, Ciuffreda M, Florio P, Longo UG, et al. Biomechanical effects of metastasis in the osteoporotic lumbar spine: a finite element analysis. BMC Musculoskelet Disord. 2018;19:38.
14. Tschirhart CE, Nagpurkar A, Whyne CM. Effects of tumor location, shape and surface serration on burst fracture risk in the metastatic spine. J Biomech. 2004;37:653–60.
15. Schoenfeld AJ, Ferrone ML, Blucher JA, Agaronnik N, Nguyen L, Tobert DG, et al. Prospective comparison of the accuracy of the New England Spinal Metastasis Score (NESMS) to legacy scoring systems in prognosticating outcomes following treatment of spinal metastases. Spine J. 2022;22:39–48.

16. Laufer I, Rubin DG, Lis E, Cox BW, Stubblefield MD, Yamada Y, et al. The NOMS framework: approach to the treatment of spinal metastatic tumors. Oncologist. 2013;18:744–51.
17. Liu JKC, Laufer I, Bilsky MH. Update on management of vertebral column tumors. CNS Oncol. 2014;3:137–47.
18. Bilsky MH, Laufer I, Fourney DR, Groff M, Schmidt MH, Varga PP, et al. Reliability analysis of the epidural spinal cord compression scale. J Neurosurg Spine. 2010;13:324–8.
19. Bilsky MH, Lis E, Raizer J, Lee H, Boland P. The diagnosis and treatment of metastatic spinal tumor. Oncologist. 1999;4:459–69.
20. Gerszten PC, Mendel E, Yamada Y. Radiotherapy and radiosurgery for metastatic spine disease: what are the options, indications, and outcomes? Spine (Phila Pa 1976). 2009;34. Available from: https://journals.lww.com/spinejournal/fulltext/2009/10151/radiotherapy_and_radiosurgery_for_metastatic_spine.11.aspx.
21. Chang EL, Shiu AS, Mendel E, Mathews LA, Mahajan A, Allen PK, et al. Phase I/II study of stereotactic body radiotherapy for spinal metastasis and its pattern of failure. J Neurosurg Spine. 2007;7:151–60.
22. Gibbs IC, Kamnerdsupaphon P, Ryu MR, Dodd R, Kiernan M, Chang SD, et al. Image-guided robotic radiosurgery for spinal metastases. Radiother Oncol. 2007;82:185–90.
23. Ryu S, Yin FF, Rock J, Zhu J, Chu A, Kagan E, et al. Image-guided and intensity-modulated radiosurgery for patients with spinal metastasis. Cancer. 2003;97:2013–8.
24. Moulding HD, Elder JB, Lis E, Lovelock DM, Zhang Z, Yamada Y, et al. Local disease control after decompressive surgery and adjuvant high-dose single-fraction radiosurgery for spine metastases: clinical article. J Neurosurg Spine. 2010;13:87–93.
25. Fisher CG, DiPaola CP, Ryken TC, Bilsky MH, Shaffrey CI, Berven SH, et al. A novel classification system for spinal instability in neoplastic disease: an evidence-based approach and expert consensus from the Spine Oncology Study Group. Spine (Phila Pa 1976). 2010;35. Available from: https://journals.lww.com/spinejournal/fulltext/2010/10150/a_novel_classification_system_for_spinal.19.aspx.
26. Fourney DR, Frangou EM, Ryken TC, DiPaola CP, Shaffrey CI, Berven SH, et al. Spinal instability neoplastic score: an analysis of reliability and validity from the spine Oncology Study Group. J Clin Oncol. 2011;29:3072–7.
27. Al Farii H, Aoude A, Al Shammasi A, Reynolds J, Weber M. Surgical management of the metastatic spine disease: a review of the literature and proposed algorithm. Glob Spine J. 2023;13:486–98.
28. Barzilai O, Versteeg AL, Sahgal A, Rhines LD, Bilsky MH, Sciubba DM, et al. Survival, local control, and health-related quality of life in patients with oligometastatic and polymetastatic spinal tumors: a multicenter, international study. Cancer. 2019;125:770–8.
29. Altaf F, Weber M, Dea N, Boriani S, Ames C, Williams R, et al. Evidence-based review and survey of expert opinion of reconstruction of metastatic spine tumors. Spine (Phila Pa 1976) Lippincott Williams and Wilkins. 2016;41:S254–61.
30. Hamad A, Vachtsevanos L, Cattell A, Ockendon M, Balain B. Minimally invasive spinal surgery for the management of symptomatic spinal metastasis. Br J Neurosurg. 2017;31:526–30.
31. Suvithayasiri S, Santipas B, Wilartratsami S, Ruangchainikom M, Luksanapruksa P. Non-fusion palliative spine surgery without reconstruction is safe and effective in spinal metastasis patients: retrospective study. Sci Rep. 2021;11:17486.
32. Rajah G, Altshuler D, Sadiq O, Nyame VK, Eltahawy H, Szerlip N. Predictors of delayed failure of structural kyphoplasty for pathological compression fractures in cancer patients. J Neurosurg Spine. 2015;23:228–32.
33. Barzilai O, McLaughlin L, Lis E, Reiner AS, Bilsky MH, Laufer I. Utility of cement augmentation via percutaneous fenestrated pedicle screws for stabilization of cancer-related spinal instability. Operative Neurosurg. 2019;16:593–9.
34. Rispoli R, Reverberi C, Targato G, D'Agostini S, Fasola G, Trovò M, et al. Multidisciplinary approach to patients with metastatic spinal cord compression: a diagnostic therapeutic algorithm to improve the neurological outcome. Front Oncol. 2022;12:902928.

16 Lumbo-Sacral Primary Tumors

Zach Pennington, Daniel Schneider, Sheng-Fu Larry Lo, and Daniel M. Sciubba

Introduction and Epidemiology

Primary vertebral column tumors comprise both benign and malignant pathologies, with prior population-level surveillance data suggesting primary vertebral column malignancies to occur at an annualized rate of 0.36–0.54 cases per 100,000 person-years [1]. Incidence increases with age, ranging from 0.38 per 100,000 person-years in young patients (20–29 years old) to 3.08 per 100,000 person-years in those aged ≥80, with a slight male predominance [1, 2]. In surgical datasets, [3–7] patients are most commonly in the 5th–7th decade of life. This trend reflects both the attrition due to mortality from other causes and the increased risks associated with surgical intervention in older patients. The exception to this is Ewing sarcoma, which disproportionately affects patients in the second and third decades of life [3].

Malignant lesions such as chordoma, chondrosarcoma, osteosarcoma, and Ewing sarcoma show differences in their age of detection and relative prognosis [2]. With the exception of Ewing sarcoma, *en bloc* resection with negative margins is considered the gold standard as it is associated with improved progression-free survival [2–9]. For Ewing sarcoma, neoadjuvant chemotherapy is critical to overall survival as it has been associated with improved survival [3], and it may additionally shrink the tumor and thereby improve the success of surgical resection.

Diagnosis and Preoperative Workup

Patients with primary lumbosacral vertebral neoplasms commonly present with non-specific symptoms, such as back pain or pelvic pain [10]. As the tumor progresses, symptoms may become more specific, prompting imaging that leads to detection of the mass. The expanding tumor may involve local neural structures, including the thecal sac and lumbosacral nerve roots, resulting in radicular pain, paresthesias, sensory loss, weakness, and/or bowel/bladder dysfunction. Additionally, erosion of the surrounding bone can cause instability of the lumbar spine (or for sacral tumors the sacroiliac joint), with resultant mechanical pain.

Once the lesion has been detected, the patient should undergo pathologic diagnosis and staging along with consideration for referral to a high-volume center due to the improved survival outcomes observed at these centers [11]. Staging imaging includes both local staging—definition

Z. Pennington
Department of Neurologic Surgery, Mayo Clinic, Rochester, MN, USA

D. Schneider · S.-F. L. Lo · D. M. Sciubba (✉)
Department of Neurosurgery, Donald and Barbara Zucker School of Medicine at Hofstra/Northwell Health, Manhasset, NY, USA
e-mail: dsciubba1@northwell.edu

A. A. Baaj et al. (eds.), *Surgery of the Lumbar Spine*, https://doi.org/10.1007/978-3-032-18097-1_16

of the anatomic relationships of the tumor to the surrounding structures—and systemic staging—evaluation of the patient's global disease burden. Local staging for lesions in the mobile spine is typically performed using the Weinstein-Boriani-Biagini system [12]. The revised eighth edition of the American Joint Committee on Cancer presented a similar local staging methodology, though it has not been used as extensively within the spine oncology community [13].

Systemic staging is critical to assess whether the morbidity of aggressive surgical resection is justified given the known negative prognostic impact of disseminated disease on survival outcomes [14, 15]. Imaging should include a computed tomography (CT) scan of the chest, abdomen, and pelvis to look for metastatic disease, given the predilection for bony sarcomas to disseminate to the lung tissue. Nuclear testing can also be employed and may help to improve the accuracy of staging [16]. Technitium-99 m (Tc99m) bone scintigraphy was previously used as a mechanism for assessing the presence of other skeletal metastases and makes use of a radioactively labeled bisphosphonate analog that is taken up by regions with high bone turnover, such as occult fractures, osteomyelitis, and malignancy. However, increasingly staging is performed with positron-emission tomography, which makes use of 18-fluorodeoxyglucose to label metabolically active cells, such as tumor cells. PET/CT has been shown to have greater sensitivity relative to bone scintigraphy [17] and can also be used to evaluate for visceral metastases.

Pathologic diagnosis should be performed via CT-guided core needle biopsy, which has been shown to have superior diagnostic accuracy relative to fine needle aspirate [18]. A sheathed needle should be considered for reduction of tumor seeding risk, and the biopsy tract should be planned along a trajectory that allows for resection of the biopsy tract as needed [8]. Repeat biopsy and biopsy of multiple sites both offer little additional diagnostic yield, but may increase the risk of seeding [9]. Should the biopsy demonstrate the lesion to be a metastatic pathology, piecemeal resection with or without local reconstruction/stabilization is reasonable and the reader is referred to Chap. 15.

Lastly, preoperative evaluation should include a general medical evaluation to determine the patient's appropriateness for surgery, along with upright 36″ radiographs. Though the primary objective of surgical management of primary vertebral column tumors is oncologic cure, consideration of the patient's native alignment is imperative as inadequate reconstruction can result in post-resection deformity and complications. This is especially true for patients undergoing total sacrectomy, where the resection creates lumbopelvic dissociation and care must be taken to restore the native spinopelvic alignment [19].

Operative Management

Resection

Where *en bloc* resection is sought, care must be taken to avoid violation of the tumor capsule. This can often involve healthy nerve root sacrifice to avoid disruption of the specimen. Tumors generally respect the disc spaces, which can be used to set the cranial and caudal bounds of the resection. For lumbo-sacral lesions (Fig. 16.1), a staged posterior-anterior approach is generally performed as this allows for anterior delivery of the specimen thereby minimizing the likelihood that nerve root sacrifice is required; such sacrifice is unavoidable with posterior specimen delivery. The posterior approach is performed first. Initial dissection of the bony elements is performed, followed by instrumentation to stabilize the spine following tumor delivery. The posterior elements are then removed at the level of the planned spondylectomy to reveal the thecal sac and associated roots. To deliver the posterior elements *en bloc* Tomita wires can be passed around the pedicles, which are then transected, allowing for delivery. However, with the rise of ultrasonic bone-cutting instruments, we increasingly rely on these tools for their precision, control, and decreased risk of inadvertent injury to adjacent structures. Nerve roots are then mobilized; those involved in the

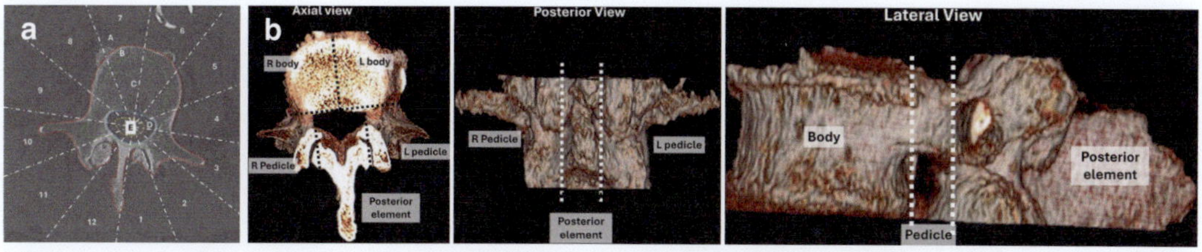

Fig. 16.1 (**a**) The Weinstein-Boriani-Biagini (WBB) system was devised to morphologically characterize primary tumor morphology and help guide surgical planning for *en bloc* resection. The system divides the vertebral body into five concentric tissue rings and 12 sectors to describe the tumoral involvement of both the load-bearing portions of the vertebra and the adjacent neurovascular structures. The tissues rings from outermost to innermost are the extraosseous soft tissues (A), superficial layers of bone (B), deep/medullary/cancellous bone (C), epidural space (D), and intradural space (E). The sectors are numbered as a clockface with sectors 12 and 1 straddling the spinous process, and the numbers proceeding clockwise, with sectors 5–8 encompassing the vertebral body, and sectors 4 and 9 encompassing the left and right pedicles. (**b**) American Joint Committee on Cancer staging for spine tumors. In the AJCC system the body is divided into left and right hemivertebrae, and the posterior elements are divided into a central spinous process/medial lamina component (posterior element) and bilateral posterolateral compartments including the transverse processes, pedicles, and lateral hemilaminae

tumor that are to be delivered with the specimen are ligated proximal to their entry into the tumor. A temporary rod is then placed unilaterally to stabilize the spine during tumor release. The psoas muscles are freed bilaterally from the vertebral column, leaving a rim of psoas muscle on the tumor to preserve a tumor-free margin. The PLL and surrounding posterior and lateral annulus of the cranial and caudal disc spaces are cut in preparation for final anterior release left for the anterior stage. A silastic sheath is placed ventral to the thecal sac and nerve roots to serve as both a protective layer as well as a surgical landmark for the second stage. This also ensures all remaining neural elements have been dissected and are free from the specimen. The final rods are then contoured and placed, and the remaining bony surfaces are decorticated, and bone graft is placed. The second, anterior, stage is then performed with the assistance of general or vascular surgery for the laparotomy and exposure of the ventral spine. Aorto-bifemoral and inferior vena-cava-bifemoral bypasses may be necessary to achieve negative margins in those patients with involvement of the great vessels [20]. The lumbar segmental vessels are sacrificed to allow for more extensive vessel mobilization. Once the great vessels have been mobilized completely, the cranial and caudal discectomies are completed along with any additional paraspinal dissection followed by *en bloc* delivery of the tumor. Reconstruction can then be performed with strut allograft, vascularized strut graft, or a titanium cage. Vascularized fibular strut autograft offers a theoretically increased chance of osseous fusion, but has been reported to have poorer weight-bearing capacity relative to distractable cages [21].

For sacral lesions (Fig. 16.2), multi-level nerve root sacrifice is often required, though the resultant morbidity must be discussed preoperatively with the patient. If there is no established rectal or anterior vasculature involvement, an all-posterior approach can be pursued [22]. This proceeds with exposure of the sacrum and lower lumbar spine; if the tumor involves the dorsal sacrum, then exposure should respect the lumbosacral fascia to preserve a capsule around the tumor. The fascia is incised cephalad to the planned cranial osteotomy, and the paraspinal muscles are elevated cranially away from their lumbopelvic insertions. L5 and S1 laminectomies are performed to expose the thecal sac (laminectomy proceeds more caudally for tumors involving only the distal sacrum), and the nerve roots are isolated. Those involved in the tumor are ligated with silk suture and osteotomies are made laterally through the alae or medial iliac wing (depending upon the extent of the tumor) to isolate the tumor specimen. The cranial osteotomy (or L5/S1 diskectomy in the case of total sacrectomy) is then performed which completes the bony releases, allowing for initial gentle ele-

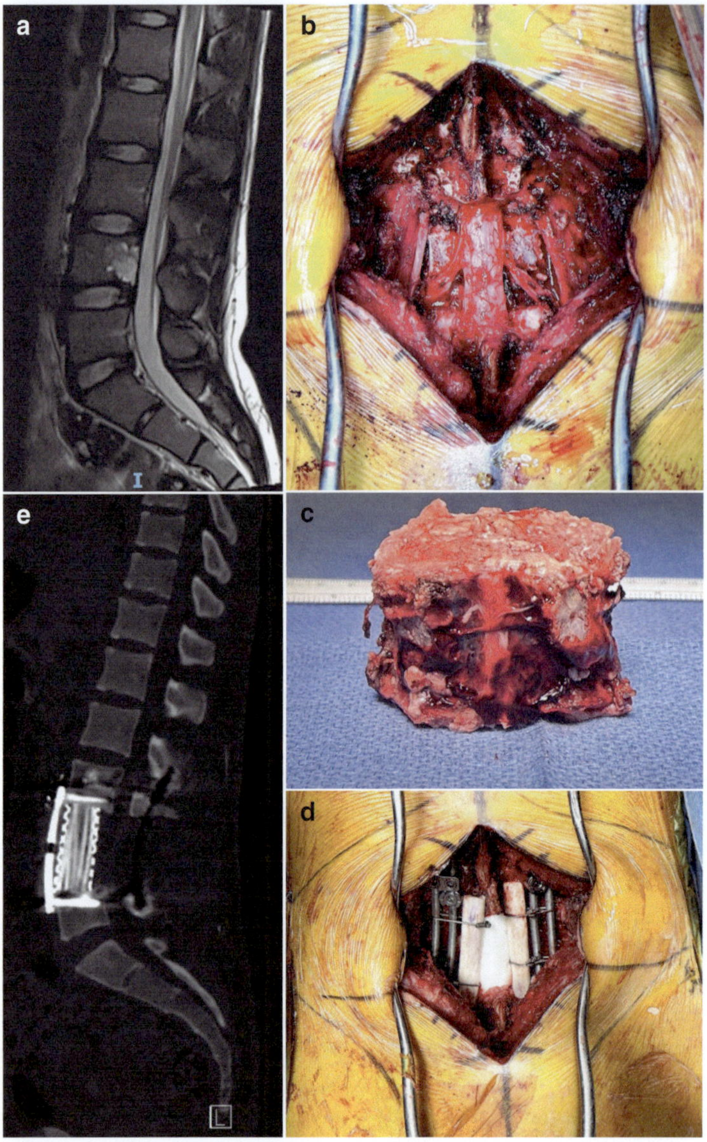

Fig. 16.2 (clockwise from top left). (**a**) Patient presented with nonspecific low back pain for which he underwent contrast-enhanced MR. T2 sagittal sequence shows T2 hyperintense mass within the posterior L4 vertebral body and minimal epidural disease. (**b**) Patient was taken for staged posterior-anterior L4 en bloc spondylectomy and circumferential L3–5 fusion. Image shows skeletonized thecal sac and L4 roots. (**c**) Specimen was delivered en bloc via an anterior approach. (**d**) Posterior reconstruction was performed with L3–5 quad rod construct posteriorly with fibular strut grafts cabled in bilaterally. (**e**) Postoperative non-contrast CT showing L4 spondylectomy defect reconstructed with titanium mesh cage and L3–5 pedicle screw construct

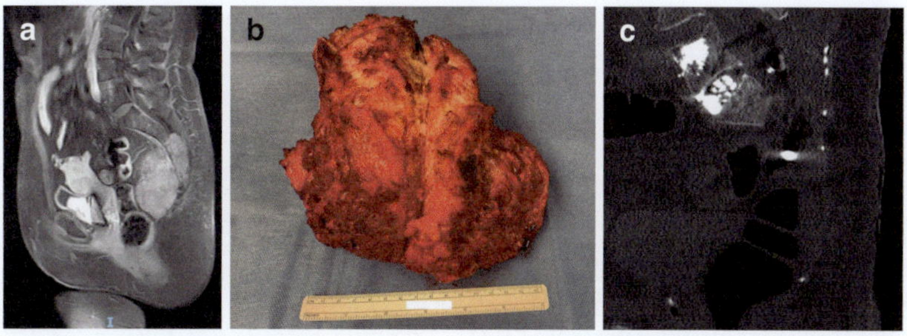

Fig. 16.3 (**a**) Patient presented to clinic with sensation of gluteal fullness and low back/buttock pain for which she underwent MR lumbosacral spine with and without contrast. Fat-suppressed, contrast-enhanced T1-weighted sequences showed a homogenously contrast-enhancing mass of the distal sacrum with presacral component compressing the rectum. Patient was offered *en bloc* high sacrectomy with S1/2 proximal osteotomy level and delivery via posterior approach. (**b**) Specimen was delivered *en bloc*. (**c**) Postoperative CT shows reconstruction with L5-pelvis instrumented fusion with L5/S1 anterior lumbar interbody fusion with integrated fixation device and cement-augmentation of L5 pedicle screws

vation of the specimen, and facilitating ventral dissection including ligation of the median sacral and potentially the internal iliac vessels. The sacrospinous and sacrotuberous ligaments are robust and must be divided to deliver the specimen although care should be taken with ventral dissection to avoid injury to the rectum. It is important to note that the sacrum is tethered by numerous soft tissues, including ligaments, periosteum, nerves, and vessels, all of which must be fully released before the specimen can be delivered (Fig. 16.3). The bony releases mark only the beginning of the procedure. Lumbopelvic reconstruction is then performed as needed. For lesions with significant ventral extent, an anterior stage is generally performed first, creating a ventral plane over the tumor, releasing the great vessels, and performing an initial diskectomy, if a total sacrectomy is to be performed [23]. A silastic sheath is also left posterior to the great vessels and acts as a protective layer and surgical landmark similar to the lumbar spine. A vertical rectus abdominis muscle (VRAM) flap may also be harvested and placed within the abdominal cavity to help with reconstruction of the soft tissue defect after posterior tumor delivery [24, 25].

Lumbopelvic Reconstruction

The sacrum serves as a keystone that facilitates the transfer of axial loads from the caudal lumbar spine to the bony pelvis. The degree of pelvic instability following sacrectomy is dictated by the extent of the sacroiliac joint that is resected [10]. Biomechanical work [26–28] has suggested that lumbopelvic reconstruction is merited where the cranial osteotomy is cephalad to the S2 level, as this is associated with significant compromise of the sacroiliac joints. The most common strategy for reconstruction is spinopelvic fixation and reconstruction of the pelvic ring, and cadaveric work by Macki et al. demonstrated that dual iliac fixation bilaterally with placement of a cross-connector offers the most stable construct [29]. Placement of a transiliac bar has also been described [23, 30] in conjunction with spinopelvic fixation to reconstruct the pelvic ring. A femoral strut graft can be placed in the bony defect to facilitate fusion and obliterate the dead space generated by specimen delivery. Mechanical complications are common though, occurring in 15–25% of patients undergoing instrumented fusion [10].

Survival, Complications, and Adjuvant Therapy

Survival

Data from the National Cancer Institute's Surveillance, Epidemiology and End Results (SEER) database shows significant variability in both overall and progression-free survival (PFS) depending upon underlying pathology. Based on these data, five-year overall survival rates have been calculated at 62% for chordoma, 55% for chondrosarcoma, 41% for Ewing sarcoma, and 18% for osteosarcoma. Data from the AOSpine Knowledge Forum Tumor registry has demonstrated similar results with median overall survival of 7.0 years for chordoma (mobile spine lesions; 6 years for sacral lesions) [4, 5], 3.6 years for Ewing sarcoma, [3] greater than 5 years for chondrosarcoma (median survival not reached within 5-year follow-up), and 6.7 years for osteosarcoma [6]. Progression-free survival is similarly variable with the AOSpine group showing median progression-free survival of 5.3 years for chordoma (4 years for sacral lesions) [4, 5] and greater than 5-years for Ewing sarcoma, chondrosarcoma, and osteosarcoma (median PFS not reached within 5-year follow-up) [3, 6, 7].

Enneking-appropriate resection—*en bloc* resection with negative margins—appears critical to survival outcomes [8, 9]. The AOSpine data show that, for chordoma, Enneking-inappropriate resection is associated with a 602% increased hazard of recurrence for mobile spine lesions [4] and 143% increased hazard for sacral lesions [5]. Similarly, the AO data for Ewing sarcoma showed patients treated with Enneking appropriate resection had overall and progression-free survival that was superior to the point that fewer than 50% of the patients died or experienced progression within the 5-year follow-up window. By comparison with those treated with Enneking-inappropriate resection, median overall and progression-free survival were 2.2 and 1.8 years, respectively [3]. For chondrosarcoma, there was a 109% increased hazard of local recurrence, though this was not significant due to low statistical power. Overall survival was not correlated with the Enneking-appropriateness of resection, though all patients in the AO series had undergone surgical resection. Like chordoma and Ewing sarcoma, osteosarcoma showed significantly greater progression-free and overall survival following Enneking-appropriate resection.

Data from the SEER registry provide similar conclusions for chondrosarcoma, with resection resulting 56% lower hazard for overall survival and 63% lower hazard for disease-specific survival [14]. Likewise, the SEER data for osteosarcoma show a robust benefit of surgery with 45% reduced hazard of overall mortality and 54% reduced hazard of disease-specific mortality [15]. For Ewing sarcoma, surgery also appears to provide benefit, [15] though to a lesser degree with surgery correlating with a 36% reduced overall mortality hazard and 31% lower disease-specific mortality hazard among patients treated with modern chemoradiation protocols. However, for chordoma, the SEER data [31] appear to only support surgical resection as improving overall survival for sacral lesions, with 52% lower hazard of overall mortality. Yet it must be acknowledged that in contrast to the AOSpine data, the SEER data do not include surgical margin, which has repeatedly been correlated with local control [6, 8, 9].

Neurological Sequelae and Complications

Given the potential of primary vertebral column malignancies to involve the adjoining thecal sac and nerve roots, *en bloc* resection may require sacrifice of one or more nerve roots. While this is considered highly morbid when the involved root is L2–4 due to the significant negative impact on ambulatory function, sacral nerve root sacrifice is more commonly performed for Enneking-appropriate resection of primary sacral malignancies. The resultant neurological sequelae vary by the level of nerve root sacrifice, but can include weakness, numbness, bowel/bladder dysfunction, and sexual dysfunction. A systematic review of the literature [32] demonstrated sparing of at least the bilateral S1 roots was associated with only minor postoperative motor dysfunction, though sparing of at least the bilateral S2 roots [and generally an S3 root] was required for normal bladder and bowel function in most patients.

Postoperative recovery is long for patients undergoing *en bloc* spondylectomy or sacrectomy, with hospital courses often comprising the better part of a month [10]. Patients also commonly require placement to an inpatient rehabilitation or skilled nursing facility prior to returning to independent living. Complications are common, with significant complications in 40–60% of patients [10, 33, 34]. Wound complications are the most common and occur in approximately one-third of patients [35, 36]. This may be partially attributed to the high incidence of sacral numbness, bowel and bladder dysfunction, and the location of the surgical site in a region subjected to pressure during sitting and lying. The loss of sensation, combined with a fresh surgical incision, impairs the patient's natural ability to unconsciously reposition and shift weight, leading to excessive strain on the incision and potential soiling without the patient's awareness. Postoperative management may include protocols such as minimizing pressure on the incision (e.g., avoiding prolonged sitting, frequent repositioning), extended use of a Foley catheter, and, in cases of significant bowel incontinence, follow-up procedures like a diverting ostomy.

Role of Adjuvant Therapies

Chordoma, chondrosarcoma, and osteosarcoma are radioresistant pathologies; however, there is a role for radiation in light of the increased availability of charged particle and focused photon radiotherapies [37]. A recent guideline from the Spine Tumor Academy recommended doses of 75.6–77.4 Gy RBE (in 1.8-2Gy fractions) for proton therapy, 24Gy in a single-fraction or 40-50Gy in five fractions for stereotactic body radiotherapy (photons), or ≥70.4Gy in 2.2–4.4Gy fractions for carbon-ion therapy. Similar guidelines have not been published for spinal osteosarcoma, though similarly high doses (68.4Gy) have been prescribed for axial locations, especially in the case of incomplete resection or an unresectable lesion [38]. Lesions that are incompletely resected or which demonstrated a poor histologic response to neoadjuvant chemotherapy are also recommended for radiotherapy, comprising 45–54Gy. Doses ≥59Gy produce no significant interval survival benefit in this patient population but do increase the risk of radiation-induced toxicities. Given the presumed risk of wound-related complications, a plurality of experts from the AOSpine Tumor Knowledge Forum recommended waiting at least 4 weeks following resection of chordoma to minimize the risk of wound-healing complications [41]. However, the need for radiotherapy must be carefully considered, as postoperative radiation-induced changes can significantly complicate any subsequent surgical resections. Some surgeons advocate for close follow-up and interval imaging in cases where a successful en bloc resection has been achieved, rather than opting for prophylactic radiation.

Chemotherapy is not a standard part of therapy for chordoma [8] or chondrosarcoma [9] given their poor responsiveness, though it can be considered a salvage therapy in those with recurrent disease. By contrast, osteosarcoma and Ewing sarcoma both benefit from chemotherapy. For osteosarcoma, chemotherapy is performed in the neoadjuvant or adjuvant setting and commonly comprises high-dose methotrexate (6-12 g/m^2), doxorubicin, and cisplatin. Ewing sarcoma benefits heavily from neoadjuvant chemotherapy, which consists of six cycles of VIDE chemotherapy (vincristine, ifosfamide, doxorubicin, and etoposide) based upon the results of the EWING-2008 and Euro-E.W.I.N.G.99 studies [39, 40].

Postoperative Surveillance

Follow-up for all patients should include regular MRI for surveillance of lesion recurrence, and in those undergoing high sacral osteotomy (above the mid-S2 level), patients should be routinely questioned about new-onset sacral pain, which may be indicative of a radiotherapy-induced fracture [42]. Serial upright radiographs and or CT scans should also be considered for those undergoing instrumentation to look for loss of correction or hardware failure.

Conclusions

Primary tumors of the lumbo-sacral spine present significant challenges due to their rarity, complex anatomy, and resistance to conventional therapies. Achieving optimal outcomes requires a comprehensive approach that integrates precise preoperative planning, skillful surgical execution, and thorough postoperative management. *En bloc* resection with negative margins remains the cornerstone of treatment, offering the best chance for long-term progression-free survival, especially in chordoma, chondrosarcoma, and osteosarcoma. However, these procedures are not without significant morbidity, underscoring the importance of careful patient selection and the specialized expertise available at high-volume centers.

References

1. Sohn S, Kim J, Chung CK, Lee N-R, Park E, Chang U-K, Sohn MJ, Kim SH. Nationwide epidemiology and healthcare utilization of spine tumor patients in the adult Korean population, 2009–2012. Neuro-Oncol Pract. 2015;2:93–100.
2. Mukherjee D, Chaichana KL, Gokaslan ZL, Aaronson OS, Cheng JS, McGirt MJ. Survival of patients with malignant primary osseous spinal neoplasms: results from the Surveillance, Epidemiology, and End Results (SEER) database from 1973 to 2003. J Neurosurg Spine. 2011;14:143–50.
3. Charest-Morin R, Dirks MS, Patel S, et al. Ewing sarcoma of the spine: prognostic variables for survival and local control in surgically treated patients. Spine (Phila Pa 1976). 2018;43:622–9.
4. Gokaslan ZL, Zadnik PL, Sciubba DM, et al. Mobile spine chordoma: results of 166 patients from the AOSpine Knowledge Forum Tumor database. J Neurosurg Spine. 2016;24:644–51.
5. Varga PP, Szövérfi Z, Fisher CG, et al. Surgical treatment of sacral chordoma: prognostic variables for local recurrence and overall survival. Eur Spine J. 2015;24:1092–101.
6. Dekutoski MB, Clarke MJ, Rose P, et al. Osteosarcoma of the spine: prognostic variables for local recurrence and overall survival, a multicenter ambispective study. J Neurosurg Spine. 2016;25:59–68.
7. Fisher CG, Versteeg AL, Dea N, et al. Surgical management of spinal chondrosarcomas. Spine (Phila Pa 1976). 2016;41:678–85.
8. Pennington Z, Ehresman J, McCarthy EF, Ahmed AKK, Pittman PD, Lubelski D, Goodwin CRR, Sciubba DM. Chordoma of the sacrum and mobile spine: a narrative review. Spine J. 2021;21:500–17.
9. Pennington Z, Ehresman J, Pittman PD, Ahmed AK, Lubelski D, McCarthy EF, Goodwin CR, Sciubba DM. Chondrosarcoma of the spine: a narrative review. Spine J. 2021;21:2078–96.
10. Feghali J, Pennington Z, Hung B, et al. Sacrectomy for sacral tumors: perioperative outcomes in a large-volume comprehensive cancer center. Spine J. 2021;21:1908–19.
11. Lazarides AL, Kerr DL, Dial BL, Steele JR, Lane WO, Blazer DG, Brigman BE, Mendoza-Lattes SA, Erickson MM, Eward WC. Does facility volume influence survival in patients with primary malignant bone tumors of the vertebral column? A comparative cohort study. Spine J. 2020;20:1106–13.
12. Hart RA, Boriani S, Biagini R, Currier BL, Weinstein JN. A system for surgical staging and management of spine tumors. A clinical outcome study of giant cell tumors of the spine. Spine (Phila Pa 1976). 1997;22:1773–82.
13. Rose PS, Holt GE, Kneisl JS. Changes to the American Joint Committee on Cancer staging system for spine tumors—practice update. Ann Transl Med. 2019;7:215.
14. Arshi A, Sharim J, Park DY, Park HY, Bernthal NM, Yazdanshenas H, Shamie AN. Chondrosarcoma of the osseous spine. An analysis of epidemiology, patient outcomes, and prognostic factors using the SEER registry from 1973 to 2012. Spine (Phila Pa 1976). 2017;42:644–52.
15. Arshi A, Sharim J, Park DY, Park HY, Yazdanshenas H, Bernthal NM, Shamie AN. Prognostic determinants and treatment outcomes analysis of osteosarcoma and Ewing sarcoma of the spine. Spine J. 2017;17:645–55.
16. Macpherson RE, Pratap S, Tyrrell H, et al. Retrospective audit of 957 consecutive 18F-FDG PET–CT scans compared to CT and MRI in 493 patients with different histological subtypes of bone and soft tissue sarcoma. Clin Sarcoma Res. 2018;8:9.
17. Byun BH, Kong C-B, Lim I, et al. Comparison of (18) F-FDG PET/CT and (99 m)Tc-MDP bone scintigraphy for detection of bone metastasis in osteosarcoma. Skeletal Radiol. 2013;42:1673–81.
18. Yao X, Gomes MM, Tsao MS, Allen CJ, Geddie W, Sekhon H. Fine-needle aspiration biopsy versus core-needle biopsy in diagnosing lung cancer: a systematic review. Curr Oncol. 2012;19:e16–27.
19. Sankey EW, Park C, Howell EP, Pennington Z, Abd-El-Barr M, Karikari IO, Shaffrey CI, Gokaslan ZL, Sciubba D, Goodwin CRR. Importance of spinal

alignment in primary and metastatic spine tumors. World Neurosurg. 2019;132:118–28.
20. Clarke MJ, Hsu W, Suk I, et al. Three-level en bloc spondylectomy for chordoma. Oper Neurosurg. 2011;68:ons325–33.
21. Bongers MER, Ogink PT, Chu KF, Patel A, Rosenthal B, Shin JH, Lee S-G, Hornicek FJ, Schwab JH. The use of autologous free vascularized fibula grafts in reconstruction of the mobile spine following tumor resection: surgical technique and outcomes. J Neurosurg Spine. 2021;34:283–92.
22. Clarke MJ, Dasenbrock H, Bydon A, Sciubba DM, McGirt MJ, Hsieh PC, Yassari R, Gokaslan ZL, Wolinsky J-P. Posterior-only approach for en bloc sacrectomy: clinical outcomes in 36 consecutive patients. Neurosurgery. 2012;71:357–64.
23. Gallia GL, Haque R, Garonzik I, Witham TF, Khavkin YA, Wolinsky JP, Suk I, Gokaslan ZL. Spinal pelvic reconstruction after total sacrectomy for en bloc resection of a giant sacral chordoma. Technical note. J Neurosurg Spine. 2005;3:501–6.
24. Asaad M, Rajesh A, Wahood W, Vyas KS, Houdek MT, Rose PS, Moran SL. Flap reconstruction for sacrectomy defects: a systematic review and meta-analysis. J Plast Reconstr Aesthetic Surg. 2020;73:255–68.
25. Reynolds JJ, Khundkar R, Boriani S, Williams R, Rhines LD, Kawahara N, Wolinsky J-P, Gokaslan ZL, Varga PP. Soft tissue and bone defect management in total sacrectomy for primary sacral tumors. Spine (Phila Pa 1976). 2016;41:S199–204.
26. Gunterberg B, Romanus B, Stener B. Pelvic strength after major amputation of the sacrum: an experimental study. Acta Orthop Scand. 1976;47:635–42.
27. Hugate RR, Dickey ID, Phimolsarnti R, Yaszemski MJ, Sim FH. Mechanical effects of partial Sacrectomy: when is reconstruction necessary? Clin Orthop Relat Res. 2006;450:82–8.
28. Yu B, Zheng Z, Zhuang X, Chen H, Xie D, Luk KDK, Lu WW. Biomechanical effects of transverse partial sacrectomy on the sacroiliac joints. An in vitro human cadaveric *i*nvestigation of the borderline of sacroiliac joint instability. Spine (Phila Pa 1976). 2009;34:1370–5.
29. Macki M, De la Garza-Ramos R, Murgatroyd AA, Mullinix KP, Sun X, Cunningham BW, McCutcheon BA, Bydon M, Gokaslan ZL. Comprehensive biomechanical analysis of three reconstruction techniques following total sacrectomy: an in vitro human cadaveric model. J Neurosurg Spine. 2017;27:570–7.
30. Gallia GL, Suk I, Witham TF, Gearhart SL, Black JH, Redett RJ, Sciubba DM, Wolinsky J-P, Gokaslan ZL. Lumbopelvic reconstruction after combined L5 spondylectomy and total sacrectomy for En bloc resection of a malignant fibrous histiocytoma. Neurosurgery. 2010;67:E498–502.
31. Zuckerman SL, Bilsky MH, Laufer I. Chordomas of the skull base, mobile spine, and sacrum: an epidemiologic investigation of presentation, treatment, and survival. World Neurosurg. 2018;113:e618–27.
32. Zoccali C, Skoch J, Patel AS, Walter CM, Maykowski P, Baaj AA. Residual neurological function after sacral root resection during en-bloc sacrectomy: a systematic review. Eur Spine J. 2016;25:3925–31.
33. Zuckerman SL, Lee S-H, Chang GJ, Walsh GL, Mehran RJ, Gokaslan ZL, Rao G, Tatsui CE, Rhines LD. Outcomes of surgery for sacral chordoma and impact of complications: a report of 50 consecutive patients with long-term follow-up. Glob Spine J. 2021;11:740–50.
34. Boriani S, Bandiera S, Donthineni R, Amendola L, Cappuccio M, De Iure F, Gasbarrini A. Morbidity of en bloc resections in the spine. Eur Spine J. 2010;19:231–41.
35. van Wulfften Palthe ODR, Tromp I, Ferreira A, Fiore A, Bramer JAM, van Dijk NC, DeLaney TF, Schwab JH, Hornicek FJ. Sacral chordoma: a clinical review of 101 cases with 30-year experience in a single institution. Spine J. 2019;19:869–79.
36. Ji T, Guo W, Yang R, Tang X, Wang Y, Huang L. What are the conditional survival and functional outcomes after surgical treatment of 115 patients with sacral chordoma? Clin Orthop Relat Res. 2017;475:620–30.
37. Pennington Z, Ehresman J, Elsamadicy AA, Shin JH, Goodwin CR, Schwab JH, Sciubba DM. Systematic review of charged-particle therapy for chordomas and sarcomas of the mobile spine and sacrum. Neurosurg Focus. 2021;50:E17.
38. Ciernik IF, Niemierko A, Harmon DC, et al. Proton-based radiotherapy for unresectable or incompletely resected osteosarcoma. Cancer. 2011;117:4522–30.
39. Whelan J, Le Deley M-C, Dirksen U, et al. High-dose chemotherapy and blood autologous stem-cell rescue compared with standard chemotherapy in localized high-risk Ewing Sarcoma: results of Euro-E.W.I.N.G.99 and Ewing-2008. J Clin Oncol. 2018;36:3110–9.
40. Kersting J, Ranft A, Bhadri V, et al. Effect of radiotherapy dose on outcome in nonmetastatic Ewing Sarcoma. Adv Radiat Oncol. 2023;8:101269.
41. Dea N, Fisher CG, Reynolds JJ, et al. Current treatment strategy for newly diagnosed chordoma of the mobile spine and sacrum: results of an international survey. J Neurosurg Spine. 2019;30:119–25.
42. Mikula AL, Pennington Z, Lakomkin N, et al. Risk factors for sacral fracture following en bloc chordoma resection. J Neurosurg Spine. 2023;39:611–7.

Lumbar Synovial Cysts

17

Patrick Kramer, Tej Azad, and Ali Bydon

Introduction

Synovial cysts of the lumbar spine are benign, extradural, cystic structures arising from the zygapophyseal joint capsule of the lumbar spine, chiefly at the levels of L4/L5 [1]. Synovial cysts were first described by Baker in the late 1800s, with spinal cord compression symptoms described later by Kao et al. in the mid 1900s [2, 3]. The advent of diagnostic imaging greatly increased the yield of diagnoses. Lumbar synovial cysts are by far the most common, accounting for 85–95% of intraspinal synovial cysts, with cervical and thoracic synovial cysts each accounting for 2–10% [4]. Estimates of the incidence of lumbar synovial cysts range widely at 0.5–7.3% based on large cohorts of lumbar spine MRI studies [5–8].

Although "synovial cysts" is the most common terminology used to describe these structures, the nomenclature varies widely in literature and has additionally been termed juxtafacet cysts, ganglion cysts, pseudocysts, lumbar intraspinal facet cysts, fibrous cysts, and cystic formations of mobile spine [2, 3, 9–15]. The nomenclature utilized may or may not be accurate to the disease process, however the terms are often used interchangeably. Nevertheless, the treatment regimen remains largely the same, and the naming convention serves primarily to designate anatomic and histological differences [1].

Pathophysiology

Pathogenesis

The pathogenesis of synovial cysts is not completely known; however, it is thought that cysts result from facet joint osteoarthritis, microinstability and hypermobility, and/or joint inflammation that results in herniation of synovium through tears in the joint capsule [14, 16, 17]. Although the exact etiology remains up for debate, there is agreement that a strong relationship exists between synovial cysts and degenerative spinal disease as a whole [18, 19]. As described by Ramhmdani et al., spinal instability is commonly associated with synovial cysts [19]. Facet arthropathy is the most common concurrent pathology, occurring in nearly 90% of patients with lumbar synovial cysts, with spondylolisthesis and degenerative disc disease each occurring in nearly half of patients [19]. Furthermore, the disease prevalence at the level of L4/L5 is indicative of instability as a primary factor contributing to the development of lumbar synovial cysts.

P. Kramer · T. Azad · A. Bydon (✉)
Department of Neurosurgery, Johns Hopkins University School of Medicine, Baltimore, MD, USA
e-mail: pkrame16@jh.edu; tazad1@jhmi.edu; abydon1@jh.edu

A. A. Baaj et al. (eds.), *Surgery of the Lumbar Spine*, https://doi.org/10.1007/978-3-032-18097-1_17

Clinical Presentation

Demographics

Spinal synovial cysts most commonly present in older populations, often in the 60 s or 70 s. Spinal synovial cysts are rare, with few cases reported in young adults, and even fewer in pediatric populations [20–22]. There is a generally reported female predominance of synovial cysts, with some reports of 1.5–2:1 ratio of females to males, although larger cohort studies have found only slight female predominance [4, 18, 23]. The fact that this is seen in the elderly population is further proof that it's an instability issue, from older diseased joints that are prone to motion.

Presenting Symptoms

A synovial cyst that extends into the spinal canal can result in intractable back pain, radiculopathy, neurogenic claudication, and/or cauda equina syndrome [19]. In a meta-analysis of over 800 spinal synovial cysts, Ramhmdani et al. report back pain and radiculopathy as the most common presenting symptoms, each affecting roughly 75% of patients [19]. Neurological deficits occurred in over half of cases and neurogenic claudication in roughly one-third. Specifically, sensory deficits range from 10–43%, motor deficits from 20–27%, and reflex abnormalities in up to 57% of patients [19]. Cauda equina syndrome is one of the rarest presentations but nevertheless may affect up to 13% of patients and generally represents some of the most severe cases, often with an acute hemorrhagic component [3, 24, 25]. Cysts may also present incidentally, as symptoms are related to volume, site, and relationship to bony and neural structures.

Neurodiagnostics

Imaging

Magnetic resonance imaging (MRI) remains the mainstay diagnostic modality for spinal synovial cysts. On MRI, synovial cysts generally appear as well-circumscribed, extradural, facet joint-adjacent structures [3]. Synovial cysts typically measure less than 22 mm but often present with dense adhesions to dura and nerve roots [3, 26]. On T1-weighted images, synovial cysts are typically dark for simple fluid but hyperintensity is seen if the fluid content in the cyst is particularly bloody or proteinaceous [3, 27]. The converse is true for T2-weighted images with bright-appearing cysts becoming partially hypointense depending on blood and protein content, with osseous bodies also affecting signal [3, 27]. (Figs. 17.1, 17.2, and 17.3) Gadolinium contrast (which is rarely used clinically to diagnose synovial cysts) may also be helpful in the diagnosis of synovial cysts as peripheral rim enhancement is common with no internal enhancement. Diagnostically, this can help confirm lesion margins, augment the identification of subtle cysts, and distinguish benign cysts from tumors [26, 28, 29]. Furthermore, signal patterns exist that are clinically relevant. For instance, cysts with low-internal signal intensity on T2-weighted images had higher rates of unsuccessful percutaneous rupture [30].

Computed tomography (CT) scans can also help identify synovial morphological features, specifically peripheral rim calcifications and internal gas content, although their primary utility lies in characterizing the bony anatomy [31]. As discussed previously, degenerative facet joint disease is a hallmark of synovial cysts, and the extent and etiology of degenerative changes can be characterized on CT. Furthermore, CT imaging is utilized frequently to guide procedures, especially for surgical approaches. CT myelography is also occasionally used in cases where an MRI cannot be obtained [32].

Histomorphological Characterization

Morphological analysis of synovial cysts reveals a range of overlapping structures that are often categorized differently. Synovial cyst characterization focuses on three elements: (1) the lining of the cystic structure, (2) the originating location

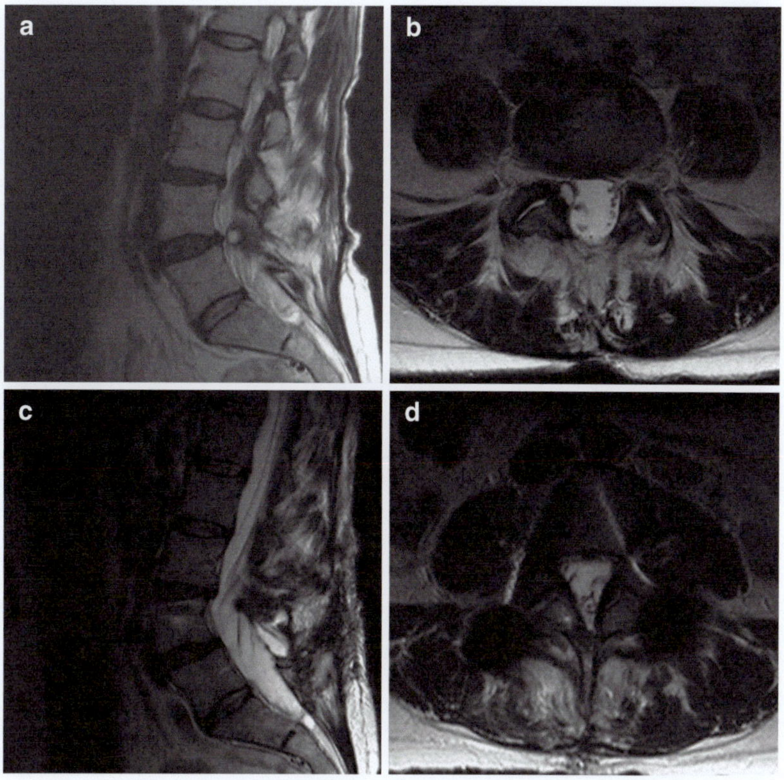

Fig. 17.1 Illustrative case 1. 51-year-old female presenting with a recurrent synovial cyst. Preoperative sagittal (**a**) and axial (**b**) T2-weighted MRI images demonstrating an 8 mm synovial cyst arising anteromedially from the right L4-L5 facet joint, abutting and mildly displacing the traversing L5 nerve root in the right lateral recess. Postoperative sagittal (**c**) and axial (**d**) T2-weighted MRI images demonstrate nonvisualization of the synovial cyst after resection and instrumentation

and involvement of the facet joint and/or ligamentum flavum, and (3) the contents of the cystic structure [33]. True synovial cysts are most well defined, characterized by focal to extensive cyst walls lined by synovial cells which either communicate directly with the facet joint or connect to it by a bursa-like channel. Conversely, lesions lacking a true synovial lining are generally categorized into pseudocysts which may have inflammatory or fibroblastic linings derived from focal degenerative changes in the ligamentum flavum. Other degenerative changes yield alternative cystic structures such as degenerative microcysts and osteophyte impingement cysts. Perhaps the most relevant differentiation is made between synovial cysts and ganglion cysts, the latter of which are not lined by synovial tissue and are filled with a myxoid, viscous, gelatinous matrix [17, 34]. Still, because of substantial morphological and histological overlap among these lesions, no universally accepted subclassification scheme has emerged. Additionally, the contents of the cysts are highly variable and not necessarily conserved across subclassifications. Empty cyst contents are common; however, myxoid, inflammatory, bloody, fibrinoid, and calcified material are also found within the cysts [33]. Nevertheless, Sabo et al. argue that there is no clinical relevance to the subclassification of synovial cysts as the treatment regimen is consistent across structures [34].

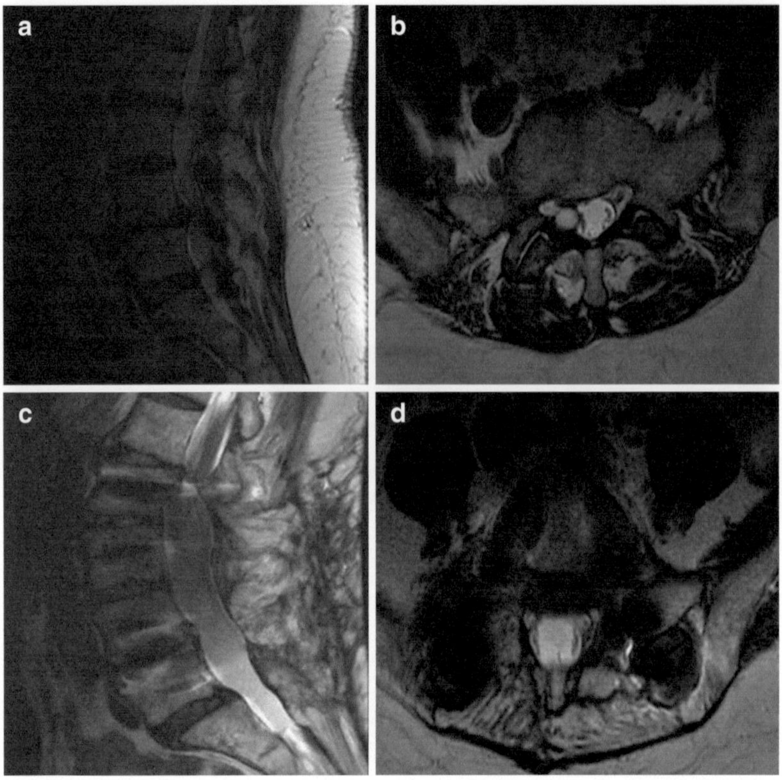

Fig. 17.2 Illustrative case 2. 69-year-old female presenting with back pain and right lower extremity radiculopathy. Preoperative sagittal (**a**) and axial (**b**) T2-weighted MRI images demonstrating a 1.0 × 0.9 × 1.7 cm hyperintense cystic structure adjacent to the anterior aspect of the right L5-S1 facet joint compatible with a synovial cyst. There is associated severe right lateral recess stenosis likely affecting and compressing the traversing right S1 nerve root. Postoperative sagittal (**c**) and axial (**d**) T2-weighted MRI images demonstrate nonvisualization of the synovial cyst after resection and instrumentation

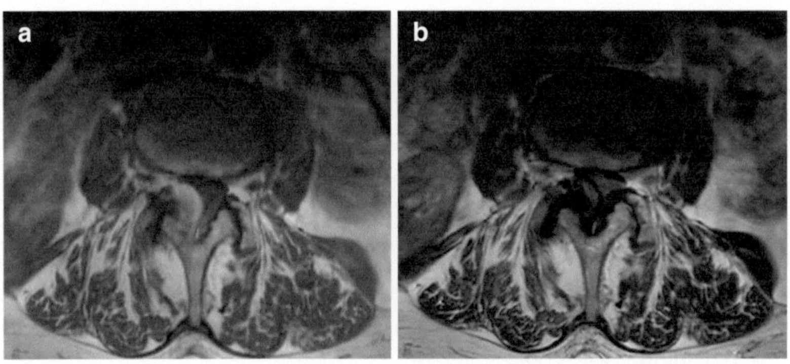

Fig. 17.3 Illustrative case 3. 80-year-old female presenting with 2 months of back pain radiating down the right leg. T1-weighted (**a**) and T2-weighted (**b**) axial MRI demonstrates a synovial cyst appearing to communicate with the medial aspect of the right facet joint at L3-L4, with intrinsic T1 shortening and T2 hypointense signal, and a rim of very dark T2 signal. There is associated effacement of the right lateral recess and anteromedial displacement of the cauda equina and impingement of the descending right-sided L4 nerve root, and near complete effacement of CSF signal.

Surgical Management

Surgical excision is the mainstay treatment for lumbar synovial cysts, especially those that present with radiculopathy, neurologic deficit, or intractable pain [16]. Open surgeries are advantageous in that macroscopic confirmation of complete cyst resection may be achieved, and appropriate exposure can ensure that all complex attachments are dissected [35]. Synovial cyst resection is often accompanied by a medial facetectomy, which may contribute to increased spinal instability. Therefore, the primary surgical dilemma is whether or not to accompany cyst resection and decompression with stabilization [35].

Surgical Techniques

Briefly, primary decompression is typically achieved with a bilateral laminectomy or hemilaminectomy depending on the size and location of the cyst and the degree of underlying bony stenosis. Visualization and discrimination of the cyst from the thecal sac and involved nerve root is chiefly important in order to remove the cyst safely, without injury to dura/root/thecal sac. Unlike a paracentral disk herniation where the traversing root is involved, in the case of a synovial cyst both traversing and exiting nerve roots should be widely decompressed as most cysts end up compressing the exiting superior root (akin to spondylolisthesis). Intraoperative monitoring of electromyography is useful to be alerted when excessive traction occurs during dissection [4, 35].

Decompression with and Without Fusion

Surgical excision with laminectomy alone is indicated for patients with no or minimal instability (no spondylolisthesis), generally more moderate symptoms, and when definitive cyst resection can be achieved [35]. Synovial cysts may be treated with bilateral laminectomy, hemilaminectomy, and/or medial facetectomy in conjunction with cyst resection. The choice to accompany surgical excision and decompression with fusion is often driven by the degree of instability (fluid in the facet joint, widening of the facet joint, spondylolisthesis) as well as back pain. Significant spondylolisthesis, evidence of hypermobility, risks of recurrence, or the necessity of a large facetectomy are all indications for fusion. Typically, patients who are selected for fusion have higher rates of preoperative neurogenic claudication and motor deficits [35]. The rates of fusion in synovial cysts vary from 16 to 40% [36–39].

In a 2010 meta-analysis, Bydon et al. identified nearly 1000 patients who had surgical excision of their synovial cysts [37]. Although more than 90% of patients experienced symptom resolution in the short-term postoperative period, recurrence of back and leg pain occurred in 22% and 13% of patients. Reoperations were required for 6% of patients who underwent decompression alone, largely due to spinal instability requiring fusion. It is thought that decompression alone may contribute to mechanical instability leading to symptom recurrence and subsequent reoperations for stabilization, although Benato et al. illustrated equivalent reoperation rates between decompression with and without fusion [35, 38]. Cyst recurrence is rare within literature, occurring in less than 2% of the cohort included in the meta-analysis (this could be attributed to underreporting due to follow-up limitations), although it should be noted that same level synovial cyst recurrence has never been reported after laminectomy and transpedicular instrumented fusion [40]. While rare, Judy et al. demonstrated a case of a synovial cyst in the setting of an interspinous fusion device, illustrating that micromotion across the joint may still lead to degenerative changes that can result in a synovial cyst [41].

Despite generally improved outcomes in decompression with fusion groups, there may be an increased risk of perioperative complications. Xu et al. demonstrated that facetectomy with instrumented fusion had longer hospitalization stays and increased rates of blood loss, incidental durotomies, infections, wound dehiscence, cerebral spinal fluid leakage, pulmonary

Table 17.1 Comparison of treatment modalities for lumbar synovial cysts

Treatment	Indications	Success rate	Recurrence risk	Complications
Conservative (PT, NSAIDs, bracing) [14, 16, 27]	Mild symptoms, incidental findings	Low (~10–20%)	Moderate	Minimal
Steroid Injection [14, 16, 27, 50, 51]	Symptom relief, poor surgical candidates	20–75% (short-term)	High	Infection, transient relief
Aspiration/Percutaneous Rupture [46–49]	Minimally invasive alternative	50–80%	Very high (~50%)	Cyst persistence, nerve irritation
Decompression (Laminectomy, Hemilaminectomy) [35–41]	Symptomatic cases with minimal instability	~90% symptom relief	Moderate (6–22%)	Dural tear, nerve damage
Decompression + Fusion [35–41]	Instability, recurrent cysts, severe degeneration	~90%	Very low	Increased surgical risks

embolism, and deep venous thrombosis [36]. These complications were nevertheless rare, and other more recent reports demonstrate approximately equivalent complication rates as surgeons became more efficient at lumbar fusions [38]. Furthermore, fusions demonstrated improved rates of radiculopathy and back pain compared to bilateral laminectomy and hemilaminectomy [38]. Because of the high rates of concurrent spondylolisthesis, decompression with fusion may be indicated in many cases [42]. (Table 17.1).

Table 17.2 Risk factors for recurrence and surgical failure [3, 37, 40, 43, 44]

Factor	Increased recurrence risk?	Increased surgical complications?
Presence of spondylolisthesis	Yes	Yes
Facet Joint Instability	Yes	Yes
Cyst Adherence to Dura	No	Yes (Dural tear risk)
Large Facetectomy Requirement	No	Yes (Instability risk)
Incomplete Resection	Yes	

Risks and Complications

The intraoperative risks are heavily dependent on the location, size, and morphology of the synovial cyst. Complete removal of the cyst may be challenging due to adherence to the dura. If a clear dural plane is visualized, the cyst may be removed entirely, however calcifications and adhesions to the theca and nerve roots may limit the resection [4]. Therefore, the primary complication associated with surgical resection is incidental dural tears which occur on average in 4% of initial surgeries, and 17% of revision surgeries [4]. Synovial cysts may also recur after resection (without fusing the source of the cyst: facet joint) as discussed previously, there have been no reports of cyst recurrence in patients who underwent concurrent decompression and instrumented fusion [37, 43, 44]. (Table 17.2).

Conservative and Procedural Treatments

Although surgical management is the most common treatment modality for synovial cysts, conservative management is indicated. It is usually utilized for patients with pain (back or leg) of less than 6–8 weeks of duration as some cysts may resolve on their own or respond to aspiration.

Conservative Management

Some have treated synovial cysts with rest, oral analgesics, physical therapy, bracing, and chiropractic care [14, 16, 27, 45]. Physical therapy techniques may include spine stabilization exercises, lower-extremity stretching, truncal musculature strengthening, and body mechanics education [16].

Percutaneous Aspiration

Synovial cysts may be treated with image-guided aspiration, which may be achieved with fluoroscopic or CT guidance. These are generally considered to be safe procedures, although the effects tend to be short-term and non-curative. Often, cysts are gelatinous and non-aspirable leaving large residual structures that can continue to compress the neural structures. Martha et al. describe a cohort of 101 patients who underwent percutaneous corticosteroid injection and cyst "rupture" for lumbar synovial cysts [46]. Cyst rupture was achieved in 81% of patients, however 55% of patients required subsequent operations, with a mean time to surgery of less than 1 year [46]. In a prospective trial of 45 patients, microsurgical resection was compared directly to percutaneous CT-guided destruction [47]. Ultimately, 60% of patients who underwent initial percutaneous aspiration required later microsurgery [47]. Cyst rupture with corticosteroid injection offered higher rates of symptom improvement than steroid injection alone [48]. Nevertheless, the operation and failure rates remain high, with some reports anywhere between 50 and 100% [4, 16, 43, 49]. (Table 17.1).

Steroid Injections

Intra-articular or epidural steroid injections are also occasionally used to treat symptoms of synovial cysts, although the efficacy is highly variable. Metellus et al. describe a series of 27 patients who underwent epidural steroid injections, with all 27 eventually requiring surgical management to relieve persistent or worsening symptoms [50]. Slipman et al. evaluated a series of spinal synovial cysts who underwent intra-articular steroid injection with a selective nerve root block [51]. Of the 14 patients in the study, only 4 patients achieved a good or excellent outcome, with half requiring subsequent surgical interventions [51]. Overall, success rates range from 20% to 75%, although most studies tend to report high failure rates [16]. (Table 17.1).

Summary

Lumbar synovial cysts are degenerative, fluid-filled outpouchings arising from the facet joints in patients in the sixth or seventh decade of life, typically driven by chronic degeneration and underlying spinal instability (facet arthropathy, facet widening, spondylolisthesis). Patients often present with constant back pain, radiculopathy, or, less commonly, features of neurogenic claudication. MRI is the primary diagnostic tool, with CT offering superior bony detail. In patients without weakness or numbness or bladder/bowel dysfunction, a trial of conservative measures is warranted (PT, injections, aspiration). Most patients fail conservative management and end up requiring definitive surgical decompression (open or tubular), with or without fusion, depending on the extent of joint degeneration and instability.

References

1. Mattei TA, Goulart CR, McCall TD. Pathophysiology of regression of synovial cysts of the lumbar spine: The "anti-inflammatory hypothesis." Med Hypotheses. 2012;79(6). https://doi.org/10.1016/j.mehy.2012.08.034.
2. Kao CC, Winkler SS, Turner JH. Synovial cyst of spinal facet. Case report. J Neurosurg. 1974;41(3) https://doi.org/10.3171/jns.1974.41.3.0372.
3. Khan AM, Girardi F. Spinal lumbar synovial cysts. Diagnosis and management challenge. Eur Spine J. 2006;15(8) https://doi.org/10.1007/s00586-005-0009-4.
4. Epstein NE. Lumbar synovial cysts: a review of diagnosis, surgical management, and outcome assessment. J Spinal Disord Tech. 2004;17(4) https://doi.org/10.1097/01.bsd.0000096267.75190.eb.
5. Janssen SJ, Ogink PT, Schwab JH. The prevalence of incidental and symptomatic lumbar synovial facet cysts. Clin Spine Surg. 2018;31(5) https://doi.org/10.1097/BSD.0000000000000648.
6. Fletcher Eyster E, Scott WR. Lumbar synovial cysts: report of eleven cases. Neurosurgery. 1989;24(1) https://doi.org/10.1227/00006123-198901000-00021.

7. Doyle AJ, Merrilees M. Synovial cysts of the lumbar facet joints in a symptomatic population: prevalence on magnetic resonance imaging. Spine (Phila Pa 1976). 2004;29(8). https://doi.org/10.1097/00007632-200404150-00010.
8. Lemish W, Apsimon T, Chakera T. Lumbar intraspinal synovial cysts: recognition and CT diagnosis. Spine (Phila Pa 1976). 1989;14(12) https://doi.org/10.1097/00007632-198912000-00016.
9. Gritzka TL, Taylor TK. A ganglion arising from a lumbar articular facet associated with low back pain and sciatica. Report of a case. J Bone Joint Surg Br. 1970;52(3) https://doi.org/10.1302/0301-620x.52b3.528.
10. Maezawa Y, Baba H, Uchida K, Furusawa N, Kubota C, Yoshizawa K. Spontaneous remission of a solitary intraspinal synovial cyst of the lumbar spine. Eur Spine J. 2000;9(1) https://doi.org/10.1007/s005860050016.
11. Lyons MK, Atkinson JLD, Wharen RE, Deen HG, Zimmerman RS, Lemens SM. Surgical evaluation and management of lumbar synovial cysts: the Mayo Clinic experience. J Neurosurg. 2000;93(1 SUPPL) https://doi.org/10.3171/spi.2000.93.1.0053.
12. Kjerulf TD, Terry DW, Boubelik RJ. Lumbar synovial or ganglion cysts. Neurosurgery. 1986;19:3. https://doi.org/10.1227/00006123-198609000-00013.
13. Houten JK, Sanderson SP, Cooper PR. Spontaneous regression of symptomatic lumbar synovial cysts. Report of three cases. J Neurosurg. 2003;99(2 Suppl):235.
14. Hemminghytt S, Daniels DL, Williams AL, Haughton VM. Intraspinal synovial cysts: natural history and diagnosis by CT. Radiology. 1982;145(2) https://doi.org/10.1148/radiology.145.2.7134440.
15. Abdullah AF, Chambers RW, Daut DP. Lumbar nerve root compression by synovial cysts of the ligamentum flavum. Report of four cases. J Neurosurg. 1984;60(3) https://doi.org/10.3171/jns.1984.60.3.0617.
16. Shah RV, Lutz GE. Lumbar intraspinal synovial cysts: conservative management and review of the world's literature. Spine J. 2003;3(6) https://doi.org/10.1016/S1529-9430(03)00148-7.
17. Wilby MJ, Fraser RD, Vernon-Roberts B, Moore RJ. The prevalence and pathogenesis of synovial cysts within the ligamentum flavum in patients with lumbar spinal stenosis and radiculopathy. Spine (Phila Pa 1976). 2009;34(23) https://doi.org/10.1097/BRS.0b013e3181b22bd0.
18. Boviatsis EJ, Staurinou LC, Kouyialis AT, et al. Spinal synovial cysts: pathogenesis, diagnosis and surgical treatment in a series of seven cases and literature review. Eur Spine J. 2008;17(6). https://doi.org/10.1007/s00586-007-0563-z.
19. Ramhmdani S, Ishida W, Perdomo-Pantoja A, Witham TF, Lo SFL, Bydon A. Synovial cyst as a marker for lumbar instability: a systematic review and meta-analysis. World Neurosurg. 2019;122 https://doi.org/10.1016/j.wneu.2018.10.228.
20. Vasani SS, Demetriades AK, Joshi SM, Yeh J, Ellamushi H. Traumatic intraspinal extradural ganglion cyst in a teenager: case report and review of the literature. Clin Neurol Neurosurg. 2007;109(1) https://doi.org/10.1016/j.clineuro.2006.03.006.
21. Gelabert-González M, Prieto-González A, María Santin-Amo J, Serramito-García R, García-Allut A. Lumbar synovial cyst in an adolescent: case report. Childs Nerv Syst. 2009;25(6) https://doi.org/10.1007/s00381-009-0833-7.
22. Kalevski SK, Haritonov DG, Peev NA. Lumbar Intraforaminal synovial cyst in young adulthood: case report and review of the literature. Glob Spine J. 2014;4(3) https://doi.org/10.1055/s-0034-1370694.
23. Indar R, Tsiridis E, Morgan M, Aldham CH, Hussein AA. Intraspinal lumbar synovial cysts: diagnosis and surgical management. Surgeon. 2004;2(3) https://doi.org/10.1016/S1479-666X(04)80074-X.
24. Kumaria A, Wood A, Gakhar HPS, Howarth SPS, Bateman AH. Facet joint cyst haematoma: a rare cause of cauda equina syndrome. Br J Neurosurg. 2023;37(4) https://doi.org/10.1080/02688697.2019.1662370.
25. Machino M, Yukawa Y, Ito K, Kanbara S, Kato F. Spontaneous hemorrhage in an upper lumbar synovial cyst causing subacute cauda equina syndrome. Orthopedics. 2012;35(9) https://doi.org/10.3928/01477447-20120822-41.
26. Apostolaki E, Davies AM, Evans N, Cassar-Pullicino VN. MR imaging of lumbar facet joint synovial cysts. Eur Radiol. 2000;10(4) https://doi.org/10.1007/s003300050973.
27. Hsu KY, Zucherman JF, Shea WJ, Jeffrey RA. Lumbar intraspinal synovial and ganglion cysts (Facet cysts): ten-year experience in evaluation and treatment. Spine (Phila Pa 1976). 1995;20(1) https://doi.org/10.1097/00007632-199501000-00015.
28. Venkatanarasimha N, Priya Suresh S. AJR teaching file: an uncommon cause of spinal canal stenosis. Am J Roentgenol. 2009;193(3 SUPPL) https://doi.org/10.2214/AJR.07.7110.
29. Lee KJX, Tan TJ, Tan EJ, Yan YY. Magnetic resonance imaging of spinal epidural lesions. Singapore Med J. 2023;64(9) https://doi.org/10.4103/singaporemedj.SMJ-2021-215.
30. Cambron SC, McIntyre JJ, Guerin SJ, Li Z, Pastel DA. Lumbar facet joint synovial cysts: does T2 signal intensity predict outcomes after percutaneous rupture? Am J Neuroradiol. 2013;34. https://doi.org/10.3174/ajnr.A3441.
31. Wang AM, Haykal HA, Lin JCT, Lee JH. Synovial cysts of the lumbar spine: CT evaluation. Comput Radiol. 1987;11(5-6) https://doi.org/10.1016/0730-4862(87)90008-4.
32. Bruder M, Cattani A, Gessler F, et al. Synovial cysts of the spine: long-term follow-up after surgical treatment of 141 cases in a single-center series and comprehensive literature review of 2900 degenerative spinal cysts. J Neurosurg Spine. 2017;27 https://doi.org/10.3171/2016.12.SPINE16756.

33. Chebib I, Chang CY, Schwab JH, Kerr DA, Deshpande V, Nielsen GP. Histopathology of synovial cysts of the spine. Histopathology. 2018;72(6) https://doi.org/10.1111/his.13465.
34. Themistoklis KM, Papasilekas TI, Boviatsis KA, et al. Spinal synovial cysts. A case series and current treatment options. J Clin Neurosci. 2018;57 https://doi.org/10.1016/j.jocn.2018.08.038.
35. Bydon M, Papadimitriou K, Witham T, et al. Treatment of spinal synovial cysts. World Neurosurg. 2013;79(2):375–80. https://doi.org/10.1016/j.wneu.2012.08.016.
36. Xu R, McGirt MJ, Parker SL, et al. Factors associated with recurrent back pain and cyst recurrence after surgical resection of one hundred ninety-five spinal synovial cysts: analysis of one hundred sixty-seven consecutive cases. Spine (Phila Pa 1976). 2010;35(10) https://doi.org/10.1097/BRS.0b013e3181bdafed.
37. Bydon A, Xu R, Parker SL, et al. Recurrent back and leg pain and cyst reformation after surgical resection of spinal synovial cysts: systematic review of reported postoperative outcomes. Spine J. 2010;10(9) https://doi.org/10.1016/j.spinee.2010.04.010.
38. Benato A, Menna G, Rapisarda A, et al. Decompression with or without fusion for lumbar synovial cysts—a systematic review and meta-analysis. J Clin Med. 2023;12(7) https://doi.org/10.3390/jcm12072664.
39. Wun K, Hashmi SZ, Maslak J, et al. The variability of lumbar facet joint synovial cyst recurrence requiring revision surgery after decompression-only and decompression/fusion. Clin Spine Surg. 2019;32(10) https://doi.org/10.1097/BSD.0000000000000870.
40. Bydon M, Lin JA, De La Garza-Ramos R, et al. The role of spinal fusion in the treatment of cervical synovial cysts: a series of 17 cases and meta-analysis. J Neurosurg Spine. 2014;21(6) https://doi.org/10.3171/2014.8.SPINE13897.
41. Judy BF, Abou-Mrad T, Bydon A. Synovial cyst in the setting of an Interspinous fusion device. World Neurosurg. 2023;179 https://doi.org/10.1016/j.wneu.2023.08.041.
42. Chen Y, Yu P, Xu H, et al. Efficacy of minimally invasive tubular approaches for management of the lumbar spinal synovial cysts: a meta-analysis. Eur J Med Res. 2023;28(1). https://doi.org/10.1186/s40001-023-01481-0.
43. Imai K, Nakamura K, Inokuchi K, Oda H. Aspiration of intraspinal synovial cyst: recurrence after temporal improvement. Arch Orthop Trauma Surg. 1998;118(1–2) https://doi.org/10.1007/s004020050323.
44. Epstein N, Baisden J. The diagnosis and management of synovial cysts: efficacy of surgery versus cyst aspiration. Surg Neurol Int. 2012;(3(4)) https://doi.org/10.4103/2152-7806.98576.
45. Swartz PG, Murtagh FR. Spontaneous resolution of an intraspinal synovial cyst. Am J Neuroradiol. 2003;24(6):1261.
46. Martha JF, Swaim B, Wang DA, et al. Outcome of percutaneous rupture of lumbar synovial cysts: a case series of 101 patients. Spine J. 2009;9(11) https://doi.org/10.1016/j.spinee.2009.06.010.
47. Schulz C, Danz B, Waldeck S, Kunz U, Mauer UM. Percutaneous CT-guided destruction versus microsurgical resection of lumbar juxtafacet cysts. Orthopade. 2011;40(7) https://doi.org/10.1007/s00132-011-1744-3.
48. Allen TL, Tatli Y, Lutz GE. Fluoroscopic percutaneous lumbar zygapophyseal joint cyst rupture: a clinical outcome study. Spine Journal. 2009;9(5) https://doi.org/10.1016/j.spinee.2008.08.008.
49. Sabers SR, Ross SR, Grogg BE, Lauder TD. Procedure-based nonsurgical management of lumbar zygapophyseal joint cyst-induced radicular pain. Arch Phys Med Rehabil. 2005;86(9) https://doi.org/10.1016/j.apmr.2004.11.051.
50. Métellus P, Fuentes S, Adetchessi T, et al. Retrospective study of 77 patients harbouring lumbar synovial cysts: functional and neurological outcome. Acta Neurochir. 2006;148(1) https://doi.org/10.1007/s00701-005-0650-z.
51. Slipman CW, Lipetz JS, Wakeshima Y, Jackson HB. Nonsurgical treatment of zygapophyseal joint cyst-induced radicular pain. Arch Phys Med Rehabil. 2000;81(7) https://doi.org/10.1053/apmr.2000.5584.

Degenerative Spondylolisthesis and Spondylolysis

18

Marisa Gandía, Diego Gordon, and Mario Taravilla-Loma

Keypoints

- Spondylolisthesis is the anterior displacement of a vertebral body, most commonly due to isthmic or degenerative causes, and is graded I to V by the Meyerding system based on the percentage of vertebral slippage.
- Symptoms range from mechanical back pain and radiculopathy to neurological deficits, with imaging (X-ray, CT, MRI) essential for diagnosis and surgical planning.
- Surgical intervention is indicated for high-grade slips, neurological compromise, progressive deformity, or failure of conservative management in symptomatic patients.
- Techniques include decompression alone, decompression with posterior spinal fusion with pedicle screws, and interbody fusion (PLIF or TLIF) to achieve stabilization and alignment. In high-grade slips, partial reduction may be attempted using gradual rod contouring and distraction with monitoring for L5 function.

M. Gandía (✉) · D. Gordon · M. Taravilla-Loma
University Hospital La Paz, Department of Neurosurgery, Madrid, Spain

Background

- *Spondylolisthesis* is defined as the subluxation of one vertebral body over another, and it constitutes a common finding in imaging studies, both in symptomatic and asymptomatic individuals [1].
- The true *prevalence* of spondylolisthesis is unknown due to its asymptomatic nature in most patients; however, it is estimated that a significant proportion of patients 65 years and older will show some evidence of degenerative lumbar spondylolisthesis, with a higher prevalence in females and an age-dependent increase [1–3].
- *Degenerative lumbar spondylolisthesis* is the term used to define the slippage of a lumbar vertebra, usually at the level of L4-L5, with an intact neural arch (no spondylolysis), and it is seldom encountered in patients younger than 50 years old [3].
- Spondylolisthesis can sometimes be *associated with spondylolysis*, a defect in the pars interarticularis, which may arise from *congenital* anomalies of the neural arch, stress fractures due to repetitive trauma, bony remodeling, or acute fractures. Spondylolysis can occur unilaterally or bilaterally, with bilateral cases more likely to progress to spondylolisthesis. This condition is usually seen in younger patients with a specific subtype of spondylolisthesis termed *isthmic*

A. A. Baaj et al. (eds.), *Surgery of the Lumbar Spine*, https://doi.org/10.1007/978-3-032-18097-1_18

spondylolisthesis, where a defect of the pars interarticularis is an obligatory finding [1].
- While many patients remain asymptomatic, spondylolisthesis can lead to *low back pain* and symptoms from neural compression *(radiculopathy* or *neurogenic claudication)* [3].

Biomechanics

- *Degenerative spondylolisthesis* is known to be *multifactorial* in origin.
  - Anatomic factors such as *facet joint orientation* can increase the risk of spondylolisthesis in the aging population, with more sagittally oriented facet joints increasing the risk of instability and consequent listhesis. A facet joint angle of more than 45 degrees was considered a major risk factor for spondylolisthesis [4], increasing the risk of instability 45-fold.
  - Additional degenerative anatomical factors, such as compromised *disk integrity* and *laxity of the anterior and posterior longitudinal ligaments*, are necessary for listhesis to occur [5]. Listhesis is not limited to the anteroposterior plane, as asymmetric involvement of the facet joints will translate into a rotational component as well.
- In *isthmic spondylolisthesis*, the major predisposing factor is *spondylolysis*, which allows the vertebral body to displace anteriorly (if bilateral pars defect).

Classification

- The most widely used grading system for spondylolisthesis is the *Meyerding classification* (Fig. 18.1). It grades the amount of subluxation of the vertebra that has slipped as a percentage relative to the vertebral body size. Most cases of spondylolisthesis are known to be grade I or grade II, which is relevant for patients treated surgically, as higher-grade spondylolisthesis is associated with a higher rate of complications [6].

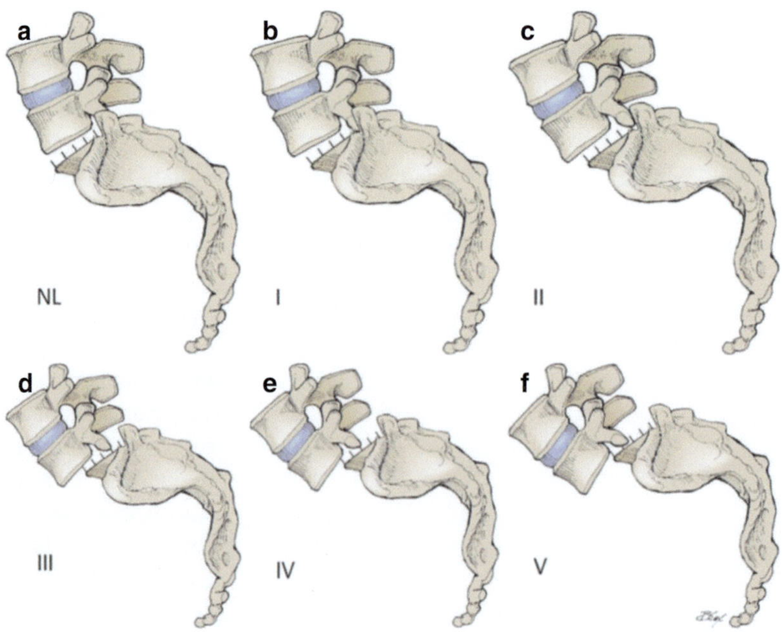

Fig. 18.1 Meyerding classification of spondylolisthesis: (**a**) Normal; (**b**) Grade I: 0–25%; (**c**) Grade II: 26–50%; (**d**) Grade III: 51–75%; (**e**) Grade IV: 76–100%; (**f**) Grade V: >100% (spondyloptosis). (Reproduced with permission from Dr. Baaj A., Mummaneni P., Uribe J., Vacaro A., Greenberg M., Handbook of Spine Surgery)

Clinical Assessment

- Although most cases of degenerative spondylolisthesis are incidental findings in asymptomatic patients [7] and the natural history of this condition is relatively benign [8, 9], low back pain and neurologic symptoms can be encountered, and deterioration occurs in a subset of patients.
- In symptomatic patients, the most common form of presentation is *low back pain associated with radicular pain or neurogenic claudication* [7].
  - *Radicular pain* is usually caused by lateral recess or foraminal stenosis. In the case of degenerative spondylolisthesis, which occurs most frequently at the L4-L5 level, the most frequently affected nerve roots are L4 (foraminal stenosis) and/or L5 (lateral recess stenosis).
  - *Neurogenic claudication* is caused by spinal stenosis.

Note: *In patients with isthmic spondylolisthesis, spinal canal stenosis is rare as the defect in the pars interarticularis means that the neural arch remains in its anatomic position as the vertebral body displaces anteriorly.

Diagnostic Workup

- X-rays
  - *Lateral oblique* radiographs in which spondylolysis can be seen as a lucency in the region of the pars interarticularis, classically a broken neck appearance of the *"Scottie dog"*. It is recommended to include right and left lateral oblique projections, as the defect may only be visible in one projection (unilateral defect) [10].
  - *Lateral standing* projections, as there is a dynamic component to the listhesis, meaning that the degree of slippage can vary significantly depending on the patient's position (standing vs. supine), or even completely reduce in the supine position [10, 11].
  - *Flexion-extension radiographs* to evaluate the degree of slippage and instability of the lumbar spine. Radiographic evidence of lumbar spinal instability is determined by the listhesis seen in flexion-extension radiographs, with a slippage of >3 mm considered abnormal and evidence of instability [12].
- CT scan to review bony anatomy.
- MRI to assess the state of the spinal canal and the neural foramina. A disk herniation is uncommon at the site of the listhesis; however, a "pseudodisc" can be seen if the disk rolls out as it is uncovered by the vertebral body above (Figs. 18.2 and 18.3).

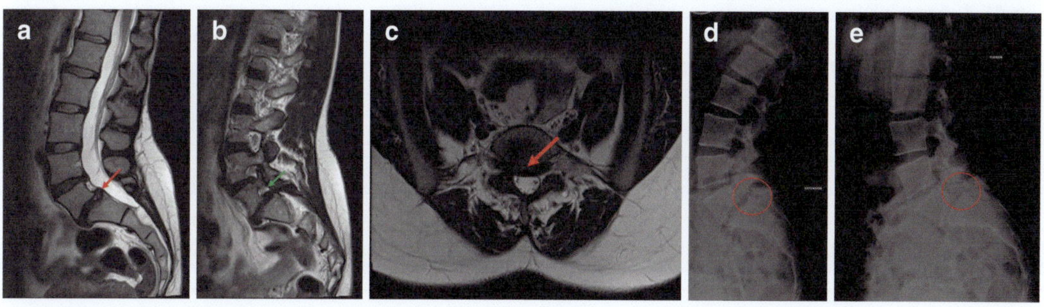

Fig. 18.2 Spondylolisthesis grade I. (**a**, **b**) T2-weighted MRI sagittal and (**c**) T2-weighted axial MRI images of the lumbar spine. (**d**). Extension and (**e**) flexion lateral X-ray. Red arrow: Pseudodisc. Green arrow: Nerve root compression by pseudodisc. Red circle shows spondylolysis

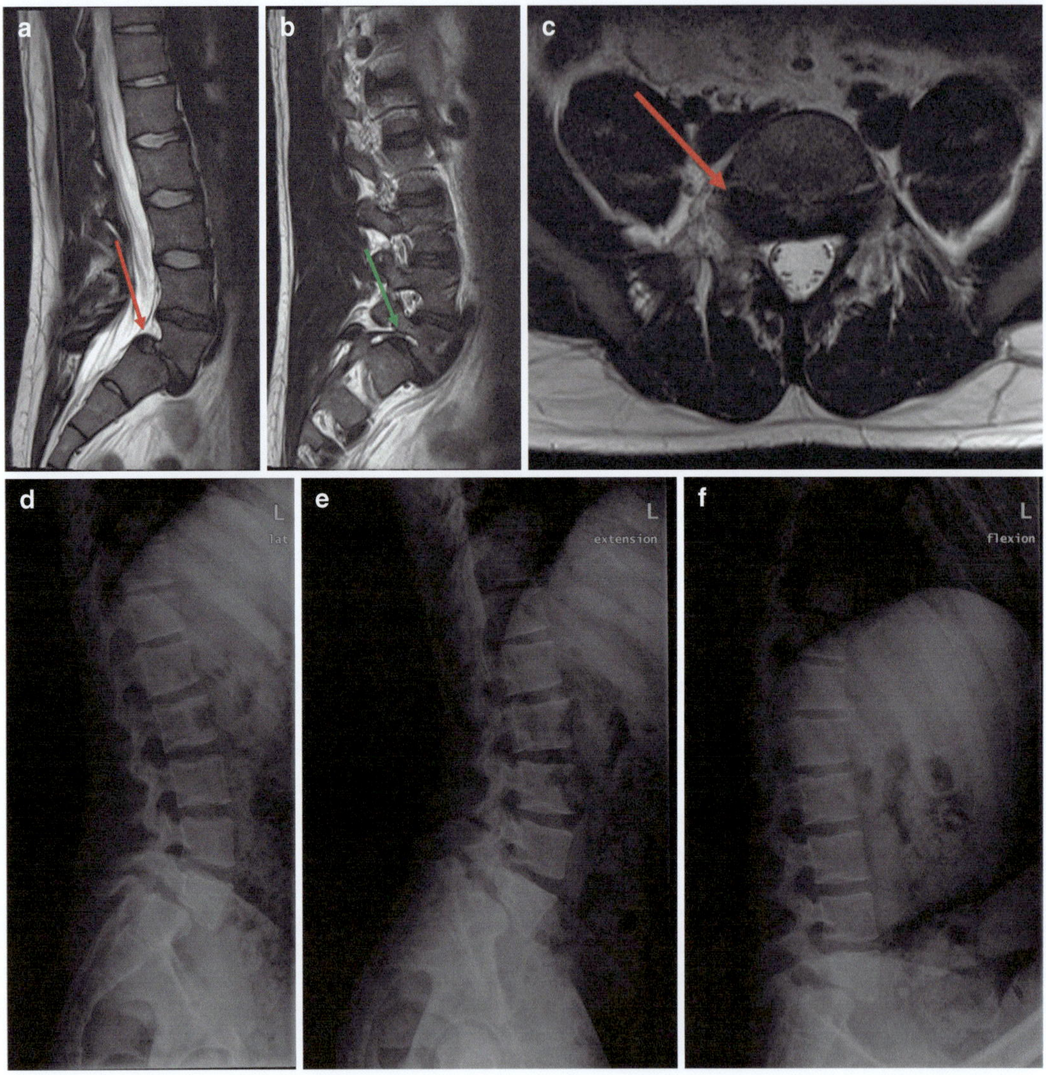

Fig. 18.3 Spondylolisthesis grade II. (**a**, **b**) T2-weighted MRI sagittal and (**c**) T2-weighted axial MRI images of lumbar spine. (**d,**) Lateral standing, (**d**) extension, and (**e**) flexion lateral X-ray. Red arrow: Pseudodisc. Green arrow: Nerve root compression by pseudodisc.

Management

Non-operative Management

A trial of conservative management is usually warranted in all patients with low back pain or lower extremity pain attributable to degenerative spondylolisthesis [13, 14]. Conservative treatment usually includes relative bed rest, a trial of NSAIDs, physical therapy, bracing, strength/postural training, and core training. It seems a reasonable option for a subset of patients without neurological symptoms at presentation, as a large proportion will improve over time [8]. However, it is important to note that in many cases surgical intervention is more effective than non-operative measures in reducing back and leg pain [9, 13–16].

Surgical Management

- Indications:
  - No improvement after 6 months of appropriately selected conservative treatment.
  - Severe neurologic symptoms (e.g., weakness/neurogenic pain that limits functional daily activities).
  - Progressive neurological deficit.

  Note: *According to the SPORT trial [16], a combined randomized cohort and observational cohort of patients with degenerative spondylolisthesis, surgical management showed better long-term results than non-operative management.

- Decompression alone (DS) versus decompression and fusion (DS + F):
  - The optimal surgical treatment remains controversial. While some authors argue that spinal decompression alone is sufficient [17, 18], many others advocate for the need of spinal fusion—a procedure that has seen a rising trend in recent years [19], despite some reports of higher morbidity associated with fusion compared to decompression alone [20, 21].
  - According to the Nordsten-DS trial, including patients with degenerative lumbar spondylolisthesis with a vertebral slip of at least 3 mm, both procedures demonstrated similar clinical outcomes after 5 years of follow-up regarding the primary endpoint (ODI) and secondary outcomes (leg and back pain, ZCQ and EQ-5D) [18].
  - The SLIP trial, comparing DS versus DS + F in patients with grade I degenerative lumbar spondylolisthesis without radiographic instability, showed that patients treated with DS + F experienced significantly greater improvement in physical health-related quality of life measured by SF-36 physical-component summary scores at 2, 3, and 4 years of follow-up. The DS group had a significantly higher cumulative reoperation rate primarily due to subsequent clinical instability [22].
  - Radiographic predictors of delayed instability after DS include a motion at spondylolisthesis of >1.25 mm, a disc height of >6.5 mm, and a facet angle of >50° [23].
- Surgical technique.
  - A common approach involves laminectomy for decompression with or without instrumented fusion. Controversy exists over the utility of correcting the slippage [22].
  - An interbody graft (TLIF, PLIF, LLIF, or ALIF) may be used to improve alignment, aid in indirect nerve root decompression by increasing disc height, and increase fusion rates [24].
    - TLIF is the most widely used due to the avoidance of neural retraction to access the intervertebral space in comparison with PLIF. LIFT randomized, controlled, non-inferiority trial found no difference regarding clinical outcomes or rate of complications between both techniques as treatment of lumbar spondylolisthesis [25].
    - ALIF is suitable for approaches to L3-S1, with more cranial levels being blocked by vascular structures [13].
    - LLIF allows access to T12-L5, with more caudal approaches blocked by the iliac crest. Some surgical pitfalls are that LLIF provides only indirect neural decompression and a higher likelihood of injury to the lumbar plexus exists when performed in caudal levels (L5-S1) [26, 27] (Table 18.1).
  - Minimally invasive approaches have proven to be as effective in single-level lumbar spondylolisthesis as traditional open approaches [28, 29]. The many advantages include reduced blood loss, decreased postoperative hospital stay, decreased postoperative pain, shorter duration of opioid therapy, reduced costs, and early return to work [31, 32] (Fig. 18.4).
  - The rate of complications in patients undergoing minimally invasive surgery (MIS) was comparable to those undergoing traditional open surgery [29].

Table 18.1 Approaches for interbody fusion suitability

Approach	Suitable for:	Not suitable if:
ALIF	L5-S1 and L3-L4, L4-L5 (upper levels can be more complex due to large vessels)	Previous abdominal surgery or scarring due to radiotherapy, morbid obesity, aortic aneurysm, or aberrant vasculature
TLIF	All of lumbar spine	Conjoined nerve roots
PLIF	All of lumbar spine	Conjoined nerve roots
LLIF	T12-L5	Previous retroperitoneal surgery, retroperitoneal scarring, need for direct neural decompression

Note that PLIF and TLIF approaches are suitable for virtually all levels

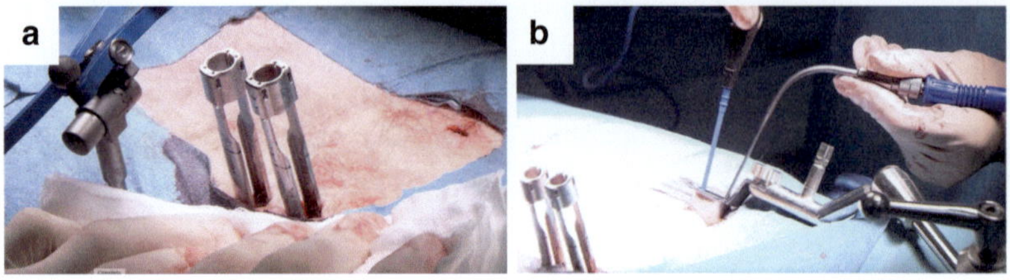

Fig. 18.4 Navigated minimally invasive spine surgery of spondylolisthesis. (**a**) Navigated percutaneous pedicle screws. (**b**) Percutaneous pedicle screws on the left side of the patient and tubular TLIF approach on the right side of the patient

– Navigation and robotics-assisted MIS had superior outcomes regarding operative blood loss, operating time, precision of screw placement, and clinical outcomes when compared to traditional MIS [33].

References

1. Wang YXJ, Káplár Z, Deng M, Leung JCS. Lumbar degenerative spondylolisthesis epidemiology: a systematic review with a focus on gender-specific and age-specific prevalence. J Orthop Transl. 2016;11:39.
2. Aoki Y, Takahashi H, Nakajima A, Kubota G, Watanabe A, Nakajima T, et al. Prevalence of lumbar spondylolysis and spondylolisthesis in patients with degenerative spinal disease. Sci Rep. 2020;10(1).
3. Jacobsen S, Sonne-Holm S, Rovsing H, Monrad H, Gebuhr P. Degenerative lumbar spondylolisthesis: an epidemiological perspective. The copenhagen osteoarthritis study.
4. Boden SD, Riew M, D4 K, Yamaguchi TP, Branch D, Schellinger, et al. Orientation of the lumbar facet joints: Association with Degenerative Disc Disease.
5. Crawford NR, Cagli S, Sonntag VK, Dickman CA. Biomechanics of grade I degenerative lumbar spondylolisthesis. Part 1: in vitro model. J Neurosurg. 2001;94(1 Suppl):45–50.
6. Sansur CA, Reames DL, Smith JS, Kojo Hamilton D, Berven SH, Broadstone PA, et al. Morbidity and mortality in the surgical treatment of 10,242 adults with spondylolisthesis Presented at the 2009 Joint Spine Section Meeting Clinical article.
7. Kalichman L, Kim DH, Li L, Guermazi A, Berkin V, Hunter DJ. Spondylolysis and spondylolisthesis. Spine. 2013;34(2):199.
8. Matsunaga S, Sakou T, Morizono Y, Masuda A, Demirtas AM. Natural history of degenerative spondylolisthesis. Pathogenesis and natural course of the slippage. Spine (Phila Pa 1976). 1990;15(11):1204–10.
9. Matsunaga S, Ijiri K, Hayashi K. Nonsurgically managed patients with degenerative spondylolisthesis: a 10- to 18-year follow-up study. J Neurosurg. 2000;93(2 Suppl):194–8.
10. Lee NJ, Mathew J, Kim JS, Lombardi JM, Vivas AC, Reidler J, et al. Flexion-extension standing radiographs underestimate instability in patients with single-level lumbar spondylolisthesis: comparing flexion-supine imaging may be more appropriate. J Spine Surg. 2021;7(1):48.
11. Bendo JA, Ong B. Importance of correlating static and dynamic imaging studies in diagnosing degenerative lumbar spondylolisthesis. Am J Orthop (Belle Mead NJ). 2001;30(3):247–50.
12. Hayes MA, Howard TC, Gruel CR, Kopta JA. Roentgenographic evaluation of lumbar spine flexion-extension in asymptomatic individuals. Spine (Phila Pa 1976). 1989;14(3):327–31.
13. Chan AK, Sharma V, Robinson LC, Mummaneni PV. Summary of guidelines for the treatment of lumbar spondylolisthesis. Neurosurg Clin N Am. 2019;30(3):353.
14. Matz PG, Meagher RJ, Lamer T, Tontz WLJ, Annaswamy TM, Cassidy RC, et al. Guideline summary review: an evidence-based clinical guideline for

the diagnosis and treatment of degenerative lumbar spondylolisthesis. Spine J. 2016;16(3):439–48.
15. Karsy M, Bisson EF. Surgical versus nonsurgical treatment of lumbar spondylolisthesis. Neurosurg Clin N Am. 2019;30(3):333.
16. Weinstein JN, Lurie JD, Tosteson TD, Hanscom B, Tosteson ANA, Blood EA, et al. Surgical versus nonsurgical treatment for lumbar degenerative spondylolisthesis. N Engl J Med. 2008;356(22):2257.
17. Chan AK, Bisson EF, Bydon M, Glassman SD, Foley KT, Potts EA, et al. Laminectomy alone versus fusion for grade 1 lumbar spondylolisthesis in 426 patients from the prospective Quality Outcomes Database. J Neurosurg Spine. 2018;30(2):234.
18. Kgomotso EL, Hellum C, Fagerland MW, Solberg T, Brox JI, Storheim K, et al. Decompression alone or with fusion for degenerative lumbar spondylolisthesis (Nordsten-DS): five year follow-up of a randomised, multicentre, non-inferiority trial. BMJ 2024.
19. Sastry RA, Chen J, Shao B, Weil RJ, Chang K, Maynard K, et al. Patterns in decompression and fusion procedures for patients with lumbar stenosis after major clinical trial results, 2016 to 2019. JAMA Netw Open. 2024;6(7).
20. Försth P, Ólafsson G, Carlsson T, Frost A, Borgström F, Fritzell P, et al. A randomized, controlled trial of fusion surgery for lumbar spinal stenosis. N Engl J Med. 2016;374(15):1413.
21. Austevoll IM, Hermansen E, Fagerland MW, Storheim K, Brox JI, Solberg T, et al. Decompression with or without fusion in degenerative lumbar spondylolisthesis. N Engl J Med. 2021;385(6):526–38.
22. Ghogawala Z, Dziura J, Butler WE, Dai F, Terrin N, Magge SN, et al. Laminectomy plus fusion versus laminectomy alone for lumbar spondylolisthesis. N Engl J Med. 2016;374(15):1424.
23. Blumenthal C, Curran J, Benzel EC, Potter R, Magge SN, Frederick J, et al. Radiographic predictors of delayed instability following decompression without fusion for degenerative Grade I lumbar spondylolisthesis Clinical article. J Neurosurg Spine. 2013;18(4):340–6.
24. Levin JM, Tanenbaum JE, Steinmetz MP, Mroz TE, Overley SC. Posterolateral fusion (PLF) versus transforaminal lumbar interbody fusion (TLIF) for spondylolisthesis: a systematic review and meta-analysis. Spine J. Elsevier Inc. 2018;18:1088–98.
25. Yee T, Zammar S, Mummaneni PV. The lumbar interbody fusion trial: TLIF or PLIF for lumbar spondylolisthesis? Lancet Region Health. 2024;43.
26. Mobbs RJ, Phan K, Malham G, Seex K, Rao PJ. Lumbar interbody fusion: techniques, indications and comparison of interbody fusion options including PLIF, TLIF, MI-TLIF, OLIF/ATP, LLIF and ALIF. J Spine Surg. 2015;1(1):2–18.
27. Rabau O, Navarro-Ramirez R, Aziz M, Teles A, Mengxiao Ge S, Quillo-Olvera J, et al. Lateral lumbar Interbody fusion (LLIF): an update. Global Spine J. 2020;10(2 Suppl):17S–21S.
28. Ali EMS, Abdeen M, Saleh MK. Minimally invasive versus mini-open transforaminal lumbar interbody fusion in managing low-grade degenerative spondylolisthesis. Acta Neurochir. 2024;166(1).
29. Lu VM, Kerezoudis P, Gilder HE, Mccutcheon BA, Phan K, Bydon M. Minimally invasive surgery versus open surgery spinal fusion for spondylolisthesis. Spine. 2017;42(3):E177.
30. Parker SL, Adogwa O, Bydon A, Cheng J, Mcgirt MJ. Cost-effectiveness of minimally invasive versus open transforaminal lumbar interbody fusion for degenerative spondylolisthesis associated low-back and leg pain over two years. World Neurosurg 2012–07;78(1–2):178.
31. Mummaneni PV, Bisson EF, Kerezoudis P, Glassman S, Foley K, Slotkin JR, et al. Minimally invasive versus open fusion for Grade I degenerative lumbar spondylolisthesis: analysis of the Quality Outcomes Database. Neurosurg Focus. 2017;43(2).
32. Kotani Y, Abumi K, Ito M, Sudo H, Abe Y, Minami A. Mid-term clinical results of minimally invasive decompression and posterolateral fusion with percutaneous pedicle screws versus conventional approach for degenerative spondylolisthesis with spinal stenosis. Eur Spine J. 2011;21(6):1171.
33. Liu C, Xu C, Liang J, Xie B. Surgical innovation: comparative efficacy of navigation-assisted modified minimally invasive Transforaminal Lumbar Interbody Fusion (MIS-TLIF) and traditional MIS-TLIF in treating low-grade isthmic spondylolisthesis in the elderly. World Neurosurg. 2024;191:e151–9.

19 Decompression Without Fusion for Lumbar Degenerative Lumber Spondylolisthesis (DLS) Decompression Without Fusion: Evidence and Technique

Clemens Weber and Ivar Magne Austevoll

Introduction

Lumbar degenerative spondylolisthesis is a common condition characterized by the forward slippage of one vertebra over another due to degenerative changes in the intervertebral discs, facet joints, and flaval ligaments, which can contribute to spinal stenosis with compression of the neural structures within the spinal canal. "Spondylolisthesis" is derived from the Greek words *σπόνδυλος* (*spondylos*), meaning vertebra, and *ολίσθησης* (*olisthesis*), a slip or a sliding. This condition is common among the elderly population, and symptomatic patients usually suffer from back and leg pain with neurogenic claudication resulting in restricted function and reduced quality of life [1]. Conservative treatment with analgesics and physical therapy is usually the initial and primary modality for symptomatic patients. Following shared decision-making, surgery can be a treatment option when conservative treatment fails.

In the last decades, surgical management for symptomatic degenerative spondylolisthesis has focused on decompression combined with instrumented fusion, which aims to relieve neural compression and stabilize the spinal segment. However, adding instrumented fusion to decompression carries some disadvantages, including increased morbidity, longer surgical time, hospital stays and recovery time and the potential development of adjacent segment disease. In recent years, decompression without fusion has gained attention as a less invasive alternative, particularly in patients where surgeons consider the spondylolisthesis to be without significant instability. This treatment option prioritizes the removal of offending structures that compress neural elements while preserving spinal motion and minimizing surgical morbidity as well as treatment costs.

Scientific Evidence

The effectiveness of decompression with or without fusion for lumbar degenerative spondylolisthesis has been a major question of debate in the field of spine surgery [2]. Following some influential publications, fusion was believed to provide superior outcomes due to its stabilizing effects for this condition [3–5]; however, recent randomized trials challenge this notion, suggesting that fusion may not be necessary in most patients with lumbar degenerative spondylolisthesis [6–9].

C. Weber (✉)
Department of Neurosurgery, Stavanger University Hospital, Stavanger, Norway
e-mail: clemens.weber@sus.no

I. M. Austevoll
Department of Orthopedic Surgery, Haukeland University Hospital, Bergen, Norway
e-mail: ivar.magne.austevoll@helse-bergen.no

A. A. Baaj et al. (eds.), *Surgery of the Lumbar Spine*, https://doi.org/10.1007/978-3-032-18097-1_19

Randomized Trials

The Spinal Laminectomy versus Instrumented Pedicle Screw (SLIP) trial was conducted at five U.S. hospitals between 2002 and 2009 and included 66 patients with single-level spondylolisthesis. Patients were not included if they had a spondylolisthesis >14 mm or dynamic motion of 3 mm or more measured on radiography. The patients' mean age was 67 years whereas 80% were females. The trial initially aimed to include 100 patients but ended up with 66 patients, of these only 57 (86%) were available for 2-years follow-up and 45 (68%) at four years. The primary outcome measure of this study was the change in the physical-component summary score of the generic 36-Item Short-Form Health Survey (SF-36). One surgeon performed 51 of the total of 66 surgeries. The study found that decompression with posterolateral instrumented fusion provided better patient-reported outcomes in terms of quality of life measured with SF-36 at two and four years postoperatively compared to decompression with laminectomy [6]. However, the study did not find significant differences in the disease-specific functional outcome measure (Oswestry Disability Index, ODI), but significantly more surgical complications, higher blood loss, longer length of procedure, and longer length of stay in patients operated with decompression and fusion. Despite the later the authors concluded that "the addition of lumbar spinal fusion to laminectomy was associated with slightly greater but clinically meaningful improvement in overall physical health-related quality of life than laminectomy alone".

The Swedish Spinal Stenosis Study (SSSS) was conducted at seven Swedish hospitals between 2006 and 2012 and included 247 patients with spinal stenosis with (n = 135) or without spondylolisthesis in one or two lumbar levels. The mean age was 67 years (79% females); 92% had 2-years follow-up and 90% had available data at five years [10]. The primary outcome of this trial was the score on the ODI 2 years after surgery. The results showed that patients undergoing decompression alone had similar patient-reported outcomes to those receiving decompression with fusion in terms of pain relief, function, and quality of life [7, 10]. The authors performed a health-economic evaluation and found that fusion was associated with additional costs of 6800 $ per patient. The authors concluded that "decompression surgery plus fusion surgery did not result in better clinical outcomes at 2 years and 5 years than did decompression surgery alone".

A randomized controlled trial from Japan included 85 patients operated with decompression alone, decompression plus fusion, or decompression plus stabilization for degenerative spondylolisthesis between 2003 and 2012. The patients had a mean age of 63 years, 58% were female, and they were recruited from two different hospitals [8, 11]. The follow-up rate at 5 years was 86%. The primary outcome measure for this trial was the score for back pain measured on a Visual Analogue Scale (VAS). The results of the study showed no significant differences among the groups at 1 and 5 years postoperatively. The authors concluded that "additional instrumentation operation for low-grade degenerative spondylolisthesis did not result in superior results to decompression alone at 1 and 5 years postoperatively".

The Norwegian degenerative spondylolisthesis and spinal stenosis (NORDSTEN) study included 267 patients randomized to decompression alone or decompression with fusion operated at 16 Norwegian hospitals between 2014 and 2017 [9, 12]. The mean age was 66 years and 69% were female. Follow-up rates were 90% after two years and 88% after five years. The primary outcome measure of this trial was a reduction of at least 30% in the ODI score. The results of this trial showed that decompression alone was noninferior to decompression with instrumented fusion regarding patient-reported outcomes such as pain, disability, symptom severity, functional status, and satisfaction with treatment both after 2 and 5 years.

One of the potential disadvantages of decompression in degenerative spondylolisthesis is the possible risk of the need for reoperation. Table 19.1 shows the long-term reoperation rates reported in the randomized trials on degenerative

Table 19.1 Summary of the four randomized controlled trials on decompression alone versus decompression with fusion for lumbar degenerative spondylolisthesis

Study	N	Mean age	Decompression technique	Primary outcome measure	Follow-up period	Follow-up rate	Reoperation rate after 2 years
Ghogawala 2016 [6]	66	67 years	Complete laminectomy (100%)	Change in SF-36 after 2 years	2 & 4 years	86% (2 years), 68% (4 years)	34% (decompression) and 7% (fusion) after 4 years
Försth 2016 [7, 10]	135	67 years	Laminectomy (82%) or bilateral, midline-preserving laminotomy (18%)	Change in ODI after 2 years	2 & 5 years	92% (2 years), 90% (5 years)	21% (decompression) and 22% (fusion) after 5 years
Inose 2018 [8, 11]	85	63 years	Decompression surgery	Change in VAS back pain	1, 5 & mean 12 years	98% (1 year), 86% (5 years)	7% (decompression) and 10% (fusion) after mean 12 years
Austevoll 2021 [9, 12]	267	66 years	Midline-preserving laminotomy (100%)	Reduction of at least 30% in ODI after 2 and 5 years	2 & 5 years	90% (2 years), 88% (5 years)	21% (decompression) and 23% (fusion) after 5 years

spondylolisthesis [6–12]. A recent analysis showed an overall reoperation rate of 9% in patients operated for degenerative spondylolisthesis, with 7% for microsurgical decompression and 10% for open laminectomy [13]. Current evidence indicates that adding fusion as a safeguard to avoid reoperations does not create any added value for patients with degenerative spondylolisthesis and might be regarded as an overcautious and unnecessary treatment [14].

Systematic Reviews and Meta-analysis

Since 2022, the available high-quality evidence has been evaluated in seven systematic reviews and meta-analyses. Six concluded evidence for decompression alone as the first choice of treatment [15–20], whereas one concluded that laminectomy with fusion was associated with superior clinical outcomes than laminectomy alone [21]. The latter, which was the only one with US authors, did not include central clinical outcomes from the Scandinavian trials in the meta-analysis [22].

Lumbar Spinal Stenosis and Degenerative Spondylolisthesis

Lumbar spinal stenosis with or without degenerative spondylolisthesis is a degenerative condition of the spine often presenting with similar signs and symptoms. The authors of the Spine Patient Outcomes Research Trial (SPORT) asked the question "if a slip matters" and concluded in their analysis of 1235 patients that lumbar spinal stenosis with and without spondylolisthesis patients have similar baseline characteristic, but different clinical outcome after surgery and therefore should be treated as two different conditions [23]. However, a secondary analysis of the NORDSTEN trials comparing patients with lumbar spinal stenosis with and without degenerative spondylolisthesis showed that the symptom burden before surgery and the clinical outcome after surgery were similar independently of a concomitant spondylolisthesis [24].

Surgical Technique

The posterior midline approach for decompression of the spinal canal is the most frequently used approach for posterior lumbar spine surgery and focuses on relieving neural compression while preserving spinal motion and avoiding the complications associated with instrumented fusion surgery [25]. Traditionally, open laminectomy was utilized, whereas in recent years less-invasive techniques preserving the posterior midline (without removal of the spinous process or the supraspinous-interspinous ligament complex) have gained more popularity with similar clinical results [26]. The following steps outline the general surgical technique of the microsurgical decompression of lumbar spinal stenosis with Degenerative lumber spondylolisthesis (DLS):decompression without fusion:

Patient Positioning and Anesthesia

Patients are positioned prone on a radiolucent table under general anesthesia. Proper positioning is crucial to maintain spinal alignment and minimize pressure on the abdomen, which helps reduce venous congestion and bleeding during surgery [27]. Fluoroscopy is utilized for localization of the targeted level and to mark the planned incision. Preoperative antibiotic prophylaxis reduces the risk of postoperative wound infection [28]. The skin is infiltrated with local anesthesia.

Operative Technique

For standard single-level surgery, a 2–3 cm midline incision is suitable in the majority of cases. The fascia is incised and subperiosteal dissection is performed to expose the spinous process, the laminae of the cranial and the caudal level, and the medial part of the facet joint. Intraoperative fluoroscopy should be used to confirm the level of surgery before the decompression. After confirmation of the level, a self-retaining retractor is placed. Midline structures, such as supra- and interspinous ligaments, should be preserved with this technique. A unilateral approach is used for over-the-top decompression, a bilateral approach for bilateral decompression. After placing the retractor, the surgery continues with a surgical microscope or surgical loupes. In general, the surgery is performed from cranial to caudal and from medial to lateral. The inferior half of the ipsilateral, cranial lamina is removed with a high-speed drill or Kerisson rongeurs. To avoid iatrogenic instability, care must be taken to preserve the pars interarticularis and the lateral half of the facet joint. The ligamentum flavum is detached from the cranial lamina and removed with Kerisson rongeurs from above the disc cranially to the level of the pedicle caudally. Due to the spondylolisthesis, the thecal sac might be lifted in the caudal part of the decompression; care should be taken to avoid accidental durotomy. After decompression of the central part of the stenosis, the ligamentum flavum and the medial part of the facet joint are removed to decompress the ipsilateral lateral recess (Fig. 19.1). When performing a cross-over (or over-the-top) decompression, the operating table should be tilted away from the surgeon. The basis of the cranial spinous process is removed with a high-speed drill, a thin-bladed chisel, or Kerisson rongeurs. Utilizing an undercutting technique, the contralateral ligamentum flavum is removed to decompress the spinal canal and the lateral recess. The extent of decompression should be controlled with a blunt probe or dissector. After obtaining hemostasis, the surgical field is irrigated thoroughly with saline solution. A postoperative drain is usually not necessary with this approach. The facia and the subcutaneous layer are sutured with 2-0 Vicryl, and the skin is closed with 3-0 Monocryl.

In patients with degenerative spondylolisthesis, a unilateral decompression with cross-over can be demanding due to the step between the two vertebrae. Therefore, a bilateral decompression can be utilized to accomplish an adequate

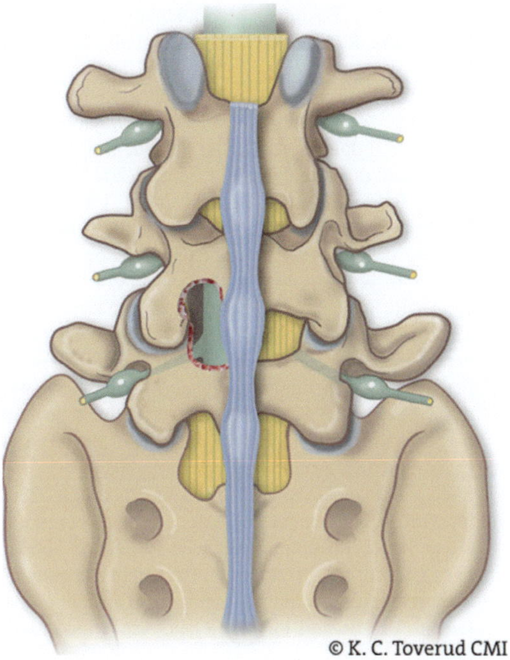

Fig. 19.1 Unilateral decompression at the L4/L5 level

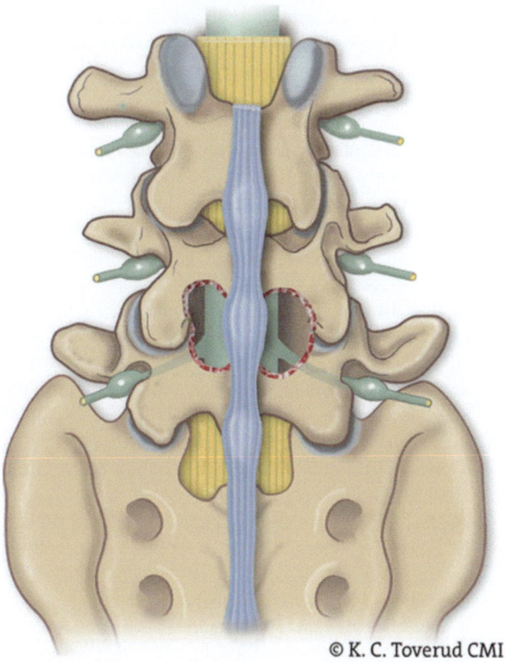

Fig. 19.2 Bilateral decompression at the L4/L5 level

decompression of the stenotic level. After decompressing the ipsilateral part of the spinal canal, the fascia is incised, subperiosteal dissection is performed, a self-retaining retractor is placed, and decompression is performed on the contralateral side (Fig. 19.2).

Alternative approaches can be utilized to decompress degenerative spondylolisthesis with spinal stenosis. Muscle-dilating tubes can be used instead of self-retaining retractors. In that case, a trans-muscular approach is used instead of the subperiosteal, midline approach described above. Endoscopic decompression is an even less invasive technique and can also be used for this condition. Both tubular and endoscopic approaches lead to similar results [29].

Postoperative Care

The goals after surgery are pain control and early mobilization. Patients operated with this technique can be mobilized within a few hours after surgery, and postoperative deep vein thrombosis prophylaxis is usually not necessary. Lumbar immobilization with a cast is usually not required. Depending on age and co-morbidities, patients can be discharged 4 to 6 hours after surgery or on postoperative day one.

References

1. Fitzgerald JA, Newman PH. Degenerative spondylolisthesis. J Bone Joint Surg Br. 1976;58(2):184–92.
2. Major surgical question has no answer. Back Lett. 2019;34(4):39–46.
3. Herkowitz HN, Kurz LT. Degenerative lumbar spondylolisthesis with spinal stenosis. A prospective study comparing decompression with decompression and intertransverse process arthrodesis. J Bone Joint Surg Am. 1991;73(6):802–8.
4. Fischgrund JS, Mackay M, Herkowitz HN, Brower R, Montgomery DM, Kurz LT. 1997 Volvo Award winner in clinical studies. Degenerative lumbar spondylolisthesis with spinal stenosis: a prospective, randomized study comparing decompressive laminectomy and arthrodesis with and without spinal instrumentation-Spine (Phila Pa 1976). 1997;22(24):2807–12.
5. Kornblum MB, Fischgrund JS, Herkowitz HN, Abraham DA, Berkower DL, Ditkoff JS. Degenerative

lumbar spondylolisthesis with spinal stenosis: a prospective long-term study comparing fusion and pseudarthrosis. Spine (Phila Pa 1976). 2004;29(7):726–33; discussion 33-4.
6. Ghogawala Z, Dziura J, Butler WE, Dai F, Terrin N, Magge SN, et al. Laminectomy plus fusion versus laminectomy alone for lumbar spondylolisthesis. N Engl J Med. 2016;374(15):1424–34.
7. Forsth P, Olafsson G, Carlsson T, Frost A, Borgstrom F, Fritzell P, et al. A randomized, controlled trial of fusion surgery for lumbar spinal stenosis. N Engl J Med. 2016;374(15):1413–23.
8. Inose H, Kato T, Yuasa M, Yamada T, Maehara H, Hirai T, et al. Comparison of decompression, decompression plus fusion, and decompression plus stabilization for degenerative lumber spondylolisthesis (DLS):decompression without fusion: a prospective, randomized study. Clin Spine Surg. 2018;31(7):E347–E52.
9. Austevoll IM, Hermansen E, Fagerland MW, Storheim K, Brox JI, Solberg T, et al. Decompression with or without fusion in degenerative lumbar spondylolisthesis. N Engl J Med. 2021;385(6):526–38.
10. Karlsson T, Forsth P, Ohagen P, Michaelsson K, Sanden B. Decompression alone or decompression with fusion for lumbar spinal stenosis: five-year clinical results from a randomized clinical trial. Bone Joint J. 2024;106-B(7):705–12.
11. Inose H, Kato T, Sasaki M, Matsukura Y, Hirai T, Yoshii T, et al. Comparison of decompression, decompression plus fusion, and decompression plus stabilization: a long-term follow-up of a prospective, randomized study. Spine J. 2022;22(5):747–55.
12. Kgomotso EL, Hellum C, Fagerland MW, Solberg T, Brox JI, Storheim K, et al. Decompression alone or with fusion for degenerative lumbar spondylolisthesis (Nordsten-DS): five year follow-up of a randomised, multicentre, non-inferiority trial. BMJ. 2024;386:e079771.
13. Muthu S, Corluka S, Buser Z, Malcolm JG, Luo Z, Gollahalli Shivashankar P, et al. Rate of reoperation following decompression-only procedure for lumbar degenerative lumber spondylolisthesis (DLS):decompression without fusion: a systematic review of literature. JB JS Open Access. 2024;9(3)
14. Peul WC, Moojen WA. Fusion for Lumbar Spinal Stenosis--Safeguard or Superfluous Surgical Implant? N Engl J Med. 2016;374(15):1478–9.
15. Abdel-Fattah AR, Bell F, Boden L, Ferry J, McCormick C, Ross M, et al. To fuse or not to fuse: the elderly patient with lumbar stenosis and low-grade spondylolisthesis. Systematic review and meta-analysis of randomised controlled trials. Surgeon. 2023;21(1):e23–31.
16. Gadjradj PS, Basilious M, Goldberg JL, Sommer F, Navarro-Ramirez R, Mykolajtchuk C, et al. Decompression alone versus decompression with fusion in patients with lumbar spinal stenosis with degenerative lumber spondylolisthesis (DLS):decompression without fusion: a systematic review and meta-analysis. Eur Spine J. 2023.
17. Huang P, Liu Z, Liu H, Yu Y, Huang L, Lu M, et al. Decompression versus decompression plus fusion for treating degenerative lumbar spinal stenosis: a systematic review and meta-analysis. Pain Pract. 2022.
18. Kaiser R, Kantorová L, Langaufová A, Slezáková S, Tučková D, Klugar M, et al. Decompression alone versus decompression with instrumented fusion in the treatment of lumbar degenerative lumber spondylolisthesis (DLS):decompression without fusion: a systematic review and meta-analysis of randomised trials. J Neurol Neurosurg Psychiatry. 2023.
19. Shen Z, Guan X, Wang R, Xue Q, Zhang D, Zong Y, et al. Effectiveness and safety of decompression alone versus decompression plus fusion for lumbar spinal stenosis with degenerative lumber spondylolisthesis (DLS) decompression without fusion: a systematic review and meta-analysis. Ann Transl Med. 2022;10(12):664.
20. Wei F-L, Zhou C-P, Gao Q-Y, Du M-R, Gao H-R, Zhu K-L, et al. Decompression alone or decompression and fusion in degenerative lumbar spondylolisthesis. EClinicalMedicine. 2022;51.
21. Shukla GG, Chilakapati SS, Matur AV, Palmisciano P, Conteh F, Onyewadume L, et al. Laminectomy with fusion is associated with greater functional improvement compared with laminectomy alone for the treatment of degenerative lumbar spondylolisthesis: a systematic review and meta-analysis. Spine (Phila Pa 1976). 2023;48(12):874–84.
22. Austevoll IM, Hellum C, Försth P. Letter to the editor regarding the paper of Shukla and colleagues on laminectomy with fusion is associated with greater functional improvement compared with laminectomy alone for the treatment of degenerative lumbar spondylolisthesis. Spine (Phila Pa 1976). 2024;49(2):E17.
23. Pearson A, Blood E, Lurie J, Tosteson T, Abdu WA, Hillibrand A, et al. Degenerative spondylolisthesis versus spinal stenosis: does a slip matter? Comparison of baseline characteristics and outcomes (SPORT). Spine (Phila Pa 1976). 2010;35(3):298–305.
24. Weber C, Hermansen E, Myklebust TA, Banitalebi H, Brisby H, Brox JI, et al. Comparison of patients operated for lumbar spinal stenosis with and without spondylolisthesis - a secondary analysis of the NORDSTEN trials. Spine (Phila Pa 1976). 2024;49:1332.

25. Ravindra VM, Senglaub SS, Rattani A, Dewan MC, Hartl R, Bisson E, et al. Degenerative lumbar Spine disease: estimating global incidence and worldwide volume. Global Spine J. 2018;8(8):784–94.
26. Nerland US, Jakola AS, Solheim O, Weber C, Rao V, Lonne G, et al. Minimally invasive decompression versus open laminectomy for central stenosis of the lumbar spine: pragmatic comparative effectiveness study. BMJ. 2015;350:h1603.
27. Derman PB, Phillips FM. Complication avoidance in minimally invasive spinal surgery. J Spine Surg. 2019;5(Suppl 1):S57–67.
28. Shaffer WO, Baisden JL, Fernand R, Matz PG, North American Spine S. An evidence-based clinical guideline for antibiotic prophylaxis in spine surgery. Spine J. 2013;13(10):1387–92.
29. Suner HI, Castano JP, Vargas-Jimenez A, Wagner R, Mazzei AS, Velazquez W, et al. Comparison of the tubular approach and uniportal interlaminar full-endoscopic approach in the treatment of lumbar spinal stenosis: our 3-year results. World Neurosurg. 2023;173:e148–e55.

20 Decompression and Fusion for Lumbar Degenerative Spondylolisthesis: Evidence-Based Medicine and Technique

Evgenii Belykh, Vadim A. Byvaltsev, Subu Magge, and Zoher Ghogawala

Spondylolisthesis was the most common indication for elective spinal fusion in the United States (45.2% in 2015) [1]. Following pivotal randomized controlled trials (RCT) published in 2016 [2, 3], the rate of surgeries for degenerative lumbar spondylolisthesis (DLS) in the United States continued to increase from 23,405 in 2016 to 37,215 in 2019 (per National Inpatient Sample that captures approximately 20% of all hospital encounters), and proportion of patients treated with fusion surgery increased from 67 to 90% [4]. The number of spinal fusion surgeries is projected to continue to increase, particularly among patients over the age of 75 [5]. Here, we evaluate the evidence behind utilization of fusion and various fusion techniques for patients with DLS.

E. Belykh
Department of Neurosurgery, Lahey Hospital and Medical Center, Burlington, MA, USA

Department of Neurosurgery, Rutgers New Jersey Medical School, Newark, NJ, USA
e-mail: Evgenii.Belykh@lahey.org

V. A. Byvaltsev
Department of Neurosurgery, Irkutsk State Medical University, Irkutsk, Russia

S. Magge · Z. Ghogawala (✉)
Department of Neurosurgery, Lahey Hospital and Medical Center, Burlington, MA, USA
e-mail: subu.n.magge@lahey.org; Zoher.Ghogawala@Lahey.org

Definition and Classifications

Degenerative lumbar spondylolisthesis is an acquired anterior displacement of one vertebra over the subjacent vertebra, associated with degenerative changes, without an associated disruption or defect in the vertebral ring [6]. The Wiltse-Neumann [7] scheme categorizes spondylolisthesis based on etiology as dysplastic, isthmic, degenerative, traumatic, pathologic, or postsurgical. The severity of spondylolisthesis is typically assessed by the degree of rostral vertebral body slip over the caudal vertebral body, measured using the Meyerding grading system: Grade I: ≤25%; II: 26–50%; III: 51–75%; IV: >75%, V: spondyloptosis [8]. Slippage of more than 3 mm or a > 5% transition of the adjacent vertebral endplates as measured on the lateral X-rays is considered pathological and may be defined as spondylolisthesis. According to the 2016 North American Spine Society (NASS) guidelines, degenerative spondylolisthesis with a slippage of 7 mm or more on upright X-rays warrants fusion [6]. While insurance companies often rely on measurements in millimeters rather than percentages [9], the specific cutoff value of 7 mm is not consistently agreed upon in the literature.

A. A. Baaj et al. (eds.), *Surgery of the Lumbar Spine*, https://doi.org/10.1007/978-3-032-18097-1_20

Pathophysiology

Degenerative lumbar spondylolisthesis is more common in patients who are older or female. The most frequently affected level is L4-L5, followed by L3-L4 and L5-S1, as the transitional anatomy of the lumbosacral area increases mechanical load on the disk. Ventral slippage narrows the central spinal canal while compensatory facet and ligamentous hypertrophy often result in lateral recess and foraminal stenosis. Diabetes, other systemic diseases, pregnancy, and decreased estrogen levels may contribute to increased ligamentous laxity and weakened collagen cross-linking. More sagittally oriented facet joints (average 33 degrees vs. 43 degrees in normal anatomy) [10], asymmetry in the sagittal orientation of facet joints (facet tropism) [10], and an increased pedicle facet angle can cause abnormal load distribution and exacerbate subluxation of the vertebral bodies.

Clinical Assessment

Morse et al. (2020) surveyed 381 members of the Lumbar Spine Research Society and Society of Minimally Invasive Spine Surgery to summarize preoperative factors impacting the decision to perform fusion for DLS [11]. While understanding these factors allows for a more detailed and individualized approach, the survey revealed substantial variation in treatment patterns and little consensus on the management of DLS. In this section, we discuss various clinical and radiographical factors to consider when selecting patients who might benefit from fusion in addition to decompression.

DLS patients typically present with central stenosis and symptoms of neurogenic claudication, which include leg and buttock cramping and a sense of muscle fatigue. Some patients also report axial low back pain, which is generally mechanical and positional. Mechanical low back pain is defined as axial back pain that worsens with axial loading and improves with unloading the spine (e.g., in the supine position). When mechanical low back pain is a significant presenting symptom, it is generally considered less appropriate for decompression alone [12].

In addition, some patients also have lumbar radiculopathy that progresses with walking. Physical examination is often normal. Sensory dysesthesias and motor weakness specific to an affected nerve root are possible. Increased age and frailty may be a factor for selecting less invasive surgical options such as minimally invasive fusion, or decompression alone. Active lifestyle, as opposed to a sedentary one, is a factor for some surgeons to favor fusion rather than decompression alone. Patients who are candidates for fusion surgery but who are actively smoking are often counseled to stop smoking, or otherwise decompression may be favored to avoid risks of nonunion.

Preoperative Imaging Considerations

Measuring spondylolisthesis on standing lateral X-rays (under the loading condition) as opposed to MRI (done flat) is usually sufficient. Although there is no standard to diagnose stable versus dynamic DLS, we believe that patients with listhesis of <7 mm on standing X-rays will benefit from flexion-extension lumbar X-rays, which in about 60% of cases allow to identify worsening listhesis >7 mm creating an argument for fusion surgery [13].

MRI scans should be evaluated carefully to assess degenerative changes, degree of spondylolisthesis, and the presence and severity of central, lateral, and foraminal stenosis at the level of listhesis, as well as at adjacent levels. Additional findings such as facet angle, tropism, and effusion should also be noted. Signs suggestive of instability, including increased slippage (Grade II

DLS), concomitant disk herniation, facet joint effusion >1.5 mm [6, 14], facet hypertrophy, interspinous fluid, vacuum phenomenon, and synovial cysts, should be considered when evaluating patients for potential instability or determining the need for fusion. Symptomatic foraminal stenosis may require more extensive bony removal for direct decompression, which could risk iatrogenic instability and therefore require fusion. Alternatively, some surgeons may opt for indirect decompression with a large footprint interbody spacer and fusion upfront to elevate foraminal height. Preserved disk height (>6.5 mm) [15] is viewed as a risk factor for increased segmental motion (as opposed to collapsed disk) that could lead to instability, restenosis, herniation, and therefore necessitate fusion, especially if increased removal of osteoligamentous complex is required for adequate decompression. Finally, assessment of bone quality using dual x-ray absorptiometry or computed tomography should be a part of the workup when fusion is considered.

Sagittal Alignment

DLS is typically associated with a loss of intervertebral disk height, reduced lumbar lordosis (LL), and a decreased sacral slope, which often leads to compensatory retrolisthesis of the upper lumbar spine segments to maintain alignment [16]. Patients with DLS tend to have a greater pelvic incidence (PI) (60 ± 10 degrees) compared to controls (52 ± 11 degrees) and anterior translation of the sagittal vertical axis (SVA) [16]. A high PI predisposes to the progression of spondylolisthesis and instability, making it an important factor to consider when selecting surgical options. The presence of laterolisthesis or scoliosis indicates global malalignment, where DLS may be a secondary compensatory mechanism for a more complex spine problem.

Several studies have demonstrated that, for single-level DLS, sagittal alignment has limited effects on the risk of adjacent segment disease or the rate of reoperations [17]. It has also been shown that for a single-level Grade I and II DLS, reduction of slippage and correction of sagittal radiographic parameters did not significantly improve clinical outcomes [18, 19]. However, there is growing interest in considering sagittal spinal parameters when planning for fusion surgeries, particularly for multilevel disease [20].

Recent data suggest that, similar to other degenerative spine conditions, a greater PI-LL mismatch and worsened SVA correlate with more severe disability and worse clinical outcomes [21]. Therefore, maintaining or restoring optimal sagittal alignment is essential to prevent iatrogenic malalignment after segmental fixation and reduce the risk of adjacent segment disease [20]. Optimal sagittal alignment parameters, derived from studies in adult spinal deformity, include PI-LL mismatch of less than 10 degrees and an SVA of less than 50 mm [22].

Nonsurgical Treatment, Natural History

Surgery is usually reserved for patients who have failed medical management which often includes pain control with non-opioid and opioid medications, physical therapy, and epidural steroid injections. While epidural steroid injections generally provide temporary relief and may not alter long-term outcomes, they may be a viable option for symptom control, particularly in patients who are not candidates for surgery [23].

Addressing the shortcomings of older studies published in 1990s such as small sample and limited geographic participation, the NIH invested 15 million dollars and sponsored The Spine Patient Outcomes Research Trial

(SPORT) to compare the effectiveness of surgical and nonsurgical treatments for various spinal pathologies, including DLS [24]. Between 2000 to 2005, patients with at least 12 weeks of symptoms related to DLS were enrolled in either a randomized cohort ($n = 304$) or an observational cohort ($n = 303$). Participants were then assigned to receive non-surgical treatments or undergo surgery, which included decompression alone or decompression combined with various fusion techniques. This study demonstrated superiority of surgery for DLS in relieving symptoms and improving patients' function [24].

Surgical Treatment

Surgical treatment is typically indicated for patients who fail to respond to medical management for over 3 months. Urgent intervention may be required in cases of severe progressive weakness or bowel and bladder dysfunction. Multiple patient factors as well as patient values should be evaluated to set appropriate goals of surgery and select proper surgical procedure from the spectrum of available options. The surgical goals include decompression of central canal and spinal nerves, robust stabilization of the segment, and correction of deformity. Selection of surgical technique is usually based on the surgeon's professional judgement and experience, as numerous techniques for decompression and spinal fusion are available. For cases involving significant segmental instability at the level of DLS, stabilization is widely recognized as one of the primary goals of surgery. However, the choice of the most effective stabilization method remains a key area of discussion. In contrast, the management of patients with DLS without instability is still a topic of significant debate. Several studies have helped guide decision-making for patients with DLS. When evaluating these studies, readers should pay attention to the studied population, severity and stability of DLS, the specific surgical techniques and interventions used for decompression and stabilization, and the outcomes that were measured (Table 20.1).

Table 20.1 Pivotal studies evaluating decompression and fusion surgeries for patients with degenerative lumbar spondylolisthesis

Study	Author, publication year	Inclusion criteria	Exclusion criteria	Techniques studied	Comments, main findings
Herkowitz and Kurz	Herkowitz and Kurz, 1991 [25]	Single-level degenerative spondylolisthesis, stenosis only at the level of spondylolisthesis	Transitional anatomy, prior lumbar surgery	Pseudo-randomized study comparing decompressive open laminectomy (removing one-half of both the cephalad and caudad laminae of the two involved vertebrae, together with bilateral medial caudal and cephalad facetectomy) and laminectomy plus fusion (intertransverse fusion with strips of corticocancellous and cancellous bone from the iliac crest 4–5 cm length).	Results in terms of relief of pain in the back and lower extremities are better in posterolateral fusion group at mean 3 years. Patients with pseudoarthrosis 9/25 (36%) still had excellent and good results.
Fischgrund et al.	Fischgrun et al., 1997 [26]	Same as above	Same as above	Same as above (laminectomy and intertransverse arthrodesis) vs. same procedure with addition of instrumentation using uniaxial posterior transpedicular screw and plate fixation	No difference in clinical outcomes at 3 years. Higher rate of pseudoarthrosis in non-instrumented group.

(continued)

Table 20.1 (continued)

Study	Author, publication year	Inclusion criteria	Exclusion criteria	Techniques studied	Comments, main findings
The Spine Patient Outcomes Research Trial (SPORT)	Weinstein et al., 2007 [24, 36]	Neurogenic claudication or radicular leg pain with associated neurologic signs, spinal stenosis, and degenerative spondylolisthesis on standing films, persistent symptoms for at least 12 weeks and had been confirmed as surgical candidates by their physicians. Patients with adjacent levels of stenosis were eligible	Isthmic spondylolisthesis	Posterior decompressive laminectomy with or without bilateral single-level fusion (iliac crest bone grafting with or without posterior pedicle-screw instrumentation). Nonsurgical protocol included usual care, active physical therapy, exercising at home, nonsteroidal anti-inflammatory agents, opioids, and injections.	As-treated effects for the combined cohorts were statistically significant in favor of surgery for all primary and secondary outcomes. Subgroup analysis of various surgical groups showed no consistent differences in clinical outcomes Among fusion groups at 4 years [36].
Spinal Laminectomy versus Instrumented Pedicle Screw (SLIP)	Ghogawala et al. 2016 [2]	Grade I lumbar spondylolisthesis (3 to 14 mm slip), lumbar stenosis, and neurogenic claudication with or without lumbar radiculopathy	Motion of >3 mm on flexion-extension radiographs; lumbar instability because of a history of mechanical low back pain with axial loading of the spine; previous lumbar spinal surgery	Complete laminectomy with partial removal of the medial facet joint (<25%) vs. lumbar laminectomy as well as implantation of pedicle screws and titanium alloy rods across the level of listhesis, with a bone graft harvested from the iliac crest	These are highly selected DLS patients without dynamic instability creating equipoise. Fusion group had a significantly greater increase in the SF-36 physical-component then decompression (15.2 vs. 9.5 points) at 2 years after surgery. Oswestry disability index change at 2, 3, and 4 years, were not significant. No pseudoarthrosis. Rate of reoperations in decompression group (34%, $n = 10$ was higher than in fusion (14%, $n = 4$). All revisions in decompression group were done for instability at index level, and none reoperations in fusion group at the index level.

Swedish Spinal Stenosis Study (SSSS)	Försth et al. 2016 [3], Karlsson et al., 2024 [37]	Pseudoclaudication in one or both legs and back pain (score on visual-analogue scale >30), 1 or 2 adjacent stenotic segments (cross-sectional area of the dural sac ≤75 mm^2) between L2 and the sacrum on magnetic resonance imaging, duration of symptoms >6 months. Degenerative spondylolisthesis was defined as at least 3 mm lysthesis.	Spondylolysis, degenerative lumbar scoliosis (cobb angle >20 degrees), history of lumbar spinal surgery for spinal stenosis or instability, stenosis not caused by degenerative changes, stenosis caused by a herniated disk, other specific spinal conditions (e.g., ankylosing spondylitis, cancer, or neurologic disorders), history of vertebral compression fractures in affected segments, psychological disorders (e.g., dementia or drug abuse) that caused the surgeon to consider participation to be inappropriate	The method used for decompression or fusion was determined by the surgeon. Fusion group: 102(90%) posterolateral fusions; 6 instrumented interbody fusions; 5 non-instrumented fusions. Autologous bone transplant from lamina or the iliac crest was used in all fusions. No bone graft substitutes. Decompression: 98 (82%) had laminectomy; 22 were bilateral laminotomies with preservation of the midline structures.	No difference in clinical outcomes in Oswestry disability index or 6-minute walk test. No differences in outcomes of lumbar stenosis patients with or without degenerative spondylolisthesis. Operating room time, blood loss, and direct costs higher with fusion. 5 years outcomes remain the same [37]
Norwegian Degenerative Spondylolisthesis and Spinal Stenosis (NORDSTEN)	Austevoll et al., 2021; [30] Kgomotso et al. 2024 [31]	At least 3 mm spondylolisthesis solely at the stenotic level on standing radiographs, regardless of whether patient presented with signs of instability, higher grade of spondylolisthesis, slippage or angulation of vertebral bodies on flexion-extension radiographs, and facet joints with increased fluid or high sagittal angle	Excessive foraminal stenosis; thoracolumbar scoliosis >20 degrees, prior surgery at the level of spondylolisthesis	Decompression with preservation of midline structures 129/132 (98%) spinous process and supraspinous, intraspinous ligaments vs. posterior decompression with or without removal of midline structures, pedicle screw fixation with bone grafting (autograft 100%, allograft 0.09%, xenograft 12%) and optional usage of interbody device (47/124 (38%).	Decompression alone was noninferior to decompression and fusion at 5 years to achieve 30% reduction in Oswestry disability index, with similar number of patients requiring additional surgery (16% vs 18%).

Decompression Alone Versus Decompression and Fusion

In 1991, Herkowitz and Kurz published a pivotal study that provided evidence in support of fusion. This pseudo-randomized study compared laminectomy with medial facetectomy to posterolateral intertransverse fusion using iliac bone graft (without instrumentation) performed by a single surgeon for the treatment of patients with single-level spinal stenosis associated with DLS [25]. Patients who underwent fusion had significantly better rates of "satisfactory" results compared to the laminectomy-only group (96% vs 44%).

The main risk of the "decompression only" approach was believed to be the progression of radiographic instability (e.g., increased spondylolisthesis or angulation on flexion-extension X-ray), which could lead to recurrent stenosis and clinical symptoms requiring reoperation. Following open laminectomy for DLS, 96% (24/25) of patients in the Herkowitz study developed progression of anterolisthesis, compared to 28% (7/25) in the posterolateral fusion group [25]. The results of this study demonstrated the clear advantage of the posterolateral fusion technique over decompression alone. Although there was still a relatively high rate of pseudoarthrosis, those patients generally did well. The primary reason for failure in the "decompression-only" group was attributed to the lack of stabilization, which led to instability-induced progression of bony and ligamentous overgrowth and subsequent symptoms of neural compression. Therefore, better surgical approaches for stabilization were developed. At that time pedicle instrumentation was gaining popularity and many advocated fixation to increase fusion rate.

In 1997, the same group published another pivotal randomized study comparing decompression plus intertransverse posterolateral fusion with iliac crest autograft ($n = 33$) to the same procedure with the addition of transpedicular screw instrumentation ($n = 35$) [26]. At two years, the noninstrumented group had a significantly higher rate of pseudoarthrosis compared to the instrumented group (55% (18/33) vs.18% (6/35)). Interestingly, clinical outcomes were equally good in both groups, with 78% (27/35) in the instrumented group and 85% (28/33) in the non-instrumented group achieving excellent and good outcomes ($p = 0.45$). This raised the question of whether solid fusion is necessarily associated with better clinical outcomes. The authors concluded that "it is true that the purpose of arthrodesis is to achieve a solid fusion, but it is also true that a good clinical outcome could be achieved without solid bony fusion" [26].

In 2004, Kornblum et al. analyzed the long-term results (average follow-up of 7.7 years) from the patients in these two studies. Although only 47 out of 118 patients could be located, those with solid fusion ($n = 22$) showed significantly better pain relief and activity improvements compared to those who developed pseudoarthrosis ($n = 25$) at the final follow-up (86% vs. 56%, $p = 0.01$) [27]. Three out of five revision surgeries in the pseudoarthrosis group underwent second operation with instrumented screw placement [27]. To address limitations of the above studies, more robust studies were performed validated patient-reported outcome measures and true randomization.

Two relevant studies appeared in the same 2016 issue of the New England Journal of Medicine: SLIP and SSSS. Ghogawala et al. published results of *Spinal Laminectomy* versus *Instrumented Pedicle Screw* (SLIP) study, which compared laminectomy alone ($n = 35$) to laminectomy with pedicle fixation and arthrodesis using iliac bone autograft ($n = 31$) in a select group of patients with single-level DLS without dynamic instability [2]. This study showed a small but clinically meaningful improvement in physical health–related qualify of life among fusion patients compared to patients treated with decompression alone. Furthermore, none of the fused patients required revision surgery at the index level although 4 (14%) required adjacent level surgery, compared to 10 reoperations in the "decompression only" group (34%) that were performed for instability at the index level. These data suggest that at least one-third of patients with Grade I DLS are unstable and would likely benefit from fusion when performing a decompression.

Försth et al. published results of the *Swedish Spinal Stenosis Study* (SSSS), which compared fusion surgery in addition to decompression surgery in patients with lumbar spinal stenosis, with or without degenerative spondylolisthesis (defined as at least a 3 mm slip) [3]. They found no significant clinical differences in outcomes at two years [3]. Additional lumbar spine surgery was performed in 22% of the patients in the fusion group and in 21% of those in the decompression-alone group. Reasons for reoperations in the fusion group included adjacent segment stenosis ($n = 13$) and pseudoarthrosis ($n = 1$). In the decompression-alone group, reoperations were performed for restenosis or foraminal stenosis at the index level ($n = 10$), back pain ($n = 1$), and adjacent segment stenosis ($n = 4$). The mean time to repeat surgery was 35 months in the fusion group and 26 months in the decompression group. Hospital stay, intraoperative blood loss, and direct surgical costs were higher in the fusion group. Notably, the authors did not use flexion-extension X-rays, questioning their reliability. Outcomes for patients with a slip of 7.4 mm or greater were not different from the overall study results when all patients were included.

In both studies, the decompression group had a higher reoperation rate at the index level, while adjacent-level stenosis was more commonly observed in the fusion group. These studies reignited academic discussion about whether fusion is necessary for patients with spinal stenosis associated with DLS and, if so, which patients benefit most from fusion. The impact of these publications varied between the United States and Europe. In the United States, from 2016 to 2019, the proportion of fusion surgeries for DLS increased from 67.4% to 90.4%, while the rates of decompression surgeries decreased from 32.6% to 9.6% [4]. In Finland, however, from 2015 to 2018, the rate of lumbar spinal fusion decreased from 34% to 30%, while decompression surgeries increased from 67% to 77% (all procedures disregarding diagnosis), excluding fractures and tumors; data calculated from incidence figure [28]. Similarly, in Denmark, from 2015 to 2018, the proportion of spinal fusions for DLS decreased from 35% to 28% [29].

In 2021, another RCT, the *Norwegian Degenerative Spondylolisthesis and Spinal Stenosis* (NORDSTEN) trial, was published [30]. This trial compared decompression preserving the supraspinous-interspinous ligament complex to decompression combined with instrumented fusion using bone graft across the level of listhesis, with optional use of interbody devices and all hardware choices left to the surgeon's discretion. Similar to the SSSS trial, the NORDSTEN trial demonstrated the non-inferiority of decompression alone for single-level DLS patients in both 2-year and 5-year outcomes [30, 31]. Similar to what was observed in the SLIP trial, the reoperation rate among the decompression alone patients in the NORDSTEN trial was higher than that of the decompression and fusion patients.

The differences in outcomes between US-based and European trials can be attributed to several factors. These include differences in studied patient populations (with US patients having higher BMI and a higher prevalence of diabetes mellitus, but lower smoking rates), variations in the pathologies studied (stable DLS in US trials vs. a mix of stable and unstable DLS in European studies), differences in surgical techniques (complete laminectomy vs. midline structure-preserving decompressions, and posterolateral vs. interbody implants), as well as variations in the primary outcome measures selected for evaluation [32].

To further investigate these differences, several publications have emerged from the large prospective, multicenter US-based Quality Outcomes Database (QOD). When comparing laminectomy alone versus laminectomy with fusion for Grade 1 DLS at one year [33] and two years [34], adjusted for factors such as age, sex, BMI, and baseline listhesis using propensity score matching, superior outcomes were observed in patients undergoing fusion in addition to decompression, particularly in the reduction of Oswestry Disability Index scores. While these QOD-based studies applied less stringent inclusion criteria (e.g., inclusion of mobile DLS and patients with higher ASA scores), they reflect real-world data from average patients presenting to US hospitals.

Surgical Techniques

Various surgical techniques for the decompression and stabilization of the lumbar spine have been developed over the past 40 years. These include anterior lumbar interbody fusion (ALIF), posterior lumbar interbody fusion (PLIF) (Fig. 20.1), transforaminal lumbar interbody fusion (TLIF) (Fig. 20.2), lateral lumbar interbody fusion (LLIF), and oblique lumbar interbody fusion (OLIF), many of which have been employed for symptomatic DLS. The development of posterior approaches to the disc to utilize endplates as a fusion surface preceded the invention of pedicle screw instrumentation, but the latter significantly contributed to the success of modern fusion techniques [35]. The choice of a surgical technique today depends on the goals of surgery, the surgeon's preference and familiarity with the method, as well as the individual patient's anatomy.

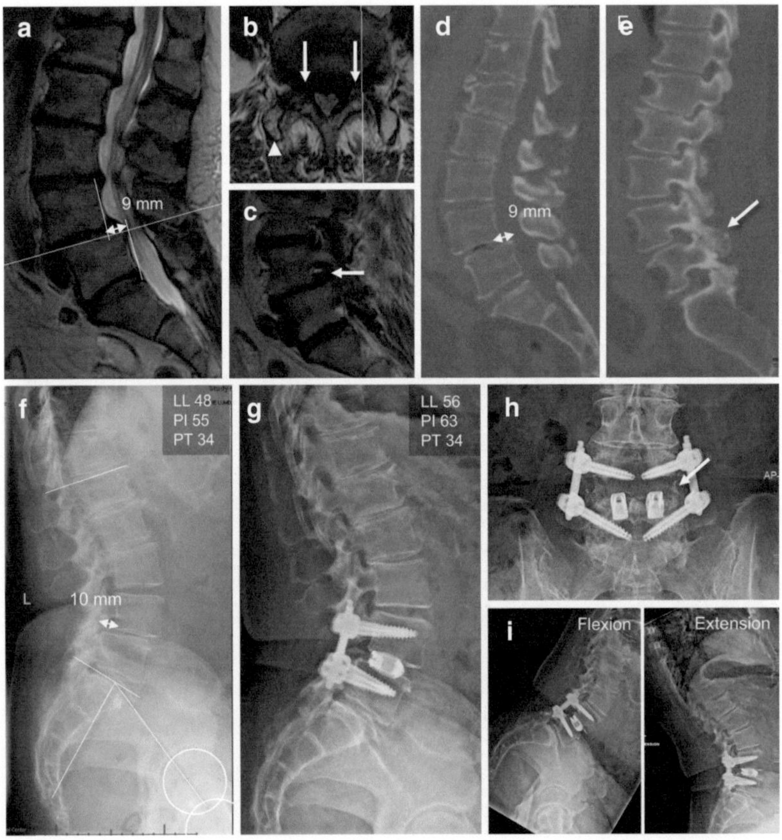

Fig. 20.1 Illustrative case of posterolateral lumbar interbody fusion (PLIF). 68 yo female with progressive back pain and bilateral leg numbness and weakness, exacerbated by walking. She has exhausted physical therapy, epidural injections and underwent L4-L5 PLIF with off-label use of rhBMP-2 into the cages and percutaneous pedicle screw instrumentation. Preoperative T2 MRI shows L4–5 Grade I spondylolisthesis (**a**) with central, bilateral lateral recess (**b**, arrows) and foraminal (**c**, arrows) stenosis, as well as facet hypertrophy (**b**, arrowhead). CT imaging redemonstrated L4-L5 slip (**d**) and facet bony overgrowth (**e**, arrow). Preoperative standing x-ray (**f**) showed global spinal alignment with slight compensatory pelvic retroflexion. Postoperative standing lateral (**g**) and anteroposterior (**h**) x-ray 6 months after surgery demonstrated preservation indirect decompression, stable hardware position, absence of segmental motion at L45 in flexion and extension (**i**), bony growth between adjacent endplates (**h**, arrow). Patient had significant improvement in her pain and returned to walking long distances

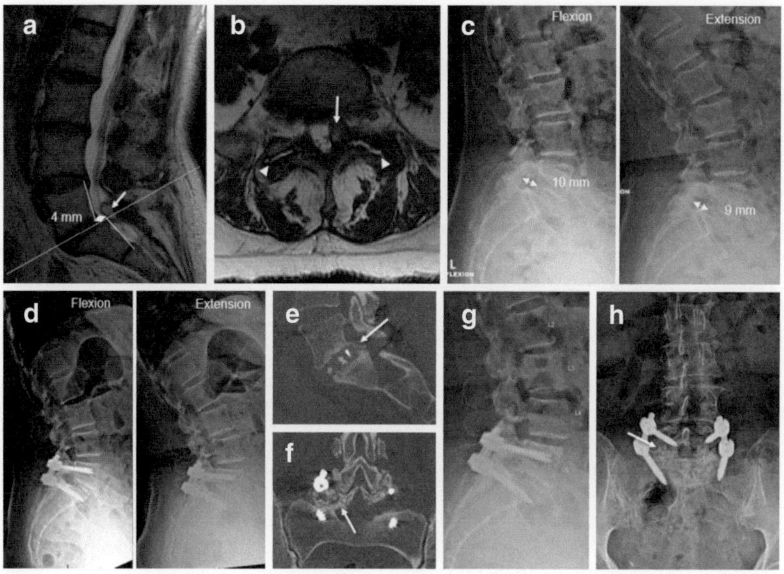

Fig. 20.2 Illustrative case of transforaminal lumbar interbody fusion (TLIF). 72 yo female with mechanical low back pain and progressive left-sided radiculopathy exacerbated by walking and relieved when lying flat, resistant to conservative treatments. Preoperative MRI demonstrated L5-S1 degenerative spondylolisthesis (**a**) with right L5-S1 disc herniation and large left L5-S1 synovial cyst (arrows) with mass effect on the left S1 nerve root (**b**) and fluid in the facet joints (arrowheads). Upright lumbar x-rays (**c**) demonstrated 1–2 mm motion with flexion-extension, and at least 5 mm difference compared to supine MRI. Patient underwent L5-S1 minimally invasive TLIF using PEEK cage, microsurgical resection of the synovial cyst. Postoperatively patient's leg and back pain significantly improved. Flexion-extension x-rays at 4 months after surgery (**d**) demonstrated restoration of disk height, stable hardware position, and no motion in L5-S1 segment. Lumbar CT at 7 months showed progressive signs of L5-S1 interbody (**e**) and right facet (**f**) fusion, no lucency of pedicle screws. Follow-up x-rays in 4 years (**g**, **h**) demonstrated good hardware position and bony fusion (arrow)

Multiple studies have failed to determine the best surgical techniques to achieve fusion that would be superior to others for DLS. An analysis of patients from the SPORT trial (n = 380) included various surgical techniques: posterolateral fusion (21%, n = 80), posterolateral instrumented fusion with pedicle screws (56%, n = 213), posterolateral instrumented fusion with pedicle screws and interbody graft (17%, n = 63, also referred to as 360° fusion), and decompression alone (6%, n = 23) [36]. The study found no significant differences in clinical outcomes among these surgical techniques for DLS [36].

The advantages and disadvantages of various lumbar fusion techniques are discussed in the following chapters. For DLS, anterior and lateral fusion techniques enable the placement of large footprint interbody devices, which facilitate indirect central canal decompression, restoration of foraminal height, realignment of the slip, and improvement in sagittal balance. Posterior approaches, on the other hand, allow for direct decompression and better visualization of neural elements. However, the benefits of indirect decompression in posterior approaches are harder to maintain, primarily due to the smaller footprint of interbody devices.

Competing Interests EB, VB, and SM have no conflicts of interest to declare that are relevant to the content of this chapter. ZG reports intellectual property in NidusAI—not related to the content of this manuscript.

References

1. Martin BI, Mirza SK, Spina N, Spiker WR, Lawrence B, Brodke DS. Trends in lumbar fusion procedure rates and associated hospital costs for degenerative

spinal diseases in the United States, 2004 to 2015. Spine (Phila Pa 1976). 2019;44(5):369–76.
2. Ghogawala Z, Dziura J, Butler WE, Dai F, Terrin N, Magge SN, et al. Laminectomy plus fusion versus laminectomy alone for lumbar spondylolisthesis. N Engl J Med. 2016;374(15):1424–34.
3. Försth P, Ólafsson G, Carlsson T, Frost A, Borgström F, Fritzell P, et al. A randomized, controlled trial of fusion surgery for lumbar spinal stenosis. N Engl J Med. 2016;374(15):1413–23.
4. Sastry RA, Chen JS, Shao B, Weil RJ, Chang KE, Maynard K, et al. Patterns in decompression and fusion procedures for patients with lumbar stenosis after major clinical trial results, 2016 to 2019. JAMA Netw Open. 2023;6(7):e2326357.
5. Heck VJ, Klug K, Prasse T, Oikonomidis S, Klug A, Himpe B, et al. Projections from surgical use models in Germany suggest a rising number of spinal fusions in patients 75 years and older will challenge healthcare systems worldwide. Clin Orthop Rel Res. 2023;481(8):1610–9.
6. Matz PG, Meagher RJ, Lamer T, Tontz WL Jr, Annaswamy TM, Cassidy RC, et al. Guideline summary review: an evidence-based clinical guideline for the diagnosis and treatment of degenerative lumbar spondylolisthesis. Spine J. 2016;16(3):439–48.
7. Wiltse LL, Newman PH, Macnab I. Classification of spondylolisis and spondylolisthesis. Clin Orthop Relat Res. 1976;117:23–9.
8. Meyerding H. Spondylolisthesis. Surg Gynecol Obstet. 1932;54:371–7.
9. Guyer R, Musacchio M, Cammisa FP Jr, Lorio MP. ISASS recommendations/coverage criteria for decompression with interlaminar stabilization - coverage indications, limitations, and/or medical necessity. Int J Spine Surg. 2016;10:41.
10. Liu Z, Duan Y, Rong X, Wang B, Chen H, Liu H. Variation of facet joint orientation and tropism in lumbar degenerative spondylolisthesis and disc herniation at L4-L5: a systematic review and meta-analysis. Clin Neurol Neurosurg. 2017;161:41–7.
11. Morse KW, Steinhaus M, Bovonratwet P, Kazarian G, Gang CH, Vaishnav AS, et al. Current treatment and decision-making factors leading to fusion vs decompression for one-level degenerative spondylolisthesis: survey results from members of the Lumbar Spine Research Society and Society of Minimally Invasive Spine Surgery. Spine J. 2022;22(11):1778–87.
12. Reitman CA, Cho CH, Bono CM, Ghogawala Z, Glaser J, Kauffman C, et al. Management of degenerative spondylolisthesis: development of appropriate use criteria. Spine J. 2021;21(8):1256–67.
13. Kashigar A, Laratta JL, Carreon LY, Bisson EF, Ghogawala Z, Yew AY, et al. Is there additional value to flexion-extension radiographs for degenerative spondylolisthesis? Spine. 2021;46(7):E458–E62.
14. Caterini R, Mancini F, Bisicchia S, Maglione P, Farsetti P. The correlation between exaggerated fluid in lumbar facet joints and degenerative spondylolisthesis: prospective study of 52 patients. J Orthop Traumatol. 2011;12(2):87–91.
15. Blumenthal C, Curran J, Benzel EC, Potter R, Magge SN, Harrington JF Jr, et al. Radiographic predictors of delayed instability following decompression without fusion for degenerative grade I lumbar spondylolisthesis. J Neurosurg Spine. 2013;18(4):340–6.
16. Barrey C, Jund J, Perrin G, Roussouly P. Spinopelvic alignment of patients with degenerative spondylolisthesis. Neurosurgery. 2007;61(5):981–6; discussion 6.
17. Toivonen LA, Mantymaki H, Hakkinen A, Kautiainen H, Neva MH. Postoperative sagittal balance has only a limited role in the development of adjacent segment disease after lumbar spine fusion for degenerative lumbar spine disorders: a subanalysis of the 10-year follow-up study. Spine (Phila Pa 1976). 2022;47(19):1357–61.
18. Oikonomidis S, Meyer C, Scheyerer MJ, Grevenstein D, Eysel P, Bredow J. Lumbar spinal fusion of low-grade degenerative spondylolisthesis (Meyerding grade I and II): do reduction and correction of the radiological sagittal parameters correlate with better clinical outcome? Arch Orthop Trauma Surg. 2020;140(9):1155–62.
19. DiMaria S, Karamian BA, Lambrechts MJ, Kanhere AP, Mangan JJ, Yen WW, et al. How does spinopelvic alignment influence short-term clinical outcomes after lumbar fusion in patients with single-level degenerative spondylolisthesis? J Craniovertebr Junct Spine. 2022;13(3):300–8.
20. Diebo BG, Balmaceno-Criss M, Lafage R, CL MD, Alsoof D, Halayqeh S, et al. Sagittal alignment in the degenerative lumbar spine. J Bone Joint Surg. 2024;106(5):445–57.
21. Thornley P, Urquhart JC, Glennie A, Rampersaud R, Fisher C, Abraham E, et al. Functional outcomes correlate with sagittal spinal balance in degenerative lumbar spondylolisthesis surgery. Spine J. 2023;23(10):1512–21.
22. Schwab FJ, Blondel B, Bess S, Hostin R, Shaffrey CI, Smith JS, et al. Radiographical spinopelvic parameters and disability in the setting of adult spinal deformity: a prospective multicenter analysis. Spine (Phila Pa 1976). 2013;38(13):E803–12.
23. Gerling MC, Bortz C, Pierce KE, Lurie JD, Zhao W, Passias PG. Epidural steroid injections for management of degenerative spondylolisthesis: little effect on clinical outcomes in operatively and non-operatively treated patients. J Bone Joint Surg Am. 2020;102(15):1297–304.
24. Weinstein JN, Lurie JD, Tosteson TD, Hanscom B, Tosteson AN, Blood EA, et al. Surgical versus nonsurgical treatment for lumbar degenerative spondylolisthesis. N Engl J Med. 2007;356(22):2257–70.
25. Herkowitz HN, Kurz LT. Degenerative lumbar spondylolisthesis with spinal stenosis. A prospective study comparing decompression with decompression and intertransverse process arthrodesis. J Bone Joint Surg Am. 1991;73(6):802–8.

26. Fischgrund JS, Mackay M, Herkowitz HN, Brower R, Montgomery DM, Kurz LT. 1997 Volvo Award winner in clinical studies. Degenerative lumbar spondylolisthesis with spinal stenosis: a prospective, randomized study comparing decompressive laminectomy and arthrodesis with and without spinal instrumentation. Spine (Phila Pa 1976). 1997;22(24):2807–12.
27. Kornblum MB, Fischgrund JS, Herkowitz HN, Abraham DA, Berkower DL, Ditkoff JS. Degenerative lumbar spondylolisthesis with spinal stenosis: a prospective long-term study comparing fusion and pseudarthrosis. Spine (Phila Pa 1976). 2004;29(7):726–33; discussion 33-4.
28. Ponkilainen VT, Huttunen TT, Neva MH, Pekkanen L, Repo JP, Mattila VM. National trends in lumbar spine decompression and fusion surgery in Finland, 1997-2018. Acta Orthop. 2021;92(2):199–203.
29. Jensen RK, Schiottz-Christensen B, Skovsgaard CV, Thorvaldsen M, Mieritz RM, Andresen AK, et al. Surgery rates for lumbar spinal stenosis in Denmark between 2002 and 2018: a registry-based study of 43,454 patients. Acta Orthop. 2022;93:488–94.
30. Austevoll IM, Hermansen E, Fagerland MW, Storheim K, Brox JI, Solberg T, et al. Decompression with or without fusion in degenerative lumbar spondylolisthesis. N Engl J Med. 2021;385(6):526–38.
31. Kgomotso EL, Hellum C, Fagerland MW, Solberg T, Brox JI, Storheim K, et al. Decompression alone or with fusion for degenerative lumbar spondylolisthesis (Nordsten-DS): five year follow-up of a randomised, multicentre, non-inferiority trial. BMJ. 2024;386:e079771.
32. Chan AK, Ghogawala Z, Mummaneni PV. Letter: is "decompression vs fusion for spondylolisthesis" the right question? Neurosurgery. 2022;90(2):e54.
33. Chan AK, Bisson EF, Bydon M, Glassman SD, Foley KT, Potts EA, et al. Laminectomy alone versus fusion for grade 1 lumbar spondylolisthesis in 426 patients from the prospective Quality Outcomes Database. J Neurosurg Spine. 2019;30(2):234–41.
34. Bisson EF, Guan J, Bydon M, Alvi MA, Goyal A, Glassman SD, et al. Patient-reported outcome improvements at 24-month follow-up after fusion added to decompression for grade I degenerative lumbar spondylolisthesis: a multicenter study using the Quality Outcomes Database. J Neurosurg Spine. 2021;35(1):42–51.
35. Fenton-White HA. Trailblazing: the historical development of the posterior lumbar interbody fusion (PLIF). Spine J. 2021;21(9):1528–41.
36. Abdu WA, Lurie JD, Spratt KF, Tosteson AN, Zhao W, Tosteson TD, et al. Degenerative spondylolisthesis: does fusion method influence outcome? Four-year results of the spine patient outcomes research trial. Spine (Phila Pa 1976). 2009;34(21):2351–60.
37. Karlsson T, Forsth P, Ohagen P, Michaelsson K, Sanden B. Decompression alone or decompression with fusion for lumbar spinal stenosis: five-year clinical results from a randomized clinical trial. Bone Joint J. 2024;106-B(7):705–12.

Lumbar Degenerative Deformity

21

Luis Felipe Colón and Han Jo Kim

Introduction

Adult degenerative lumbar deformity encompasses a spectrum of conditions affecting the alignment of the adult spine. These include: adult degenerative lumbar scoliosis (ADLS), deformity secondary to a degenerative spondylolisthesis, and flatback deformity or fixed sagittal imbalance. Degenerative spondylolisthesis and flatback are covered in separate chapters and will not be discussed. ADLS is a three-dimensional deformity of the spine due to progressive, asymmetric degeneration of the structural elements leading to malalignment. It is defined by a coronal cobb angle of greater than 10° [1–3]. Distinct from other idiopathic forms of scoliosis, this pathology is more commonly encountered by spine surgeons, particularly with the aging and increasing elderly population [2, 4, 5]. The prevalence has been reported to be as high as 68% in an elderly adult healthy population [5, 6]. It is more common in females, likely due to post-menopausal osteoporosis which contributes to further progression [7]. In less than ten years, 10% of the population in industrialized societies will be older than 65 years of age [1]. With this growing population and focus on quality of life, ADLS has become a notable healthcare concern with increasing attention on its clinical course and treatment. Recent advancements in instrumentation and surgical techniques have led to significant improvements in outcomes following management of this challenging condition. In this chapter, we will discuss the natural history, evaluation, and treatment of ADLS, including a section on the authors' preferred surgical management.

L. F. Colón (✉) · H. J. Kim
Complex Spine and Scoliosis Center, Hospital for Special Surgery, New York, NY, USA
e-mail: fcolon@txorthopaedic.com

Etiology/Natural History

ADLS occurs de novo in skeletally mature patients with previously straight spines unaffected by other forms of scoliosis (e.g., idiopathic). The natural history of de novo lumbar scoliosis is poorly understood. However, one hypothesis is that it often begins with degeneration at a lumbar disc space and is most commonly seen in the lumbar spine where the incidence of degenerative disc disease is high [8, 9]. This asymmetric degeneration of the disc space sets off a cascade of facet degeneration, osteophyte formation, and myopathy, which then leads to segmental wedging, loss of lumbar lordosis, sagittal imbalance, and decreased motion. The process is further complicated by spinal structural changes from osteoarthritis and spondylosis such as facet joint and ligamentum hypertrophy, disc protrusions, and vertebral listhesis. These may lead to neural compression from central canal

A. A. Baaj et al. (eds.), *Surgery of the Lumbar Spine*, https://doi.org/10.1007/978-3-032-18097-1_21

stenosis causing neurogenic claudication or subarticular/neuroforaminal stenosis leading to radiculopathy [2, 9, 10]. Unfortunately, most of the studies reporting on the risk factors and natural progression of lumbar scoliosis curves were done on patients with idiopathic, rather than degenerative scoliosis [11, 12].

ADLS curves tend to progress on average 3° per year [13]. Certain factors are thought to predict progression of scoliosis—curve more than 30° at presentation, apical vertebral rotation more than 30°, lateral listhesis greater than 6 mm, an inter-crest line through L5, and the presence of degenerative disc disease at L5/S1 [8, 13, 14]. However, some of these factors are extrapolated from literature on the natural progression of patients with untreated idiopathic scoliosis, rather than degenerative scoliosis [12].

The genetic and regulatory mechanisms affecting ADLS have been a popular topic for recent investigations. Several studies provide insight into aberrant biomechanical mechanisms that may affect the development of the disease process [14–17]. Some have highlighted the involvement of abnormal angiogenesis and autophagy-mediated angiogenesis in the disease process. The analysis of blood samples of patients with ADLS has found differentially expressed genes such as ubiquitin A-52 residue ribosomal protein fusion product 1 (UBA52) which is related to ubiquitination. Another potential process found in the genetic analysis of tissue samples in patients with ADLS is disruption of the extracellular matrix in the discs and facet joints [14, 16]. Cleaved C-propeptide (CPII) is a marker for type II collagen synthesis (nucleus pulposus) and C2C—a three-quarter fragment of collagen—is a marker for collagen degradation; both have been found to be elevated in patients with ADLS, suggesting both increased collagen synthesis and degradation. Alterations in collagen levels may predispose patients to ADLS [14, 15]. Additional studies have identified other core genes and regulatory mechanisms associated with ADLS, such as LTF, DEFA1B, SLC2A4, DEFA1, FDFT1, etc. [17]. These genes may provide insight into molecular mechanisms and contribute to alternative therapeutic therapies as they are related to the pathogenesis of inflammatory and degenerative conditions.

The clinical presentation of patients with ADLS ranges from asymptomatic to severely disabled. Signs and symptoms of neural compression present with claudication or radiculopathy; whereas sagittal and coronal imbalance lead to back pain, ambulatory intolerance, and cosmetic concerns. The concavity of the main curve or fractional curve distal to the main curve can lead to severe foraminal stenosis, and 97% of patients with ADLS present with symptoms of radiculopathy while seeking treatment [18]. While treatment of idiopathic scoliosis focuses on the halting of progression, the management of ADLS faces the challenge of addressing both the progressive deformity and often neural compromise. Additionally, these patients often present later in life with medical comorbidities and frailty from years of decreased function. All these factors are important considerations when developing a treatment plan for patients due to the increased morbidity of this patient population when surgical intervention is pursued.

Classifications

ADLS is complex and poorly understood, yet knowledge of its progression and treatment is constantly evolving. The primary goal in treatment of ADLS is relief of pain and disability; thus, classifications used to describe it need to identify features predictive of those two components. There are several systems that have attempted to classify the condition. Aebi et al. [1] developed a simple classification dividing adult scoliosis into type I—primary degenerative or de novo scoliosis—the focus of this chapter; type II—progressive idiopathic scoliosis of adult life; and type III—secondary degenerative scoliosis. This initial classification failed to incorporate the major predictor of pain in the ADLS population. About a year later, a clinical impact classification for adult scoliosis based on radiographic markers for disability was developed by Schwab and colleagues and found to correlate with patient-reported outcomes and operative treatment [6].

Further modifications of this classification and updated research in outcomes based on spinopelvic parameters led to an updated Scoliosis Research Society-Schwab Adult Spinal Deformity (SRS-Schwab ASD) classification to reflect this data [19, 20]. The two primary components of the classification include coronal curve type and sagittal modifiers, which are graded by the severity of the deformity. This classification provided a major advancement in classifying these patients, but it has some major limitations. It does not provide clear indications on surgical tactics and level selection for patients undergoing fusion procedures. Additionally, it does not clearly differentiate truly de novo adult scoliosis from adolescent or adult idiopathic scoliosis with secondary degeneration. To address some of these deficiencies, Berjano and Lamartina developed a classification to guide surgical treatment by comparing the symptomatic segments to the apical segments of the curve [21]. In their classification, a type I segment disease is out of the apex of the curve, type II segments are present at the apex, type III refers to extensive segmental disease both in and out of the apex, and type IV has a component of imbalance that often requires more aggressive surgical corrections.

Nonoperative Treatment

Conservative treatment should initially be pursued and maximized in all patients in the absence of progressive neurologic deficit. A rigorous protocol may benefit some patients and even if it fails to relieve their symptoms, the increased activity may help patients endure the physiologic demands of surgery and required postoperative protocols. Above all, patients should focus on improving modifiable risk factors known to increase the risk or worsen ADLS, such as obesity and inactivity [14]. Nonoperative modalities include:

- Physical therapy—focusing on strengthening of paraspinal and abdominal core musculature, stretching to increase hip and knee range of motion, and increasing cardiovascular endurance.
- Medications—such as nonsteroidal anti-inflammatory medications and nerve modulating medications (e.g., gabapentin, pregabalin); although these should be used judiciously and cautiously due to their side-effect profile.
- Avoidance of painful activities.
- Selective corticosteroid injections and pain management interventions.
- Complementary and alternative medicine—such as chiropractic manipulation and adjustment, acupuncture, and massage therapy.

Bracing is generally not recommended in this patient population as it is poorly tolerated, discourages use of core muscles, and can lead to unnecessary expenses in the cost of treatment. Although nonoperative treatment has a much lower cost associated than with operative treatment [22], it leads to less improvement in quality-adjusted life years at 5-year follow-up and patients generally fail to improve in terms of pain and disability [23, 24]. Many patients fail an extensive trial of nonoperative treatment and go on to require surgery. Lower baseline patient recorded outcome measures (PROMs) and lumbar lordosis have been found to be associated with failure of nonoperative management requiring future surgery [25].

Pre-surgical Evaluation

Previous chapters have focused on the initial evaluation of patients with lumbar spine pathology. The history and physical exam are critical, including the nature of the patient's back pain, if present, and level of disability compared to their baseline. A detailed neurologic exam must be conducted, correlated with imaging, and documented. Appropriate imaging is critical for preoperative planning. Full standing preoperative spine radiographs that include distally to the femoral heads, proximally to C7 and ideally C2 as the distance from the C2 plumb line to the planned UIV has been found to predict mechanical complications in ADLS surgery [26]. All classifications begin with assessment of full-length standing AP and lateral spine radiographs. The authors prefer to utilize EOS imaging when possible due to the lower radiation dose and inclusion of full bilateral lower extremities. Bending and supine films are used to assess the flexibility of the deformity, which aid in surgical planning. This is particularly useful for the Lamartina classification when differentiating between types (i.e., Types III and IV), when determining which levels to include in a fusion and whether more aggressive osteotomies are required for sagittal and coronal correction. Proper radiographic analysis with the addition of further advanced imaging can allow for proper parameter measurements and planning level selection, location of potential interbody fusion, and choice of spinal osteotomy planning where indicated. An MRI of the lumbar spine should be ordered to evaluate degree of stenosis and sites of neural compression, but these findings should be correlated with the patients' symptoms and physical exam. If the patient is unable to obtain an MRI for any reason, such as those who have more dated pacemakers, a CT myelogram should be obtained to evaluate for neural compression. Additionally, a CT scan of the thoracic and lumbar spine is used for planning instrumentation, particularly when free-hand techniques are employed, and to assess bone quality. Most of these patients have multiple comorbidities which require preoperative clearance. Patients with osteoporosis should undergo evaluation of their bone health with consideration of treatment to improve their bone quality prior to undergoing surgery, particularly when a longer fusion is planned. Preoperative improvements in bone quality can improve intraoperative factors such as blood loss and prevent postoperative complications, such as proximal junctional kyphosis and failure [27, 28].

Surgical Treatment

Surgery is offered to patients who fail conservative management or have significant progression of their disease. The surgical management goals of ADLS include: deformity correction, reduction of axial back pain, and neurologic element decompression. The challenge with operative management lies in selecting the correct procedure—including level selection—for the right patient. Even with the increase in adult deformity surgery with the aging population and recent increase in literature regarding this topic, there is no consensus for many of the nuances in treating these patients.

While surgery for scoliosis in younger patients, such as those with idiopathic scoliosis, is often done to halt deformity or cosmesis, surgery for ADLS is often performed for pain and disability [21, 29]. The indications for operative management include progression of symptoms after failed extensive nonoperative therapy, progressive deformity causing severe disability, inability to do activities of daily living, or progressive neurologic deficit with clear evidence of compression on imaging. After all required investigations, medical clearances, and extensive discussion of risks and benefits are completed with patients and their families, a surgeon must decide which procedures are required to achieve their goals and minimize complications. Silva et al. developed a classification with six levels of operative treatment for patients with ADLS [13], they include:

1. Level I—decompression alone
2. Level II—decompression and limited fusion
3. Level III—decompression and lumbar curve instrumented fusion
4. Level IV—decompression with anterior and posterior instrumented fusion
5. Level V—thoracic instrumentation and fusion extension
6. Level VI—spinal osteotomies for deformity correction

After deciding which level of operative treatment to pursue to achieve the goals of surgery, a surgeon is faced with the next set of challenging decisions which include proximal and distal level selection, whether to include pelvic fixation in the fusion, and where interbody fusions may be needed. The more involved the operative plan, the higher the rate of complications [30]. A patient with a stable deformity from an ankylosed spine or large bridging osteophytes with primarily radicular or claudicatory symptoms may be a candidate for decompression alone, particularly if they have comorbidities that increase their risk of a large construct or correction. This must be weighed against the risk of increased instability and deformity progression from an isolated decompression procedure without fusion [31].

The Lamartina classification provides additional guidance when developing a surgical plan after the symptomatic levels are determined during imaging and clinical workup:

1. Type I: localized non-apical level—single level decompression with or without fusion can be done
2. Type II: localized apical level—selective fusion is possible, but should include the cranial and caudal aspects of the apex
3. Type III: extensive disease located at and outside of the apex—fusion should include the entire curve and extended as needed
4. Type IV: imbalance often requiring osteotomy for correction

There are several approaches to treat deformity correction in ADLS, including anterior, posterior, and combined anterior-posterior approaches, which may be staged or done during the same operative episode. Anterior-only approaches allow release of the anterior longitudinal ligament which can assist in providing effective sagittal plane correction while also directly addressing deformity due to disc collapse. However, they are associated with significant morbidity inherent to the approach [32]. Combined approaches have been advocated by some, especially when the construct crosses the lumbosacral junction. Anterior lumbar interbody fusion between L4-S1 has been shown to provide greater segmental correction with inconsistent data on whether it protects against pseudoarthrosis [33–35]. Posterior-only approaches have become increasingly common due to improved fixation via three-column transpedicular instrumentation and the advancement in spinal osteotomy techniques which allow for effective curve correction without anterior releases [36, 37].

When choosing to perform a larger operation for deformity correction, the upper instrumented (UIV) vertebra should be stable and neutral. Correcting an entire lumbar curve usually requires the UIV to be at the upper lumbar or lower thoracic spine. When the UIV is at the thoracic level, it should be at T10 or below, or well above T6, to not end at the apex of the thoracic kyphosis. When correcting a lumbar curve, the proximal and distal instrumented levels should be stable—bisected by the CSVL, and the construct should not end at a level affected by adjacent listhesis. It is important to include the entire lumbar curve in the planned fusion and instrument cranial to the upper end vertebra in order to decrease the risk of adjacent segment disease and further complications [38]. However, recent studies suggest there may be no benefit to instrumenting to lower thoracic spine rather than L1 or in between these [39, 40], although this is dependent on the curve magnitude and morphology. Instrumentation and fusion to the upper thoracic spine should be highly considered in patients who require correction of sagittal imbalance that affects the thoracolumbar junction and distal thoracic spine—particularly patients with hyperkyphosis of the thoracic and thoracolumbar spines. This must be weighed against the higher risk for perioperative complications, pseudoarthrosis, and need for revision [41].

There are several types of interbody fusion techniques that can be used for the treatment of ADLS. Interbody fusion, in the form of either anterior lumbar interbody fusion (ALIF), lateral lumbar interbody fusion (LLIF), posterior lumbar interbody fusion (PLIF) or transforaminal lumbar interbody fusion (TLIF), may be employed when long-segment constructs cross the lumbosacral junction to mitigate the risk for pseudoarthrosis. Although interbody fusion at L5/S1 has been shown to increase biomechanical strength of the construct at L5/S1 [42], this has not been shown to significantly affect global sagittal alignment [9]. Pelvic fixation is recommended for long-segment fusions crossing the lumbosacral junction. Spinal osteotomies are the workhorse for posterior deformity correction. Schwab and colleagues developed a comprehensive classification system for osteotomies that nicely illustrates the required cuts and amount of correction possible with each type [37].

Facetectomies (Grades I and II) are often done to initially increase the flexibility of the spine. Smith-Peterson described a posterior column osteotomy (PCO) for the correction of flexion deformities in rheumatoid arthritis [43]. These technically fall under grade II in the Schwab classification and can obtain up to 10° of correction per level performed in the lumbar spine due to the disc height and mobility. More rigid deformities that require larger corrections often require additional bony resection—such as with a pedicle subtraction osteotomy (PSO, Schwab grade III) or vertebral column resection (VCR, Schwab grade V). One can also do an asymmetric PSO to add coronal plane correction when a deformity or imbalance is present (Fig. 21.1). The choice of technique to obtain correction during surgery depends on several factors such as severity of the deformity, coronal and sagittal balance, flexibility of the deformity, status of the disc spaces, and surgeon ability. The recent increase in minimally invasive techniques have popularized the use of anterior column reconstruction via the use of interbody grafts with release of the anterior longitudinal ligament to manipulate the spine [44]. Regardless of a surgeon's preferred surgical technique, the goals of surgery do not change. The priority remains to treat the patient's disability by appropriately decompressing the neurological elements and realigning the spine to where to an energetically favorable and functional state for day-to-day activities.

The fractional curve must be carefully evaluated during preoperative evaluation as this is often a generator of foraminal stenosis and radiculopathy from the concavity of the curve [45]. Failure to appropriately address the fractional curve during surgical management can make sagittal and coronal correction challenging while also increasing the risk for adjacent segment degeneration requiring revision surgery. It has been suggested that fractional curves 15° or greater should be included in the fusion construct during correction of ADLS [46].

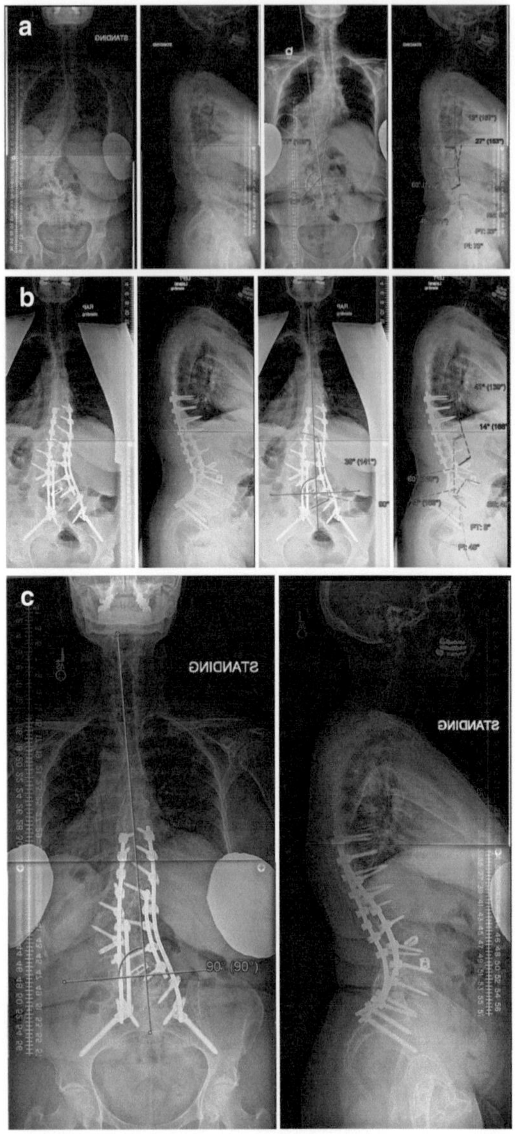

Fig. 21.1 (**a**) 67-year-old patient who presented with a 77° lumbar curve, apex at the left at L2 (**b**) She had failed extensive conservative measures and underwent a T8-pelvis fusion with an asymmetric PSO at L2 and TLIFs at L2/3 and L3/4. (**c**) 5-year postoperative radiographs demonstrating maintenance of correction, successful fusion as well as adequate coronal and sagittal balance

One of the most common postoperative complications after surgical correction of ADLS is proximal junctional kyphosis [47, 48]. Several risk factors increase the risk of PJK, including osteoporosis and poor bone quality [49]. Many studies have reported on the utility of measuring Hounsfield units (HU) on a preoperative CT at the UIV and UIV + 1 [50]. A cutoff value of 120 HU was found to significantly predict increased risk of PJK and a HU value of 160 or more can further decrease the risk of developing PJK. There has been increasing attention in the prevention of PJK in this population with certain techniques being employed with varying support from the literature. Aside from bone health optimization, another strategy is cement augmentation of the UIV and UIV + 1 [51, 52], which provides a biomechanical advantage by buffering axial compressive forces and may prevent the development of PJK (Fig. 21.2). This and other techniques to prevent

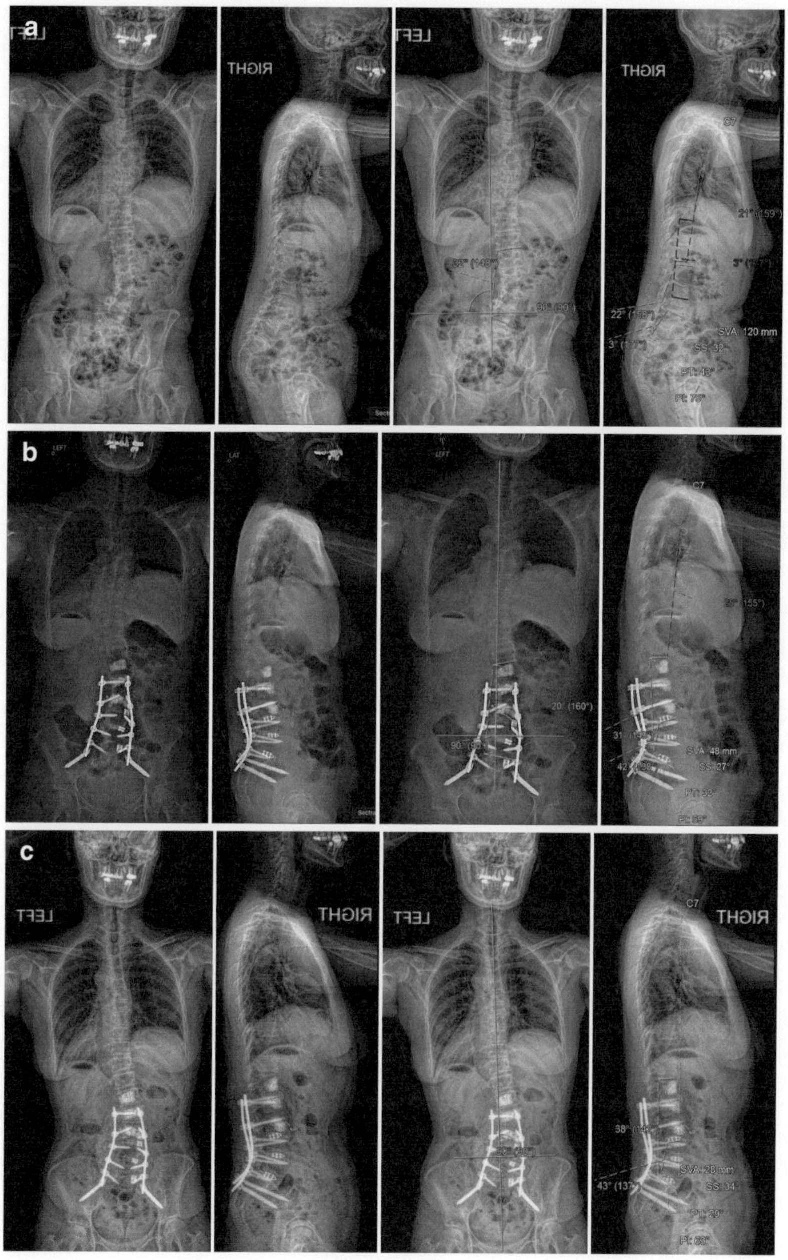

Fig. 21.2 (**a**) 63-year-old patient presenting with a lumbar curve measuring 32° with apex on the right and sagittal imbalance. She had multi-level listhesis, central and neuroforaminal stenosis. (**b**) She underwent L2 to pelvis PSF with L3-S1 TLIF and laminectomies. Additionally, she had cement augmentation of the upper two vertebrae and UIV + 1. These are her radiographs prior to discharge on postoperative day 3. (**c**) 2-year postoperative radiographs demonstrate maintenance of correction as well as coronal and sagittal balance

PJK have been found to be cost-effective while maintaining alignment postoperatively [53].

Sagittal Alignment

The progressive deformity of ADLS often leads to sagittal imbalance and increased disability. The global spinal axis strongly correlates with health-related quality of life (HRQOL) measures. SRS-Schwab defined goal alignment targets that correlate with HRQOL measures: PT < 20°, PI-LL < 10°, and SVA < 4 cm. However, these have not been proven to be consistent in predicting outcomes for this patient population [54]. In part because the "normal" values for these parameters change with advancing patient age and varying PI [55]. The C2 tilt is one of the only measures that has consistently been shown to have minimal variation and be an ideal measure for sagittal balance when evaluating asymptomatic individuals with non-diseased spines [56]. There has been a recent focus on the use of different measurements, such as vertebral pelvic angles (VPAs) [57]. The importance of VPAs has been emphasized considering a normal spine achieves sagittal balance by responding to changes in position and alignment through pelvic tilt and VPAs. These novel targets can be modifiable during surgery and are more easily measured with an intraoperative lateral radiograph while the patient is still prone. The L1PA has been found to correlate with functional outcome scores and associated with pelvic tilt in adult deformity patients. It accounts for the magnitude and distribution of lumbar lordosis and is strongly associated with the PI. Additionally, L1PA has the benefits of being a direct measure of spinopelvic alignment, having a strong association with PI and LL, and being directly modifiable during surgery. It can be easily obtained with just a lateral lumbar fluoroscopic radiograph. The T4 pelvic angle (T4PA) is within 4° of the L1PA and, thus, there has been a recent focus on the T4 minus L1 pelvic angles (T4-L1PA). The T4PA is only modifiable when fusion constructs extend into the upper thoracic spine (T1–5). The sagittal alignment targets for L1PA come from the formula $PI \times 0.5 - (19° +/- 2°)$ and the T4-L1PA mismatch should fall between −3° and 1°. Deviation from these normal values in either direction has been found to increase the risk of mechanical failures in long deformity constructs [58]. Despite careful analysis and detailed planning of a patient's alignment on imaging, one must take into account the patient's complaints and keep in mind the consistent goal of getting the patient's head over the pelvis and bringing them back to the cone of economy. Additionally, one must consider the patient's age, comorbidities, tolerance to rehabilitation, and personal goals when choosing a surgical tactic.

Authors Preferred Treatment

The authors prefer addressing these deformities through an all-posterior approach with a freehand pedicle-screw insertion technique. Since most of these procedures are invasive and require long constructs, we prefer to avoid any additional morbidity and surgical time that is necessarily added when an anterior approach is included. Anterior fusion via TLIF is done in certain levels that may have foraminal stenosis necessitating decompression that would compromise bone stock necessary to achieve fusion. TLIFs can also be done to aid in the correction of focal deformities and rotatory subluxation and spondylolisthesis. Additionally, TLIF may be utilized in patients at increased risk for nonunion at the fractional curve level such as active smokers or patients with osteoporotic bone. Most of the correction lies in the use of osteotomies. Flexible deformities, defined by at least 30% correction on supine [59, 60] and bending films, may be addressed with PCOs. Stiff deformities often require larger bone resections, such as with a PSO. In patients with coronal imbalance in addition to sagittal plane deformities, an asymmetric PSO at or near the apex or the curve allows significant correction in both planes, as seen in the case demonstrated in Fig. 21.1. If the L5/S1 disc space appears healthy and has not had a previous decompression, L5 could be considered as the LIV for the construct. Otherwise, fusions are extended to the sacrum and supplemented with pelvic fixation in order to decrease the stress on the implant-bone interface throughout the construct and to minimize the risk for L5-S1 pseudarthrosis. After all instrumentation is placed, osteotomies and releases are completed, the correction is performed via rod placement. The rods are initially secured distally to the pelvic fixation and fractional curve level. The convex side of the lumbosacral fractional curve is corrected first in an attempt to horizontalize L4 with compression in order to preserve or generate sufficient lordosis. The rods are then sequentially secured to the screws proximally and cantilevered slowly—ensuring to share the load as to not increase the risk for screw pullout during correction. After the rods are fully secured, intraoperative 36-inch cassette flat plate radiographs are taken to evaluate the correction and obtain coronal and sagittal measurements.

Conclusion/Summary

ADLS is of growing interest to spine surgeons and the health community due to its prevalence in a growing elderly population because of improved care and increased longevity. Nonoperative management has limited utility for patients wanting to improve their quality of life. There are no uniform guidelines for the surgical management of this condition. In part, due to the variability of each patient's clinical presentation and deformity. No one curve is equal to another. Treatment must be individualized to each patient based on their health, curve characteristics, and goals.

References

1. Aebi M. The adult scoliosis. Eur Spine J. 2005;14(10):925–48.
2. Ploumis A, Transfledt EE, Denis F. Degenerative lumbar scoliosis associated with spinal stenosis. Spine J. 2007;7(4):428–36.
3. Wong E, Altaf F, Oh LJ, Gray RJ. Adult degenerative lumbar scoliosis. Orthopedics. 2017;40(6):e930–e9.
4. Dagdia L, Kokabu T, Ito M. Classification of adult spinal deformity: review of current concepts and future directions. Spine Surg Relat Res. 2019;3(1):17–26.
5. Schwab F, Dubey A, Gamez L, El Fegoun AB, Hwang K, Pagala M, et al. Adult scoliosis: prevalence, SF-36, and nutritional parameters in an elderly volunteer population. Spine (Phila Pa 1976). 2005;30(9):1082–5.
6. Schwab F, Farcy JP, Bridwell K, Berven S, Glassman S, Harrast J, et al. A clinical impact classification of scoliosis in the adult. Spine (Phila Pa 1976). 2006;31(18):2109–14.
7. Urrutia J, Diaz-Ledezma C, Espinosa J, Berven SH. Lumbar scoliosis in postmenopausal women: prevalence and relationship with bone density, age, and body mass index. Spine (Phila Pa 1976). 2011;36(9):737–40.
8. Kotwal S, Pumberger M, Hughes A, Girardi F. Degenerative scoliosis: a review. HSS J. 2011;7(3):257–64.
9. Murata Y, Takahashi K, Hanaoka E, Utsumi T, Yamagata M, Moriya H. Changes in scoliotic curvature and lordotic angle during the early phase of degenerative lumbar scoliosis. Spine (Phila Pa 1976). 2002;27(20):2268–73.
10. Herkowitz HN, Kurz LT. Degenerative lumbar spondylolisthesis with spinal stenosis. A prospective study comparing decompression with decompression and intertransverse process arthrodesis. J Bone Joint Surg Am. 1991;73(6):802–8.
11. Weinstein SL. Natural history. Spine (Phila Pa 1976). 1999;24(24):2592–600.
12. Ascani E, Bartolozzi P, Logroscino CA, Marchetti PG, Ponte A, Savini R, et al. Natural history of untreated idiopathic scoliosis after skeletal maturity. Spine (Phila Pa 1976). 1986;11(8):784–9.
13. Silva FE, Lenke LG. Adult degenerative scoliosis: evaluation and management. Neurosurg Focus. 2010;28(3):E1.
14. Petrosyan E, Fares J, Lesniak MS, Koski TR, El Tecle NE. Biological principles of adult degenerative scoliosis. Trends Mol Med. 2023;29(9):740–52.
15. Hwang DW, Kim KT, Lee SH, Kim JY, Kim DH. Association of COL2A1 gene polymorphism with degenerative lumbar scoliosis. Clin Orthop Surg. 2014;6(4):379–84.
16. Lee JS, Shin JK, Goh TS. Interleukin 6 gene polymorphism in patients with degenerative lumbar scoliosis: a cohort study. Eur Spine J. 2018;27(3):607–12.
17. Zhu A, Liu Y, Liu Y. Identification of key genes and regulatory mechanisms in adult degenerative scoliosis. J Clin Neurosci. 2024;119:170–9.
18. Fu KM, Rhagavan P, Shaffrey CI, Chernavvsky DR, Smith JS. Prevalence, severity, and impact of foraminal and canal stenosis among adults with degenerative scoliosis. Neurosurgery. 2011;69(6):1181–7.
19. Bess S, Schwab F, Lafage V, Shaffrey CI, Ames CP. Classifications for adult spinal deformity and use of the Scoliosis Research Society-Schwab adult spinal deformity classification. Neurosurg Clin N Am. 2013;24(2):185–93.
20. Schwab F, Ungar B, Blondel B, Buchowski J, Coe J, Deinlein D, et al. Scoliosis Research Society-Schwab

adult spinal deformity classification: a validation study. Spine (Phila Pa 1976). 2012;37(12):1077–82.
21. Berjano P, Lamartina C. Classification of degenerative segment disease in adults with deformity of the lumbar or thoracolumbar spine. Eur Spine J. 2014;23(9):1815–24.
22. Carreon LY, Glassman SD, Lurie J, Shaffrey CI, Kelly MP, Baldus CR, et al. Cost-effectiveness of operative versus nonoperative treatment of adult symptomatic lumbar scoliosis an intent-to-treat analysis at 5-year follow-up. Spine (Phila Pa 1976). 2019;44(21):1499–506.
23. Bridwell KH, Glassman S, Horton W, Shaffrey C, Schwab F, Zebala LP, et al. Does treatment (nonoperative and operative) improve the two-year quality of life in patients with adult symptomatic lumbar scoliosis: a prospective multicenter evidence-based medicine study. Spine (Phila Pa 1976). 2009;34(20):2171–8.
24. Kelly MP, Lurie JD, Yanik EL, Shaffrey CI, Baldus CR, Boachie-Adjei O, et al. Operative versus nonoperative treatment for adult symptomatic lumbar scoliosis. J Bone Joint Surg Am. 2019;101(4):338–52.
25. Clohisy JCF, Smith JS, Kelly MP, Yanik EL, Baldus CR, Bess S, et al. Failure of nonoperative care in adult symptomatic lumbar scoliosis: incidence, timing, and risk factors for conversion from nonoperative to operative treatment. J Neurosurg Spine. 2023;39(4):498–508.
26. Yoshida G, Ushirozako H, Hasegawa T, Yamato Y, Kobayashi S, Yasuda T, et al. Preoperative and postoperative sitting radiographs for adult spinal deformity surgery: upper instrumented vertebra selection using sitting C2 plumb Line distance to prevent proximal junctional kyphosis. Spine (Phila Pa 1976). 2020;45(15):E950–E8.
27. Harris AB, Wang KY, Mo K, Kebaish F, Raad M, Puvanesarajah V, et al. Bone mineral density T-score is an independent predictor of major blood loss in adult spinal deformity surgery. Glob Spine J. 2024;14(1):153–8.
28. Yagi M, Ohne H, Konomi T, Fujiyoshi K, Kaneko S, Komiyama T, et al. Teriparatide improves volumetric bone mineral density and fine bone structure in the UIV+1 vertebra, and reduces bone failure type PJK after surgery for adult spinal deformity. Osteoporos Int. 2016;27(12):3495–502.
29. Bess S, Boachie-Adjei O, Burton D, Cunningham M, Shaffrey C, Shelokov A, et al. Pain and disability determine treatment modality for older patients with adult scoliosis, while deformity guides treatment for younger patients. Spine (Phila Pa 1976). 2009;34(20):2186–90.
30. Transfeldt EE, Topp R, Mehbod AA, Winter RB. Surgical outcomes of decompression, decompression with limited fusion, and decompression with full curve fusion for degenerative scoliosis with radiculopathy. Spine (Phila Pa 1976). 2010;35(20):1872–5.
31. Kelleher MO, Timlin M, Persaud O, Rampersaud YR. Success and failure of minimally invasive decompression for focal lumbar spinal stenosis in patients with and without deformity. Spine (Phila Pa 1976). 2010;35(19):E981–7.
32. Smith JA, Deviren V, Berven S, Bradford DS. Does instrumented anterior scoliosis surgery lead to kyphosis, pseudarthrosis, or inadequate correction in adults? Spine (Phila Pa 1976). 2002;27(5):529–34.
33. Cummins DD, Clark AJ, Gupta MC, Theologis AA. Anterior lumbar interbody fusion versus transforaminal lumbar interbody fusion for correction of lumbosacral fractional curves in adult (thoraco)lumbar scoliosis: a systematic review. N Am Spine Soc J. 2024;17:100299.
34. Dorward IG, Lenke LG, Bridwell KH, O'Leary PT, Stoker GE, Pahys JM, et al. Transforaminal versus anterior lumbar interbody fusion in long deformity constructs: a matched cohort analysis. Spine (Phila Pa 1976). 2013;38(12):E755–62.
35. Meyers AJ, Wick JB, Rodnoi P, Khan A, Klineberg EO. Does L5-S1 anterior lumbar interbody fusion improve sagittal alignment or fusion rates in long segment fusion for adult spinal deformity? Global Spine J. 2021;11(5):697–703.
36. Dorward IG, Lenke LG. Osteotomies in the posterior-only treatment of complex adult spinal deformity: a comparative review. Neurosurg Focus. 2010;28(3):E4.
37. Schwab F, Blondel B, Chay E, Demakakos J, Lenke L, Tropiano P, et al. The comprehensive anatomical spinal osteotomy classification. Neurosurgery. 2014;74(1):112–20; discussion 20.
38. Cho KJ, Suk SI, Park SR, Kim JH, Jung JH. Selection of proximal fusion level for adult degenerative lumbar scoliosis. Eur Spine J. 2013;22(2):394–401.
39. Guppy KH, Chang R, Fennessy J, Prentice HA, Harris JE, Ho AL, et al. Incidence rates and risks for reoperations for nonunion and adjacent level disease: stopping at L1 versus T10/T11/12. Spine (Phila Pa 1976). 2025.
40. Kim YJ, Bridwell KH, Lenke LG, Rhim S, Kim YW. Is the T9, T11, or L1 the more reliable proximal level after adult lumbar or lumbosacral instrumented fusion to L5 or S1? Spine (Phila Pa 1976). 2007;32(24):2653–61.
41. O'Shaughnessy BA, Bridwell KH, Lenke LG, Cho W, Baldus C, Chang MS, et al. Does a long-fusion "T3-sacrum" portend a worse outcome than a short-fusion "T10-sacrum" in primary surgery for adult scoliosis? Spine (Phila Pa 1976). 2012;37(10):884–90.
42. Kostuik JP, Valdevit A, Chang HG, Kanzaki K. Biomechanical testing of the lumbosacral spine. Spine (Phila Pa 1976). 1998;23(16):1721–8.
43. Smith-Petersen MN, Larson CB, Aufranc OE. Osteotomy of the spine for correction of flexion deformity in rheumatoid arthritis. Clin Orthop Relat Res. 1969;66:6–9.
44. Uribe JS, Schwab F, Mundis GM, Xu DS, Januszewski J, Kanter AS, et al. The comprehensive anatomical spinal osteotomy and anterior column realignment classification. J Neurosurg Spine. 2018;29(5):565–75.

45. Campbell PG, Nunley PD. The lumbosacral fractional curve in adult degenerative scoliosis. Neurosurg Clin N Am. 2023;34(4):537–44.
46. Bridwell KH. Selection of instrumentation and fusion levels for scoliosis: where to start and where to stop. Invited submission from the Joint Section Meeting on Disorders of the Spine and Peripheral Nerves, March 2004. J Neurosurg Spine. 2004;1(1):1–8.
47. Glattes RC, Bridwell KH, Lenke LG, Kim YJ, Rinella A, Edwards C 2nd. Proximal junctional kyphosis in adult spinal deformity following long instrumented posterior spinal fusion: incidence, outcomes, and risk factor analysis. Spine (Phila Pa 1976). 2005;30(14):1643–9.
48. Lazaro B, Sardi JP, Smith JS, Kelly MP, Yanik EL, Dial B, et al. Proximal junctional failure in primary thoracolumbar fusion/fixation to the sacrum/pelvis for adult symptomatic lumbar scoliosis: long-term follow-up of a prospective multicenter cohort of 160 patients. J Neurosurg Spine. 2023;38(3):319–30.
49. Kim HJ, Upfill-Brown A, Hirase T. The evaluation, prevention, and management of proximal junctional kyphosis and failure. J Am Acad Orthop Surg. 2025;33:e1477.
50. Yao YC, Elysee J, Lafage R, McCarthy M, Louie PK, Alshabab BS, et al. Preoperative hounsfield units at the planned upper instrumented vertebrae may predict proximal junctional kyphosis in adult spinal deformity. Spine (Phila Pa 1976). 2021;46(3):E174–E80.
51. Ghobrial GM, Eichberg DG, Kolcun JPG, Madhavan K, Lebwohl NH, Green BA, et al. Prophylactic vertebral cement augmentation at the uppermost instrumented vertebra and rostral adjacent vertebra for the prevention of proximal junctional kyphosis and failure following long-segment fusion for adult spinal deformity. Spine J. 2017;17(10):1499–505.
52. Kebaish KM, Martin CT, O'Brien JR, LaMotta IE, Voros GD, Belkoff SM. Use of vertebroplasty to prevent proximal junctional fractures in adult deformity surgery: a biomechanical cadaveric study. Spine J. 2013;13(12):1897–903.
53. Passias PG, Krol O, Williamson TK, Bennett-Caso C, Smith JS, Diebo B, et al. Proximal junctional kyphosis and failure prophylaxis improves cost efficacy, while maintaining optimal alignment, in adult spinal deformity surgery. Neurosurgery. 2025;97:410.
54. Faraj SSA, De Kleuver M, Vila-Casademunt A, Holewijn RM, Obeid I, Acaroglu E, et al. Sagittal radiographic parameters demonstrate weak correlations with pretreatment patient-reported health-related quality of life measures in symptomatic de novo degenerative lumbar scoliosis: a European multicenter analysis. J Neurosurg Spine. 2018;28(6):573–80.
55. Protopsaltis TS, Soroceanu A, Tishelman JC, Buckland AJ, Mundis GM Jr, Smith JS, et al. Should sagittal spinal alignment targets for adult spinal deformity correction depend on pelvic incidence and age? Spine (Phila Pa 1976). 2020;45(4):250–7.
56. Hills J, Lenke LG, Sardar ZM, Le Huec JC, Bourret S, Hasegawa K, et al. The T4-L1-hip Axis: defining a normal sagittal spinal alignment. Spine (Phila Pa 1976). 2022;47(19):1399–406.
57. Protopsaltis TS, Lafage R, Smith JS, Passias PG, Shaffrey CI, Kim HJ, et al. The lumbar pelvic angle, the lumbar component of the T1 pelvic angle, correlates with HRQOL, PI-LL mismatch, and it predicts global alignment. Spine (Phila Pa 1976). 2018;43(10):681–7.
58. Hills J, Mundis GM, Klineberg EO, Smith JS, Line B, Gum JL, et al. The T4-L1-hip axis: sagittal spinal realignment targets in long-construct adult spinal deformity surgery: early impact. J Bone Joint Surg Am. 2024;106(23):e48.
59. Lin JD, Osorio JA, Baum GR, Menger RP, Reid PC, Dyrszka MD, et al. A new modular radiographic classification of adult idiopathic scoliosis as an extension of the Lenke classification of adolescent idiopathic scoliosis. Spine Deform. 2021;9(1):175–83.
60. Lovecchio F, Elysee JC, Lafage R, Varghese J, Bannwarth M, Schwab F, et al. The impact of preoperative supine radiographs on surgical strategy in adult spinal deformity. J Neurosurg Spine. 2022;36(1):71–7.

22 High-Grade Spondylolisthesis

Maile Curbo and Eric Klineberg

Introduction and Classification

High-grade spondylolisthesis is a severe spinal deformity that can present in children, adolescents, and adults. Spondylolisthesis is the displacement of one vertebral body over another. Spondylolisthesis was first described in 1782 by Herbiniaux, who reported difficulty in labor and delivery of a patient with complete dislocation of L5 over S1 [1]. Many reported cases were made in the 1800s; however, in 1888, Neugebauer recognized that a bony defect at the pars interarticularis allowed for the anterior translation of the vertebral body [2]. In 1932, Meyerding recognized the importance of spondylolisthesis and its role in back pain and disability [3]. He created a grading system based on the percentage of slippage of the proximal vertebral body over the distal vertebral body. The classification describes that a grade 1 spondylolisthesis correlates with a 0–25% slip, grade 2 is 25–50%, grade 3 is 50–75%, and grade 4 is 75–100%. High grade-spondylolisthesis is comprised of Meyerding grade 3 and grade 4 slips [3].

In 1976, Wiltse described a classification based on the underlying etiology causing the individual patient's spondylolisthesis [4]. There are five main categories. Dysplastic spondylolisthesis describes any congenital abnormality of the sacrum or the L5 arch that allows for spondylolisthesis. The L5 arch or the sacrum cannot support the spinal column's anterior pull, and the slip occurs and progresses. This is commonly associated with spina bifida [5]. The next category, isthmic spondylolisthesis, describes defects in the pars interarticularis, which can be further subclassified into lytic, elongated, and acute fractures [6]. Lytic is associated with repetitive activities in athletes, causing fatigue fractures. Elongation is similarly related to repetitive

M. Curbo · E. Klineberg (✉)
UTHealth Houston, McGovern Medical School, Department of Orthopaedic Surgery, Houston, TX, USA
e-mail: Maile.E.Curbo@uth.tmc.edu; Eric.Klineberg@uth.tmc.edu

A. A. Baaj et al. (eds.), *Surgery of the Lumbar Spine*, https://doi.org/10.1007/978-3-032-18097-1_22

trauma; however, subsequent healing causes elongation of the pars. Lastly, the acute fracture subtype is a direct result of trauma and results in traumatic spondylolisthesis. Type 3 is degenerative spondylolisthesis. The pars interarticularis remains intact, while intersegmental instability causes facet joint degeneration. This allows for worsened instability and is often combined with sagittally oriented facets, allowing for slippage [7]. Type 4 is a traumatic fracture of the posterior elements that allows for spondylolisthesis. Type 5 describes pathologic spondylolisthesis that causes destruction of the posterior spinal elements from bone disease. Examples of this can include arthrogryposis, Paget's disease, or metastatic disease. Lastly, type 6 describes post-surgical iatrogenic causes of spondylolisthesis [4].

Epidemiology

Spondylolisthesis has an overall reported incidence of 4 to 6% in childhood and 5 to 10% in adults. Children most commonly have isthmic spondylolisthesis at L5 to S1. In adults, the degenerative spondylolisthesis type predominates with higher rates at L4 to L5 [8, 9]. While spondylolisthesis is a common diagnosis, only 11.3% of adults diagnosed with spondylolisthesis fall into grade 3 and grade 4 [10].

Spinopelvic Parameters and Alignment

Global spine alignment and neutral sagittal plane alignment are critical when evaluating and treating patients with lumbar spinal deformity. Maintenance and restoration of sagittal balance are pertinent for improved clinical outcomes and function [11–13]. Pelvic and sacral morphology is closely related to global spine alignment and must be evaluated in patients with high-grade spondylolisthesis.

Roussouly and his team evaluated spinopelvic balance in patients with high- versus low-grade spondylolisthesis and created a classification system to describe the findings. Patients with low-grade spondylolisthesis are subclassified as having high PI (>60 degrees) or low PI (<45 degrees). Patients with a high PI have pars spondylolysis secondary to a tension failure. In contrast, those with a low PI have pars failure via the "nutcracker" effects, which causes impingement of posterior elements during extension [14, 15].

Conversely, patients with high-grade spondylolisthesis almost always have an elevated PI. These patients are categorized into balanced versus unbalanced pelvis. Patients with a balanced pelvis have low pelvic tilt and high sacral slope. Patients with an unbalanced pelvis have a high PT and low SS secondary to pelvis retroversion [14, 15]. The pelvis retroversion contributes to hamstring tightness, knee contractures, and crouched gait [16].

Clinical Presentation

Axial back pain is the most common presenting symptom in patients with spondylolisthesis [17]. Mechanical axial back pain can be secondary to multiple factors, including facet joint degeneration, axial pain from sagittal imbalance, discogenic back pain, or pain from the pars interarticularis, particularly in those with isthmic spondylolisthesis [11, 18].

Neurologic symptoms are also prevalent in patients presenting with spondylolisthesis. While both low- and high-grade spondylolisthesis can cause radiculopathy of the exiting nerve root due to foraminal stenosis, high-grade spondylolisthesis can also cause neurogenic claudication secondary to central stenosis. The central stenosis at these levels may also cause radiculopathy of the traversing nerve root [17, 19].

Children have been described to present with flattened lumbar lordosis and heart-shaped buttocks due to the vertical alignment of the sacrum. They often have hamstring tightness and knee contractures to maintain a neutral sagittal alignment and can be quantified utilizing the popliteal angle [16, 20].

Imaging Strategies

High-grade spondylolisthesis should be evaluated utilizing whole spine standing AP and lateral radiographs. Spinopelvic parameters, including sagittal balance, pelvic tilt, pelvic incidence, and sacral slope, should be assessed (Fig. 22.1). The etiology of the spondylolisthesis can often be noted on radiographs. Supine radiographs can be utilized to predict the correction that may be expected with positioning. Flexion and extension views may be used to evaluate the dynamic stability of the slip, though this is often of less value in patients with high-grade spondylolisthesis.

Magnetic resonance imaging (MRI) is essential in evaluating patients with high-grade spondylolisthesis. Determining the regions of compression in the spine is paramount to address any neurologic deficits the patient may have. Central, lateral recess, and foraminal stenosis can all be evaluated on MRI (Fig. 22.2). The discs at the adjacent levels should be assessed for degenerative changes and considered when determining fusion levels.

Computed tomography is often valuable for patients with high-grade spondylolisthesis to fur-

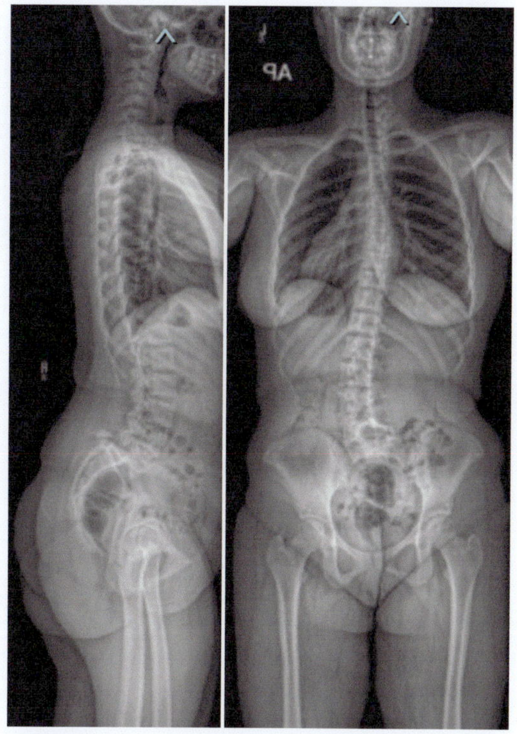

Fig. 22.1 Anterior/posterior and lateral standing X-rays of a patient with a grade 4 isthmic spondylolisthesis. Note the anterior translation, and loss of lumbar lordosis from L4-S1 due to the listhesis and resultant lumbosacral kyphosis

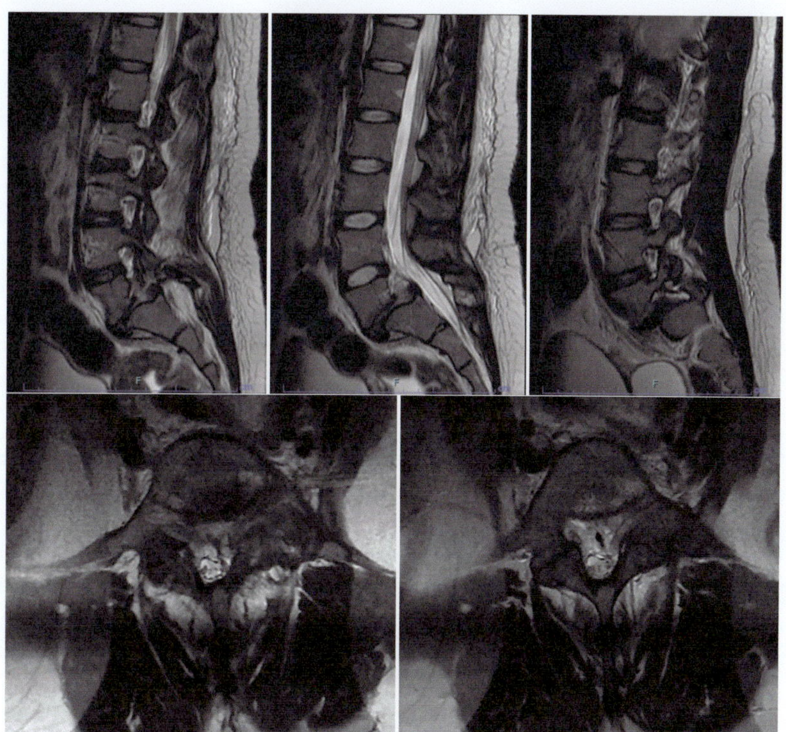

Fig. 22.2 Sagittal and axial T2-weighted MRI images demonstrating severe foraminal stenosis of the L5 nerve root due to high-grade spondylolisthesis. Note also that there is partial reduction of the spondylolisthesis on the supine imaging

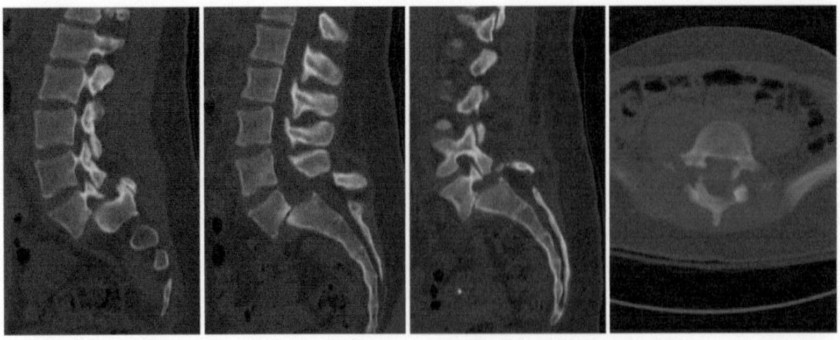

Fig. 22.3 Selected computed tomography images detailing bony anatomy for preoperative planning. This allows for evaluation of the pedicular anatomy for implant placement and detailed anatomy of the posterior elements when performing dissection and decompression. Also note that there is some flexibility of the 5/1 disc space, with slight improvement in the kyphotic angle, with maintained anterior slip at L5/S1

ther evaluate dysplastic elements and to assess the dimensions of the pedicles for screw fixation, particularly at L5 (Fig. 22.3) [21].

Conservative Treatment

Many studies have evaluated the efficacy of operative and nonoperative management of high-grade spondylolisthesis. This is a controversial topic, and the related studies are often confounded by the inability to stratify patients based on etiology.

While there are excellent natural history studies for low-grade spondylolisthesis and its role in nonoperative management, fewer studies depict the natural history of high-grade spondylolisthesis [22]. Harris and Weinstein discussed long-term outcomes in nonoperative and operative management in high-grade spondylolisthesis in young patients (ages 10–25 years old at diagnosis). 11 patients were treated nonoperatively, and after 18 years of follow-up, 36% were symptom-free, 55% had mild symptoms, and one patient had significant symptoms. Within this study, it was noted that skeletally immature patients were less likely to have a successful long-term outcome when treated nonoperatively [23]. Pizzutillo et al. followed 12 patients (aged 6–21 years) with high-grade spondylolisthesis, and only one patient (8%) improved with nonoperative management. The remaining eleven patients (92%) required surgical intervention [24]. While nonoperative management in high-grade spondylolisthesis has a limited role, physical therapy focused on hamstring stretching and core strengthening can assist with symptomatic management. Bracing has not been shown to improve outcomes in patients with high-grade spondylolisthesis [25].

While low-grade, stable spondylolisthesis can most often be treated nonoperatively in adults, there may be a role for nonoperative management in more high-grade slips. Provided the patient remains neurologically stable, conservative management can be initiated. This is predominantly guided by symptom management. Axial low back pain can be managed with physical therapy, anti-inflammatory medication, or prescription, non-opioid medication. Intra-articular facet injections, medial branch blocks, or radiofrequency ablation may also be utilized. When the spondylolisthesis causes neurologic compression secondary to central or foraminal stenosis, epidural steroid injections can be employed to assist with symptom management [26].

Operative Treatment

Patients with high-grade spondylolisthesis are usually symptomatic and have a high likelihood of failing nonoperative management and, thus, typically progress into operative management.

They are also much more likely to undergo progression of their spondylolisthesis and require surgical intervention. Risk factors for progression include young age at presentation, high slip angle, and dysplastic spondylolisthesis [17].

The goals in surgical management of high-grade spondylolisthesis include restoring the lumbosacral lordosis, improving neurologic function, and restoring the lumbosacral junction's ability to withstand shear forces. This is accomplished by restoring the posterior tension band and providing anterior column support [27].

Fusion and the Role of Reduction

Restoring the posterior tension band via fusion is critical. Low-grade spondylolisthesis can be treated with in-situ fusion relatively reliably [28, 29]. However, controversy exists when determining the role of reduction. Without reduction, high-grade spondylolisthesis treated with in-situ fusion is prone to pseudoarthrosis or progression of the slip [30, 31, 34]. The interbody graft has also been theorized to be under tension without a reduction performed, increasing the likelihood of pseudoarthrosis [32]. However, a study by Poussa et al. showed better functional results at 15 years of follow-up in adolescents with high-grade slips when fused in situ compared to reduction and fusion. The limitations of this study were the small patient population and lack of anatomic reduction [33]. Other studies have described reserving reduction for patients with an unbalanced pelvis and performing in situ fusion without reduction in patients with balanced deformities. The most considerable risk in reduction involves the potential injury to the L5 nerve root during the reduction via a traction mechanism and compression of the L5 nerve root after reduction by the lumbosacral ligament. The neurologic injury most often occurs in the terminal 50% of slip reduction and has led many authors to advocate for partial reduction techniques [34–36]. The critical point for reduction is that reduction of lumbar lordosis is most important, while decreasing the grade of slip may lead to neurologic traction injury. Achieving normal spinopelvic parameters may lead to improved long-term outcomes.

Interbody Selection

Anterior column support may be helpful to correct the lordosis for high-grade spondylolisthesis to facilitate deformity correction and fusion mass formation. Without anterior column support, there is an increased rate of nonunion and loss of correction [27]. Anterior or posterior lumbar interbody fusions have been described. While anterior lumbar interbody fusion has been shown to achieve a higher rate of correction of lumbar lordosis compared to posterior techniques, an additional approach, aberrant anatomy, and risk of damage to the superior hypogastric plexus, particularly in young males, must be considered [37]. Often placement of a graft may not be possible with an anterior approach, in which case anterior longitudinal ligament resection and then placement of allograft bone in the disc space will allow for release and fusion of the disc space without structural support (Fig. 22.4). This can still help achieve anterior fusion.

Reduction Techniques

Many reduction techniques have been described in the literature, including casting, Harrington rod placement, and external fixator placement [33, 34]. Decompression should be performed before reduction to allow for direct visualization of the nerve roots during the reduction [34]. The disc space should be prepared; in some cases, a sacral dome osteotomy and resection may be performed [38]. Pedicle screws are then placed. The interbody graft can then be placed, and distraction can be attained by utilizing a lamina spreader or Cobb elevator to lever open the intervertebral space [34]. Harrington rods, pre-contoured plates, and Schanz pins have all been described as adjuvant tools to assist in reduction [33, 34]. Placement of the iliac bolts and then rotating a lordotic rod onto the L5 and S1 screws is also helpful and can allow for restoration of the lordo-

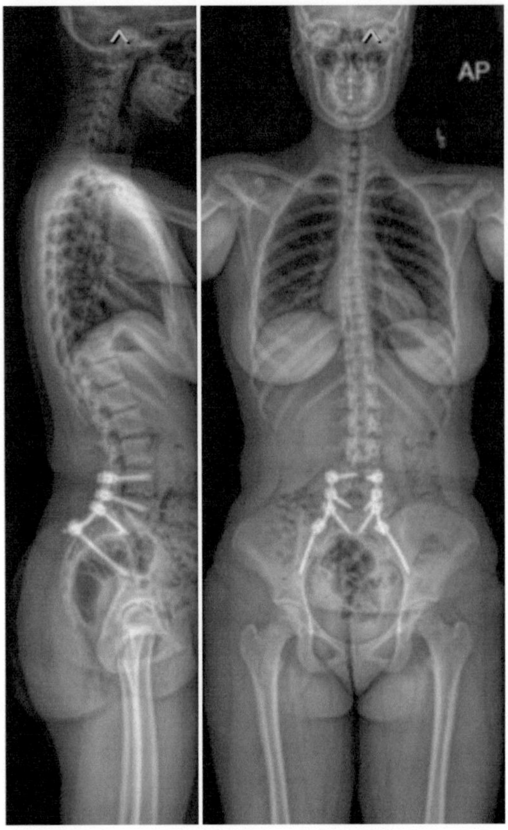

Fig. 22.4 Anterior/posterior and lateral standing X-rays of the same patient in Fig. 22.1. The high-grade spondylolisthesis has been surgically treated with anterior/posterior surgical release and realignment. This involved an anterior longitudinal resection and partial reduction anteriorly. An interbody cage could not be placed safely due to insufficient reduction after anterior exposure and release. This was immediately followed by posterior decompression and fusion from L4-pelvis with release of the L5 nerve roots into the pelvis. Restoration of lordosis is the goal of the procedure as is reduction of the slip to a grade 1 only, to prevent neural tension. Note the relaxed posture of the thoracic and pelvic version due to restoration of the lumbosacral lordosis

sis with reduction of the slip angle. It is imperative to perform the reduction incrementally with continual evaluation of the L5 nerve root to ensure it remains free of compression and tension. Rods can then be placed into the pedicle screws, and the reduction confirmed on fluoroscopic imaging [34]. The L5 nerve can also be stimulated to ensure that the threshold does not increase indicating a traction injury. Often palpation and inspection of the root is the only clue that a traction injury may occur, and often this injury can present in a delayed fashion, 2–3 days post-operatively.

Complications

Complications in high-grade spondylolisthesis are significantly higher than that of low-grade spondylolisthesis. Complications as high as 50–60% in operatively treated adult and pediatric patients have been reported [39]. Neilsen reported a 40% reoperation rate in adolescent patients within 5 years of index surgery [40]. Neurologic deficits, pseudoarthrosis, and adjacent segment disease often complicate these surgeries. Infection, dural tears, and epidural hematomas can also complicate the surgery.

As discussed previously, neurologic deficits can occur, particularly with the L5 nerve root, during spondylolisthesis reduction. Adequate decompression with direct visualization of the nerve root, neuromonitoring, incremental reduction, and appropriate reduction goals can help avoid nerve root compression [39]. Additionally, postoperatively careful examination of the nerve and resultant pain is important to follow. The senior author usually has the patient kept with knees and hips flexed for the first week when in bed to minimize nerve stretch during the early post-operative period. If pain or weakness develops late, treatment with a short course of steroids is helpful in symptom management.

Pseudoarthrosis has been reported at rates of up to 20% [41]. This risk can be partially mitigated by ensuring appropriate preoperative optimization, particularly in adult patients. Intraoperative factors such as bone graft utilization, anterior column interbody under compression, meticulous preparation of endplates, and additional posterior fusion can help decrease pseudoarthrosis rates. Reduction has been reported to decrease pseudoarthrosis rates by allowing for compressive forces in the interbody and increasing surface area for fusion [41].

Adjacent-level disease is another common disease with reported rates of 25–30%. Older age, laminectomy, and osteoporosis are risk factors for adjacent segment disease. Restoration of sagittal imbalance is critical in preventing adjacent segment disease and should be addressed appropriately in the index procedure [42].

Conclusion

High-grade spondylolisthesis is a controversial topic in the literature. Many surgical techniques may be employed in treating high-grade spondylolisthesis. Restoration of sagittal balance, adequate decompression of neurologic elements, and restoration of the lumbosacral anatomy to support the spinal column are paramount when attempting surgical management of high-grade spondylolisthesis. While varied modalities exist to attain these goals, posterior instrumented fusion and anterior column support utilizing interbody grafts have shown reliable results and should be considered when operating on high-grade spondylolisthesis. The role of reduction is controversial, but it can promote improved sagittal alignment and fusion rates especially when the surgeon focuses on the lordosis restoration rather than the listhesis. Spinopelvic restoration should be considered when managing a patient with high-grade spondylolisthesis.

References

1. Herbiniaux G. Traite sur divers accouchemens laborleux et sur les polypes de la matrice. Bruxelles: JL DeBoubers; 1782.
2. Capener N. Spondylolisthesis. Br J Surg. 1932;19:374–86.
3. Meyerding HW. Spondylolisthesis. J Bone Jt Surg. 1931;13:39–48.
4. Wiltse LL, Newman PH, Macnab I. Classification of spondylolysis and spondylolisthesis. Clin Orthop. 1976;117:23–9.
5. Amuso SJ, Mankin HJ. Hereditary spondylolisthesis and spina bifida. J Bone Joint Surg. 1967;49A:507–13.
6. Wiltse LL, Widell EH Jr, Jackson DW. Fatigue fracture: the basic lesion is isthmic spondylolisthesis. J Bone Joint Surg Am. 1975;57:17–22.
7. Dai LY. Orientation and tropism of lumbar facet joints in degenerative spondylolisthesis. Int Orthop. 2001;25:40–2.
8. Turner RH, Bianco AJ Jr. Spondylolysis and spondylolisthesis in children and teenagers. J Bone Joint Surg. Am. 1971;53:1298–306.
9. Fredrickson BE, Baker D, McHolick WJ, Yuan HA, Lubicky JP. The natural history of spondylolysis and spondylolisthesis. J Bone Joint Surg Am. 1984;66:699–707.
10. Kalichman L, Kim DH, Li L, Guermazi A, Berkin V, Hunter DJ. Spondylolysis and spondylolisthesis: prevalence and association with low back pain in the adult community-based population. Spine. 2009;34(2):199–205.
11. Haddas R, et al. Balance effort, cone of economy, and dynamic compensatory mechanisms in common degenerative spinal pathologies. Gait Posture. 2021;89:67–73.
12. Glassman SD, et al. The impact of positive sagittal balance in adult spinal deformity. Spine. 2005;30:2024–9.
13. Mac-Thiong JM, et al. Can C7 plumbline and gravity line predict health-related quality of life in adult scoliosis? Spine. 2009;34:519–27.
14. Mac-Thiong J, Duong L, Parent S, et al. Reliability of the spinal deformity study group classification of lumbosacral spondylolisthesis. Spine. 2012;37(2):E95–E102.
15. Labelle H, Mac-Thiong JM, Roussouly P. Spinopelvic sagittal balance of spondylolisthesis: a review and classification. Eur Spine J. 2011;20 Suppl 5 (Suppl 5):641–6.
16. Herring JA, Bradford DS. Severe spondylolisthesis. J Pediatr Orthop. 1985;5:737–9.
17. Cavalier R, Herman MJ, Cheung EV, Pizzutillo PD. Spondylolysis and spondylolisthesis in children and adolescents: I. Diagnosis, natural history, and nonsurgical management. J Am Acad Orthop Surg. 2006;14(7):417–24.
18. Varlotta GP, Lefkowitz TR, Schweitzer M, et al. The lumbar facet joint: a review of current knowledge: part II: diagnosis and management. Skeletal Radiol. 2011;40:149–57.
19. Halperin N, Copeliovitch L, Schachner E. Radiating leg pain and positive straight leg raising in spondylolysis in children. J Pediatr Orthop. 1983;3:486–90.
20. Oetgen M, Blakemore L. Clinical evaluation of pediatric patient with spondylolisthesis. Spondylolisthesis. 2023;2:49–58.
21. Tang C, Liao YH, Tang Q, Ma F, Wang Q, Zhong DJ. What is the difference in pedicle morphology of the fifth lumbar vertebra between isthmic and degenerative L5–S1 spondylisthesis? An anatomic study of 328 patients via multi-slice spiral computed tomography. Eur Spine J. 2021;30(8):2301–10.
22. Beutler WJ, et al. The natural history of spondylolysis and spondylolisthesis: 45-year follow-up evaluation. Spine (Phila Pa 1976). 2003;28(10):1027–35.
23. Harris IE, Weinstein SL. Long-term follow-up of patients with grade-III and IV spondylolisthesis. Treatment with and without posterior fusion. J Bone Jt Surg Am. 1987;69(7):960–9.

24. Pizzutillo PD, Hummer CD. Nonoperative treatment for painful adolescent spondylolysis or spondylolisthesis. J Pediatr Orthop. 1989;9(5):538–40.
25. O'Sullivan PB, Phyty GD, Twomey LT, Allison GT. Evaluation of specific stabilizing exercise in the treatment of chronic low back pain with radiologic diagnosis of spondylolysis or spondylolisthesis. Spine (Phila Pa 1976). 1997;22(24):2959–67.
26. Frymoyer JW. Degenerative spondylolisthesis: diagnosis and treatment. JAAOS. 1994;2(1):9–15.
27. Molinari RW, Bridwell KH, Lenke LG, Baldus C. Anterior column support in surgery for high-grade, isthmic spondylolisthesis. Clin Orthop Relat Res. 2002;394:109–20.
28. DeWald RL, et al. Severe lumbosacral spondylolisthesis in adolescents and children. Reduction and staged circumferential fusion. J Bone Jt Surg Am. 1981;63(4):619–26.
29. Johnson JR, Kirwan EO. The long-term results of fusion in situ for severe spondylolisthesis. J Bone Jt Surg Br. 1983;65(1):43–6.
30. Grzegorzewski A, Kumar SJ. In situ posterolateral spine arthrodesis for grades III, IV, and V spondylolisthesis in children and adolescents. J Pediatr Orthop. 2000;20(4):506–11. 22.
31. Molinari RW, Bridwell KH, Lenke LG, Ungacta FF, Riew KD. Complications in the surgical treatment of pediatric high-grade, isthmic dysplastic spondylolisthesis. A comparison of three surgical approaches. Spine (Phila Pa 1976). 1999;24(16):1701–11.
32. Hanley EN Jr, Levy JA. Surgical treatment of isthmic lumbosacral spondylolisthesis. Analysis of variables influencing results. Spine (Phila Pa 1976). 1989;14(1):48–50.
33. Poussa M, et al. Treatment of severe spondylolisthesis in adolescence with reduction or fusion in situ: long-term clinical, radiologic, and functional outcome. Spine. 2006;31(5):583–90.
34. Shuffebarger HL. High dysplastic spondylolisthesis: anatomic reduction. The Harms/Shuffebarger technique. In: DeWald RL, Bridwell KH, editors. The textbook of spinal surgery. 3rd ed. Philadelphia: Lippincott Williams & Wilkins; 2011. p. 660–7.
35. Boachie-Adjei, Oheneba et al. Partial lumbosacral kyphosis reduction, decompression, and posterior lumbosacral transfixion in high-grade isthmic spondylolisthesis: clinical and radiographic results in six patients. Spine 2002; 27(6): E161–8.
36. Petraco DM, Spivak JM, Cappadona JG, Kummer FJ, Neuwirth MG. An anatomic evaluation of L5 nerve stretch in spondylolisthesis reduction. Spine. 1996;21(10):1133–8.
37. Lightsey H, et al. ALIF versus TLIF for L5-S1 isthmic spondylolisthesis: ALIF demonstrates superior segmental and regional radiographic outcomes and clinical improvements across more patient-reported outcome measures. Spine. 2022;47(11):808–16.
38. Min K, et al. Sacral dome resection and single-stage posterior reduction in the treatment of high-grade high dysplastic spondylolisthesis in adolescents and young adults. Eur Spine J. 2012;21(6):S785–91.
39. Gonçalves Barsotti CE, Aguiar Lira RC, Andrade RM, Torini AP, Ribeiro AP. L5 radiculopathy after formal reduction of high-grade SDSG type 5 and 6 L5-S1 isthmic spondylolisthesis with 2-year follow-up. Int J Spine Surg. 2021;15(4):645–53.
40. Nielsen E, et al. 40% reoperation rate in adolescents with spondylolisthesis. Spine Deform. 2020;8(5):1059–67.
41. Hirase T, et al. Instrumented versus noninstrumented spinal fusion for degenerative lumbar spondylolisthesis: a systematic review. Clin Spine Surg. 2022;35(5):213–21.
42. Matsumoto T, Okuda S, Maeno T, Yamashita T, Yamasaki R, Sugiura T, et al. Spinopelvic sagittal imbalance as a risk factor for adjacent-segment disease after single-segment posterior lumbar interbody fusion. J Neurosurg Spine. 2017;26(4):435–40.

Lumbar Spondylodiscitis

23

Marc Khalifé, Jean-Baptiste Odent, Thomas Volpé, and Michaël Thy

Introduction and Etiology

Infectious spondylodiscitis (IS) is the infection of the intervertebral disc and the contiguous vertebral bodies, mainly from hematogenous contamination, starting in the vertebral endplate. IS is a rare condition, more frequent in the elderly, but is more and more frequently diagnosed as population ages and diagnostic methods improve. In the United States, its rate is estimated between 2 and 7 cases/100.000/year.

Microbiologically, Staphylococcus aureus is the most frequently found germ (40% of spondylodiscitis cases). The mode of contamination, as well as the patient's condition, influence the type of bacteria responsible for the infection. Thus, when spondylodiscitis is secondary to endocarditis (25% of cases), streptococci and enterococci are the germs most frequently found. Conversely, when spondylodiscitis is secondary to a genitourinary or digestive infection, Gram-negative bacilli (mainly Escherichia coli) are more frequently isolated. The latter germs are also frequently found in elderly patients, as well as in drug addicts.

In some cases, with rates varying according to studies and geographic areas, IS may be tubercular: "Pott's disease". Fungal IS are very rare, mainly caused by Candida spp., and favored by immunodepression or previous broad-spectrum antibiotic treatment. In around 10% of cases, no infectious agent is identified.

M. Khalifé (✉) · J.-B. Odent
Department of Orthopaedic Surgery, Hôpital Européen Georges-Pompidou, AP-HP, Paris, France

Université Paris-Cité, Paris, France
e-mail: marc.khalife@aphp.fr; jeanbaptiste.odent@aphp.fr

T. Volpé · M. Thy
Université Paris-Cité, Paris, France

Department of Infectious and Tropical Diseases, Bichat-Claude Bernard Hospital, AP-HP, Paris, France
e-mail: thomas.volpe@aphp.fr; michael.thy@aphp.fr

Diagnosis

The diagnosis of IS can be clinically challenging as symptoms are not specific, explaining a mean delay in diagnosis of 30 days. All clinical suspicions of IS must lead to a complete imaging and biological workup. The lumbar region is the most commonly affected by IS (50–70%), then thoracic (23–35%) and cervical, more rarely. Multiple synchronous locations can be found, particularly in cases of Pott's disease, the tuberculous affection of the spine [1].

Clinical Symptoms

The clinical presentation of IS may vary and symptoms usually are insidious and non-specific in the early stages. The only constant symptom is

A. A. Baaj et al. (eds.), *Surgery of the Lumbar Spine*, https://doi.org/10.1007/978-3-032-18097-1_23

the low back pain, often progressive with an inflammatory component. Neurological impairment, that may reveal the disease, must be thoroughly looked for, spanning from neurologic pain in the lower limbs to cauda equina syndrome. Infectious signs are inconstant and are a sign of bacteriemia.

In addition to looking for the infection entry, it is important to identify synchronous bacterial affections such as septic arthritis or endocarditis, especially in group-B Streptococcus infections [2]. In case of Pott's disease, other locations of tuberculosis must be looked for.

Imaging

When IS is suspected, a CT-scan and an MRI must be ordered. The MRI is highly sensitive (>95%) and specific (>90%) to diagnose IS, identify complications (spinal cord compression, epiduritis, paravertebral abscess, and facet arthritis), and rule out differential diagnoses such as inflammatory disc degeneration and spondylarthritis [3]. Abnormalities suggestive of IS are an inflammatory signal of the disc and adjacent vertebral endplates: hyper-T2 and hypo-T1 with enhancement after gadolinium injection and an irregular appearance of the endplates [4] (Fig. 23.1). In case of contraindication, an 18-FDG PET/CT-scanner can be ordered, with similar sensitivity and specificity [5].

CT-scan brings valuable information regarding the extent of vertebral body osteolysis and mechanical stability of the spine (Fig 23.2). In Pott's disease, vertebral osteomyelitis is usually not centered on the disc as in pyogenic bacteria, but on the vertebral body itself. CT-scan is also useful in the preoperative assessment to determine the size of implants, the extent of fixation, and the need for circumferential stabilization.

Conventional radiography is not relevant for the diagnosis of IS as X-rays are usually normal in the early stages of the disease. After 2 to 3 weeks, the first sign of infection to appear is an irregular and blurry aspect of the endplates. However, X-rays are useful for the assessment of spinal alignment during follow-up as they are performed in erect position.

Biology

The elevation of CRP is almost constant (>90% of cases) and bears a diagnostic and prognostic significance. Indeed, it has been shown that a CRP > 150 mg/L was an independent risk factor for neurological impairment and CRP > 100 mg/L

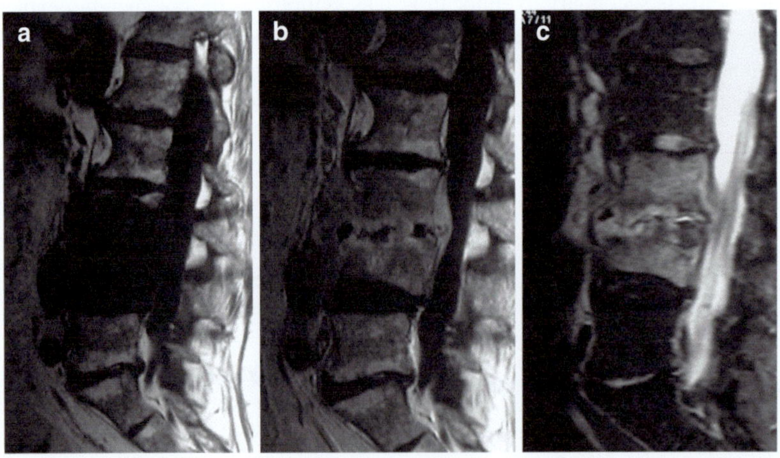

Fig. 23.1 Characteristic MRI images of an L3-L4 IS. (**a**) T1-weighted symmetric hyposignal of the endplates extending to the vertebral bodies. (**b**) After gadolinium injection, marked enhancement of hyposignal zones in T1-weighted images. (**c**) STIR-weighted hypersignal of the endplates and bodies centered on the disc. (From Dubost et al., in Encylopédie Médico-Chirurgicale [6])

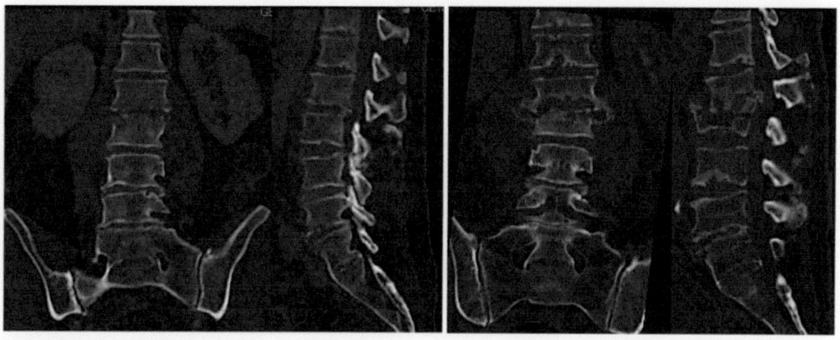

Fig. 23.2 Coronal and sagittal images of a destructive IS causing segmental kyphosis and instability

at admission was associated with higher mortality rates [7, 8]. Conversely, a higher white blood cells count (neutrophils) is inconstant (one third of cases).

Apart from very rare situations where antibiotic treatment must be started in emergency (septic shock, associated meningitis), it is required to identify the bacteria responsible for the IS before undertaking treatment. Performing at least two pairs of aerobic and anaerobic blood cultures detects around 90% of bacteremia, whether the patient has fever or not [9, 10]. In case of sterile blood cultures, a disco-vertebral biopsy must be performed before antibiotic treatment or ideally after a two-week antibiotic-free period. A second biopsy can be ordered if the first one was not able to identify the bacteria. Molecular biology methods can be useful for complementing conventional culture methods, particularly in patients pre-exposed to antibiotics, or for detecting rare germs that do not develop in conventional culture (targeted PCR for Mycoplasma, Trophyrema whippleii, Coxiella burnetti, Bartonella henselae…).

Treatment

Medical

A multidisciplinary management of vertebral osteomyelitis is recommended, accounting for clinical findings, comprehensive imaging evaluation of the spine, and bacteriological sampling. Treatment of IS mainly involves medical management with prolonged systemic antibiotic therapy targeting the pathogen responsible for the infection, for 6 weeks but can be extended to 12 weeks in case of multi-resistant bacteria or epidural/paraspinal abscess [11]. Without instability signs on imaging workup and if pain is controlled, bed rest or bracing are not recommended [10]. Bracing can be useful if it allows early mobilization of a painful patient [12].

In a minority of cases, estimated around 8% of patients in the literature, surgical intervention is required [13–15].

Surgical

Surgical management of IS is indicated after failure of medical management or in cases of complications: neurological impairment (6% of cases), mechanical instability, or kyphotic deformity. It is generally accepted that urgent surgical decompression is required if neurological deficits develop [16–18]. Open laminectomy and removal of the epidural abscess is the gold standard procedure associated with bacteriological sampling, irrigation, and debridement. If there is an important osteolysis or if a large facetectomy is performed, pedicle screw fixation must be considered in addition to the laminectomy (Fig. 23.3).

There is less consensus on the indication for surgical treatment of IS without neurological deficit. Some studies have shown that 44% of patients with IS develop spinal deformity, with a mean increase in segmental kyphosis of 16° [19, 20]. These post-infectious deformities can lead to a significant reduction in quality of life. Inspired by the SINS score, Schömig et al. proposed a score to help assess the instability in the setting of IS [21].

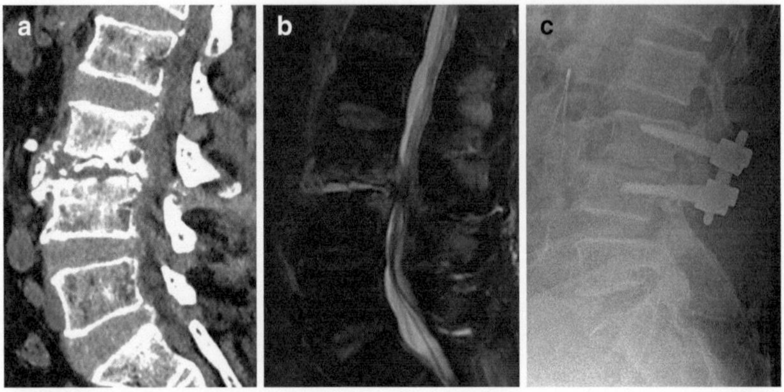

Fig. 23.3 Preoperative sagittal CT-scan (**a**) and MRI (**b**) images of an L3-L4 IS. Postoperative lateral X-ray after L3-L4 laminectomy and fusion (**c**)

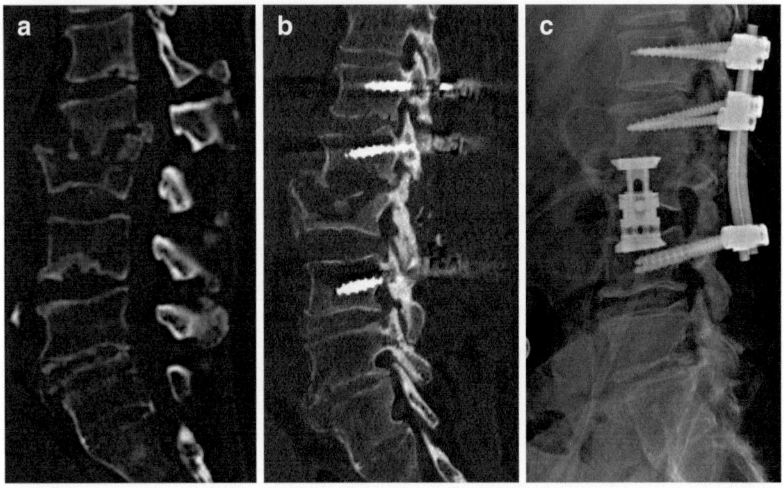

Fig. 23.4 Osteoporotic 73-year-old male with L2-L3 spondylodiscitis with major osteolysis. Preoperative sagittal CT-scan (**a**), after laminectomy and posterior fixation (**b**), and after corpectomy (**c**)

For the least osteolytic lesions, if bracing seems inadequate (elderly, obese patients) and no decompression is required, a percutaneous fixation of the adjacent vertebra can be indicated, to prevent the onset of kyphosis. For the most severe vertebral body lyses, corpectomy procedure can be indicated (depending on patients' conditions). The corpectomy is usually performed after posterior laminectomy and fusion with pedicle screw construct as these severe lesions often associate osteolysis and cauda equina compression (Fig. 23.4).

Conclusion

IS, the infection of the intervertebral disc and the contiguous vertebral bodies, is to be managed in a multidisciplinary fashion, accounting for clinical findings, comprehensive imaging evaluation of the spine, and bacteriological sampling. Its treatment is usually medical with prolonged antibiotic therapy. However, in cases of failure of conservative management or complications occurrence (neurological deficit, mechanical instability, or kyphosis), surgery is indicated.

References

1. Krogsgaard MR, Wagn P, Bengtsson J. Epidemiology of acute vertebral osteomyelitis in Denmark: 137 cases in Denmark 1978–1982, compared to cases reported to the National Patient Register 1991–1993. Acta Orthop Scand. 1998;69:513–7. https://doi.org/10.3109/17453679808997789.
2. Mulleman D, Philippe P, Senneville E, et al. Streptococcal and enterococcal spondylodiscitis (vertebral osteomyelitis). High incidence of infective endocarditis in 50 cases. J Rheumatol. 2006;33:91–7.

3. Herren C, Jung N, Pishnamaz M, et al. Spondylodiscitis: diagnosis and treatment options. Dtsch Arztebl Int. 2017; https://doi.org/10.3238/arztebl.2017.0875.
4. Varma R, Lander P, Assaf A. Imaging of pyogenic infectious spondylodiskitis. Radiol Clin North Am. 2001;39:203–13. https://doi.org/10.1016/S0033-8389(05)70273-6.
5. Georgakopoulos A, Pneumaticos SG, Sipsas NV, Chatziioannou S. Positron emission tomography in spinal infections. Clin Imaging. 2015;39:553–8. https://doi.org/10.1016/j.clinimag.2015.04.002.
6. Dubost J-J, Tournadre A, Soubrier M, Ristori J-M. Spondylodiscite infectieuse non tuberculeuse. EMC. 2006;1:1–11. https://doi.org/10.1016/s0246-0521(06)41700-9.
7. Bhavan KP, Marschall J, Olsen MA, et al. The epidemiology of hematogenous vertebral osteomyelitis: a cohort study in a tertiary care hospital. BMC Infect Dis. 2010;10:158. https://doi.org/10.1186/1471-2334-10-158.
8. Lemaignen A, Ghout I, Dinh A, et al. Characteristics of and risk factors for severe neurological deficit in patients with pyogenic vertebral osteomyelitis. Medicine (Baltimore). 2017;96:e6387. https://doi.org/10.1097/MD.0000000000006387.
9. Aagaard T, Roed C, Dragsted C, Skinhøj P. Microbiological and therapeutic challenges in infectious spondylodiscitis: a cohort study of 100 cases, 2006–2011. Scand J Infect Dis. 2013;45:417–24. https://doi.org/10.3109/00365548.2012.753160.
10. Lacasse M, Derolez S, Bonnet E, et al. 2022 SPILF - Clinical Practice guidelines for the diagnosis and treatment of disco-vertebral infection in adults. Infect Dis Now. 2023;53:104647. https://doi.org/10.1016/j.idnow.2023.01.007.
11. Spondylodiscites infectieuses primitives, et secondaire un à geste intra-discal, sans mise en place de matériel. Med Mal Infect. 2007;37:573–83. https://doi.org/10.1016/j.medmal.2007.03.007.
12. Nasto LA, Colangelo D, Mazzotta V, et al. Is posterior percutaneous screw-rod instrumentation a safe and effective alternative approach to TLSO rigid bracing for single-level pyogenic spondylodiscitis? Results of a retrospective cohort analysis. Spine J. 2014;14:1139–46. https://doi.org/10.1016/j.spinee.2013.07.479.
13. Rutges JPHJ, Kempen DH, van Dijk M, Oner FC. Outcome of conservative and surgical treatment of pyogenic spondylodiscitis: a systematic literature review. Eur Spine J. 2016;25:983–99. https://doi.org/10.1007/s00586-015-4318-y.
14. Lew DP, Waldvogel FA. Osteomyelitis. Lancet. 2004;364:369–79. https://doi.org/10.1016/S0140-6736(04)16727-5.
15. Carragee EJ. Pyogenic vertebral osteomyelitis. J Bone Joint Surg Am. 1997;79:874–80. https://doi.org/10.2106/00004623-199706000-00011.
16. Gouliouris T, Aliyu SH, Brown NM (2010) Spondylodiscitis: update on diagnosis and management. J Antimicrob Chemother. 65:iii11–24. https://doi.org/10.1093/jac/dkq303.
17. Guerado E, Cerván AM. Surgical treatment of spondylodiscitis. An update. Int Orthop. 2012;36:413–20. https://doi.org/10.1007/s00264-011-1441-1.
18. Eismont FJ, Bohlman HH, Soni PL, et al. Pyogenic and fungal vertebral osteomyelitis with paralysis. J Bone Joint Surg Am. 1983;65:19–29.
19. Rezai AR, Woo HH, Errico TJ, Cooper PR. Contemporary management of spinal osteomyelitis. Neurosurgery. 1999;44:1018–25. https://doi.org/10.1097/00006123-199905000-00047.
20. Srinivasan D, Terman SW, Himedan M, et al. Risk factors for the development of deformity in patients with spinal infection. Neurosurg Focus. 2014;37:E2. https://doi.org/10.3171/2014.6.FOCUS14143.
21. Schömig F, Li Z, Perka L, et al. Georg schmorl prize of the German spine society (DWG) 2021: Spinal Instability Spondylodiscitis Score (SISS)—a novel classification system for spinal instability in spontaneous spondylodiscitis. Eur Spine J. 2022;31:1099–106. https://doi.org/10.1007/s00586-022-07157-3.

Postoperative Spinal Infections

24

Vincent Raymaekers, Maarten Wissels, and Sven Bamps

Introduction

Postoperative spinal infections (PSIs) or surgical site infections (SSIs) are a significant complication following spinal surgeries, contributing to patient morbidity, extended hospital stays, and increased healthcare costs [1, 2]. These infections are a primary concern for spine surgeons due to their complexity in management and potential for treatment failure. Although advances in surgical techniques, instrumentation, and infection prevention strategies have reduced the overall incidence of PSIs, they remain a critical issue in postoperative care [3].

The incidence of PSIs ranges widely between 2% and 5%, depending on different factors such as the type of surgery, the presence of instrumentation, and patient comorbidities. Infection rates in surgically treated spinal injuries have been reported to be higher up to 10–15% [2, 4–6]. Infections are less common in non-instrumented procedures, since instrumentation significantly increases the risk due to the potential for bacterial colonization on the implanted hardware. In cases where the infection involves the hardware, treatment becomes more complex, requiring both medical and surgical interventions [7].

PSIs are associated with considerable healthcare costs, with estimates of treatment expenses around $15,000 to $30,000 of direct medical costs per case, depending on the severity of the infection and the need for prolonged care. These infections also lengthen hospital stays, further compounding to this financial burden [1, 8, 9]. While they remain relatively infrequent in many patient groups, the associated costs, both direct and indirect, make prevention and early intervention crucial.

V. Raymaekers
Department of Neurosurgery Jessa Hospital, Hasselt, Belgium

Faculty of Medicine and Life Sciences, Hasselt University, Hasselt, Belgium

Faculty of Medicine and Health Sciences, University of Antwerp, Antwerp, Belgium

M. Wissels
Department of Neurosurgery Jessa Hospital, Hasselt, Belgium

Study and Research Center Neurosurgery Virga Jesse, Hasselt, Belgium
e-mail: maarten.wissels@jessazh.be

S. Bamps (✉)
Department of Neurosurgery Jessa Hospital, Hasselt, Belgium

Faculty of Medicine and Life Sciences, Hasselt University, Hasselt, Belgium

Study and Research Center Neurosurgery Virga Jesse, Hasselt, Belgium
e-mail: Sven.Bamps@jessazh.be

A. A. Baaj et al. (eds.), *Surgery of the Lumbar Spine*, https://doi.org/10.1007/978-3-032-18097-1_24

Classification of SSI After Spinal Surgery

SSI after spinal surgery can be categorized based on two primary features: the use of spinal instrumentation and the depth of the infection.

Superficial SSIs remain limited to the skin and/or subcutaneous tissues, often presenting within the first week or two after surgery. These infections are generally easier to treat and often involve standard wound care and a course of antibiotics. However, deep infections involve the tissues below the fascia, including muscles or even the spine itself, such as discitis (infection of the intervertebral disc) or osteomyelitis (infection of the vertebral bone).

Non-instrumented procedures, such as spinal decompressions or microdiscectomies, generally have lower infection rates. The infection rate in lumbar discectomies is reported below 1% [10]. Recent advances in endoscopic lumbar discectomies have even reduced these infections rated to 0,001% in a recent cohort study by Mahan et al. [11]. Moreover, infections after non-instrumented surgeries are usually easier to treat because they typically do not involve deep-seated biofilms or hardware colonization. In contrast, instrumented procedures involving implantation of hardware such as screws, rods, or cages carry a higher risk of infection, ranging from 1% to 10% [7, 12]. Margaryan et al. performed a prospective study showing that 98% of infections in spinal instrumented surgery were acquired during surgery in contrast to delayed hematogenous infection [13]. The presence of foreign material increases the likelihood of bacterial colonization, especially with organisms that can form biofilms on the surface of implants. The majority of infections after instrumented surgery are early-onset acute infections. However, hardware infections can occur months to years after the initial surgery, manifesting as a low-grade, late-onset infection [7].

Common Causative Bacteria

The microbiological profile of spinal SSI is dominated by skin flora, with *Staphylococcus aureus* being the most common pathogen. In acute postoperative cases, these highly virulent microbes (*Staphylococcus aureus* and *Streptococcus* spp.) are responsible for the commonly purulent infection. Methicillin-resistant *Staphylococcus aureus* (MRSA) infections are particularly concerning due to their resistance to standard antibiotic treatments and their association with more severe infections [14].

In cases of delayed-onset infections, less virulent microbes are the culprits for chronic postoperative spinal implant infections leading to loosening of the instrumentation and neurological deterioration. For example, *Staphylococcus epidermidis*, a coagulase-negative staphylococcus, is associated with biofilm formation on spinal instrumentation. This bacterium is less virulent but more difficult to eradicate due to its slow-growing nature and ability to adhere to implant surfaces [2, 7]. Next, *Cutibacterium acnes* can be responsible for late-onset infections. The isolation of *C. Acnes* required prolonged incubation of the microbiological samples up to more than a week [15]. Gram-negative organisms, including *Escherichia coli* and *Pseudomonas aeruginosa*, can also cause infections, especially in patients with certain risk factors such as prolonged hospital stays or those with compromised immune systems [14].

Risk Factors and Prevention

Postoperative spinal infections (PSIs) can arise from several risk factors that are present before, during, and after surgery. Identifying these factors helps spine surgeons implement tailored prevention strategies to minimize infection risks. These risk factors can be seen as the combination of the impact of the surgical act and the patient's health status.

A large number of studies have found that increased operative time is associated with an increased risk of SSI following spine surgery due to prolonged tissue exposure and greater blood loss [16, 17]. The use of spinal instrumentation increases the risk of SSI due to potential bacterial adhesion, particularly from pathogens like *Staphylococcus epidermidis* and *Cutibacterium acnes*. Poor surgical technique and excessive soft tissue manipulation, particularly in obese patients, can lead to tissue ischemia further raising the likelihood of infection [16].

Patient-specific comorbidities altering the immune function play a significant role in increasing the likelihood of SSI. Advanced age and obesity have been identified as a risk factor.

De la Garza-Ramos et al. found that obesity (BMI >30 kg/m^2) is related to a risk ratio of 3,11 for SSI after lumbar fusion surgery [18]. Next, (uncontrolled) diabetes mellitus, malnutrition (low serum albumin levels (<3.5 mg/dL)), or chronic immunosuppressive treatment all influence a patient's immune response and further complicate wound healing exacerbating the risk for SSI. Smoking, nicotine in specific, leads to peripheral vasoconstriction and tissue hypoxia and decreased wound collagen production, resulting in an increased vulnerability to infections. Lastly, in the postoperative phase, prolonged hospital/ICU stays, poor wound care, and improper drain management increase infection risks [17, 19].

Prevention strategies involve a multifaceted approach. Preoperatively, optimizing patient health by controlling diabetes and encouraging smoking cessation can significantly reduce infection risks. Prophylactic antibiotic therapy tends to be beneficial for spinal surgery, even when expected infection rates are low based on a meta-analysis by Barker et al. [20]. Antibiotics should be administered within an hour before incision, in consultation with the infectiology department based on your local resistance pattern (e.g., first-generation cephalosporins, cefazolin 2 g) in both instrumented and non-instrumented spinal procedures. Clindamycin or vancomycin can be administered in case of allergy to cephalosporins or penicillin [21, 22]. Intraoperative measures, such as minimizing tissue damage, sterile environment, education of nursing on sterility, double gloving, and irrigation with povidone-iodine solution, have proven to lower infection rates [23, 24]. Finally, postoperative monitoring of inflammatory markers, proper drain management, and early mobilization are crucial in preventing infections [16, 19].

Clinical Presentation and Diagnosis

SSI after spinal surgery can manifest with a range of clinical symptoms depending on the timing, depth, and severity of the infection. Early recognition and accurate diagnosis are essential for initiating prompt treatment.

The onset of postoperative spinal infections can vary significantly. In general, infections may present early (within 30 days of surgery) or late (weeks, months, or even years post-surgery). Early infections are often associated with superficial wound infections or deep infections that occur within the first few weeks postoperatively. In contrast, delayed infections, particularly in cases involving spinal instrumentation, may manifest months to years after surgery due to biofilm formation on the hardware. Superficial infections typically occur within the first few weeks following surgery. They are characterized by localized symptoms, which include redness (erythema) around the surgical wound, swelling or induration at the incision site, warmth over the affected area, purulent drainage, and in some cases, wound dehiscence. These infections are often easier to detect due to their obvious external signs, allowing for earlier intervention.

Deep infections, which extend into deeper tissues such as muscles, bones, or intervertebral discs, present with more severe, and often systemic symptoms. Patients may experience intense back pain that is disproportionate to the expected postoperative recovery, fever (which may be absent in chronic cases), night sweats, and general malaise. Neurological symptoms, such as radiculopathy or myelopathy, may also be present if an epidural abscess is compressing neural structures. Deep infections, including conditions like discitis or osteomyelitis, often present later and require a high index of suspicion due to their more insidious onset [25, 26].

Important biochemical markers in diagnosing PSIs are elevated white blood cell (WBC) counts and C-reactive protein (CRP). Elevated WBC is common in acute infections but can be normal in delayed or low-grade infections. CRP typically peaks within the first few days after surgery and normalizes within a few weeks, therefore persistently high levels may indicate infection. A negative CRP is no exclusion criterion for spinal infections, as chronic low-grade infections could have no systemic inflammation. In patients with signs of systemic infection or sepsis (such as fever or rigors), blood cultures should be taken [12, 27, 28].

One of the key elements in the diagnosis and treatment of SSI after spinal surgery is proper tissue sampling and bacteriological studies before the administration of antibiotics. Wound cultures should be taken for superficial infections if no surgical debridement is anticipated. In suspected deep infections, definitely in the case of instrumented spinal surgery, deep tissue biopsies are necessary both from the subcutaneous tissue and beneath the fascia [2]. The PRO-IMPLANT foundation assembled guidelines on postoperative spinal implant infection, based on the European Bone and Joint Infection Society criteria for periprosthetic joint infection. They advise that two out of three tissue samples or sonication fluids should be obtained and positive for bacterial growth. Moreover, histopathology should be performed to confirm peri-implant inflammation [7]. If surgery is not immediately indicated, a CT-guided biopsy can be performed to obtain samples (ex. spondylodiscitis). Gram staining and cultures should be obtained before antibiotic administration to avoid false-negative results. Biofilm-forming bacteria, such as *S. epidermidis* and *C. acnes*, may require extended culture times [13, 15].

The diagnosis of SSI after spine surgery can be supported by different Imaging modalities. Magnetic resonance imaging (MRI) is considered the gold standard for detecting spinal infections, with high sensitivity and specificity (>90%). Early MRI findings include bone marrow edema, disc space narrowing, and enhancement of infected tissues on contrast-enhanced sequences (Fig. 24.1a, b). It is valuable in detecting epidural abscesses and determining the extension of infection into neighboring soft tissues. MRI is effective in distinguishing between infection and postoperative changes [29].

Next, computed tomography (CT) scans are useful for detecting bone destruction, hardware loosening, or pseudoarthrosis, especially in cases where MRI is contraindicated. X-rays may reveal hardware failure, bone destruction, or sagittal imbalance in the later stages of infection but are less sensitive in the early phase. Finally, nuclear medicine scans (e.g., Technetium-99 m and indium-111 leukocyte scans) can be helpful when MRI is unavailable or inconclusive, though their

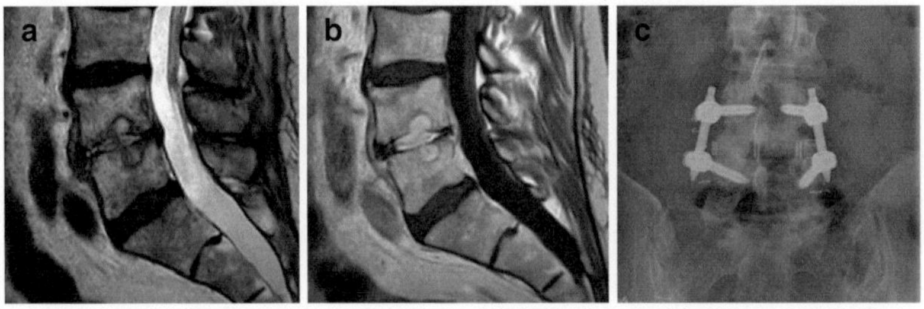

Fig. 24.1 Magnetic resonance imaging (MRI) as golden standard for the detection of spinal infections. (**a**) MRI T2 image showing discitis L4-L5 with end plate destruction and bone marrow oedema. (**b**) MRI T1 image showing contrast enhancement in the intervertebral disc between L4-L5, indicating the diagnosis of discitis. (**c**) X-ray of a patient with intractable pain and spinal instability treated with extreme lateral interbody fusion (XLIF) and percutaneous pedicle screw fixation

specificity is limited in some specific cases of trauma or cancer. Lastly, an FDG-PET scan can differentiate between infection and inflammation in the early postoperative period [30, 31].

Treatment of Postoperative Spinal Infections

Postoperative spinal infections (PSIs) present significant challenges to both patients and spine surgeons. The goal of treatment is to eliminate infection, preserve spinal function/stability, and minimize patient morbidity. The approach to treatment depends on the severity of the infection, the presence of instrumentation, and the patient's clinical status (Fig. 24.2). Both non-operative and operative treatments have a role, and the decision-making process requires careful consideration of several factors.

Conservative Treatment

Non-operative management can be effective for certain types of spinal SSIs, particularly in cases where the infection is superficial. Non-operative treatment typically consists of antibiotic therapy tailored to the specific organism isolated from cultures, alongside close monitoring of the patient's wound healing and clinical status.

In superficial wound infections limited to the skin and subcutaneous tissues, local wound care and empirical antibiotic treatment targeting skin flora (e.g., *Staphylococcus aureus*) can be sufficient. These infections may not require reoperation, especially if there is no deep tissue involvement or hardware in place. Antibiotics should be initiated based on the most likely pathogens, and then adjusted once culture results are available. Infections presenting within the first few weeks of surgery that do not involve spinal instrumentation or deep tissues (e.g., discitis or osteomyelitis) can often be managed non-operatively. In case deep tissues are involved in case of spondylodiscitis, conservative treatment is primarily considered. This typically involves prolonged antibiotic therapy (6–12 weeks) following pathogen identification via blood cultures or CT-guided biopsy. An infection disease specialist should always be consulted in spinal SSI to tailor the antimicrobial treatment to a specific case.

Surgical Treatment

While non-operative management can be effective for superficial infections and certain early infections, there are limits to its success. Persistent or worsening infections after failure of non-operative measures, spinal instability, neuro-

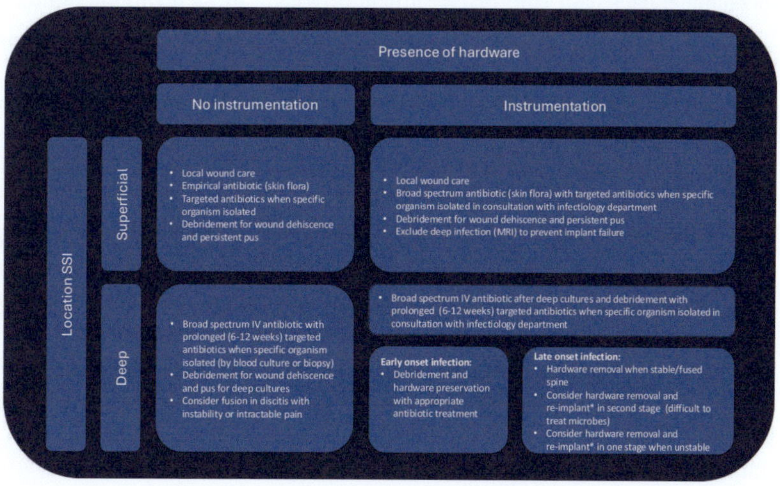

Fig. 24.2 A decision framework for managing surgical site infections (SSIs) post-spinal surgery, categorizing infections based on the depth of the infection (superficial vs. deep) and the presence of hardware

logical deficits, evidence of deep infection, particularly those involving spinal instrumentation generally require surgical intervention. The presence of spinal implants complicates the surgical decision-making.

In non-instrumented spinal surgery, a surgical revision is performed for superficial wound infections with wound dehiscence and recurrent purulent secretions. During surgery, opening of the fascia can be considered when the infection is suspected to have spread below the fascia, for example, when there is evidence on MRI. During surgical debridement of the wound, thorough cleaning of any purulent material with the removal of necrotic tissue is important. Depending on the findings during surgery, primary wound closure may be performed [27, 32]. In cases of significant wound breakdown or persistent infection, a VAC device can be applied to promote wound healing by removing exudate and stimulating the formation of granulation tissue. VAC therapy is particularly useful in high-risk patients with large, non-healing wounds [33].

In case of osteomyelitis or discitis, patients often present with unbearable pain during mobilization. As mentioned earlier, the primary treatment is conservative with antibiotics. In some cases, progressive discitis is associated with uncontrollable pain, inflammatory parameters, and the development of spinal instability [34, 35]. Here, surgical treatment can be considered to establish local source control by decreasing the infectious load and stabilizing the spine to reduce mechanical back pain. Surgical treatment options for spondylodiscitis include posterior pedicle screw stabilization and/or interbody fusion with thorough debridement of the infected intervertebral disc [36]. Recent advances in minimally invasive spine surgery such as extreme lateral interbody fusion (XLIF) and percutaneous screws allow for adequate source control and spinal stabilization with decreased burden for the patients (Fig. 24.1c). In a recent multicenter case series, Raymaekers et al. concluded that XLIF topped off with a percutaneous pedicle screw fixation might be a feasible choice to surgically treat patients with spondylodiscitis with fast and important improvement in VAS [37].

Neurological deficits resulting from the spinal SSI, caused by an epidural abscess compressing neural structures, are an absolute indication for immediate surgical treatment to decompress the spinal cord or involved nerve roots from the abscess.

Cases of extensive deep infections, particularly those involving spinal instrumentation or leading to spinal instability, more aggressive surgical intervention.

Infections involving spinal instrumentation present unique challenges. The presence of hardware increases the risk of biofilm formation, which can make the infection more resistant to antibiotics and complicate treatment. In some cases of early infection, especially if the hardware is still providing mechanical stability, it may be possible to retain the instrumentation while managing the infection with a combination of surgical debridement and prolonged antibiotic therapy. Retaining the hardware may be preferred in cases where the infection is diagnosed early (within 30 days of surgery) or the spinal fusion is incomplete, and removing the hardware would lead to instability. In case of potential loosening of the instrumentation, hardware retention might not be a good idea [7, 25, 28, 36]. When the instrumentation is removed, pedicle screws are always removed whereas intervertebral cages are usually retained, unless the infection is not contained by antibiotic treatment.

In cases of late-onset infections, particularly those involving biofilm formation or loosening of hardware, removal of the hardware is often necessary. In some cases, the infected hardware is removed in a first surgery, followed by a period of antibiotic therapy. After the infection is controlled, re-instrumentation can be performed in a second surgery or can be omitted when fusion is obtained. In other cases, removal of the infected hardware and placement of new instrumentation can be performed in the same surgery, provided the infection is adequately controlled, and the patient's clinical condition allows it. This approach minimizes the period of instability but carries a higher risk of recurrent infection if the infection is not fully eradicated [7, 34, 38].

Conclusion

Postoperative spinal infections pose a substantial challenge for spine surgeons due to the potential for severe complications and the high cost of treatment. The prevention of PSIs relies on a combination of preoperative patient optimization, strict intraoperative protocols, and postoperative monitoring. Early diagnosis and timely intervention are key to improving patient outcomes. For deep infections, especially those involving spinal instrumentation, a multidisciplinary approach that includes infectious disease specialists, radiologists, and spine surgeons is essential for effective management. Continued research into infection prevention, diagnosis, and treatment modalities will be critical to advancing the field and improving patient care.

References

1. Whitmore RG, Stephen J, Stein SC, Campbell PG, Yadla S, Harrop JS, et al. Patient comorbidities and complications after spinal surgery: a societal-based cost analysis. Spine (Phila Pa 1976). 2012;37(12):1065–71.
2. Parchi PD, Evangelisti G, Andreani L, Girardi F, Darren L, Sama A, et al. Postoperative spine infections. Orthop Rev (Pavia). 2015;7(3):5900.
3. Urquhart JC, Gurr KR, Siddiqi F, Rasoulinejad P, Bailey CS. The impact of surgical site infection on patient outcomes after open posterior instrumented thoracolumbar surgery for degenerative disorders. J Bone Joint Surg Am. 2021;103(22):2105–14.
4. Blam OG, Vaccaro AR, Vanichkachorn JS, Albert TJ, Hilibrand AS, Minnich JM, et al. Risk factors for surgical site infection in the patient with spinal injury. Spine (Phila Pa 1976). 2003;28(13):1475–80.
5. Attenello J, Allen RT. Postoperative spine infections. Semin Spine Surg. 2019;31(4):100754.
6. Weinstein MA, McCabe JP, Cammisa FP Jr. Postoperative spinal wound infection: a review of 2,391 consecutive index procedures. J Spinal Disord. 2000;13(5):422–6.
7. Karczewski D, Schnake KJ, Osterhoff G, Spiegl U, Scheyerer MJ, Ullrich B, et al. Postoperative spinal implant infections (PSII)-a systematic review: what do we know so far and what is critical about it? Global Spine J. 2022;12(6):1231–46.
8. Blumberg TJ, Woelber E, Bellabarba C, Bransford R, Spina N. Predictors of increased cost and length of stay in the treatment of postoperative spine surgical site infection. Spine J. 2018;18(2):300–6.
9. Campbell PG, Yadla S, Nasser R, Malone J, Maltenfort MG, Ratliff JK. Patient comorbidity score predicting the incidence of perioperative complications: assessing the impact of comorbidities on complications in spine surgery. J Neurosurg Spine. 2012;16(1):37–43.
10. Mastronardi L, Rychlicki F, Tatta C, Morabito L, Agrillo U, Ducati A. Spondylodiscitis after lumbar microdiscectomy: effectiveness of two protocols of intraoperative antibiotic prophylaxis in 1167 cases. Neurosurg Rev. 2005;28(4):303–7.
11. Mahan MA, Prasse T, Kim RB, Sivakanthan S, Kelly KA, Kashlan ON, et al. Full-endoscopic spine surgery diminishes surgical site infections – a propensity score-matched analysis. Spine J. 2023;23(5):695–702.
12. Kasliwal MK, Tan LA, Traynelis VC. Infection with spinal instrumentation: review of pathogenesis, diagnosis, prevention, and management. Surg Neurol Int. 2013;4(Suppl 5):S392–403.
13. Margaryan D, Renz N, Bervar M, Zahn R, Onken J, Putzier M, et al. Spinal implant-associated infections: a prospective multicentre cohort study. Int J Antimicrob Agents. 2020;56(4):106116.
14. Lazennec JY, Fourniols E, Lenoir T, Aubry A, Pissonnier ML, Issartel B, et al. Infections in the operated spine: update on risk management and therapeutic strategies. Orthop Traumatol Surg Res. 2011;97(6, Supplement):S107–S16.
15. Bémer P, Corvec S, Tariel S, Asseray N, Boutoille D, Langlois C, et al. Significance of Propionibacterium acnes-positive samples in spinal instrumentation. Spine (Phila Pa 1976). 2008;33(26):E971–6.
16. Zhang L, Li EN. Risk factors for surgical site infection following lumbar spinal surgery: a meta-analysis. Ther Clin Risk Manag. 2018;14:2161–9.
17. Yao R, Zhou H, Choma TJ, Kwon BK, Street J. Surgical site infection in spine surgery: who is at risk? Global Spine J. 2018;8(4 Suppl):5s–30s.
18. De la Garza-Ramos R, Bydon M, Abt NB, Sciubba DM, Wolinsky JP, Bydon A, et al. The impact of obesity on short- and long-term outcomes after lumbar fusion. Spine (Phila Pa 1976). 2015;40(1):56–61.
19. Peng X-Q, Sun C-G, Fei Z-G, Zhou Q-J. Risk factors for surgical site infection after spinal surgery: a systematic review and meta-analysis based on twenty-seven studies. World Neurosurg. 2019;123:e318–e29.
20. Barker FG 2nd. Efficacy of prophylactic antibiotic therapy in spinal surgery: a meta-analysis. Neurosurgery. 2002;51(2):391–400; discussion −1.
21. Dobzyniak MA, Fischgrund JS, Hankins S, Herkowitz HN. Single versus multiple dose antibiotic prophylaxis in lumbar disc surgery. Spine. 2003;28(21):E453.
22. Abola MV, Lin CC, Lin LJ, Schreiber-Stainthorp W, Frempong-Boadu A, Buckland AJ, et al. Postoperative prophylactic antibiotics in spine surgery: a propensity-matched analysis. J Bone Joint Surg Am. 2021;103(3):219–26.
23. Tanner J, Parkinson H. Double gloving to reduce surgical cross-infection. In: Cochrane Database Syst Rev, vol. 3; 2002. p. Cd003087.

24. Chang FY, Chang MC, Wang ST, Yu WK, Liu CL, Chen TH. Can povidone-iodine solution be used safely in a spinal surgery? Eur Spine J. 2006;15(6):1005–14.
25. Sarraj M, Alqahtani A, Thornley P, Koziarz F, Bailey CS, Freire-Archer M, et al. Management of deep surgical site infections of the spine: a Canadian nationwide survey. J Spine Surg. 2022;8(4):443–52.
26. Lener S, Hartmann S, Barbagallo GMV, Certo F, Thomé C, Tschugg A. Management of spinal infection: a review of the literature. Acta Neurochir. 2018;160(3):487–96.
27. Dowdell J, Brochin R, Kim J, Overley S, Oren J, Freedman B, et al. Postoperative spine infection: diagnosis and management. Global Spine J. 2018;8(4 Suppl):37s–43s.
28. Collins I, Wilson-MacDonald J, Chami G, Burgoyne W, Vinayakam P, Berendt T, et al. The diagnosis and management of infection following instrumented spinal fusion. Eur Spine J. 2008;17(3):445–50.
29. Dhodapkar MM, Patel T, Rubio DR. Imaging in spinal infections: current status and future directions. N Am Spine Soc J. 2023;16:100275.
30. Raghavan M, Lazzeri E, Palestro CJ. Imaging of spondylodiscitis. Semin Nucl Med. 2018;48(2):131–47.
31. Gratz S, Dörner J, Oestmann JW, Opitz M, Behr T, Meller J, et al. 67Ga-citrate and 99Tcm-MDP for estimating the severity of vertebral osteomyelitis. Nucl Med Commun. 2000;21(1):111–20.
32. Hegde V, Meredith DS, Kepler CK, Huang RC. Management of postoperative spinal infections. World J Orthop. 2012;3(11):182–9.
33. Kumar N, Hui SJ, Ali S, Lee R, Jeyachandran P, Tan JH. Vacuum assisted closure and local drug delivery systems in spinal infections: a review of current evidence. N Am Spine Soc J. 2023;16:100266.
34. Rutges JPHJ, Kempen DH, van Dijk M, Oner FC. Outcome of conservative and surgical treatment of pyogenic spondylodiscitis: a systematic literature review. Eur Spine J. 2016;25(4):983–99.
35. Ahsan K, Hasan S, Khan SI, Zaman N, Almasri SS, Ahmed N, et al. Conservative versus operative management of postoperative lumbar discitis. J Craniovertebral Junct Spine. 2020;11(3):198.
36. Campbell DH, Dowling TJ III, Hah R, Alluri RK, Wang JC. Surgical strategies for spinal infections: a narrative review. N Am Spine Soc J. 2023;16:100293.
37. Raymaekers V, Roosen G, Put E, Vanvolsem S, Achahbar SE, Meeuws S, et al. Extreme lateral Interbody fusion as a feasible treatment for thoracolumbar spondylodiscitis: a multicenter Belgian case-series. World Neurosurg. 2023;172:e299–303.
38. Palmowski Y, Bürger J, Kienzle A, Trampuz A. Antibiotic treatment of postoperative spinal implant infections. J Spine Surg. 2020;6(4):785–92.

List of Relevant Scientific Papers

39. Levi AD, Dickman CA, Sonntag VK. Management of postoperative infections after spinal instrumentation. J Neurosurg. 1997;
40. Olsen MA, Mayfield J, Lauryssen C. Risk factors for surgical site infection in spinal surgery. J Neurosurg. 2003;
41. Mirovsky Y, Floman Y. Management of deep wound infection after posterior lumbar interbody fusion with cages. J Spinal Disord Tech. 2007;
42. Picada R, Winter RB. Postoperative deep wound infection in adults after posterior lumbosacral spine fusion with instrumentation. J Spinal Disord. 2000;
43. Singh K. Rechtine G. Rothman-Simeone The Spine: Postoperative spine infections; 2006.
44. Calderone RR, Garland DE. Cost of medical care for postoperative spinal infections. Orthop Clin North Am. 1996;
45. McPhee IB, Williams RP. Factors influencing wound healing after surgery for metastatic disease of the spine. Spine. 1998;
46. Rechtine GR. Postoperative wound infection after instrumentation of thoracic and lumbar fractures. J Orthop Trauma. 2001;
47. Blam OG, Vaccaro AR. Risk factors for surgical site infection in the patient with spinal injury. Spine. 2003;
48. Olsen MA, Nepple JJ. Risk factors for surgical site infection following orthopaedic spinal operations. J Bone Joint Surg Am. 2008;
49. Perry JW, Montgomerie JZ. Wound infections following spinal fusion with posterior segmental instrumentation. Clin Infect Dis. 1997;
50. Ho C, Sucato DJ. Risk factors for delayed infections following spinal fusion. Spine. 2007;
51. Clark CE, Shufflebarger HL. Late-developing infection in instrumented idiopathic scoliosis. Spine. 1999;
52. Sweet FA, Roh M. Infections in posterior lumbar spinal fusion: postoperative deep wound infections in adults. Spine J. 2011;
53. Olsen MA. Risk factors for deep wound infection following spinal fusion procedures. J Neurosurg Spine. 2008;
54. Fang A, Hu SS. Risk factors for infection after spinal surgery. Spine. 2005;
55. Muschik M, Luck W. Implant removal for late-developing infection after instrumented posterior spinal fusion. Eur Spine J. 2004;
56. Bank M, Graziano GP. Postoperative infections following spinal fusion. Clin Spine Surg. 2017;
57. Wimmer C, Gluch H. Infection risk factors in spine surgery: a review. J Spinal Disord. 1998;

58. Abdul-Jabbar A, Takemoto S. Risk factors for surgical site infections following spinal surgery. J Neurosurg Spine. 2012;
59. Levi AD. Diagnosis and management of postoperative spinal infections. J Neurosurg Spine. 1997;
60. Rubinstein E. Prophylactic cephazolin in spinal surgery: a double-blind placebo-controlled trial. J Bone Joint Surg (Br). 1994;
61. Stambough JL. Surgical site infections after spinal fusion procedures. Clin Orthop Relat Res. 2013;
62. McGirt MJ. Minimally invasive spine surgery and reduced infection rates. J Neurosurg Spine. 2011;
63. Sutherland AG. Postoperative infection following lumbar decompression. Spine. 2004;
64. Khan NR. Prophylactic use of vancomycin powder in spinal surgery. J Neurosurg Spine. 2015;

25 Lumbar Open and Tubular Microdiscectomy

Yazid Maghrabi, Fatimah A. Alghabban, and Saleh S. Baeesa

Introduction

Lumbar disc herniation is a prevalent condition that often leads to significant morbidity, including lower back pain, sciatica, and sensory or motor deficits, resulting from nerve root compression [1–4]. While conservative treatments such as physical therapy, analgesics, and epidural steroid injections are initially employed, surgery is indicated when these methods fail after 6 weeks [5, 6]. Historically, open microdiscectomy has been the standard surgical approach for lumbar disc herniation, particularly in complex or recurrent cases [7]. This technique provides the surgeon with a large operative field and clear visualization, essential for managing complicated cases such as multilevel herniations or spinal instability, which may involve scar tissue and anatomical distortions from previous surgeries [8, 9].

The evolution of spine surgery has witnessed a shift toward minimally invasive techniques driven by the desire to reduce tissue trauma, operative blood loss, and postoperative recovery times [10]. Tubular microdiscectomy, introduced as a less invasive alternative to open procedures, has gained prominence for smaller, single-level herniations. The tubular technique employs a smaller incision and specialized instrumentation to minimize disruption to surrounding tissues while achieving comparable decompression of the neural elements [11, 12]. While initially limited to simple herniations, recent advancements in surgeon experience and instrumentation have expanded the indications of tubular microdiscectomy to more complex cases, including recurrent herniations and larger disc protrusions [12].

The purpose of this chapter is to examine both lumbar open microdiscectomy and tubular microdiscectomy techniques in depth. Through a comprehensive review of operative techniques, postoperative care, and patient outcomes, this chapter aims to provide insight into the benefits and limitations of each surgical method. Special attention is given to comparing their clinical outcomes and complications, which are critical in informing the choice of the appropriate surgical technique based on patient-specific factors.

Y. Maghrabi
Neurosciences Department, King Abdulaziz Medical City, Ministry of the National Guard-Health Affairs, Jeddah, Saudi Arabia

F. A. Alghabban
Neurosurgery Department, King Abdulaziz Speciality Hospital, Taif, Saudi Arabia

S. S. Baeesa (✉)
Department of Neurosciences, King Faisal Specialist Hospital and Research Centre, Jeddah, Saudi Arabia
e-mail: salehbaeesa@gmail.com

A. A. Baaj et al. (eds.), *Surgery of the Lumbar Spine*, https://doi.org/10.1007/978-3-032-18097-1_25

Indications and Patients' Selection

The diagnosis of lumbar disc herniation is established through a comprehensive patient history, clinical examination, and appropriate imaging studies [5, 6]. Surgical intervention is generally considered only after 6 weeks of failed conservative management unless the leg pain is intolerable and/or associated with significant motor deficit, which typically includes physical therapy, analgesics, and epidural steroid injections [5, 6].

The choice of surgical technique depends on several factors, including the size and complexity of the herniation, patient comorbidities, and patient preference. Open microdiscectomy is commonly indicated for large or complex herniations that require more extensive surgical exposure and thorough decompression [9]. Furthermore, recurrent lumbar disc herniation often warrants open microdiscectomy due to the presence of scar tissue and anatomical changes, which necessitate enhanced visualization to safely remove scar tissue without causing further damage [8]. Additionally, multilevel disc herniations or spinal instability are more effectively addressed with the open microdiscectomy technique, given the need for a larger operative field and greater visibility [13].

In contrast, tubular microdiscectomy is typically indicated for simple, single-level, small to moderate herniations, as it minimizes trauma to the surrounding tissues and facilitates quicker recovery [14]. As the learning curve for tubular microdiscectomy improves, its indications are expanding to include more complex cases, such as recurrent disc herniations, fusion surgeries, and even larger disc herniations [12]. A helpful decision on which methods to choose is outlined in Fig. 25.1.

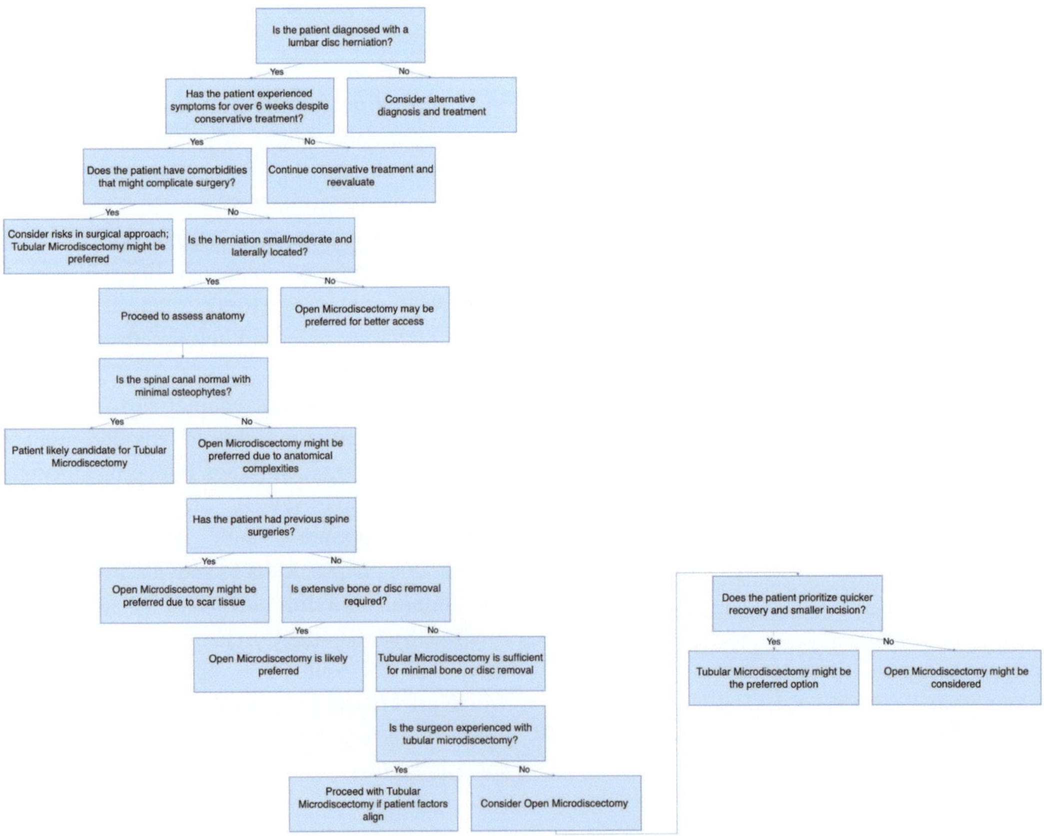

Fig. 25.1 A decision-making flowchart for selecting between tubular microdiscectomy and open microdiscectomy in patients diagnosed with lumbar disc herniation

Operative Technique

Lumbar Open Microdiscectomy

Under general anesthesia, the patient is positioned prone on a Wilson frame, which helps to keep the abdomen free and opens the interlaminar space at the index level. The index level is localized using lateral projections of intraoperative fluoroscopy. In morbidly obese patients, anteroposterior projections may be used to confirm the midline, as palpating spinous processes can be challenging.

A wide area is prepared and draped, with the surgeon standing on the affected side. A midline incision of 1.3–1.9 cm is made, and blunt dissection is performed to reach the lumbosacral fascia. Finger palpation of the spinous processes helps to identify the midline, and monopolar electrocautery is used to open the fascia and carry out subperiosteal dissection.

Once the exposure is completed, lateral intraoperative fluoroscopy is again used to confirm the index level, and a frame-based retractor is applied. The microscope is then brought into the field to begin bony work and expose the disc space. Under microscopic guidance, two-thirds of the cephalad lamina and one-third of the caudal lamina are removed using a combination of a high-speed burr and a Kerrison rongeur. This allows for decompression of the lateral recess and removal of the ligamentum flavum, exposing the thecal sac. The thecal sac is gently retracted medially using a nerve hook retractor to reveal the index disc space (Fig. 25.2a).

Before opening the disc space, the epidural venous plexus is coagulated using bipolar electrocautery. An incision is made in the annulus fibrosus with an 11-blade, and the herniated nucleus pulposus is removed using a combination of a Kerrison rongeur, pituitary forceps, and various curettes. Adequate decompression is confirmed by probing in all directions with blunt instruments, such as a Penfield dissector or a Woodson elevator.

Closure is performed by suturing the lumbar fascia with 0 Vicryl, followed by 2-0 Vicryl sutures for the subcutaneous layer, and a running 3-0 Prolene for the skin. Intramuscular injection of bupivacaine (Marcaine) is administered to reduce postoperative pain.

A randomized controlled trial by Guo et al. comparing closed drainage versus non-drainage in single-level microdiscectomy found that closed drainage reduces postoperative low-grade fever and decreases pain at the operation site. However, it had no effect on postoperative complication rates or clinical outcomes [15].

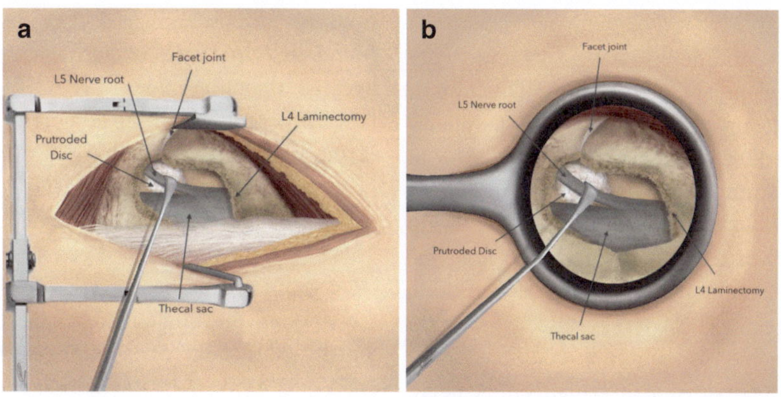

Fig. 25.2 (**a**) An artistic illustration depicting an open posterior microdiscectomy of the L4/5 disc, showing the L4 laminectomy, L5 nerve root, thecal sac, and the protruded disc being removed. (**b**) An artistic illustration depicting a tubular microdiscectomy of the L4/5 disc, using a small incision and a tubular retractor to access and remove the herniated disc with minimal tissue disruption

Lumbar Tubular Microdiscectomy

Under general anesthesia, the patient is positioned prone on the Wilson frame, allowing the abdomen to remain free and opening the interlaminar space at the index level. The index level is localized using lateral projections of intraoperative fluoroscopy. In morbidly obese patients, anteroposterior projections may be used to confirm the midline, as palpation of the spinous processes can be challenging.

A wide area is prepared and draped, and the surgeon stands on the affected side. A 22-gauge needle is inserted along a trajectory that precisely bisects the index disc space. A stab incision of 1.6 cm is made, with the needle tip centered in the incision. A guidewire is then inserted, piercing the lumbar fascia along the same trajectory. After the guidewire passes the lumbar fascia, the first tubular retractor is inserted, and the guidewire is removed. The initial dilator is then used to detect the lamina to ensure proper docking. The first dilator is sequentially replaced with the second, third, and fourth dilators, and the trajectory is confirmed using intraoperative fluoroscopy. Following confirmation, a 16-mm tubular retractor of the appropriate length is inserted over the fourth dilator and docked onto the bone. A fixable arm is attached to the operating table on the same side as the surgeon.

The operating microscope is brought into the field. Soft tissue is removed using monopolar electrocautery, and hemostasis is achieved with bipolar or monopolar electrocautery. The inferior edge of the lamina is identified, and hemilaminectomy is performed using a high-speed drill. The lamina is removed until the insertion of the ligamentum flavum becomes visible. A ball-tip dissector is then used to carefully separate the ligamentum flavum from the underlying dura, and the ligamentum flavum is resected using a Kerrison rongeur. Resection is continued until the traversing nerve root is visualized. A nerve root retractor is used to protect the nerve root and expose the index disc level (Fig. 25.2b).

The epidural venous plexus is coagulated using bipolar electrocautery, and free disc fragments are removed. In cases of contained herniation, an incision is made in the annulus fibrosus using a bayonetted 15-blade. Decompression is performed with various pituitary forceps and curettes. Adequate decompression is confirmed when a ball-tip dissector can pass freely beneath the traversing nerve root and the thecal sac without resistance.

A gelfoam soaked with Depo-Medrol is sprayed over the nerve root. A single Vicryl 0 suture is done to approximate the lumbar fascia, and a single 2-0 Vicryl suture of the subcutaneous tissue. Skin is closed with 3-0 Vicryl Rapide [11].

Postoperative Care

Patients may be discharged on the same day or the following day if they meet the discharge criteria, which include adequate pain control, tolerating oral intake, and normal voiding. Early mobilization is typically encouraged for all patients to promote recovery [16].

Outcome and Complications

Clinical Outcome

A multicenter prospective study by Rajamani et al., comparing 2-year outcomes and complications of various lumbar discectomy techniques, found that in terms of surgical outcomes, the average operative time was 54.12 min in the tubular discectomy group compared to 66.28 min in the open microdiscectomy group ($P < 0.05$) [17]. Blood loss was significantly lower in the tubular microdiscectomy group, averaging 16.41 cc, compared to 59.44 cc in the open group ($P < 0.05$) [17]. The average hospital stay was 1.8 days in the tubular microdiscectomy group and 1.7 days in the open microdiscectomy group [17].

Regarding functional outcomes, there was no significant difference in the 2-year visual analog score (VAS) for back pain, leg pain, and the Oswestry Disability Index (ODI) between the two groups ($P > 0.05$) [17]. However, in the immediate postoperative period and at 6 months postoperatively, the tubular group showed slight superiority in VAS back pain and ODI scores compared to the open group ($P < 0.05$) [17].

A systematic review and meta-analysis by Li et al. found no significant difference in operative time ($P > 0.05$), blood loss ($P > 0.05$), or hospital length of stay ($P > 0.05$) [18]. Moreover, there was no significant difference in functional outcomes, including VAS for back pain, leg pain, and ODI ($P > 0.05$) [18].

Another systematic review and meta-analysis by Wang et al. also found no statistically significant difference in VAS scores between the tubular and conventional microdiscectomy groups ($P > 0.05$) [19]. However, pooled analysis of the ODI revealed a statistically significant advantage for the tubular group at 1 year postoperatively ($P < 0.05$) [19]. Secondary outcomes such as operation time, intraoperative blood loss, and hospital stay duration were similar between the groups ($P > 0.05$) [19].

Long-term results from a randomized controlled trial by Overdevest et al. demonstrated no statistically significant differences in functional outcomes, including VAS back pain, VAS leg pain, and the Roland disability score, during a five-year follow-up between the tubular and conventional groups ($P > 0.05$) [14]. Additionally, there was no significant difference in the rate of postoperative recovery between the groups ($P > 0.05$) [14].

Complications Profile

Complications that can arise in lumbar open microdiscectomy and lumbar tubular microdiscectomy most commonly include unintended durotomy, nerve root injury, and wrong-level surgery [20]. Additional complications include postoperative wound hematoma, superficial or deep wound infection, and cerebrospinal fluid (CSF) leaks [20]. Other medical complications, such as deep vein thrombosis (DVT), urinary tract infection (UTI), and urinary retention, have also been reported [20]. Increases in neurological deficits, whether motor or sensory, are rare [20]. The recurrence rate at the same level is similar between the two techniques [20].

A meta-analysis of randomized controlled trials by Overdevest and colleagues found no statistically significant difference in postoperative complication rates between the two techniques ($P > 0.05$) [14]. Furthermore, the reoperation rate was similar between the two techniques [14]. Similarly, a meta-analysis by Zhang et al. found no statistically significant difference in reoperation rates ($P > 0.05$) or the incidence of dural tears between the techniques ($P > 0.05$) [21]. They also noted that the recurrence rate between the two techniques showed no statistical significance [21].

Conversely, a large observational study of 797 patients comparing tubular discectomy ($n = 339$) and open discectomy ($n = 211$) found that the incidence of incidental durotomy was lower in the tubular discectomy group (4% vs. 8% in the open discectomy group, $P = 0.04$) [22]. Wound complications, including infection, were also lower in the tubular discectomy group (3% vs. 9% in the open discectomy group, $P < 0.01$) [22]. However, the reoperation rate was similar between the two groups (7% vs. 7%, $P = 0.95$) [22].

Conclusion

In conclusion, while both techniques provide effective solutions for lumbar disc herniation, the choice of surgical approach should be guided by patient-specific factors, including the complexity of the herniation and patient comorbidities. Open microdiscectomy remains the gold standard for large and complex herniations, while tubular microdiscectomy offers a less invasive option and faster recovery for simpler cases. Future advancements in minimally invasive spine surgery, combined with surgeon expertise, are expected to further expand the indications for tubular microdiscectomy, thereby enhancing its applicability in complex spinal conditions.

Acknowledgement We sincerely thank Dr. Fatimah A. Alghabban, a Senior Neurosurgery Resident, for providing Fig. 25.2 illustrations for this publication. These illustrations have substantially enhanced the clarity and educational value of the content.

References

1. Amin RM, Andrade NS, Neuman BJ. Lumbar disc herniation. Curr Rev Musculoskelet Med. 2017;10(4):507–16.
2. Frymoyer JW. Back pain and sciatica. N Engl J Med. 1988;318(5):291–300.
3. Koes BW, van Tulder MW, Peul WC. Diagnosis and treatment of sciatica. BMJ. 2007;334(7607):1313–7.
4. Kreiner DS, Hwang SW, Easa JE, Resnick DK, Baisden JL, Bess S, et al. An evidence-based clinical guideline for the diagnosis and treatment of lumbar disc herniation with radiculopathy. Spine J. 2014;14(1):180–91.
5. Bailey CS, Rasoulinejad P, Taylor D, Sequeira K, Miller T, Watson J, et al. Surgery versus conservative care for persistent sciatica lasting 4 to 12 months. N Engl J Med. 2020;382(12):1093–102.
6. Davison MA, Lilly DT, Moreno J, Bagley C, Adogwa O. A comparison of successful versus failed nonoperative treatment approaches in patients with degenerative conditions of the lumbar spine. J Clin Neurosci. 2021;86:71–8.
7. Li W-S, Yan Q, Cong L. Comparison of endoscopic discectomy versus non-endoscopic discectomy for symptomatic lumbar disc herniation: a systematic review and meta-analysis. Global Spine J. 2022;12(5):1012–26.
8. Chen P, Hu Y, Li Z. Percutaneous endoscopic transforaminal discectomy precedes interlaminar discectomy in the efficacy and safety for lumbar disc herniation. Biosci Rep. 2019;39(2)
9. Watters WC 3rd, Mirkovic S, Boss J. Treatment of the isolated lumbar intervertebral disc herniation: microdiscectomy versus chemonucleolysis. Spine (Phila Pa 1976). 1988;13(3):360–2.
10. Drossopoulos PN, Sharma A, Ononogbu-Uche FC, Tabarestani TQ, Bartlett AM, Wang TY, et al. Pushing the limits of minimally invasive spine surgery—from preoperative to intraoperative to postoperative management. J Clin Med. 2024;13(8):2410.
11. Clark AJ, Safaee MM, Khan NR, Brown MT, Foley KT. Tubular microdiscectomy: techniques, complication avoidance, and review of the literature. Neurosurg Focus. 2017;43(2):E7.
12. Staartjes VE, de Wispelaere MP, Miedema J, Schröder ML. Recurrent lumbar disc herniation after tubular microdiscectomy: analysis of learning curve progression. World Neurosurg. 2017;107:28–34.
13. Barber SM, Nakhla J, Konakondla S, Fridley JS, Oyelese AA, Gokaslan ZL, et al. Outcomes of endoscopic discectomy compared with open microdiscectomy and tubular microdiscectomy for lumbar disc herniations: a meta-analysis. J Neurosurg Spine. 2019;31(6):802–15.
14. Overdevest GM, Peul WC, Brand R, Koes BW, Bartels RH, Tan WF, et al. Tubular discectomy versus conventional microdiscectomy for the treatment of lumbar disc herniation: long-term results of a randomised controlled trial. J Neurol Neurosurg Psychiatry. 2017;88(12):1008–16.
15. Guo H, Wang B, Ji Z, Gao X, Zhang Y, Yuan L, et al. Closed drainage versus non-drainage for single-level lumbar discectomy: a prospective randomized controlled study. BMC Musculoskelet Disord. 2020;21(1):484.
16. Baaj AA, et al. Open and minimally invasive spinal lumbar microdiskectomy. In: Baaj AA, Mummaneni P, Uribe JS, editors. Handbook of spine surgery. 2nd ed. Thieme; 2015.
17. Rajamani PA, Goparaju P, Kulkarni AG, Bhojraj SY, Rajasekaran S, Chhabra HS, et al. A 2-year outcomes and complications of various techniques of lumbar discectomy: a multicentric retrospective study. World Neurosurg. 2021;156:e319–e28.
18. Li X, Chang H, Meng X. Tubular microscopes discectomy versus conventional microdiscectomy for treating lumbar disk herniation: systematic review and meta-analysis. Medicine (Baltimore). 2018;97(5):e9807.
19. Wang Y, Liang Z, Wu J, Tu S, Chen C. Comparative clinical effectiveness of tubular microdiscectomy and conventional microdiscectomy for lumbar disc herniation: a systematic review and network meta-analysis. Spine (Phila Pa 1976). 2019;44(14):1025–33.
20. Sonawane DV, Chobing H, Kolur SS, Chandanwale A, Jawale SA, Ansari NAFA, et al. Conventional versus tubular microdiscectomy for lumbar disc herniation: a prospective randomized study. Indian Spine J. 2024;7(1):59–65.
21. Zhang T, Guo N, Wang K, Gao G, Li Y, Gao F, et al. Comparison of outcomes between tubular microdiscectomy and conventional microdiscectomy for lumbar disc herniation: a systematic review and meta-analysis of randomized controlled trials. J Orthop Surg Res. 2023;18(1):479.
22. Evaniew N, Bogle A, Soroceanu A, Jacobs WB, Cho R, Fisher CG, et al. Minimally invasive tubular lumbar discectomy versus conventional open lumbar discectomy: an observational study from the Canadian spine outcomes and research network. Global Spine J. 2023;13(5):1293–303.

Lumbar Endoscopic Decompression

26

Abhinav K. Sharma, Don Young Park, and Peter B. Derman

Techniques, Indications, and Approaches in Lumbar Endoscopic Decompression

Endoscopic spine surgery (ESS) is gaining traction due to advancements that enable effective decompression of neural structures under direct visualization through smaller incisions [1–3]. As a subset of minimally invasive spine (MIS) surgery, ESS involves insertion of an endoscope through a small skin incision [4]. The endoscope provides magnified visualization via a high-definition camera and display. Full endoscopic spine surgery (FESS), or uniportal endoscopy, utilizes a single channel for both viewing and operating, while unilateral biportal endoscopy (UBE), also known as biportal endoscopic spine surgery (BESS), features separate channels for viewing and instrument manipulation [1] (Fig. 26.1). Both techniques leverage continuous irrigation to maintain space between tissue planes and facilitate clear visualization. ESS is being applied to decompression procedures as well as lumbar interbody fusion, showing comparable effectiveness to traditional open surgical methods with less surgical morbidity and faster recovery [5–10].

Given the single portal utilized in FESS, viewing and instrument manipulation must be performed in a collinear manner [11, 12]. Deployable curved or angled instruments allow for off-axis tissue manipulation, and angled lenses facilitate visualization of structures that are not directly in line with the endoscope. Beveled working cannulas can be used as retractors while maintaining a working space. In contrast, unilateral biportal endoscopy (UBE) decouples the camera from the instruments. This allows for more flexibility of motion and the introduction of standard spine surgery instruments as they do not need to fit down the narrow working portal of a uniportal endoscope. However, UBE necessitates more extensive tissue dissection as a space must be created to permit visualization and tissue manipulation in a non-contained space [13]. Navigation can be used in establishing orientation, trajectory, and targets during endoscopic procedures, but standard intraoperative fluoroscopy is more frequently employed instead [14].

In lumbar spine FESS, there are two primary approaches: the interlaminar (posterolateral) approach and the transforaminal (extraforaminal) approach [11, 12]. For the purposes of maximizing efficiency and minimizing surgical footprint, both approaches aim to minimize osseous resection by utilizing existing bony windows. The choice between these methods depends on ana-

A. K. Sharma · D. Y. Park
Department of Orthopaedic Surgery, University of California, Irvine, Orange, CA, USA
e-mail: donyp@hs.uci.edu

P. B. Derman (✉)
Texas Back Institute, Plano, TX, USA

A. A. Baaj et al. (eds.), *Surgery of the Lumbar Spine*, https://doi.org/10.1007/978-3-032-18097-1_26

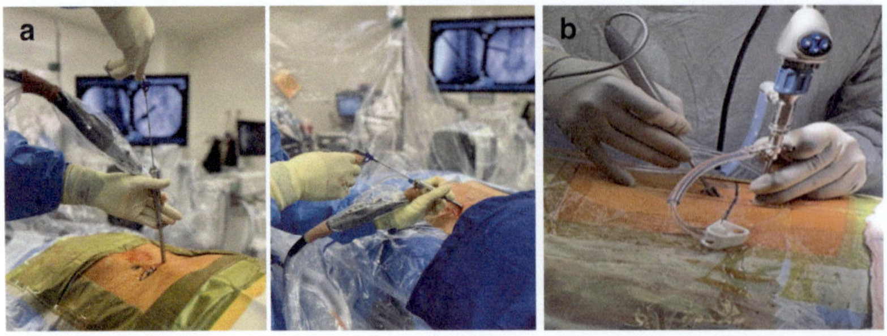

Fig. 26.1 (**a**) Surgeonhand positioning for uniportal spinal endoscopy, demonstrating coupling of the spinal endoscope and surgical instruments with the non-dominant hand maneuvering the endoscope and dominant hand holding the instruments through a single working channel. The interlaminar approach is seen in the left panel, and the transforaminal approach on the right. (**b**) Dual portal spinal endoscopy with an endoscopic viewing portal and a separate working portal. Right-handed surgeons typically stand on the left side of the patient (opposite for left-handed surgeons). The surgeon's left hand should hold the endoscope, and the right hand should hold the surgical instruments

tomical constraints present at the specific spinal level as well as the surgeon's preference [11, 12]. The interlaminar approach may be more intuitive during the early learning curve, as its procedural steps and access to the spinal canal closely resemble those of tubular and open surgical techniques.

The interlaminar approach is commonly used for treating central and paracentral disc herniations at L5-S1 and is often favored for addressing central and lateral recess stenosis due to dorsal spondylosis across all lumbar levels [11, 12]. This approach traverses the interlaminar space, which becomes progressively smaller at cephalad lumbar levels. While the L5-S1 interlaminar window is typically sufficiently large to permit access to the spinal canal without necessitating bone removal, a hemilaminotomy is typically necessary to enlarge the window at L4-5 and above [11, 12].

The transforaminal approach is suitable for treating foraminal and far lateral pathology in the lumbar spine and at the lumbosacral junction. It can also be used to access ventral sources of canal compression at the L4-L5 level and above, but the iliac crest makes this difficult at L5-S1 [11, 12]. The transforaminal technique utilizes Kambin's triangle, a defined safe working zone bound by the exiting nerve root as the cranial/lateral boundary, the superior endplate of the caudal lumbar segment as the inferior boundary, and the traversing nerve root as the medial boundary [14]. Surgeons can access anatomical structures through this triangular zone while minimizing risk.

For UBE, the interlaminar approach is the workhorse technique. The added space necessary to introduce instruments in a separate trajectory from the endoscope makes it more difficult to work within and through the confined environment of the foramen with UBE. Transforaminal UBE is therefore less frequently performed. Fortunately, the ability to utilize standard spine instruments (e.g., high-speed burrs and large Kerrisons/graspers) makes the necessary posterior bone resection for interlaminar UBE more efficient. Pathologies such as migrated and sequestered lumbar disc herniations, lumbar spinal stenosis, synovial cysts, and extradural and intradural tumors can be successfully treated with UBE [15–18].

Operating Room Set-Up

For ESS, patients can be positioned either prone or in the lateral decubitus position. When in the prone position, a Jackson table with a Wilson frame attachment may be used, allowing the patient to be positioned in relative kyphosis to enhance access to posterior interosseous corridors. The C-arm is placed on the opposite side of the table from the surgeon and moved toward the head of the bed after localization and endoscope docking. The endoscopic monitor should be positioned directly in front of the surgeon for optimal visibility and ergonomic support. For transforaminal approaches, care should be taken to prep and drape widely on the side of the approach to ensure that the skin entry point is not excluded.

Interlaminar Technique in FESS for Lumbar Decompression

Preoperative Planning and Localization

Once the patient is positioned, prepped, and draped, the entry point is localized. The ideal trajectory to the disc level is not directly in-line with the disc space, but instead in a slightly caudal-to-cranial direction to maximally exploit the interlaminar window and minimize the need for bony resection. This can be established based on intraoperative fluoroscopic imaging (Fig. 26.2). A perfect anteroposterior (AP) fluoroscopic image of the target level is obtained to ensure neutral rotation. The C-arm is angled caudally—about 5° for upper lumbar segments and 15° for lower segments—until the spinous processes of the vertebrae about the level of interest are centered over the disc space. Finally, the incision is marked overlying the interlaminar window, approximately midway between the spinous process and the facet joint.

Technical Tips for Decompression Using the Interlaminar Approach

Local anesthetic is injected with caution to avoid entering the spinal canal. An erector spinae or other similar regional block can also be used for this and other endoscopic approaches. A 1-cm longitudinal incision is made with an 11-blade scalpel, extending through the fascia. The initial dilator is then carefully advanced to the trailing edge of the lamina of the cranial vertebrae at the spinolaminar junction. AP fluoroscopic imaging is used to confirm the correct positioning of the initial dilator before proceeding with the placement of subsequent dilators.

The endoscopic cannula is advanced, dilators removed, and the endoscope inserted. Electrocautery and micropituitary rongeurs are used to expose the trailing edge of the cranial lamina at the spinolaminar junction, which serves as an osseous landmark. The endoscope and cannula are directed caudally over the interlaminar window, providing visualization of the ligamentum flavum. If necessary, a burr may be used to perform an ipsilateral hemilaminotomy and medial facetectomy or even to work over-the-top to the contralateral side if a unilateral laminotomy for bilateral decompression (ULBD) is planned. It is crucial to preserve at least 1-cm of the pars interarticularis and half of the facet joint to minimize the risk of iatrogenic instability.

A blunt-tipped endoscopic scissor can be used to create an opening in the ligamentum flavum or

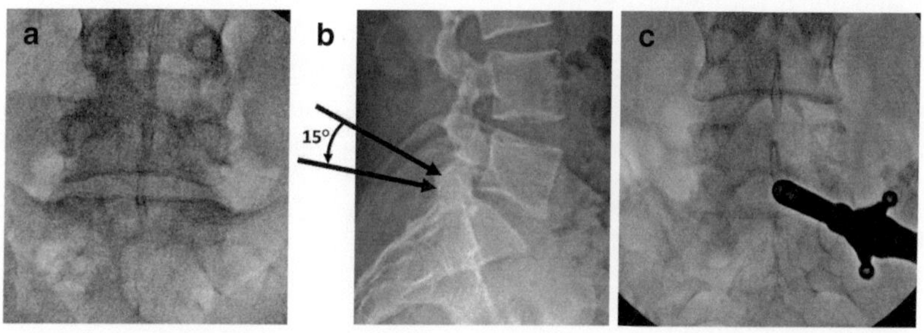

Fig. 26.2 Intraoperative fluoroscopy images demonstrating localization and docking for the interlaminar uniportal approach on the right at L5-S1. (**a**) The L5 lamina largely overlies the interlaminar window on an AP image in line with the disc space. (**b**) A slightly caudal-to-cranial trajectory with the fluoroscopy beam and subsequent docking facilitates access. (**c**) An AP image with the endoscope in place; note how the L5-S1 interlaminar window is more apparent in this trajectory

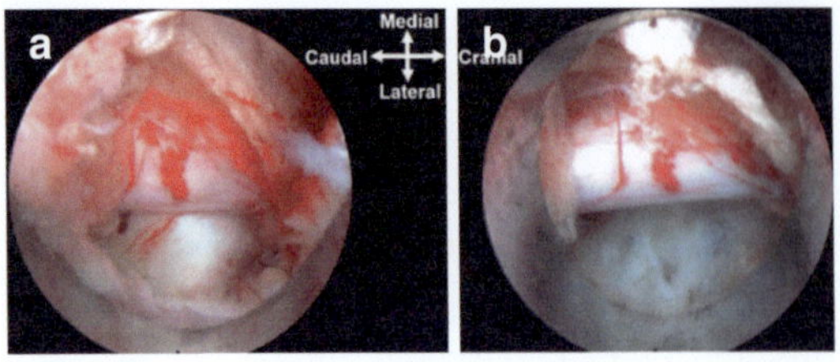

Fig. 26.3 Intraoperative endoscopic images before (**a**) and after (**b**) disc material has been removed during a right L5-S1 uniportal interlaminar discectomy. The traversing right S1 nerve root is seen running from left-to-right across these images with the disc space below. Prior to discectomy, herniated disc material is seen pressing up against the nerve root (**a**). Once this has been removed, ample space is observed ventrally (**b**). The appearance of the "Derman shadow" beneath the neural elements is one cue that appropriate decompression has been achieved

it can be detached from the lamina with a blunt probe if a hemilaminotomy has been performed. Once this tissue plane has been traversed, the hydrostatic pressure of the irrigation fluid rushes into the canal and retracts the neural elements away. The ligamentum flavum can then be excised with a Kerrison or micropituitary rongeur. The traversing nerve root is carefully visualized and mobilized, while any epidural vessels are cautiously cauterized. To address ventral pathology, the endoscopic working cannula is advanced lateral to the traversing nerve root with the bevel facing medially. A preliminary discectomy can be performed if herniated disc material is encountered at this stage. The cannula is then rotated 180°, retracting the traversing nerve root and thecal sac medially to provide circumferential protection and facilitate safe ventral decompression. Any additional herniated disc material can be removed with a micropituitary rongeur, and hard ventral pathology, if present, can be safely drilled down. Decompression of the neural elements is confirmed through palpation, direct visualization, and fluoroscopic imaging, ensuring all areas of pathology are adequately addressed (Fig. 26.3).

Transforaminal Technique in FESS for Lumbar Decompression

Preoperative Planning and Localization

Preoperative planning to understand anatomical constraints is crucial. The position of the exiting nerve root within the foramen should be assessed on parasagittal magnetic resonance imaging (MRI) cuts to determine the safety of a direct approach to Kambin's triangle. In the event of a severely collapsed disc space with less than 1 cm pedicle-to-pedicle distance, a transforaminal approach is typically not advisable; and restoration of foraminal height (potentially via interbody fusion) may be necessary to adequately re-establish foraminal dimensions. If sufficient up-down space is present, rostro-caudal approach angle and incision distance from the midline are planned on preoperative imaging and depend on the site of pathology and the patient's body habitus. An approximately 30° rostro-caudal trajectory is typically effective for facilitating docking and access to foraminal pathology, although a steeper angle may be necessary for caudally migrated disc herniations and a flatter angle for central or cranially-migrated pathology. Preoperative axial imaging can be used to plot out the planned trajectory and the distance from midline at which it exits the skin. A more lateral starting point is utilized in larger patients and for more medial pathology. It is important to ensure that the starting point is not sufficiently lateral to endanger the retroperitoneal space. In the event of a low-lying nerve or when substantial osseous resection is planned, employing the alternative trans-superior articular process (SAP) approach may be prudent (described in section "Technical tips for decompression using the transforaminal approach").

There are a variety of valid localization methods, one of which is presented here. Localization begins with obtaining a precise AP fluoroscopic image of the superior end plate of the caudal vertebral body. A radiopaque object is then used to mark key points on the skin, including the midline, the superior endplate, and the ipsilateral pedicle. Following this, a lateral fluoroscopic image is captured, positioning the radiopaque object according to the premeasured inclination angle, ensuring its tip is at the junction of the superior edge of the pedicle and the superior end plate of the caudal vertebra. The incision is made at the intersection of the inclination line from the lateral image and the vertical line marked at the predetermined distance from the midline on the AP image.

Technical Tips for Decompression Using the Transforaminal Approach

Local anesthetic is injected along the chosen trajectory under fluoroscopic guidance, taking care to avoid inadvertent dural puncture. An erector spinae or other similar regional block can also be used. A long spinal needle is inserted initially onto the lateral aspect of the facet joint and then carefully advanced to rest on bone just above the ipsilateral pedicle of the caudal vertebra. The tip of the needle should never cross the medial pedicular line at the operative level to avoid canal entry at this stage and incidental durotomy. A guidewire is then placed through the spinal needle, and a one-centimeter transverse skin incision is made with an 11-blade scalpel. Sequential dilators are placed. Reaming can be performed to plane down the non-articular undersurface of the SAP and superior aspect of the caudal pedicle but should be avoided if there is any concern for a low-lying nerve root. A beveled tubular working cannula is introduced with the bevel facing ventrally against the disc space. As long as the tip of the bevel is positioned against the posterior annulus and ventral to the neural elements, it can be advanced medial to the medial pedicular line. After confirming the position fluoroscopically, the dilators are removed, and the endoscope is inserted.

If the alternative trans-SAP approach is to be utilized, a jamshidi is placed through a 1-centimeter incision at the planned starting point and malleted into the SAP of the caudal vertebra just above the pedicle. A guidewire is placed, the jamshidi removed, and dilators followed by the working cannula and endoscope are placed. Instead of docking within the foramen, this allows for "shallow docking" on the lateral aspect of the facet joint. Reaming can therefore be performed more safely or a burr to be used to expand the dimensions of the foramen before inserting anything into the foramen itself. The ability to perform this foraminoplasty and then enter the foramen under direct visualization makes this the preferred transforaminal approach for many surgeons when there is concern regarding the position of the exiting nerve root or the absence of sufficient space to accommodate it and the working channel.

Connective tissue within the foramen is excised using a combination of electrocautery and pituitary rongeurs. The bony arch that extends along the superior border pedicle to the ventral surface of the superior articular process of the caudal vertebra is the primary osseous landmark (Fig. 26.4). Once this area is identified, the specific pathology of the patient guides the subsequent steps of the procedure, allowing for targeted intervention based on the individual anatomical and pathological considerations. Care should be taken to avoid excessive manipulation or retraction of the dorsal root ganglion in the cranial aspect of the foramen as this could result in postoperative pain or even neurologic deficits.

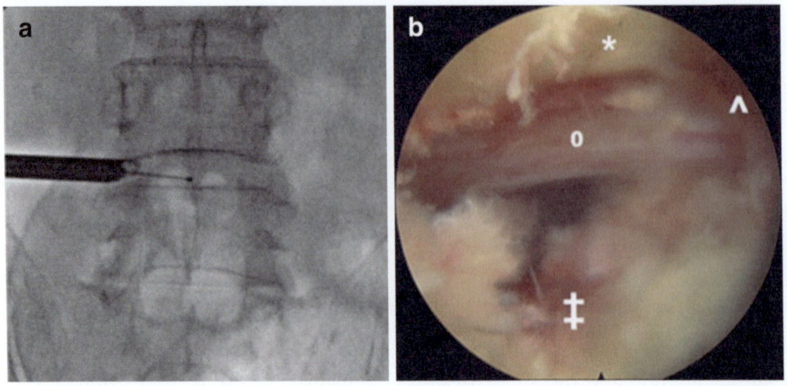

Fig. 26.4 A left-sided L4–5 transforaminal uniportal approach. (**a**) The working cannula is seen entering the foramen with a ball-tipped probe extended to midline in the ventral epidural space. (**b**) Endoscopic view through the foramen with key anatomic structures indicated. Cranial is to the left. ^ superior aspect of the L5 pedicle, * undersurface of the L5 superior articular process, ^{0} traversing right L5 nerve root, ‡ L5-S1 disc space

Interlaminar Unilateral Biportal Endoscopic Technique for Lumbar Decompression

Preoperative Planning and Localization

A true AP image is first obtained by positioning the C-arm parallel to the disc space at the surgical level. The midline, medial pedicle line, and disc space are marked on the skin (Figs. 26.5 and 26.6). Skin incisions are made along the medial pedicle line above and below the target disc space [19, 20]. For UBE, typical incisions consist of a 3–4 mm stab incision for the endoscope and a 7–8 mm incision for the working portal, which also functions as the outflow portal for endoscopic irrigation. These two incisions are aligned along the medial pedicle line and spaced approximately 2–3 cm apart, depending on the soft tissue thickness from the skin to the target area [19, 20].

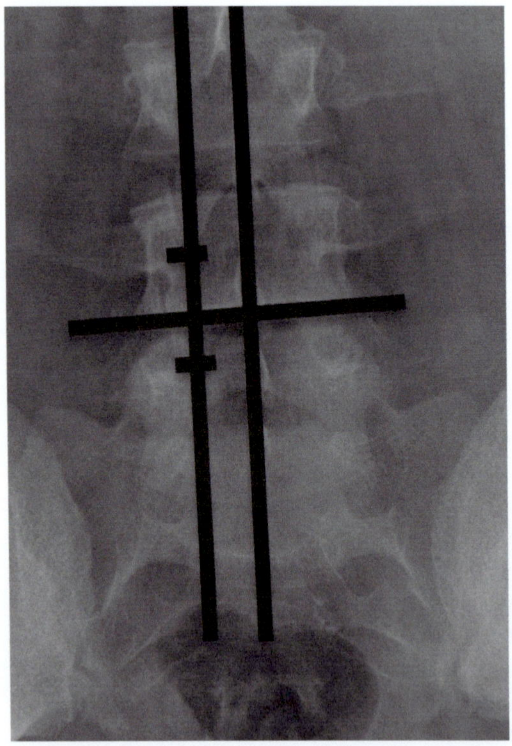

Fig. 26.5 An AP x-ray is used to determine the locations for the working and viewing portals, centered on the disc space line and in line with the medial pedicle line. The cranial and caudal incisions are planned along the pedicles, respectively, targeting the spinolaminar junction of the cranial lamina

Technical Tips for Unilateral Biportal Endoscopic Decompression

The target area for interlaminar decompression at the spinal levels of interest in UBE is at the spinolaminar junction, which is the junction of the

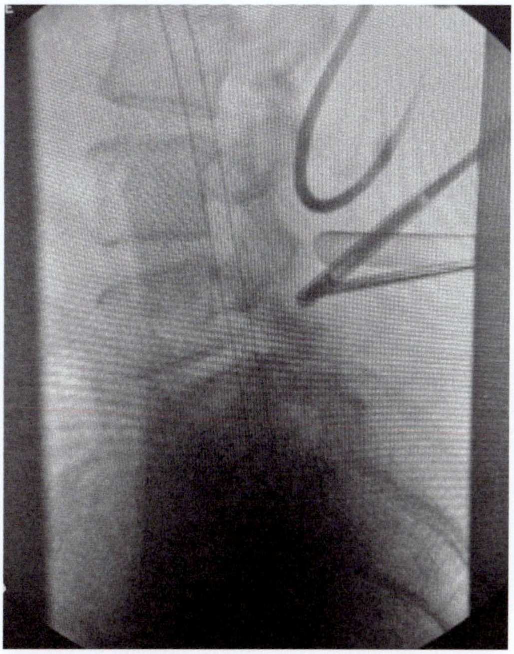

Fig. 26.6 A lateral fluoroscopic x-ray is used to determine the trajectories for the working and viewing portals (aiming both to the target area) and to verify the correct spinal level

spinous process and caudal laminar margin of the superior vertebra [19, 20]. Serial dilators are employed to separate the paraspinal muscles and the lumbodorsal fascia, ensuring that the outflow tract remains patent with an outflow cannula. Maintaining constant and proper outflow is paramount in the UBE technique to ensure that hydrostatic pressure does not increase excessively within the epidural space or within the paraspinal muscle compartment.

An arthroscopic system equipped with either a 0° or 30° scope is used for the procedure. For right-handed surgeons, the UBE technique is more straightforward with the endoscope held in the left hand and surgical instruments in the right hand. Left-sided approaches are therefore easier for right-handed surgeons. As right-handed surgeons progress through the learning curve, performing UBE on the right side becomes more natural.

A 3–4 mm high-speed diamond burr or a 4 mm bone cutting shaver is used to initiate decompression by drilling the ipsilateral lamina from its lower margin starting at the spinolaminar junction. The hemilaminotomy is continued cranially and medially until the origin of the ligamentum flavum and midline raphe are encountered [19, 20]. The ipsilateral ligamentum flavum is completely released from the cranial attachments. If bilateral decompression is to be performed, the undersurface of the spinous process base is then drilled until the contralateral ligamentum flavum is exposed. The cranial attachment of the contralateral ligamentum flavum is then detached [19, 20]. Drilling continues on the contralateral undersurface until the lateral recess is nearly reached [19, 20]. The contralateral ligamentum flavum is detached from its attachment on the lamina [19, 20].

The ipsilateral cranial margin of the lower vertebra's lamina is then drilled, and the ligamentum flavum is detached from its caudal attachment point bilaterally [19, 20]. This allows for circumferential release of the ligamentum, facilitating en bloc removal. At this point, the hypertropic superior articulating process is partially resected on both sides with Kerrison rongeurs to decompress the traversing nerve roots [19, 20]. During the decompression, the medial aspect of the facet joint is carefully drilled to preserve the facet joint as much as possible, reducing the risk for iatrogenic instability [19, 20]. If a disc herniation is present, nerve root retractors can be utilized to gently retract the neural elements while a discectomy is performed [19, 20]. At the conclusion of the procedure, the neural elements should be free and mobile (Fig. 26.7). Meticulous hemostasis can be accomplished with coagulation of epidural veins with radiofrequency wands as well as placement of bone wax to bleeding cancellous bony surfaces. Once careful hemostasis is complete, a suction drain tube may be inserted to facilitate fluid drainage and potentially reduce the risk of symptomatic epidural hematoma (Fig. 26.8).

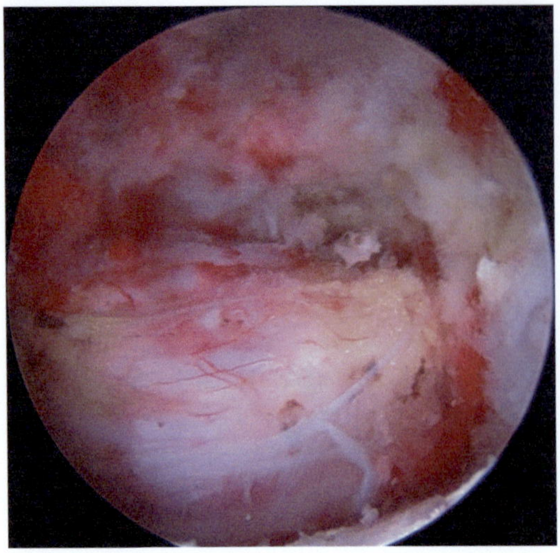

Fig. 26.7 Endoscopic view of the decompressed spinal canal at the conclusion of a bilateral UBE decompression

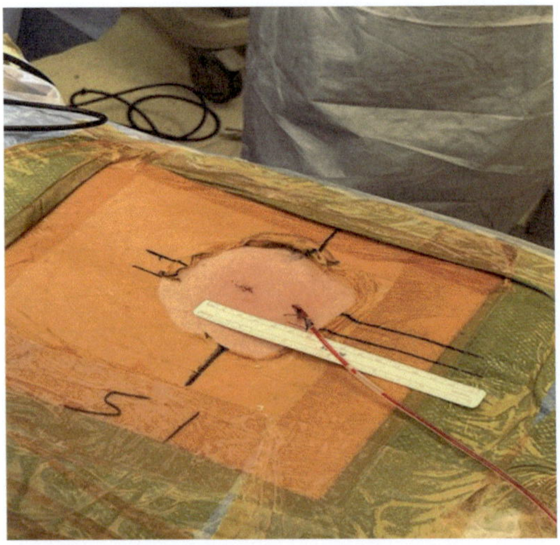

Fig. 26.8 A photograph of the surgical field taken after incision closure and drain placement for a UBE case

Conclusion

ESS encompasses both FESS and UBE approaches, which provide access to a variety of lumbar spinal pathologies while minimizing damage to the surrounding soft tissues. They provide at least non-inferior long-term outcomes compared to traditional open and tubular methods but with more rapid recovery. Although there is a learning curve associated with adopting these techniques, proper training, careful planning, and meticulous execution can lead to excellent outcomes.

References

1. Hofstetter CP, Ahn Y, Choi G, et al. AOSpine consensus paper on nomenclature for working-channel endoscopic spinal procedures. Global Spine J. 2020;10:111S–21S.
2. Simpson AK, Lightsey HM, Xiong GX, Crawford AM, Minamide A, Schoenfeld AJ. Spinal endoscopy: evidence, techniques, global trends, and future projections. Spine J. 2022;22:64–74.
3. Ohara Y. Full endoscopic spine surgery with image-guided navigation system as "hybrid endoscopic spine surgery": a narrative review. World Neurosurg. 2023;179:45–8.
4. Stone BK, Paradkar R, Anderson GM, Daniels A, Iyer S, Derman PB, Telfeian AE, Basques B. Development of an endoscopic spine surgery program. JB JS Open Access. 2023;8(e22):00152.
5. Park S-M, Song K-S, Kim H-J, et al. Comparing the efficacy and safety of minimally invasive biportal endoscopic spine surgery versus conventional microscopic discectomy in single-level lumbar herniated intervertebral disc (ENDO-BH trial): a multicenter, prospective, randomized controlled equivalence trial study protocol. Trials. 2022;23:172.
6. Chung AS, McKnight B, Wang JC. Scientific view on endoscopic spine surgery: can spinal endoscopy become a mainstream surgical tool? World Neurosurg. 2021;145:708–11.
7. Ahn J-S, Lee H-J, Choi D-J, Lee K-Y, Hwang S-J. Extraforaminal approach of biportal endoscopic spinal surgery: a new endoscopic technique for transforaminal decompression and discectomy. J Neurosurg Spine. 2018;28:492–8.
8. Min W-K, Kim J-E, Choi D-J, Park EJ, Heo J. Clinical and radiological outcomes between biportal endoscopic decompression and microscopic decompression in lumbar spinal stenosis. J Orthop Sci. 2020;25:371–8.
9. Heo DH, Son SK, Eum JH, Park CK. Fully endoscopic lumbar interbody fusion using a percutaneous unilateral biportal endoscopic technique: technical note and preliminary clinical results. Neurosurg Focus. 2017;43:E8.
10. Shen J. Fully endoscopic lumbar laminectomy and Transforaminal lumbar Interbody fusion under local anesthesia with conscious sedation: a case series. World Neurosurg. 2019;127:e745–50.
11. Derman PB. Introduction to endoscopic spine surgery. Contemp Spine Surg. 2021;22:1.

12. Perfetti DC, Derman PB. Uniportal endoscopic lumbar decompression: Interlaminar and transforaminal techniques and outcomes. Semin Spine Surg. 2024;36:101080.
13. Ahn Y, Lee S. Uniportal versus biportal endoscopic spine surgery: a comprehensive review. Expert Rev Med Devices. 2023;20:549–56.
14. Liounakos JI, Basil GW, Urakawa H, Wang MY. Intraoperative image guidance for endoscopic spine surgery. Ann Transl Med. 2021;9:92.
15. Kang T, Park SY, Park GW, Lee SH, Park JH, Suh SW. Biportal endoscopic discectomy for high-grade migrated lumbar disc herniation. J Neurosurg Spine. 2020;33:360–5.
16. Leyendecker J, Sofoluke N, Hofstetter CP, Konakondla S. Full endoscopic resection of large bilateral synovial cysts in lumbar spine. Neurosurg Focus Video. 2024;10:V7.
17. Brown HL, Kumar S. Transforaminal endoscopic decompression of facet cysts by interventional pain physicians. Cureus. 2021;13:e18308.
18. Kim S, Bendardaf R, Ali M, Kim H, Heo E, Lee S. Unilateral biportal endoscopic tumor removal and percutaneous stabilization for extradural tumors: technical case report and literature review. Front Surg. 2022;9:863931.
19. Pao J-L, Lin S-M, Chen W-C, Chang C-H. Unilateral biportal endoscopic decompression for degenerative lumbar canal stenosis. J Spine Surg. 2020;6:438.
20. Park DK, Weng C, Zakko P, Choi D-J. Unilateral Biportal endoscopy for lumbar spinal stenosis and lumbar disc herniation. JBJS Essent Surg Tech. 2023;13(e22):00020.

Lumbar Endoscopy, Beyond Degenerative Decompression

27

Vincent Hagel and Kai-Uwe Lewandrowski

Introduction

Extradural and intradural spinal tumors, spinal infections, tethered cord syndrome, and intradural/perineural cysts are relatively rare compared to degenerative diseases like disc herniation and stenosis. Despite their rarity, these conditions can present significant challenges due to their complex nature and the delicate structures involved. Advances in diagnostic imaging have improved the detection and characterization of these pathologies, allowing for more targeted and individualized treatment plans. As surgical techniques evolve, there is a growing interest in minimally invasive approaches that aim to reduce patient recovery time and enhance surgical precision. These advancements offer new hope for effectively managing these intricate spinal conditions while minimizing the impact on patients' overall well-being.

V. Hagel (✉)
Asklepios Hospital Lindau, Spine Center, Lindau, Germany
e-mail: v.hagel@asklepios.com

K.-U. Lewandrowski
Division Personalized Pain Research and Education, Center for Advanced Spine Care of Southern Arizona, Tucson, AZ, USA

Department of Orthopaedic Surgery, University of Arizona, Banner Medical Center, Tucson, AZ, USA

Department of Orthopaedics, Fundación Universitaria Sanitas, Bogotá D.C., Colombia

Department of Orthopedics at Hospital Universitário Gaffree Guinle, Universidade Federal do Estado do Rio de Janeiro, Rio de Janeiro, Brazil
e-mail: business@tucsonspine.com

Intradural Pathologies

The authors' preferred surgical management of intradural conditions requires introducing an endoscope into the intradural space. Although endoscopic intradural procedures were described several decades ago [1–3], it took significant time to develop endoscopes specifically for various intradural conditions. Building on this pioneering work, it is now possible to address selected intradural mass lesions [4, 5], tethered cord syndrome [6, 7], and intradural cysts [8, 9] using endoscopic techniques. However, performing intradural procedures endoscopically remains uncommon. Conventional methods often lead to significant access trauma when treating these pathologies. Many surgeons still rely on extensive approaches, including muscle dissection extending up to two levels above and below the target area, as well as laminectomy or even multilevel laminectomies, even for small intradural lesions [10, 11].

Regarding intradural mass lesions, these approaches have been linked to a high rate of gross-total resection [11, 12]. Yet, the question arises whether similarly high rates of complete

A. A. Baaj et al. (eds.), *Surgery of the Lumbar Spine*, https://doi.org/10.1007/978-3-032-18097-1_27

resection can be achieved with less invasive techniques. This shift in approach could potentially result in fewer immediate postoperative complications, faster patient mobilization, shorter rehabilitation periods, and a lower risk of long-term instability. The term "minimally invasive technique" usually refers to the use of retraction systems, such as tubular retractors, in conjunction with microscopic or endoscopic visualization. In contrast, this chapter will present the application of the full-endoscopic technique.

Infections

Spinal infections primarily involve spondylodiscitis and epidural abscesses. The increasing prevalence of comorbid conditions—such as malignancy, diabetes mellitus, immunodeficiency, renal insufficiency, and substance abuse—as well as factors like injections and the use of immunosuppressive medications, has led to a higher incidence of these infectious diseases. To reduce mortality rates, which currently range from 3% to 25%, a rapid diagnostic and therapeutic workflow is essential [13–15]. Since these infections often occur in older patients with multiple comorbidities, adopting a highly effective yet minimally invasive treatment approach could provide significant benefits.

Tethered Cord Syndrome

Tethered cord syndrome is a neurological disorder caused by the abnormal attachment of the spinal cord to surrounding tissues, limiting its movement within the spinal column [6]. This condition often results from congenital defects but can also be due to spinal injuries or surgeries. Symptoms typically include back pain, leg weakness, sensory disturbances, and bladder or bowel dysfunction [7]. Traditionally, treatment involves surgical untethering to free the spinal cord. Endoscopic techniques, including intradural cord release, are gaining attention as a minimally invasive alternative. These methods offer the potential for reduced recovery times and decreased surgical trauma by allowing precise visualization and targeted release of tethering structures. Implementing endoscopic techniques could enhance surgical outcomes by minimizing tissue disruption and promoting quicker healing. Early diagnosis and intervention remain crucial to prevent irreversible neurological damage and to improve long-term prognoses.

Surgical Technique

Indications/Contraindications

There are only limited studies on the full-endoscopic treatment of extra−/intradural lesions and spinal infections. Therefore, careful and cautious selection of suitable cases is advised. The primary limitations of endoscopic techniques, both uniportal and biportal, compared to traditional methods, include the technical design with typically a single working channel, limited range of motion, inadequate instruments, and specific complications. These disadvantages may be mitigated by the less invasive nature and potential benefits of endoscopy, such as high magnification, irrigation leading to clearer vision, and improved washout of inflammatory factors in spondylodiscitis, or reduced cerebrospinal fluid (CSF) loss in intradural pathologies.

Technical Insights

Various full-endoscopic approaches to the lumbar spine are available, including transforaminal, transpedicular, interlaminar, and translaminar (Fig. 27.1) approaches, along with interlaminar contralateral variations. For extradural pathologies such as tumors and infections, any of these approaches may be appropriate, depending on the individual anatomy and the location and extent of the lesion. However, for intradural pathologies, the interlaminar/translaminar approach and its variations are preferred. Balancing the extent of osteoligamentous decompression to preserve the facet joint and maintain the segment's stability

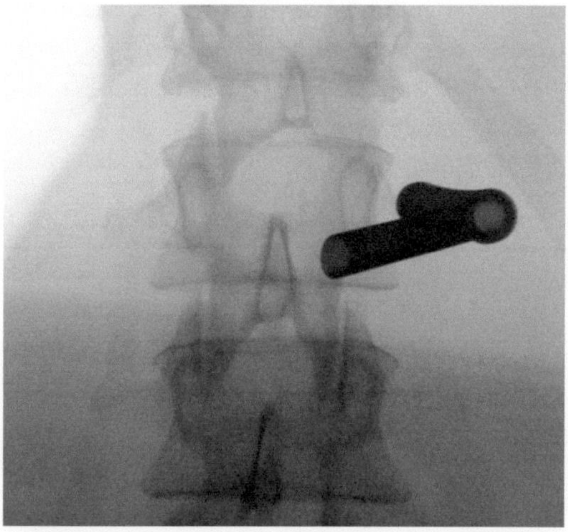

Fig. 27.1 Fluoroscopic confirmation of working sleeve position in a translaminar approach. The image illustrates a fluoroscopic view of the lumbar spine, verifying the correct positioning of the working sleeve. (Image source [16])

and function is always a consideration when ensuring adequate exposure.

Today, endoscopes are available in various sizes. Larger endoscopes are designed for effective osteoligamentous decompression, while smaller ones offer superior mobility. Although osteoligamentous decompression is essential during the approach, enhanced mobility may be more critical during the treatment of the actual pathology. Therefore, selecting the appropriate endoscope should be based on the specific characteristics of each case.

Endoscopy in Spinal Oncology

Endoscopic techniques in spinal oncology are still in the developmental phase, primarily documented through case reports detailing their use for various interventions. For instance, biopsies have been performed using endoscopes in cases involving large B-cell non-Hodgkin lymphoma and pediatric paraganglioma [17, 18]. Endoscopy has also been employed as an adjunct in open surgeries, particularly in thoracic pathologies [19]. Debulking procedures have been reported, providing benefits such as resolved radicular pain in cases of sacral metastasis and bilateral decompression [20–22]. In addition, endoscopic definitive resections have been documented for pathologies such as meningioma and osteoblastoma [5, 23, 24]. This evolving field shows promise in offering less invasive options for managing spinal tumors (Table 27.1).

Intradural Definitive Resection

Osteoligamentous decompression exposes the dura (Fig. 27.2a). After sufficient exposure, the dura is carefully incised (Fig. 27.2b). Currently, no dedicated instrument exists for performing an intentional durotomy, leaving the execution to the surgeon's discretion. Unlike traditional microsurgery, where tack-up stitches minimize epidural bleeding due to continuous cerebrospinal fluid (CSF) loss, this technique is not applicable in a full-endoscopic approach. In full-endoscopic procedures, continuous irrigation provides counterpressure, potentially mitigating CSF loss and reducing epidural space expansion (Fig. 27.2c). Continuous irrigation also increases pressure within the epidural space, minimizing bleeding occurrence. Besides controlling bleeding, tack-up stitches help separate the dura, improving visualization of neural structures and the lesion. Unfortunately, no suitable dura retraction system is currently available for full-endoscopic techniques. Meanwhile, the beveled working sleeve can be used for dura retraction (Fig. 27.2d). It is crucial to carefully position the working sleeve to avoid inadvertent compression of neural structures.

Once the tumor is exposed, attached structures must be dissected. However, suitable sharp dissectors and scissors are currently unavailable. Existing instruments such as blunt dissectors (Fig. 27.3a) and nerve hooks (Fig. 27.3b) only permit limited dissection. For meningiomas, after separating the tumor from neural structures, precise dissection at its dural origin is crucial. Extensive dural resection should be minimized due to limited options for full-endoscopic dural repair or closure. Following the dissection along the dura, the inner dural surface must be coagu-

Table 27.1 Applications of endoscopic techniques in spinal oncology interventions [25]

Intervention	Authors	Patients (n)	Additional information
Biopsy	Konakondla et al. (2020) [17]	1	Large B-cell non-Hodgkin lymphoma
	Konakondla et al. (2021) [18]	1	Pediatric; paraganglioma
Adjunct during open surgery	McLain (2001) [19]	9	Thoracic pathology
Debulking	Telfeian et al. (2015) [20] and Telfeian et al. (2020) [21]	4	Resolved radicular pain
	Tsai et al. (2018) [22]	1	Sacral metastasis
	Gao et al. (2019) [23]	1	Bilateral decompression
Definitive resection	Senturk et al. (2019) [5]	1	Meningioma
	Newman et al. (2020) [24]	1	Osteoblastoma

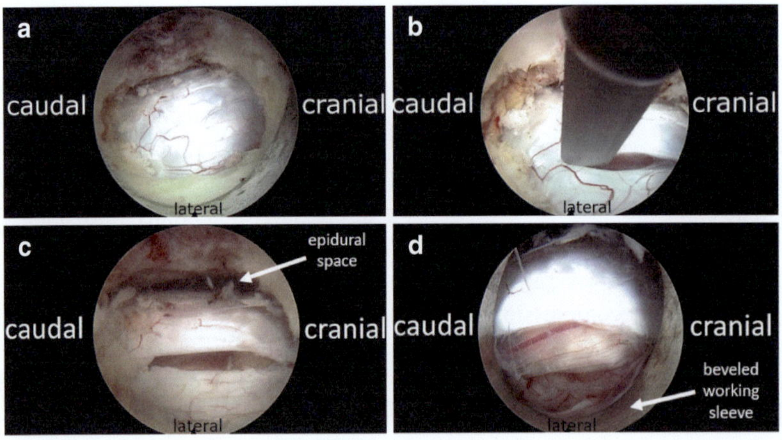

Fig. 27.2 The sequence illustrates key steps in intradural definitive resection. (**a**) The dura is exposed following osteoligamentous decompression. (**b**) An incision is made in the dura, performed at the surgeon's discretion. (**c**) Continuous irrigation during the procedure minimizes cerebrospinal fluid loss, leading to only a minimal increase in epidural space. (**d**) The beveled working sleeve is employed for dura retraction, ensuring optimal visualization while avoiding compression of neural structures. (Image source [16])

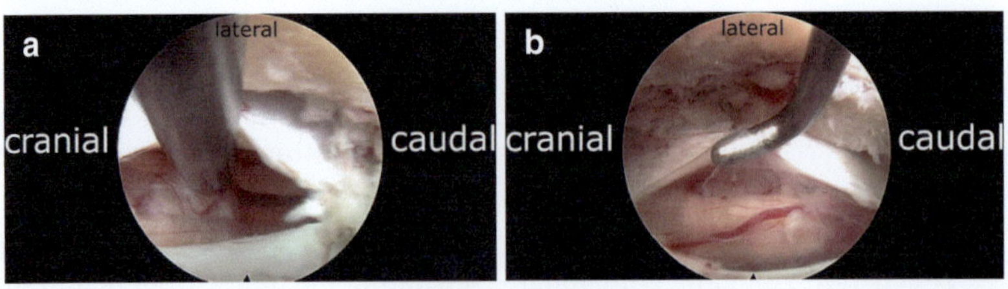

Fig. 27.3 The image sequence shows tumor dissection techniques using available instruments. (**a**) The blunt dissector is employed to carefully separate the tumor from surrounding structures, while (**b**) the nerve hook assists in precise manipulation and further dissection of attached tissues. These tools, though limited, are integral in managing pathologies such as meningiomas and schwannomas due to the current lack of more specialized instruments. (Image source [16])

lated to achieve at least a Simpson grade II resection, indicating complete tumor removal with additional coagulation of its dural attachment.

In the case of a schwannoma, as shown in Figs. 27.4 and 27.5, it is critical to identify the tumor's originating rootlet after carefully dissecting the surrounding neural structures (Fig. 27.5a). Given the limitations of the available instruments, preserving the structure and function of the rootlet while separating it from the tumor is often not possible. Therefore, it is necessary to coagulate and excise the tumor's originating rootlet (Fig. 27.5b, c). Once circumferential dissection of the tumor is achieved, it can be safely extracted using forceps (Fig. 27.5d).

After tumor removal, dural closure should be attempted (Fig. 27.6). However, achieving effective dural closure may not always be as reliable as in traditional microsurgery. Yet, the question arises if dural closure needs to be as water-tight as in traditional techniques. The minimally invasive nature of this approach could potentially lower the risk of complications such as meningocele, cerebrospinal fluid (CSF) fistula, and infec-

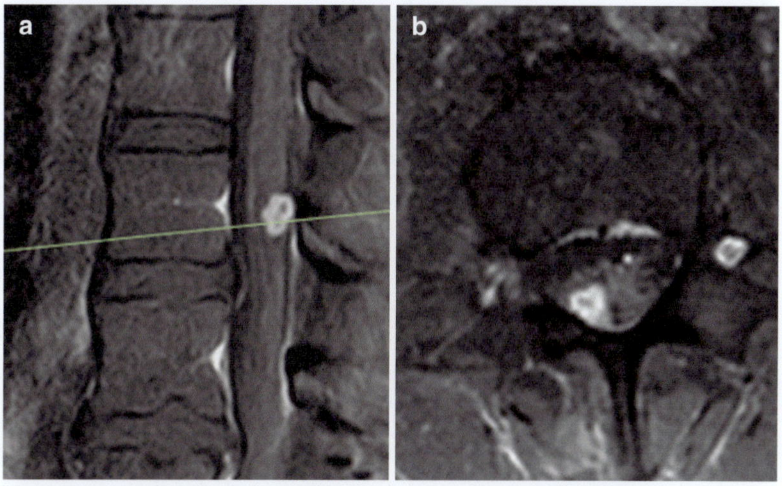

Fig. 27.4 Contrast-enhanced T1-weighted MRI images depict an intradural schwannoma at the L1 level. (**a**) The sagittal view highlights the tumor's location and size within the spinal canal. (**b**) The axial view provides a cross-sectional perspective, illustrating the relationship of the schwannoma to adjacent neural structures. (Image source [16])

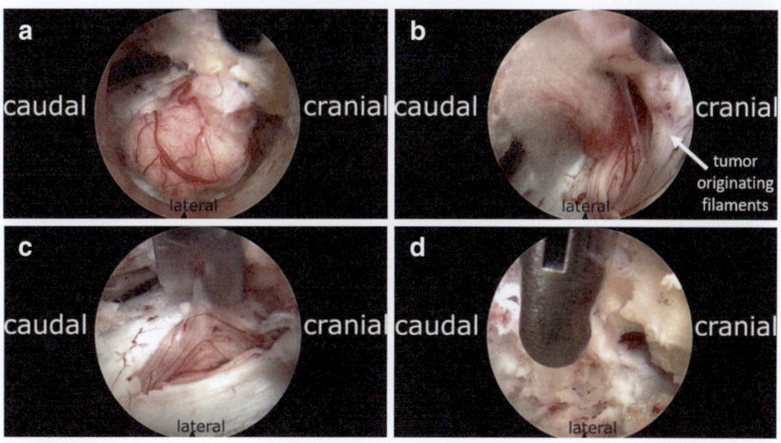

Fig. 27.5 The sequence illustrates the surgical steps for schwannoma removal. (**a**) The tumor is first relocated outside of the dura. (**b**) The neural structure from which the tumor originates is coagulated using bipolar coagulation. (**c**) The coagulated filament is carefully cut. (**d**) Finally, the completely detached tumor is removed using forceps, completing the resection process. (Image source [16])

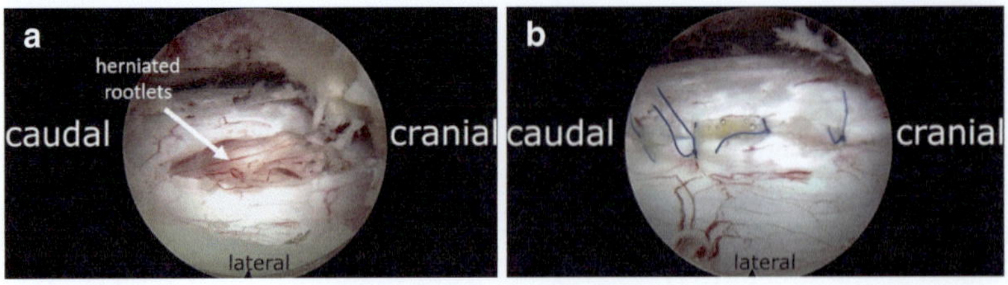

Fig. 27.6 The images depict the dural repair process following tumor removal. (**a**) The herniation of rootlets through the dural defect is visible. (**b**) Dural closure is performed using patches and sutures to effectively seal the defect and possibly prevent complications such as cerebrospinal fluid leakage. (Image source [16])

tion. This assumption is based on the endoscopic approach creating minimal dead space and the readaptation of soft tissue upon retraction of the working sleeve, which may reduce the likelihood of CSF leakage, thereby decreasing the risk of CSF fistulas and infections. In the demonstrated case, dural closure is performed using patches and sutures (Fig. 27.6b).

Discussion

Intradural Lesions

Tredway et al. were among the first to introduce a minimally invasive technique for the removal of intradural mass lesions in 2006 [2]. Since then, several studies have demonstrated the feasibility and effectiveness of such minimally invasive approaches [3–7]. Moreover, research by Ogden et al. [26] and Xie et al. [27] has shown that minimally invasive techniques for intradural tumor removal not only decrease postoperative complications but also lead to less spinal instability and deformity compared to traditional methods, as supported by finite element analyses.

A comparative study by Wong et al. in 2015, along with several subsequent investigations, highlights significant advantages of minimally invasive techniques (excluding full-endoscopic methods) for the removal of intradural-extramedullary spine tumors [28]. These studies report benefits such as reduced intraoperative blood loss, decreased necessity and shorter duration for postoperative lumbar drain placement, improved ASIA (American Spinal Injury Association) scores, and shorter hospital stays [2, 6, 10, 11]. These compelling results emphasize the need for further exploration of minimally invasive approaches, including full-endoscopic techniques, in the treatment of intradural tumors.

As of this writing, there are only three studies specifically focused on the full-endoscopic removal of intradural tumors, of which two are case reports. The case reports titled "Percutaneous Full-Endoscopic Removal of Lumbar Intradural Extramedullary Tumor via Translaminar Approach" published by Şentürk in 2019 [5] and "Full-Endoscopic Resection of a Lumbar Intradural Tumor (Schwannoma): Video Case Report and Description of the Surgical Technique" published by Hagel in 2024 [16] concluded that selective cases performed by experienced surgeons may yield positive outcomes for the removal of intradural-extramedullary mass lesions. Additionally, in 2018, Dhandapani et al. compared 15 "microendoscopic" cases with 16 "pure-endoscopic" cases and found no significant difference in clinical improvement or radiological confirmation of complete removal, which was achieved in all patients [29].

Tethered Cord Syndrome

The standard surgical procedure for untethering the spinal cord involves a multilevel laminectomy, dural opening, and identification and sectioning of the filum [6, 7]. However, some studies indicate that minimally invasive microscopic techniques using tubular and expandable retractors can achieve the same outcomes as traditional open surgeries [30, 31]. Surgical interventions for lipomyelomeningocele carry significant risks, including scar formation, nerve damage, and cerebrospinal fluid leakage [32, 33]. In certain cases, the specific morphology of the lipomyelomeningocele may allow for an ultra-minimal invasive endoscopic approach. Telfeian et al. reported a case where a working channel endoscope was used to locate the filum terminale [7], followed by the introduction of endoscopic instruments to remove it from the intrathecal space. This case highlights the potential benefits of minimally invasive spine techniques in managing tethered cord syndrome, offering advantages such as reduced pain, decreased risk of cerebrospinal fluid leakage, and minimized scarring [7].

Infections

Minimally invasive techniques for treating spondylodiscitis and epidural abscesses are emerging as safe and effective alternatives to traditional surgical methods. Evidence supports that endoscopic approach for thoracolumbar spondylodiscitis is a reliable technique, yielding satisfactory clinical outcomes and a high rate of pathogen identification [34]. In a study with 34 patients, Yu et al. demonstrated the feasibility of full-endoscopic methods for treating spondylodiscitis, epidural abscesses, and psoas abscesses [35]. Similarly, Kang et al. reported findings from a cohort of 13 patients, highlighting the viability of the biportal full-endoscopic approach for spinal epidural abscess intervention [36]. These minimally invasive procedures offer benefits such as reduced blood loss, shorter hospital stays, and quicker normalization of C-reactive protein (CRP) levels [37, 38].

The referenced studies primarily focus on endoscopic management of spondylodiscitis and short-distance epidural abscesses. However, for long-distance epidural abscesses, a case report by Hagel et al. suggests using two simultaneous approaches, one endoscopic and the other non-endoscopic. This method aims to create a continuous pressure gradient across the epidural space between the two access points, facilitating effective drainage [39]. These minimally invasive techniques, however, have limitations in access and mobility, which may restrict the extent of surgical debridement and potentially lead to inadequate bacterial load reduction. Therefore, until more high-quality studies are available, the full-endoscopic approach should be reserved for selected cases and performed by experienced surgeons only.

Conclusions

Despite promising results from a few studies on full-endoscopic treatment of extra- and intradural non-degenerative pathologies, the available instruments for dural opening, retraction, dissection, and mobilization remain limited. This is because the industry has primarily focused on treating degenerative pathologies. Additionally, certain inherent risks exist in full-endoscopic spine surgery, particularly when working intradurally, such as severe headache, seizure, and visual disturbance. Therefore, the use of endoscopic techniques for non-degenerative pathologies should be carefully considered by experienced surgeons. While literature and the authors' experience suggest positive outcomes, the limited number of patients treated is a significant drawback. Furthermore, short follow-up periods restrict the ability to draw meaningful conclusions about mid-term and long-term results. To establish more robust evidence, further studies are essential—preferably prospective and randomized—comparing full-endoscopic techniques with traditional approaches.

References

1. Tanaka T, Sakamoto T, Koyama T, Watanabe K, Tanaka T, Murata K. Endoscopic treatment of symptomatic spinal subarachnoid cysts. AJR Am J Roentgenol. 1997;169(6):1719–20.
2. Pool JL. Myeloscopy: intraspinal endoscopy. Surg Clin North Am. 1957;37(5):1401–2.
3. Endo T, Tominaga T. Use of an endoscope for spinal intradural pathology. J Spine Surg. 2020;6(2):495.
4. Parihar VS, Yadav N, Yadav YR, Ratre S, Bajaj J, Kher Y. Endoscopic management of spinal intradural

extramedullary tumors. J Neurol Surg Part A Cent Eur Neurosurg. 2017;78(03):219–26.
5. Şentürk S, Ünsal ÜÜ. Percutaneous full-endoscopic removal of lumbar intradural extramedullary tumor via translaminar approach. World Neurosurg. 2019;125:146–9.
6. Woods KR, Colohan AR, Yamada S, Yamada SM, Won DJ. Intrathecal endoscopy to enhance the diagnosis of tethered cord syndrome. J Neurosurg Spine. 2010;13(4):477–83.
7. Telfeian AE, Punsoni M, Hofstetter CP. Minimally invasive endoscopic spinal cord untethering: case report. J Spine Surg. 2017;3(2):278.
8. Endo T, Takahashi T, Jokura H, Tominaga T. Surgical treatment of spinal intradural arachnoid cysts using endoscopy. J Neurosurg Spine. 2010;12(6):641–6.
9. Mauer UM, Gottschalk A, Kunz U, Schulz C. Arachnoscopy: a special application of spinal intradural endoscopy. Neurosurg Focus. 2011;30(4):E7.
10. Gu R, Liu JB, Xia P, Li C, Liu GY, Wang JC. Evaluation of hemilaminectomy use in microsurgical resection of intradural extramedullary tumors. Oncol Lett. 2014;7(5):1669–72.
11. Goodarzi A, Clouse J, Capizzano T, Kim KD, Panchal R. The optimal surgical approach to intradural spinal tumors: laminectomy or hemilaminectomy? Cureus. 2020;12(2)
12. Seppälä MT, Haltia MJ, Sankila RJ, Jääskeläinen JE, Heiskanen O. Long-term outcome after removal of spinal schwannoma: a clinicopathological study of 187 cases. J Neurosurg. 1995;83(4):621–6.
13. Hsu T-L, Yang C-J, Pao J-L. Salmonella spondylodiscitis and epidural abscess successfully treated with unilateral biportal endoscopic discectomy and debridement: a rare case report. J Int Med Res. 2022;50(3):03000605221085405.
14. Iida K, Yoshikane K, Tono O, Tarukado K, Harimaya K. The effectiveness of a percutaneous endoscopic approach in a patient with psoas and epidural abscess accompanied by pyogenic spondylitis: a case report. J Med Case Rep. 2019;13:1–6.
15. Sales JG, Tabrizi A, Elmi A, Soleimanpour J, Gavidel E. Adolescence spinal epidural abscess with neurological symptoms: case report, a lesson to be re-learnt. Med J Islam Repub Iran. 2013;27(1):38.
16. Hagel V, Isseldyk FV. Full-endoscopic resection of a lumbar Intradural tumor (schwannoma): video case report and description of the surgical technique. Neurospine. 2024;21(4):1096–9.
17. Konakondla S, Sofoluke N, Xia J, Grant R, Telfeian AE, Hofstetter CP, et al. Transforaminal endoscopic approach for large-sample tumor biopsy using beveled working channel for core technique: a technical note. World Neurosurg. 2020;141:346–51.
18. Konakondla S, Nakhla J, Xia J, Barber SM, Fridley JS, Oyelese AA, et al. A novel endoscopic technique for biopsy and tissue diagnosis for a paraspinal thoracic tumor in a pediatric patient: a case report. Int J Spine Surg. 2021;14(s4):S66–70.
19. McLain R. Spinal cord decompression: an endoscopically assisted approach for metastatic tumors. Spinal Cord. 2001;39(9):482–7.
20. Telfeian AE, Choi DB, Aghion DM. Transforaminal endoscopic surgery under local analgesia for ventral epidural thoracic spinal tumor: case report. Clin Neurol Neurosurg. 2015;134:1–3.
21. Telfeian AE, Oyelese A, Fridley J, Doberstein C, Gokaslan ZL. Endoscopic surgical treatment for symptomatic spinal metastases in long-term cancer survivors. J Spine Surg. 2020;6(2):372.
22. Tsai S-H, Wu H-H, Cheng C-Y, Chen C-M. Full endoscopic interlaminar approach for nerve root decompression of sacral metastatic tumor. World Neurosurg. 2018;112:57–63.
23. Gao Z, Wu Z, Lin Y, Zhang P. Percutaneous transforaminal endoscopic decompression in the treatment of spinal metastases: a case report. Medicine (Baltimore). 2019;98(11):e14819.
24. Newman WC, Vaynrub M, Bilsky MH, Laufer I, Barzilai O. Full endoscopic resection of a lumbar osteoblastoma. J Neurosurg Spine. 2020;33(2):252–5.
25. Ali R, Hagan MJ, Shaaya E, Leary OP, Feler J, Bajaj A, et al. Endoscopic techniques for spinal oncology: a systematic literature review. Int J Spine Surg. 2022;
26. Ogden AT, Bresnahan L, Smith JS, Natarajan R, Fessler RG. Biomechanical comparison of traditional and minimally invasive intradural tumor exposures using finite element analysis. Clin Biomech. 2009;24(2):143–7.
27. Xie T, Qian J, Lu Y, Chen B, Jiang Y, Luo C. Biomechanical comparison of laminectomy, hemilaminectomy and a new minimally invasive approach in the surgical treatment of multilevel cervical intradural tumour: a finite element analysis. Eur Spine J. 2013;22:2719–30.
28. Wong AP, Lall RR, Dahdaleh NS, Lawton CD, Smith ZA, Wong RH, et al. Comparison of open and minimally invasive surgery for intradural-extramedullary spine tumors. Neurosurg Focus. 2015;39(2):E11.
29. Dhandapani S, Karthigeyan M. "Microendoscopic" versus "pure endoscopic" surgery for spinal intradural mass lesions: a comparative study and review. Spine J. 2018;18(9):1592–602.
30. Warder DE. Tethered cord syndrome and occult spinal dysraphism. Neurosurg Focus. 2001;10(1):1–9.
31. Potts MB, Wu J-C, Gupta N, Mummaneni PV. Minimally invasive tethered cord release in adults: a comparison of open and mini-open approaches. Neurosurg Focus. 2010;29(1):E7.
32. Arai H, Sato K, Okuda O, Miyajima M, Hishii M, Nakanishi H, et al. Surgical experience of 120 patients with lumbosacral lipomas. Acta Neurochir. 2001;143:857–64.
33. Kanev PM, Lemire RJ, Loeser JD, Berger MS. Management and long-term follow-up review of children with lipomyelomeningocele, 1952–1987. J Neurosurg. 1990;73(1):48–52.

34. Giordan E, Liu Y, Suvithayasiri S, Russo S, Lee C, Hasan GA, et al. Endoscopic treatment of thoraco-lumbar spondylodiscitis: a systematic review and meta-analysis. World Neurosurg. 2024;189:296–306.
35. Yu C-H. Full-endoscopic debridement and drainage treating spine infection and psoas muscle abscess. J Spine Surg. 2020;6(2):415.
36. Kang T, Park SY, Lee SH, Park JH, Suh SW. Spinal epidural abscess successfully treated with biportal endoscopic spinal surgery. Medicine (Baltimore). 2019;98(50):e18231.
37. Fu T-S, Wang Y-C, Lin T-Y, Chang C-W, Wong C-B, Su J-Y. Comparison of percutaneous endoscopic surgery and traditional anterior open surgery for treating lumbar infectious spondylitis. J Clin Med. 2019;8(9):1356.
38. Hagel V, Dymel F, Werle S, Barrera V, Farshad M. Combined endoscopic and microsurgical approach for the drainage of a multisegmental thoracolumbar epidural abscess: illustrative case. J Neurosurg Case Lessons. 2023;6(19)
39. Farshad M, Stauffer A, Zipser CM, Kheram N, Spirig JM, Widmer J, et al. An experimental model for fluid dynamics and pressures during endoscopic lumbar discectomy. Neurospine. 2024;21(3):745.

Complication Management in Lumbar Endoscopy

28

Alexandre Simonin

Introduction

Endoscopic spine surgery (ESS) has been implemented in many spine centers as the standard. As such, not only ortho- and neurosurgeons use them in their daily practice, but young surgeons are also trained in ESS, sometimes without previous microsurgical experience in lumbar spine diseases. Although ESS has been proven to be safe and effective [1–3, 5, 6], surgeons should be aware that severe complications may still occur, despite the most minimally invasive feature of the technique.

We will start the chapter by detailing general complications and their management, before focusing on specific complications related to the interlaminar and the transforaminal approaches. Complication avoidance is very important during the steep learning curve of ESS, and will be emphasized in this chapter.

General Complications

Instruments

ESS is performed by using waterflow running through an endoscope, at the end of which a high definition camera and powerful LED permit to transmit visual information to a screen. Although every technical feature is of importance, the waterflow pressure represents the main technical aspect that can produce complications, along with the radiofrequency (RF) probe used for coagulation, if not set adequately. Generally, a pressure pump is recommended in order to limit the water inflow if a certain pressure has been measured inside the surgical field. Using gravity is a simpler and cheaper way to build pressure, but it is not adaptive to epidural pressure. Several complications have been described in relation to water pressure: damage to the nerve roots, headaches, postoperative neck pain, seizures, strokes, etc. [2, 7–10]. However, a definitive pressure limit has not been clearly identified. Generally, authors recommend a pressure between 4 cm H20 (2 mmHg) and 30 cm H20 (22 mmHg) [7–10]. The pressure can be higher when the surgeon works outside of the spinal canal, but should be lower in the epidural space, and as low as possible in the intradural space (or in case of inadvertent dural tear).

The RF probe is used in a bipolar "coagulation" mode, especially around neural structures. However, monopolar "cut" mode may be used for muscle bleeding and facet thermal ablation, for example. It may be dangerous to use the "cut" mode near neural structures.

The surgeon uses instruments that go through the working channel of the endoscope (uniportal)

A. Simonin (✉)
Sion Cantonal Hospital, Sion, Switzerland
e-mail: alexandre.simonin@hopitalvs.ch

A. A. Baaj et al. (eds.), *Surgery of the Lumbar Spine*, https://doi.org/10.1007/978-3-032-18097-1_28

or through another working port (biportal). In uniportal ESS, the endoscope is introduced inside a working cannula. It is important to consider the working cannula as a distinct surgical instrument, as it may injure structures that are not visible on the screen. This occurs when the endoscope is introduced further than the working cannula, for example, while decompressing the recess of a nerve root. It is recommended to “zoom out” regularly and pull back the working cannula away from neural structures.

The endoscopic drill is a must to perform ESS beyond simple interlaminar or transforaminal disc herniations. It permits to expand the indications, but is quite hard to master. First, because the endoscopic surgeon cannot rest his hand on the patient, the drill will be “floating” in the working cannula of the endoscope. As such, we advise to drill in a medio-lateral, or cranio-caudal direction, from the depth to the surface. Resting the little finger on the working cannula also helps for stability. This avoids inadvertent “plunging” toward neural structures. Round drills permit a maximum vision of the drilling, and diamond burrs are more forgiving.

Type of Anesthesia

In ESS, many complications happen when the surgeon is actually not seeing what he is currently doing. This is typically the case during the transforaminal approach before placing the endoscope, but also during the initial part of the interlaminar approach. Inadvertent lesions of the neural structures may happen during the approach (placement of the introducer, working cannula, endoscope). Some authors advocate to perform ESS as an awake surgery [4, 11]. However, weaning off neuromuscular blocking agents since the start of the procedure may help in monitoring neural compromise even under general anesthesia [11]. Any muscle twitch during the approach should prompt an immediate stop of the current move.

Wrong Site Surgery

Also probably less common than in microscopic surgery, wrong site (wrong level or side) surgery may still happen in ESS. It may be more common in thoracic or cervical pathologies, but it may still happen in the lumbar region, especially when addressing the foramen. X-ray guidance should be used until the pathology is identified. For difficult cases, for example, L5-S1 foraminoplasty, also called transforaminal endoscopic lumbar foraminotomy (TELF), navigation may be used, especially for the beginner endoscopic surgeon. In case of wrong site surgery, identification during the procedure and change to the correct level is better than delayed identification.

Honest communication to the patient is mandatory.

Dural Tear

Dural tears represent the most common complication in ESS, with reported rates ranging from 0% to 8.6%, overall 2.7% [2]. Inadvertent dural tears may be a frightening complication for the beginner ESS surgeon, and is a common reason for a conversion to microscopic surgery. However, according to most of the authors and previous experiences, it may be easier to manage endoscopically.

Because most of the paraspinal muscles are preserved, they slide back after removal of the endoscope and working cannula. Thus, the surgical cavity shrinks at the end of the procedure, and cerebrospinal fluid (CSF) does not accumulate, decreasing the chances of wound leakage. Generally, converting to an open procedure in case of dural tear is not recommended, because it will only raise chances for a wound leakage. This is mostly accepted for small dural tears.

When a dural tear occurs during ESS, we generally recommend to:

- Set the water pressure to the lowest value, and keep the jet away from the intradural compartment if possible.
- Assess the damage to the dura and/or rootlets. If a small dural tear without exteriorization of the rootlets is identified, no conversion is needed, but the procedure should be finished as early as possible.
- If rootlets are exposed, they should be repositioned in the dural sac. This is mainly to prevent reherniation of rootlets postoperatively, which could be a reason for intractable neurogenic pain [2–4]. To do this, a combination of instruments and "on-off" play with the waterflow should be used. Typically, the water flow is stopped, the RF probe (without cautery) is then used to push the rootlets back in the dural sac, using intermittent water flow to clear the bleeding if needed. A piece of Tachosil® may be used to cover a defect, using a rongeur to place it through the working channel of the endoscope. The piece of Tachosil should be fairly small, and barely held by the rongeur, because the most difficult part will be to detach it from the rongeur to place it at the right position. Intradural placement ("double layer") of a patch has been proposed by authors [2, 7] in order to prevent rootlets reherniation. However, because it partially dissolves intradurally, the chemical effect and potential adherence to the rootlets is unknown [3]. Bioabsorbable dural clips have been designed for easier dural closure, mostly for biportal endoscopy, but they may clip the rootlets and subsequent removal may be challenging. Suturing instruments with knot pusher may also be used.

In summary, only if the endoscopic surgeon cannot perform repositioning of the rootlets endoscopically, conversion to microscopy is recommended.

Bleeding

Profuse bleeding is another common cause of conversion to open surgery for the beginner endoscopic surgeon. It may be a challenge during surgery, but also could create a postoperative epidural hematoma, which remains the most common cause of return to the OR after ESS [2], ranging between 0% and 1% of cases. Most of the time, continuous irrigation prevents blurred vision, and the patency of saline outflow is especially important for biportal ESS [11–14].

There are different types of bleeding events that may occur:

- Soft tissue bleeding. A muscular or subcutaneous bleeder occurs. We advise to stay in position with the endoscope (left hand) in order to keep the suspected bleeder in the field, "zoom in", meaning advance the endoscope close to the bleeder to visualize, and consider raising pump pressure. If despite those maneuvers the bleeding point is not identified, the RF probe should be inserted toward the end of the endoscope working channel, and gradually withdrawn in a corkscrew manner while cauterizing to maximize the chance of coagulating the bleeder. If this does not work, consider administration of thrombin agents (e.g., Surgiflo® or Floseal®) through the working channel of the endoscope. For maximum efficacy, waterflow should be stopped just before injecting the thrombin agent, and wait 2–3 minutes before continuing.
- Bone bleeding. It usually occurs while drilling. The most efficient way is to continue until cortical bone is found, because bleeders consist of emissary veins running through the spongious bone. A diamond burr could be used to lower the risk of spongious bone bleeding, but reverse use of a classic burr may

represent an effective (and cheaper) alternative.

- Bone wax may be applied, mostly in biportal ESS. In uniportal ESS, it is slightly harder, because wax will stick to the working channel if applied through the endoscope. Therefore, we recommend placing the bone wax on a dissector, and enter the working channel in a reverse position. It may also be placed on the burr of the drill.
- Epidural bleeding. Careful coagulation of the epidural vessel is recommended. If diffuse, at the end of a decompression procedure, thrombin agent injection as stated before will be the most efficient management. Finally, drainage has been recommended by some authors in case of profuse epidural bleeding to prevent postoperative hematoma [2, 7].

Infection

Infection rate is probably the most important difference in favor of ESS compared to microscopic procedures. Surgical site infections range between 0.001% and 0.1% between studies [2, 3, 7], which appears to be much lower than microscopic series. Infections should be treated the same way, with evacuation of the infected material and intravenous antibiotics.

Insufficient Decompression

A commonly cited complication of ESS is insufficient decompression of the disc material in lumbar disc herniation or ligamentum flavum in canal stenosis. This seems to be correlated to the surgeon's learning curve [7] and improves with the number of cases. It may be explained by the "zoom effect", meaning that the surgeon has a precise (and often 15–25° angle) view of a very narrow surgical site. Thus, it is difficult to assess the entire pathology, especially the contralateral flavum when performing the cross-over flavectomy in LE-ULBD. For disc herniations, it may be useful to measure the sequester removed (in a syringe) and compare the volume with preoperative MRI.

Specific Complications

Interlaminar Approach

During full-endoscopic IELD, the goal is to reach and remove a disc fragment compressing a nerve root through the interlaminar window. This involves cutting the yellow ligament with endoscopic scissors and placing the endoscope in the epidural space. To avoid damage to the neural structures, the endoscopic surgeon has to take care of:

- Cutting the yellow ligament carefully laterally, because the epidural fat (and space) is less laterally and inadvertent dural tear may happen.
- Avoid building pressure on the dural sac and cauda equina rootlets by blocking the water outflow
- Generally avoid entering the canal with the working cannula (so-called "turning maneuver") especially in cases of narrow central canal (stenosis, congenital, median disc herniation). Based on our experience, postoperative cauda equina syndrome may happen when entering an 8 mm working cannula in a $\leq$ 1.5 cm central canal. It is safe and effective to keep the working cannula in the posterior epidural space, and use a rongeur to perform the sequestrectomy.

Transforaminal Approach

The transforaminal approach was initially the first ESS procedure described [7]. It consists of entering through the Kambin's triangle, which is limited by the exiting nerve root. Therefore, it is at risk during this approach. Several points may help to avoid postoperative dysesthesia (POD) or motor weakness:

- Tailor the entrypoint and trajectory to each specific situation. An L5-S1 transforaminal approach is very different from L1-2. The MRI may show the best entrypoint and trajectory to avoid entering the peritoneum, kidney, etc.

- Think about the outside-in technique in narrow foramen. One can choose to start the procedure from the disc (inside-out technique) or start from the superior articulating process (SAP, outside-in technique). The latter is safer, because the procedure starts posterior from the exiting nerve root, and then goes inside Kambin's triangle. This is generally recommended for foraminoplasty (enlarging the foramen by drilling the SAP) or for disc herniations with narrow foramen. The inside-out technique permits faster identification of the disc space, especially if methylene blue stain is used (discography). However, it may accelerate disc degeneration [7] and if the approach is performed too laterally or cranially, the exiting nerve root may be damaged (Fig. 28.1).
- Assess the patient's nerve root function with conscious sedation, or at least without neuromuscular blocking agents if performed under general anesthesia.

Other specific complications include retroperitoneal hematoma (Fig. 28.2). This may happen if the approach is performed too anteriorly at the disc level. It can usually be managed conservatively, with close monitoring in an intermediate care unit. Because the retroperitoneal space has a very low pressure, a considerable amount of blood may accumulate before reaching hemostasis. An endovascular embolization may be attempted in severe cases. Open procedures may lead to massive blood losses and are rarely recommended [11]. Finally, it is common to inject methylene blue while performing the "inside-out" technique. It is metabolized by the kidneys and urine may be stained in blue, which may surprise the patient and the surgeon, but does not harm.

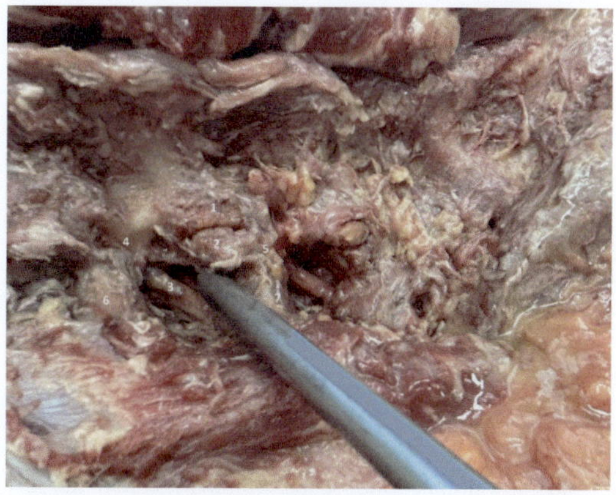

Fig. 28.1 Anatomical Institute of Fribourg, Switzerland. Cadaver view, left side L4-5 transforaminal approach. 1: inferior articular process of L4; 2: superior articular process of L5; 3: exiting nerve root (L4); 4: L4 pedicle; 5: L5 pedicle; 6: L4 transverse process; 7: L5 transverse process

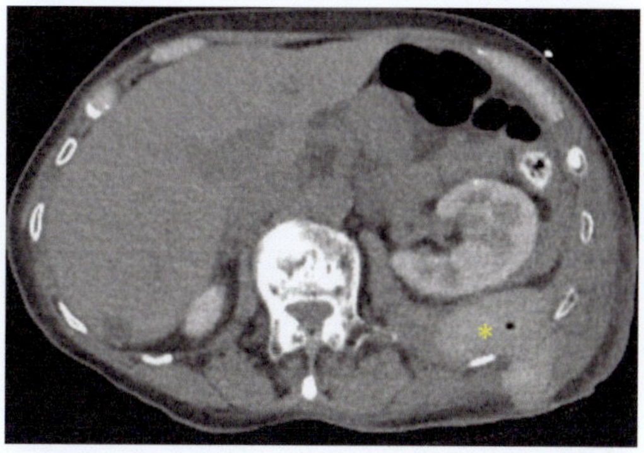

Fig. 28.2 Postoperative CT-scan after a transforaminal approach. A large retroperitoneal hematoma (*) due to an intercostal artery injury is displacing the left kidney anteriorly. An embolization was attempted, but unsuccessful. Patient was monitored and managed conservatively. Two units of blood were given with subsequent favorable evolution

Acknowledgments I would like to thank Dr. Jean-Yves Fournier, Head of the department, who mentored my endoscopy journey.

References

1. Hofstetter CP, Ahn Y, Choi G, et al. Aospine consensus paper on nomenclature for working-channel endoscopic spinal procedures. Global Spine J. 2020;10(2 Suppl):111S–21S.
2. Ju CI, Lee SM. Complications and management of endoscopic spinal surgery. Neurospine. 2023;20(1):56–77.
3. Kim HS, Sharma S, Wu P, et al. Complications and limitations of endoscopic spine surgery and percutaneous instrumentation. Indian Spine J. 2020;3(1):78.
4. Telfeian AE, Sastry R, Oyelese A, et al. Awake, transforaminal endoscopic lumbar spine surgery in octogenarians: case series. Pain Physician. 2022;25(2):E255–62.
5. Kapetanakis S, Gkasdaris G, Angoules AG, Givissis P. Transforaminal percutaneous endoscopic discectomy using transforaminal endoscopic spine system technique: pitfalls that a beginner should avoid. World J Orthop. 2017;8(12):874–80.
6. Wang B, He P, Liu X, Wu Z, Xu B. Complications of unilateral biportal endoscopic spinal surgery for lumbar spinal stenosis: a systematic review of the literature and meta-analysis of single-arm studies. Orthop Surg. 2023;15(1):3–15.
7. Kwon WK, Hur JW. Overview and prevention of complications during fully endoscopic lumbar spine surgery. J Minim Invasive Spine Surg Tech. 2023;8(2):136–44.
8. Fan N, Yuan S, Du P, et al. Complications and risk factors of percutaneous endoscopic transforaminal discectomy in the treatment of lumbar spinal stenosis. BMC Musculoskelet Disord. 2021;22(1):1041.
9. Farshad M, Stauffer A, Zipser CM, et al. An experimental model for fluid dynamics and pressures during endoscopic lumbar discectomy. Neurospine. 2024;21(3):745–52.
10. Hong YH, Kim SK, Hwang J, et al. Water dynamics in unilateral biportal endoscopic spine surgery and its related factors: an in vivo proportional regression and proficiency-matched study. World Neurosurg. 2021;149:e836–43.
11. Ahn Y. Transforaminal percutaneous endoscopic lumbar discectomy: technical tips to prevent complications. Expert Rev Med Devices. 2012;9(4):361–6.
12. Hagan MJ, Remacle T, Leary OP, et al. Navigation techniques in endoscopic spine surgery. Biomed Res Int. 2022;2022:8419739.
13. Park DY, Upfill-Brown A, Curtin N, et al. Clinical outcomes and complications after biportal endoscopic spine surgery: a comprehensive systematic review and meta-analysis of 3673 cases. Eur Spine J. 2023;32(8):2637–46.
14. Zhuang HX, Guo SJ, Meng H, Lin JS, Yang Y, Fei Q. Unilateral biportal endoscopic spine surgery for lumbar spinal stenosis: a systematic review and meta-analysis. Eur Rev Med Pharmacol Sci. 2023;27(11):4998–5012.

Open Transforaminal Lumbar Interbody Fusion (TLIF)

29

Fernando Padilla-Lichtenberger, A. Guiroy, F. Landriel, and J. Emmerich

Introduction

The transforaminal lumbar interbody fusion (TLIF) is a surgical technique in which bilateral anterior column support can be achieved through a unilateral posterolateral approach, and also posterolateral fusion is accomplished after pedicle screws placement. The circumferential fusion, now referred to as 360° fusion, was initially demonstrated by Kim [1], Kozak [2], and Grob [3] as a procedure that significantly enhanced fusion rates and clinical outcomes in the lumbosacral spine. Despite its advantages, one of the primary challenges has been the lack of safe and effective surgical techniques for this procedure. Traditional approaches have included sequential anterior and posterior fusions, as well as posterior lumbar interbody fusion combined with simultaneous posterolateral fusion. However, the prolonged operative time and heightened risks associated with the sequential methods have limited their widespread implementation.

In 1982, Harms and Rolinger [4] presented a series of 41 cases utilizing a transforaminal posterior approach for anterior lumbar interbody fusion. They performed an osteotomy of the pars interarticularis and the inferior articular facet, granting access to the disc space with minimal retraction of the dural sac and nerve roots. They suggested the placement of bone graft and titanium mesh into the disc space that previously had been distracted using pedicle screw instrumentation. This technique enabled them to avoid the anterior approach, thereby reducing the associated morbidity and complications.

The TLIF is a well-established surgical technique employed to address various degenerative lumbar spine conditions. The TLIF has the potential to achieve a circumferential fusion with reduced neural retraction and neurologic risk in an unstaged operation.

In 2001, Rosenberg & Mummaneni [5] published a retrospective study that demonstrated the safety, advantages, and surgical efficacy of the technique, and also proposed some modifications of the TLIF with pedicle screws fixation that are used nowadays.

F. Padilla-Lichtenberger (✉)
Spine Surgery Department, Université de Montréal, Montreal, QC, Canada

A. Guiroy
Spine Surgery Department, Clínica de Cuyo, Mendoza, Argentina

F. Landriel
Department of Neurological Surgery, Hospital Italiano de Buenos Aires, Buenos Aires, Argentina
e-mail: federico.landriel@hospitalitaliano.org.ar

J. Emmerich
Department of Neurological Surgery, Children's Hospital La Plata, La Plata, Argentina

A. A. Baaj et al. (eds.), *Surgery of the Lumbar Spine*, https://doi.org/10.1007/978-3-032-18097-1_29

Indications

Lowe et al. [6] described the main indications of the TLIF. Mainly, it is indicated for patients with anterior column deficiencies accompanied by chronic mechanical pain due to degenerative disc disease, recurrent disc herniation, and/or spondylolisthesis. The primary indications for performing this procedure include:

- Symptomatic Degenerative Disc Disease: Patients with significant disc degeneration leading to chronic back pain and radiculopathy.
- Lumbar Spondylolisthesis: Both isthmic and degenerative spondylolisthesis can benefit from stabilization and fusion. Kwon et al. assessed 35 consecutive cases of TLIF in patients with isthmic spondylolisthesis [7]. Their findings showed that TLIF effectively enhanced disc space height and reduced anterolisthesis, with a more anterior placement of the interbody cage being ideal for restoring lordosis.
- Relative indication for surgery in the case of recurrent disc herniations, depending on the surgeon preference and the presence of instability.
- Pseudoarthrosis: The TLIF procedure may yield a higher rate of successful arthrodesis since the anterior graft is subjected to compressive loading. It is also suitable for patients with multiple comorbidities that could impact fusion success, such as obesity, smoking, diabetes, or previous failed fusions, as it offers circumferential fusion via a posterior-only approach. Furthermore, TLIF can help address pseudoarthrosis cases [6].

Surgical Technique

Preoperative Time

Preoperative Planning: Careful selection of the surgical approach based on the patient's anatomy and pathology is crucial; the need of a posterior decompression, or a bilateral facetectomy with lordosis restoration is key.

Intravenous antibiotics are administered and a Foley catheter is placed. Patients are positioned prone on a radiolucent table. Protective padding and pillows are placed to prevent pressure injuries. Trichotomy is performed if necessary, followed by a thorough wash of the area. The surgical level is then marked using fluoroscopy. Next, surgical antisepsis is conducted with iodopovidone or chlorhexidine, applied four times. Finally, it is recommended to use an antimicrobial incision surgical drape.

Surgical Time

The TLIF typically involves seven steps: (1) posterior midline approach; (2) the pedicle screws placement; (3) bony decompression stage that varies between patients and their needs; (4) discectomy and endplate preparation; (5) the interbody fusion; (6) the rods placement, construct compression and posterolateral fusion; and (7) finally the closure.

Step 1: Posterior Lumbar Approach and Decompression

A standard midline incision is made through the skin and subcutaneous layers, with careful subperiosteal dissection of the laminae. Then, dissection is continued laterally until the articular facets and transverse processes are exposed. Both the transverse process and pars interarticularis at the upper and lower levels should be completely exposed, taking care to avoid damaging the capsule of the upper facet joint while identifying the landmarks for the upper pedicle screw (Fig. 29.1). An intraoperative lateral fluoroscopy verifies the correct exposed level.

Step 2: Pedicle Screws Placement

Before bony decompression, pedicle screw fixation is performed, using a combination of anatomic landmarks and fluoroscopic guidance. Pedicle screws are inserted using standard techniques. The entry point is defined by the mammillary tubercle, marking the junction of the transverse process, superior facet, and vertebral isthmus. The lateral-to-medial angle generally

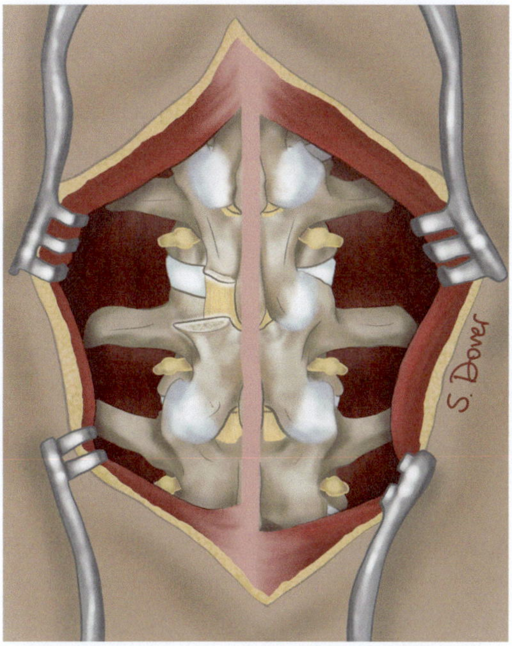

Fig. 29.1 Surgical exposure after a classic posterior midline approach with a left facetectomy. Look at the relationships between the thecal sac, the exiting nerve root, and the disc

ranges from 5° to 20° from L1 to L5, increasing by 5° at each level. The cranio-caudal angle should remain parallel to the pedicle, which can be located with a Woodson probe or through intraoperative fluoroscopy.

Step 3: Facetectomy and/or Laminectomy

The decompression process should be preoperatively planned according to the patient's specific needs, evaluating whether a complete laminectomy is necessary for spinal canal stenosis or if a bilateral facetectomy is warranted to restore lordosis [8] or address bilateral symptoms [9]. The procedure begins with a medial/descending facetectomy on the side of the symptoms, which involves resecting the inferior articular process of the upper vertebra (L4) for a TLIF at L4/L5. An osteotome or high-speed drill can be utilized to section the vertebral isthmus over the exiting nerve root at the lower edge of the upper pedicle (L4). If a laminectomy is not performed, a sagittal cut in the lamina is made prior to sectioning the vertebral isthmus. The exiting nerve root should be identified and protected. A Leksell rongeur is used to remove the medial facet en bloc, which is then utilized as an autograft for fusion. The ligamentum flavum is separated with an angled curette and subsequently resected with a Kerrison, exposing the dural sac and the exiting nerve root caudal to the L4 pedicle. Dissection is continued laterally, and a foraminotomy may be performed if necessary. Next, the lateral/ascending facetectomy is carried out at the caudal level (L5) until the pedicle of that vertebra is reached. A pedicle-to-pedicle exposure is performed, and the disc space is identified. Finally, any small osteophytes are drilled if present (Fig. 29.1).

Step 4: Discectomy and Endplates Preparation

After identifying the posterior longitudinal ligament and annulus, blunt dissection with a Penfield dissector is used to release any adhesions between the disc and neural elements. Hemostasis is then achieved using bipolar cautery or hemostatic materials. An annulotomy in a rectangular fashion is performed with a No. 11 or No. 15 blade. The nucleus pulposus is removed with pituitary forceps to expose the endplates. A total discectomy is attempted, taking care not to injure the anterior longitudinal ligament. Curettes are used to prepare the endplates, without violating the subchondral bone. Sequential dilation of the disc space should be accomplished with serial dilators. It is recommended to leave the cage trials in place for about 3 min to allow for disc space expansion. Fluoroscopy should be used to assess the correct position of the dilators, and determine whether a larger or smaller prosthesis is needed. Care must be taken to follow the sagittal plane of the interspace in order to avoid damaging the endplate. Once this is decided, morselized bone graft is placed in syringes of 1–3 ml to enhance fusion.

Step 5: Interbody Fusion

It is recommended to measure the height of the disc to be treated during the preoperative assessment. If the height is significantly reduced,

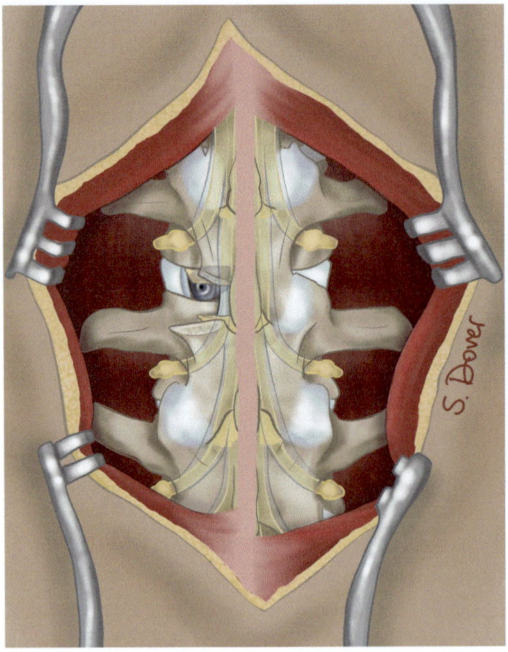

Fig. 29.2 After the discectomy, the cage is introduced in the discal space, with previous sequential dilation of the disc space

the immediately superior disc can serve as a reference for determining the size of the interbody cage, which may be constructed from titanium or PEEK. After testing with the trial cage, the interbody graft should be filled with autograft, allograft, or another fusion substrate. Harvesting cancellous autograft from the iliac crest is advised. Subsequently, the cage is gently "shifted" toward the contralateral side by alternately rotating it around its longitudinal axis using a forked impactor (Fig. 29.2). It is essential to begin adjusting the cage medially as it settles into the disc space, aiming to position the mesh across the vertebral body, crossing the midline, and advancing anteriorly to improve lordosis [9]. Fluoroscopy is key to assess the correct placement of the cage.

Step 6: Rods Placement, Construct Compression, and Posterolateral fusion

At this stage, the first step is to decorticate the transverse processes to provide support for the posterolateral fusion. Rods should be measured, cut, and bent into the appropriate lordosis, and then secured in the pedicle screws. The screws are then tightened, compressing the heads to generate additional lordosis. Finally, the bone graft is placed at the level of the intertransverse space, which has been previously decorticated, with special care taken to avoid allowing bone chips to fall into the defects from the laminectomy/facetectomy (Fig. 29.3). A final anteroposterior and lateral X-ray shows the results obtained with the cage, screws, and rods position (Fig. 29.4).

Step 7: Closure

An extensive wash with sterile saline is performed, followed by meticulous hemostasis. The closure is done at the muscular level and the thoracolumbar fascia, followed by the subcutaneous layer, and finally the epidermis is sutured. A surgical drain may be left in place if deemed necessary by the surgeon.

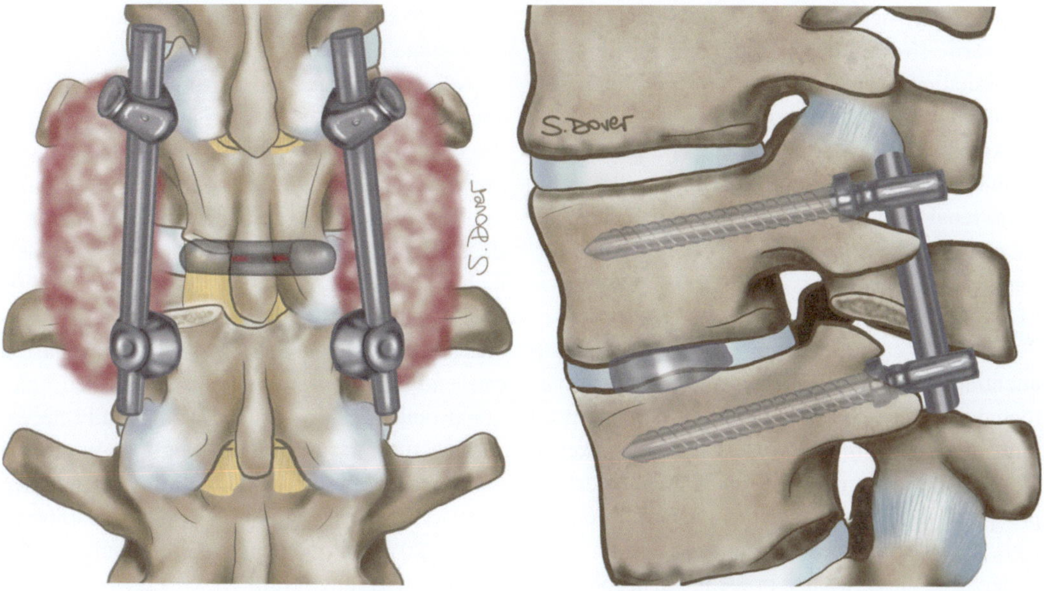

Fig. 29.3 Anteroposterior and lateral views of the TLIF construct with the cage and anterior fusion, the screws and rods, and the posterolateral fusion

Fig. 29.4 X-rays of an Open L4-L5 Tlif. (**a**) Preop with 10° of segmental lordosis; (**b**) Lateral postop with 26° of segmental lordosis; (**c**) Anteroposterior final view

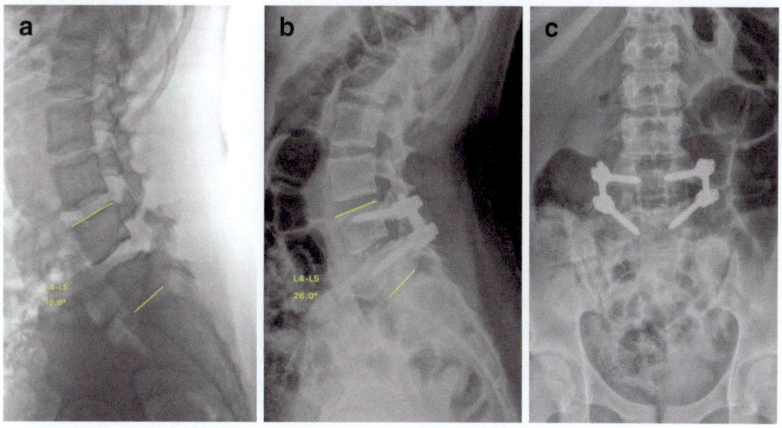

Complications

As with any surgical procedure, the TLIF carries the risk of complications; however, the overall complication rate is relatively low [10]. These complications can be categorized as minor or major, and either acute/perioperative or delayed.

Among the minor acute complications, incidental durotomy occurs in up to 16–19% of cases [10–12]. Typically detected during surgery, this dural defect can often be repaired successfully. The rate of postoperative meningitis is less than 1%. Other minor complications include hematomas (2%) [12], wound issues (less than 5%) [10], such as superficial infections (<3%) [12] or wound dehiscence, as well as transient root injuries due to retraction, which occur in about 7–13% of cases [10, 11]. Pedicle screw or cage misplacement are usually detected during the surgical procedure, and can be corrected. The majority of the screw's misplacement are asymptomatic, without the need of a reoperation [12].

Additionally, neuropathies or pressure injuries may arise from improper patient positioning, necessitating careful attention to decubitus protection.

Among the more serious acute complications, significant vascular injury—such as to the vena cava, renal vein, or aorta—represents a rare but catastrophic risk, particularly if the anterior longitudinal ligament is violated during discectomy [12].

Delayed complications warrant particular attention. Non-surgical delayed complications include deep venous thrombosis (DVT) and pulmonary embolism. Yamasaki et al. reported a 32% of DVT after a lumbar fusion [13]. Effective preoperative risk management includes prophylactic treatment and early diagnosis. For patients undergoing these surgical procedures, prophylactic measures against DVT commonly involve the use of intermittent pneumatic compression devices and graduated compression stockings. Additionally, early mobilization and postoperative anticoagulant therapy is typically recommended for those at high risk [13].

Surgical delayed complications, notably pseudoarthrosis and adjacent segment disease, are quite important. This type of complication occurs more frequently in patients with spinal deformity, including sagittal or coronal imbalance, and patients who have undergone more than 1 level of fusion [12]. Rates of lumbosacral pseudarthrosis have been reported between 3% and 24% for constructs that extend to the pelvis using contemporary instrumentation [14]. This condition can result in persistent pain, failure of the instrumentation, loss of surgical correction, and further progression of the deformity. Particularly with TLIF, pseudoarthrosis can result from inadequate preparation of the endplates, compromising the essential irrigation and metabolism of the disc. Thus, meticulous handling of endplate preparation is crucial to maintain their integrity, especially in osteoporotic patients, where the use of blunt distractors is recommended to reduce the risk of injury. Surgeons should also pay careful attention to the sagittal orientation of the endplates as viewed on intraoperative imaging, ensuring this alignment is preserved throughout the procedure. Nonunion at the fusion site may necessitate revision surgery [14, 15].

Adjacent segment disease (ASD) refers to symptomatic degenerative changes that occur at the levels adjacent to those that have undergone previous surgical intervention, particularly after lumbar arthrodesis [16]. This condition can manifest through various pathologic processes, including disc degeneration, listhesis, instability, herniated nucleus pulposus, stenosis, and compression fractures. ASD is concerning because it can lead to increased pain and diminished functional outcomes post-surgery, potentially necessitating further surgical intervention. While the prevalence of asymptomatic degenerative changes following lumbar arthrodesis can be as high as 20%, the incidence of symptomatic ASD is reported to range from 1.9% to 2.7% [16].

Why Is TLIF Superior to a Classic Posterolateral Fusion?

Theoretically, one of the key advantages of TLIF is its ability to achieve circumferential (360°) fusion, in contrast to merely providing a posterolateral fusion. The placement of an anterior interbody graft not only increases disc space height but also strengthens the integrity of the anterior column, thereby enhancing the overall stability of the construct. The endplates surrounding the graft offer a significant surface area that promotes effective graft fusion. Moreover, the interbody distraction increases neuroforaminal height, potentially alleviating nerve root compression. Glassman et al. [17] were the first to demonstrate a clinical benefit of TLIF vs. posterolateral fusion in patients treated for spondylolisthesis, in which TLIF generated more favorable ODI outcomes than PSF for patients with spondylolisthesis.

Restoration of Lordosis with TLIF

There has been considerable debate surrounding the effects of TLIF on lumbar curvature, particularly regarding its potential to induce either lordosis or kyphosis. Initially, TLIF was often viewed as a procedure that promoted kyphosis [18, 19]. Particularly, when compared to the powerful anterior lumbar interbody fusion (ALIF), the lordosis restoration and disc high is not so much restored as with TLIF [20]. However, recent evidence suggests this perspective is not entirely accurate. Numerous studies have shown that, when performed with proper surgical techniques and meticulous carpentry, TLIF can indeed achieve lordosis. Liu et al. demonstrated that TLIF can function as either a lordosing or kyphosing procedure [21], emphasizing that anterior cage placement is crucial for maximizing lordosis. This positioning allows for more effective posterior screw compression. Additionally, patient-specific preoperative characteristics, such as the preoperative pelvic incidence minus lumbar lordosis (PI-LL), were greater in cases where TLIF resulted in lordosis than those resulting in kyphosis.

To address this controversy, Jagannathan et al. [22] introduced a technique that involves laminectomy and bilateral total facetectomies, along with segment compression, representing a distinctive approach to TLIF. The authors highlighted several factors contributing to their improvements in lumbar lordosis: the execution of bilateral facetectomies enabled intraoperative adjustments akin to a Smith-Peterson osteotomy, and the use of a larger interbody graft, positioned as anteriorly as possible, acted as a fulcrum between the anterior and middle thirds of the vertebral body. This strategy aimed to enhance lordotic potential, increase the construct's overall stiffness, and reduce strain on the rods.

Conclusion

The TLIF is a powerful tool in the spine surgeon's arsenal for treating various lumbar pathologies. The TLIF offers a high fusion rate (>95%) similar to anterolateral approaches [23]. The use of classic TLIF may be limited in patients with rigid coronal and kyphotic deformities. In these cases, achieving correction in both the coronal and sagittal planes may require the TLIF described by Jagannathan [22] combined with bilateral facetectomy or osteotomies to effectively address the deformities. While it offers significant benefits, careful attention to surgical technique and postoperative management is essential to optimize outcomes and minimize complications.

References

1. Kim SS, Denis F, Lonstein JE, Winter RB. Factors affecting fusion rate in adult spondylolisthesis. Spine. 1990;15:979–84.
2. Kozak JA, O'Brien JP. Simultaneous combined anterior and pos-terior fusion: an independent analysis of a treatment for the disabled low-back pain patient. Spine. 1990;15:322–8.
3. Grob D, Scheier HJ, Dvorak J, Siegrist H, Rubeli M, Joller R. Circumferential fusion of the lumbar and lumbosacral spine. Arch Orthop Trauma Surg. 1991;111:20–5.
4. Harms J, Rolinger H. A one-stage procedure in operative treat-ment of spondylolistheses: dorsal traction-reposition and anterior fusion [in German]. Z Orthop Ihre Grenzgeb. 1982;120:343–7.
5. Rosenberg WS, Mummaneni PV. Transforaminal lumbar interbody fusion: technique, complications, and early results. Neurosurgery. 2001;48(3):569–75.
6. Lowe TG, Tahernia AD, O'Brien MF, Smith DA. Unilateral transforaminal posterior lumbar interbody fusion (TLIF): indications, technique, and 2-year results. J Spinal Disord Tech. 2002;15(1):31–8. https://doi.org/10.1097/00024720-200202000-00005.
7. Kwon BK, Berta S, Daffner SD, et al. Radiographic analysis of transforaminal lumbar interbody fusion for the treatment of adult isthmic spondylolisthesis. J Spinal Disord Tech. 2003;16:469–76.
8. Yson SC, Santos ER, Sembrano JN, Polly DW Jr. Segmental lumbar sagittal correction after bilateral transforaminal lumbar interbody fusion. J Neurosurg Spine. 2012;17(1):37–42. https://doi.org/10.3171/2012.4.SPINE111013.
9. Vialle EN, Ramos GZ, Hinojosa FL, Guiroy A, Rocha LGDD, Arruda AO. Correlation between cage positioning and lumbar lordosis in transforaminal lumbar Interbody fusion (TLIF). Rev Bras Ortop (Sao Paulo). 2022;57(5):821–7. Published 2022 Oct 10.
10. Potter BK, Freedman BA, Verwiebe EG, Hall JM, Polly DW Jr, Kuklo TR. Transforaminal lumbar interbody fusion: clinical and radiographic results and complications in 100 consecutive patients. J Spinal Disord Tech. 2005;18(4):337–46.
11. Mehta VA, McGirt MJ, Garcés Ambrossi GL, et al. Trans-foraminal versus posterior lumbar interbody fusion: comparison of surgical morbidity. Neurol Res. 2011;33(1):38–42.
12. Kurra S, Lavelle WF, Silverstein MP, Savage JW, Orr RD. Long-term outcomes of transforaminal lumbar interbody fusion in patients with spinal stenosis and

degenerative scoliosis. Spine J. 2018;18(6):1014–21. https://doi.org/10.1016/j.spinee.2017.10.063.
13. Yamasaki K, Hoshino M, Omori K, et al. Prevalence and risk factors of deep vein thrombosis in patients undergoing lumbar spine surgery. J Orthop Sci. 2017;22(6):1021–5.
14. Dinizo M, Srisanguan K, Dolgalev I, Errico TJ, Raman T. Pseudarthrosis and rod fracture rates after Transforaminal lumbar Interbody fusion at the caudal levels of long constructs for adult spinal deformity surgery. World Neurosurg. 2021;155:e605–11.
15. Villavicencio AT, Burneikiene S, Bulsara KR, et al. Perioperative complications in transforaminal lumbar interbody fusion versus anterior-posterior reconstruction for lumbar disc degeneration and instability. J Spinal Disord Tech. 2006;19:92–7.
16. Yee TJ, Terman SW, La Marca F, Park P. Comparison of adjacent segment disease after minimally invasive or open transforaminal lumbar interbody fusion. J Clin Neurosci. 2014;21(10):1796–801. https://doi.org/10.1016/j.jocn.2014.03.010.
17. Glassman SD, Carreon LY, Ghogawala Z, Foley KT, McGirt MJ, Asher AL. Benefit of Transforaminal lumbar Interbody fusion vs posterolateral spinal fusion in lumbar spine disorders: a propensity-matched analysis from the national neurosurgical quality and outcomes database registry. Neurosurgery. 2016;79(3):397–405.
18. Hsieh PC, Koski TR, O'Shaughnessy BA, et al. Anterior lumbar interbody fusion in comparison with transforaminal lumbar interbody fusion: implications for the restoration of foraminal height, local disc angle, lumbar lordosis, and sagittal balance. J Neurosurg Spine. 2007;7(4):379–86.
19. Dorward IG, Lenke LG, Bridwell KH, et al. Transforaminal versus anterior lumbar interbody fusion in long deformity constructs: a matched cohort analysis. Spine (Phila Pa 1976). 2013;38(12):E755–62.
20. Watkins RG 4th, Hanna R, Chang D, Watkins RG 3rd. Sagittal alignment after lumbar interbody fusion: comparing anterior, lateral, and transforaminal approaches. J Spinal Disord Tech. 2014;27(5):253–6.
21. Liu J, Duan P, Mummaneni PV, et al. Does transforaminal lumbar interbody fusion induce lordosis or kyphosis? Radiographic evaluation with a minimum 2-year follow-up. J Neurosurg Spine. 2021;35(4):419–26.
22. Jagannathan J, Sansur CA, Oskouian RJ Jr, et al. Radiographic restoration of lumbar alignment after transforaminal lumbar interbody fusion. Neurosurgery. 2009;64(5):955–64.
23. Schroeder GD, Kepler CK, Millhouse PW, et al. L5/S1 fusion rates in degenerative spine surgery: a systematic review comparing ALIF, TLIF, and axial Interbody arthrodesis. Clin Spine Surg. 2016;29(4):150–5.

30 Posterior Lumbar Interbody Fusion: MIS

Avelino Parajón, Angela Carrascosa, and Jose Antonio Gutiérrez

Introduction

Minimally invasive lumbar interbody fusion includes mainly MIS TLIF (the most widespread technique and the one we will focus on this chapter) and PLIF transforaminal lumbar interbody fusion.

PLIF was developed by Cloward in the 1950s (the first PLIF surgery performed by him in 1943) [1]. As an alternative to that technique in 1982 Harms and Rolinger introduced TLIF, with less need of neural retraction, what means less risk of dural tears and neurological deficit [2]. The same year Magerl first reported the use of percutaneous pedicle screws in conjunction with an external fixator—although he had been working on that since 1970s [3]. In the 1990s–2000s K Foley and other authors developed tubular approaches for decompression and MIS TLIF as an alternative to open techniques [4, 5]. It is interesting to point out that at the moment these techniques were introduced, the surgical procedure was done with endoscopic assistance. Due to the lack of popularity of endoscopy between spine surgeons at that time and the superiority of microscopes for visualization and illumination at that time, the technique became more popular under microscopic visualization; and nowadays thanks to the technical improvement in endoscopes, the endoscopic version of MIS TLIF (endolif) is gaining interest in the spine surgery community [6].

There are different ways to perform an MIS TLIF, according to the type of retractor used (mounted on the screws, valve retractor, tubular rigid, expandable, McCulloch type, etc.); depending on the use of fluoroscopy, navigation, robotics; with microscopic or exoscopic. Visualization, and some other variations.

There are two basic and common steps in all MIS TLIF surgeries, no matter the skin incision, retractor, image system, or implants used:

- Decompression, discectomy, and cage insertion
- Pedicular screws (MIS or percutaneous)

These 2 steps can be done inserting first the cage and later the screws or inserting the screws and then the cage. Inserting the cage first has some disadvantages: a new scan will be needed to navigate the screws (if navigation is used), and the air in the surgical field will worsen the accuracy in AP fluoroscopy if X-rays are used. For these reasons, we prefer to insert the screws first.

MIS TLIF can be done:

- "Pure" MIS TLIF, or percutaneous, through the multifidus fibers (this is the way tubular microsurgical approach is done).

A. Parajón (✉) · J. A. Gutiérrez
Department of Neurosurgery, Hospital Universitario Ramón y Cajal, Madrid, Spain

A. Carrascosa
Department of Neurosurgery, Hospital Universitario San Carlos, Madrid, Spain

A. A. Baaj et al. (eds.), *Surgery of the Lumbar Spine*, https://doi.org/10.1007/978-3-032-18097-1_30

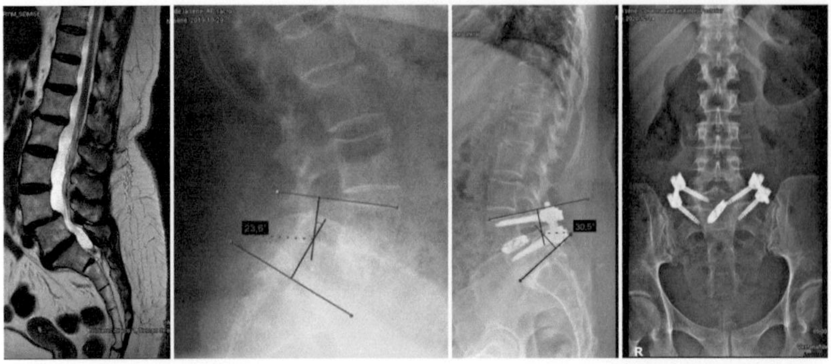

Fig. 30.1 Pre- and postoperative images of a patient with lumbar degenerative spondylolisthesis treated with MIS TLIF with expandable cage

- "Mini Open" or Wiltse approach, between multifidus and longissimus muscles [7].

Indications and Contraindications for MIS TLIF

Indications

- Segmental instability caused by grade I or II spondylolisthesis (Fig. 30.1)
- Lumbar disc re-herniation (with instability)
- Degenerative disc disease causing discogenic low back pain
- Dynamic foraminal stenosis

Relative Contraindications

- High-grade spondylolisthesis
- Severe osteoporosis
- More than 2-level disease (high risk of postop flat back spine)

Evidence

There is Class II and Class III evidence of the advantage of MIS TLIF: faster recovery, improved perioperative pain, less blood loss, and lower infection rates. Minimally invasive spine surgery results in less collateral tissue damage by focusing on the use of muscle-splitting retractors, limiting the width of the surgical corridor, and avoiding disruption of tendon attachment of key muscles [8, 9]. Minimally invasive TLIF fusion and complication rates are similar or better than open TLIF procedures [10].

MIS TLIF—Tubular Microsurgical Technique

From all the different ways to do an MIS TLIF, we will describe here the tubular microsurgical technique as standardized by the AOSpine MIS Task Force [11, 12], which is the common way we have been doing it for the last 10 years.

The rationale for the tubular access, which is a transmuscular access, is minimize trauma to the muscle and tendons, minimizing iatrogenic instability, producing less postoperative pain, lower infection rates, and early recovery.

Surgical main steps in MIS TLIF (Fig. 30.2):

1. OR set up and patient positioning
2. Incision location
3. Screws/K-wires insertion
4. Tubular dilators and tubular retractor insertion
5. Opening of the facet capsule
6. Resection of inferior facet
7. Resection of superior facet
8. Resection of ligamentum flavum
9. Discectomy
10. Bone graft

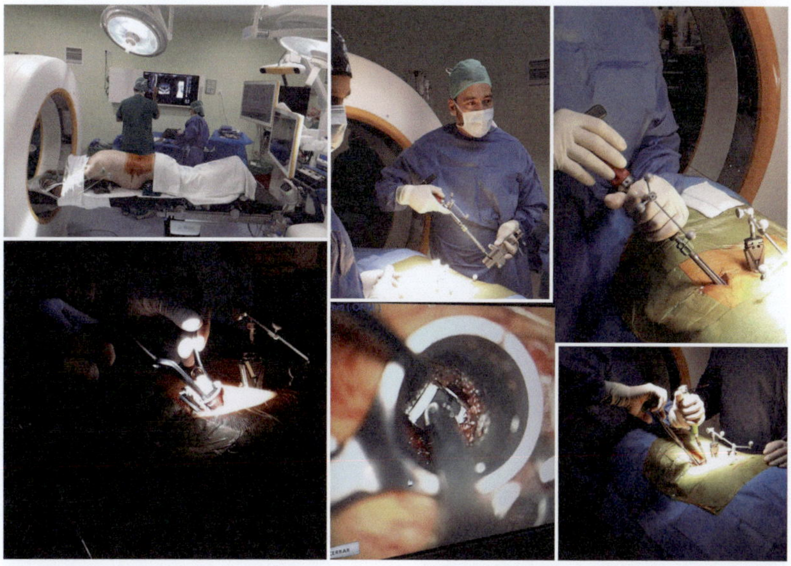

Fig. 30.2 3D navigated tubular microsurgical MIS TLIF. From upper left to right: position of the patient and OR setup; calibration of screwdriver; screw insertion. From down left to right: tubular microsurgical decompression, cage insertion, final tightening of rods and locks. In this case reference array was positioned in the spinous processes

11. Structural implant
12. Additional decompression if required
13. Ipsilateral screws insertion (in the case K-wires are used)
14. Rods and locks
15. Closure

1. OR set up and patient positioning.

   OR set up depends on size, shape of the OR, and additional technology to be used in the surgery (X-rays, navigation, robotics, neurophysiology, microscope, exoscope, endoscope). The patient should be positioned prone on a mattress with a hollow at the center to accommodate the abdomen and reduce pressure on the inferior vena cava. Alternatively, other support systems can be used like cushions under the chest and iliac crest in order to help correct lumbar lordosis, Jackson table, etc. Arms are abducted and placed on lateral support (don't abduct the arms more than 90°). The legs are slightly elevated. Then the patient is draped exposing the lumbar spine.

2. Incision location.

   If navigation is used, at this moment reference array must be inserted. Star can be positioned on the spinous process through a small midline incision or on the iliac crest with one or two pins, depending on the navigation system used, specific surgical case or preferences of the surgeon (Fig. 30.3). Then scan can be done for navigation.

   If X-rays are used, skin landmarks are marked: midline, discs, and pedicles at the levels to be fused using AP and lateral fluoroscopy.

3. Screws/K-Wires insertion.

   Contralateral screws are inserted first using either navigation/robotics or AP and lateral fluoroscopy. On the ipsilateral side we prefer to drop just the K-wires at this point. With some of the modern implants and at some levels like 4–5 is possible to insert also ipsilateral screws and there will be enough space to drop a tube between them.

4. Tubular dilators and tubular retractor insertion.

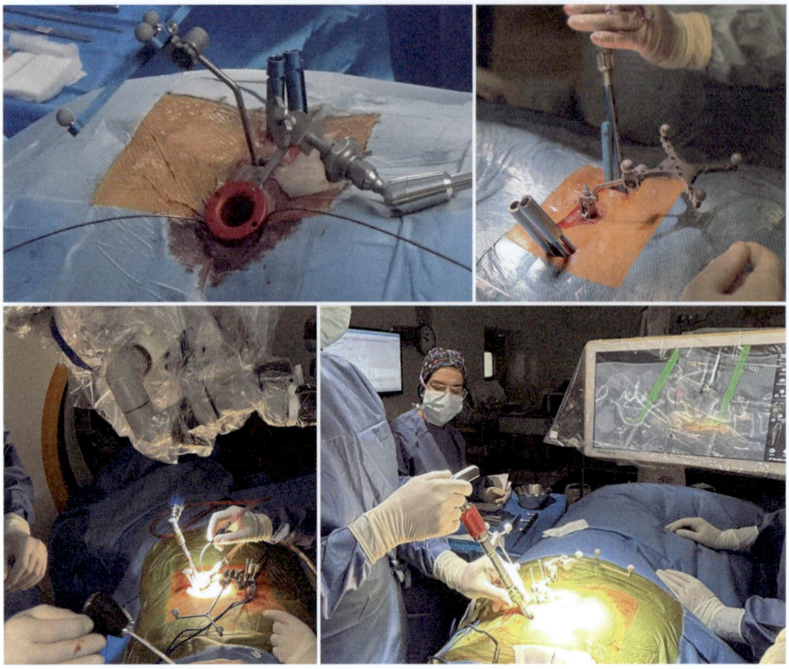

Fig. 30.3 Reference array can be attached to the spinous process through a small midline incision or can be inserted with one or two pins on the iliac crest

Location of the entry point and ideal trajectory (on top of facet joint over interarticular line) with aid of navigation or fluoroscopy; sometimes an additional medial fascial incision is needed. Sequential dilators are inserted dilating the paravertebral (multifidus) muscles down to the level of the lamina-facet joint; and final tubular retractor. For an MIS TLIF or MIS PLIF most common size of the tube is 22 mm diameter, but 18 mm is enough.

5. Opening of the facet capsule.

   At this point microscope (or exoscope) is brought into the surgical field. Microscope is preferred over surgical loupes for different reasons, like coaxial lighting, better 3D visualization due to interpupillary distance, better visualization for the assistant and team, recording, and fluorescence options [13]. Exoscope can be an alternative to microscope and has some advantages like ergonomics and more amplitude for hand movements. The remaining soft tissue over the bone is removed using the long monopolar (bipolar is an option but usually takes longer time) and facet capsule is identified and opened using a high-speed drill with attached 3 mm fluted matchstick burr.
6. Resection of the inferior facet.

   Drill and Kerrison punch are used to remove the inferior facet of the cranial vertebra. An osteotome can be an alternative, but through a tubular retractor it can be risky.
7. Resection of the superior facet.

   Similar procedure is used to resect the superior facet of the inferior vertebra.
8. Resection of ligamentum flavum.

   Ligamentum flavum is resected at its lateral part with a 2 or 3 mm Kerrison. A bayonetted hook with a ball tip is useful to dissect the ligament from adherences to the dura. Epidural bleeding is controlled with bipolar coagulation and local hemostatic agents.
9. Discectomy.

   Disc is incised with an 11-blade lancet. Disc is removed with straight and angled pituitary rongeurs, curettes, sharp paddle distractors, box cutters, and other disc shavers.

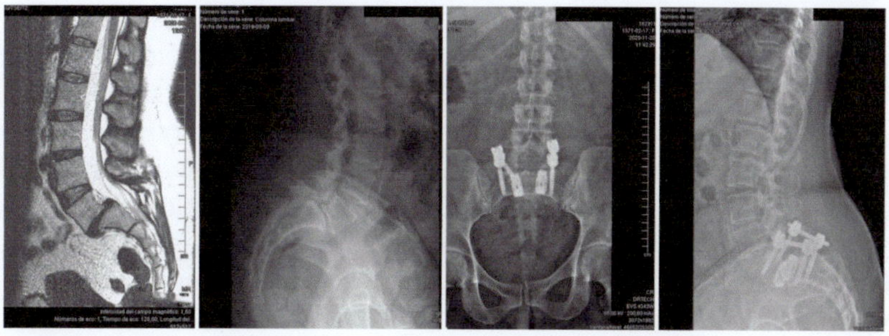

Fig. 30.4 Pre- and postoperative images of a patient with lumbar spondylolisthesis with lisis treated with MIS PLIF with expandable cages

Rasps and curettes can be used to decorticate endplates. Be careful in older or osteoporotic patients not to damage endplates. A thorough discectomy is a crucial step for decompression in many cases, to avoid complications and to ensure fusion.

10. Bone graft.

    Fusion can't rely on the small amount inside the cages. So filling the disc space with bone graft is essential. We prefer to put the bone graft prior to the insertion of the cage in the case of a straight one (also with PLIF cages) and to put the bone graft after the cage insertion if a banana type is used.

11. Cage insertion.

    A trial can be used but usually we prefer to measure the adequate size of the definitive cage on the preop images and with the pointer of the navigation system.

    The cage can be a straight one in oblique position, or a banana cage anteriorly placed. Theoretically banana cages can help gaining lordosis, but straight cages are easier to insert through a tube.

12. Additional decompression.

    In the case bilateral decompression is required, resection of ipsilateral and contralateral laminae and ligamentum flavum can be done as in a tubular "over the top" decompression [14]. For contralateral side tilting the tube and table is necessary.

13. Ipsilateral screws are inserted using the previously left in place K-wires.
14. Rods and locks.

    Rod size is measured using the tools provided by the company of the implants usually. Navigation and preoperative planning can help as well in this decision.

    Insert the appropriately sized pre-lordosed rods below the fascia until they are fully seated into each screw head and ensure the tip of the rod protrudes out of both screw heads. Insert a set screw into each head and tighten them capturing the rod. Connect the counter-torque wrench to the end of each screw for final tightening. The rod holder can also be used as counter-torque. Free the rod from the holder after the final tightening. Control scan is done at this point in the case navigation is used. Lateral and AP fluoroscopy is an alternative for final checking.

15. Closure of the wound in the standard way.

In PLIF the tube needs to be positioned more medially, over the inferior border of the upper lamina of the segment to be operated. Thus, the entrance point for the implant will be medial to the TLIF one. More retraction of the dural sac medially is needed and cages are inserted bilaterally (shorter than the TLIF ones) (Fig. 30.4).

Fusion and Bone Graft

Similar fusion rates have been described in MIS TLIF as in open TLIF [10]. The success of MIS-TLIF and MIS PLIF relies on a solid interbody fusion since a posterolateral fusion is difficult to achieve given the limited exposure. Different types of grafts and fusion enhancers can be used including local cortico-cancellous autologous bone from laminectomy and facetectomy, harvested autologous bone graft from iliac crest, allograft bone, bone substitutes (hydroxyapatite, ceramics), demineralized bone matrix, and recombinant human bone morphogenetic protein (rhBMP). Autologous local bone offers some advantages: lower cost, easy to harvest; iliac crest advantages are the same, but includes the disadvantage of donor site complications; allografts from processed cadaveric bone have advantages of abundant material supply and the avoidance of harvesting complications, yet they bear the risk of infectious disease transmission (extremely low risk) as well as the risk for immunologic reaction. Overall fusion rates for MIS TLIF are high regardless of graft material used. Utilization of autologous local bone in combination with both bone extenders and rhBMP showed the highest fusion rate (98.8%) at 12-month follow-up in a meta-analysis published in 2017 [15]. In the same study isolated use of local bone resulted in the lowest fusion rate (91.8% at 12 months) and the highest fusion rate without the use of BMP was seen with autologous local bone plus bone extender (93.1%).

Types of Interbody Cages

MIS TLIF and PLIF cages can be titanium or PEEK (polyether ether ketone) made (also PEEK with a titanium covering and PEKK (polyetherketoneketone)). Titanium offers immediate stability and better osteointegration; however, titanium implants have an increased risk of subsidence [16, 17]. This risk can be reduced when using 3D printed titanium, highly porous and can increase in elderly or osteoporotic patients.

Regarding the shape of the cages, cages can be straight bullet type or banana type. Through a rigid tube bullet cages are easier to insert, but also have a higher risk of migration. Banana cages are trickier at the insertion, but theoretically, when placed very anteriorly have the potential to increase segmental lordosis.

Expandable cages are relatively new. Some studies have shown a long-lasting restoration of disc height and foraminal height with them [18]. Improvement of lordosis with expandable cages is controversial in terms of evicendence-based medicine, but they may be a good tool to prevent complications such as dural tears or root damage due to excessive retraction [19, 20].

Complications and Disadvantages of MIS TLIF: How to Avoid Them

- Impossibility to insert the cage: not being able to put the cage into the disc space. Ensuring a complete discectomy and making a good preparation and distraction of the space can help in preventing it.
- Cages subsidence into vertebral body: careful endplate preparation and avoiding sharp instruments in osteoporotic bone help to avoid this. We recommend using fluoroscopy when expanding a TLIF cage.
- Cage pull out (movement of the cage into the canal/foramen): banana cages have less probability of pull out and screws compression maneuver after final placement are good options to prevent pull out. Cage migration is related to unilateral cages (usually we don't use bilateral in MIS TLIF), bullet-shaped cages, osteoporotic bone, inadequate endplates preparation, undersized cages (width), and over distraction [21].
- Nerve root damage (mainly transverse nerve root). This can be avoided by complete resection of facets and using nerve retractors to protect neural structures during cage instruction. Intraoperative neuromonitoring can also help in preventing neural injuries.
- Pseudoarthrosis: use enough bone graft in the disc space, consider bone substitutes.
- Inability to gain or maintain lordosis. This is one of the main critics to MIS TLIF. There are many studies that have shown anterior and lateral approaches are better to provide lordosis to the lumbar spine [22]. With unilateral approach, MIS TLIF technique is difficult to resect facets bilaterally. There are some strate-

gies that may help in gaining lordosis: expandable cages, bilateral approach with two tubes (increases surgical time and complications risk), partial resection of contralateral facets through an "over the top" approach, bending the rods, and patient selection (in some cases MIS TLIF may be not the best option for a one or two level lumbar decompression and fusion if lordosis is a main surgical goal) [23].

- Screw malposition. Navigation is the best tool to increase the accuracy of implants position being able to reduce malposition rate to a minimum [24, 25]. Other advantages of navigation are reduction in dose radiation for the surgical team and choosing better size and trajectories for the implants [26, 27].

Ambulatory MIS TLIF

Standardization of the surgical technique of MIS TLIF has led to the development of specific educational tools like apps or simulators to train this technique [28] and together with the development of new technologies and postoperative protocols like ERAS has open the door to making MIS TLIF an outpatient surgery.

In certain patients, MIS TLIF can be done as an ambulatory procedure. There are some predictors of prolonged length of stay after lumbar interbody fusion, like age, body mass index, ASA classification, comorbidities (diabetes mellitus, HTN, cardiac), and operative time [29]. Patient selection is crucial when planning an ambulatory MIS TLIF: age younger than 75, BMI less than 35, good social support, preoperative ODI no higher than 50, patient education, standardized surgical technique, use of navigation—robotics, tubular or endoscopic approach have been proposed as favorable for making this procedure ambulatory [30].

Tips for MIS LTIF Surgery

- Use microscope (exoscope or endoscope are alternatives).
- High-speed drills can facilitate the surgery.
- Tubular retractors are commonly used, require the surgeon to become familiar with them.
- Optimize fusion rates by spending time with the discectomy and endplates preparation and grafting.
- Navigation is a good tool to prevent complications. Makes surgery easier and faster. Robotics is an alternative.
- Train with simulators/apps/cadaver labs. It will make surgeries easier and safer.

References

1. Cloward RB. The treatment of ruptured lumbar intervertebral discs by ventral body fusions. J Neurosurg. 1953;10(2):154–68.
2. Harms J, Rolinger H. Die operative Behandlung der Spondylolisthese durch dorsale Aufrichtung und ventral Verblockung. Z Orthop. 1982;120:343–7.
3. Magerl F. External skeletal fixation on the lower thoracic and the lumbar spine. In: Uhthoff HK, editor. Current concepts of external fixation of fractures. Berlin: Springer Verlag; 1982. p. 353–66.
4. Smith MM, Foley KT. Microendoscopic discectomy: the first 100 cases. Neurosurgery. 1998;43(3)
5. Foley KT, Holly LT, Schewneder JD. Minimally invasive lumbar fusion. Spine. 2003;28(Suppl25):S26–35.
6. Wagner R, Haefner M. Uniportal endoscopic lumbar interbody fusion. Neurospine. 2020;17(Suppl1):S120–8.
7. Wiltse L, Bateman JG, Hutchinson RH, Nelson WE. The paraspinal sacrospinalis-splitting approach to the lumbar spine. J Bone Joint Surg. 1968;50(5):919–26.
8. Skovrlj B, Belton P, Zarzour H, Qureshi SA. Perioperative outcomes in minimally invasive lumbar spine surgery: a systematic review. World J Orthop. 2015;6(11):996–1005.
9. Parker SL, Adogwa O, Witham TF, Aaronson OS, Cheng J, McGirt MJ. Post-operative infection after minimally invasive versus open transforaminal lumbar interbody fusion (TLIF): literature review and cost analysis. World Neursourg. 2011;54(1):33–7.
10. Wu RH, Fraser JF, Härtl R. Minimal acces verus open transforaminal lumbar interbody fusion. Meta-analysis of fusion rates. Spine. 2010;35(26):2273–81.
11. Schmidt FA, Wong T, Kirnaz S, Taboada N, Assaker R, Hofstetter C, Kim JS, Parajón A, Taylor P, Assous M, Härtl R. Development of a curricurlum for minimally invasive spine surgery (MISS). Global Spine J. 2020;20(2 Suppl):122S–5S.
12. Härtl R, Gelb D: Step by step guide: key steps in a MIS TLIF procedure. AOSpine Intl, Duebendorf, 2020.

13. Parajón A, Hernandez RN, Kirnaz S, Korge A. Technology: Microscope in MISS. Chapter 9. In: Härtl R, Navarro- Ramírez R, editors. Essential step by step techniques for minimally invasive spinal surgery. New York: Thieme; 2022.
14. Parajón A, Härtl R: Step by step guide: minimally invasive tubular approaches to lumbar spine decompression and dural repair- surgical techniques. AOSpine Intl, Duebendorf 2020.
15. Parajón A, Alimi M, Navarro-Ramírez R, Chirstos P, Torres-Campa JM, Moriguchi Y, Lang G, Härtl R. Minimally invasive transforaminal lumbar interbody fusion: meta-analysis of the fusion rates. What is the optimal graft material? Neurosurgery. 2017;81:958–71.
16. Singhatanadgige W, Tangchitcharoen N, Kerr SJ, Tanasansomboon T, Yingsakmongkol W, Kotheeranurak V, Limhongkul W. A comparison of polyethereherketone and titanium-coated PEEK in minimally invasive transforaminal lumbar interbody fusion: a randomized clinical trial. World Neurosurg. 2022;168:e471–9.
17. Seaman S, Kerezoudis P, Bydon M, Torner JC, Hichon PW. Titanium vs PEEK interbody fusion: meta-analysis and review of the literature. J Clin Neurosci. 2017;44:23–9.
18. Hawasli AH, Khalifeh JM, Chatrath A, Yarbrough CK, Ray WZ. Minimally invasive transforaminal lumbar interbody fusion with expandable versus static interbody devices: radiographic assessment of sagittal segmental and pelvic parameters. Neurosurg Focus. 2017;43(2):E10.
19. Yee TJ, Joseph JR, Terman WW, Park P. Expancable vs static cages in transforaminal lumbar interbody fusion: radiographic comparison of segmental and lumbar sagittal angles. Neurosurgery. 2017;81(1):69–74.
20. Alvi M, Kurian SY, Wahood W, Goyal A, Elder BD, Bydon M. Assessing the difference in clinical and radiologic outcomes between expandable cage and nonexpendable cage among patients undergoing minimally invasive transforaminal interbody fusion: a systematic review and meta-analysis. Word Neurosurg. 2019;127:596–606.
21. Duncan JW, Bailey RA. An analysis of fusion cage migration in unilateral and bilateral fixation with transforaminal lumbar interbody fusion. Euro J Spine. 2013;22:439–45.
22. Uribe JS, Myhre SL, Ypussef JA. Preservation or restoration of segmental and regional spinal lordosis using minimally invasive interbody fusion techniques in degenerative lumbar conditions. Spine. 2016;41(85):S50–8.
23. Liu J, Duan P, Mummaneni PV, Xie R, Dong y, Berven S, Chou D. Does transforaminal lumbar interbody fusion induce lordosis or kyphosis? Radiographic evaluation with a minimum 2-year follow-up. J Neurosurg Spine. 2021;35:419–26.
24. Shin BJ, James AR, Njoku IU, Härtl R. Pedicle screw navigation: a systematic revies and meta-analysis of perforation risk for computer- navigated versus freehand insertion. J Neurosurg Spine. 2012;17:113–22.
25. Verma R, Krishan S, Haendmayer K, Mohsen A. Functional outcome of computer- assisted spinal pedicle screw placement: a systematic review and meta-analysis of 23 studies including 5992 pedicle screws. Eur Spine J. 2010;19:370–5.
26. Kim CW, Lee YP, Taylor W, Oygar A, Kim WK. Use of navigation-assisted fluoroscopy to decrease radiation exposure during minimally invasive spine surgery. Spine J. 2008;8:584–90.
27. Luther N, Iorgulescu B, Geannette C, Gebhard H, Saleh T, Tsiouris A, Härtl R. Comparison of navigated versus non-navigated pedicle screw placement in 260 patients and 1434 screws. Screw accuracy, screw size and the complexity of surgery. J Spinal Disord Tech. 2015;28:E298. E303
28. Aderman J, GeiBler N, Bernal LE, Kotzsh S, Korb W. Development and validation of an artificial wetlab training systeme for the lumbar discectomy. Eur Spine J. 2014;23(9):1978–83.
29. Kobayashi K, Ando K, Kato F, Kanemura T, Sato K, Hachiya Y, Matsubara Y, Kamiya M, Sakai Y, Yagi H, Shijo R, Ishiguro N, Imagama S. Predictors of prolonged length of stay after lumbar interbody fusion: a multicenter study. Global Spine Surg. 2019;9(5):466–72.
30. Kim CW. MIS TLIF, EndoTLIF and the ability of navigation/robotics to enable spinal surgery in an ambulatory care setting. Global Spine J. 2022;12(25):34S–9S.

Lateral Lumbar Interbody Fusion

31

Rodrigo Amaral, Gabriel Pokorny,
Jullyene Pokorny, Fernando Marcelino,
Igor Barreira, Rafael Moriguchi, and Luiz Pimenta

Historical Overview and Brief Description

Lateral interbody fusion (LLIF), introduced by Luiz Pimenta and Willian Taylor and with a case series first published in 2006, has evolved into a versatile tool in minimally invasive spine surgery. The transpsoas approach allows the implantation of cages of different dimensions and lordotic angles, facilitating the restoration of disc height and segmental lordosis [1, 2]. This restoration is crucial not only for relieving neural compression but also for reestablishing sagittal alignment and optimizing the biomechanical distribution of loads in the lumbar spine [3].

The choice of technique depends on the level affected, the patient's anatomy, and the surgeon's experience. In general, LLIF is preferred between levels T12 and L5. In all cases, the selection of the technique should consider the safest and most effective access route on the basis of the evaluation of adjacent anatomical structures, such as the great vessels, the lumbar plexus, and the topography of the psoas muscle [4].

Despite the clear benefits, appropriate patient selection is essential to ensure the success of the lateral approach. There are well-established contraindications, such as the presence of previous ipsilateral retroperitoneal surgeries, which can alter the natural anatomical planes, increasing the risk of injury to key structures during dissection. Active retroperitoneal infections, abscesses, or areas of intense fibrosis can also make safe access impossible. Careful analysis of clinical and surgical history, associated with high-resolution imaging, is essential for identifying such risk factors [4, 5].

Brief Description of the Surgical Technique

Patient Positioning and Correct Level Localization

The patient was placed under anesthesia in the lateral decubitus position at 90° to the table. The patient was secured below the iliac crest, thoracic region, and greater trochanter to the knee. The table is bent slightly to increase the space between the iliac crest and ribs for spine access. The position was confirmed with fluoroscopic images. *Importantly*, EMG monitoring is required when traversing the psoas muscle to avoid lumbar plexus injury. An incision is made via two Kirschner wires over the targeted disc, and lateral fluoroscopic images were obtained. The first line is drawn anteroposteriorly at the index level center, and the second line is drawn superoinferiorly across the center of the vertebral bodies. A skin incision was made at the marked intersections,

R. Amaral · G. Pokorny · J. Pokorny (✉) ·
F. Marcelino · I. Barreira · R. Moriguchi · L. Pimenta
Instituto de Patologia da Coluna, São Paulo, Brazil
e-mail: lpimenta@patologiadacoluna.com.br

A. A. Baaj et al. (eds.), *Surgery of the Lumbar Spine*, https://doi.org/10.1007/978-3-032-18097-1_31

followed by a fascia incision. The initial dilators are guided to the psoas muscle. The lateral-abdominal layers were opened sequentially until the retroperitoneal fat was reached.

Retroperitoneal Space Work and Retractor Placement

After reaching the retroperitoneal space, the index finger is used to dissect through the retroperitoneal fat, sweeping the finger both deep and back up toward the skin and opening the retroperitoneal space above the psoas muscle. Care was taken not to perforate the peritoneum. The surgeon's index finger will now guide the placement of the first dilator over the psoas and protect the abdominal structures from inadvertent injuries. After proper positioning is confirmed, sequential dilators through the psoas muscle fibers are introduced via neural guidance attached to the dilators for EMG monitoring of the relative distance of the lumbar plexus.

After dilator insertion, an expandable retractor is placed. The retractor should always be attached to the table to avoid unwanted movement; it is also important to attach the retractor to the posterior third of the intervertebral disc with a shim through the posterior blade. With the working portal opened and the correct positioning checked by fluoroscopic imaging, disc removal, endplate preparation, and implant placement are ready to start.

Discectomy, Endplate Preparation, and Interbody Cage Placement

Discectomy begins with the opening of the disc annulus, and then the nucleus pulposus is removed with rongeurs. Meticulous preparation of the disc space is paramount to a good fusion process, and it includes removal of all the disc material and scraping of the cartilaginous endplates, which may hinder fusion between the implant and the vertebral bodies. With the aid of a Cobb elevator, the contralateral annulus is disrupted, which enables parallel endplate distraction and the placement of a large implant reaching the ring apophysis bilaterally. The anterior and posterior portions of the disc with longitudinal ligaments must be preserved to maintain ligamentotaxis and indirect neural decompression. Minimal endplate scraping maximizes support and reduces cage subsidence [6].

Supplementation

After the operative wound is closed in a standard fashion, the patient can be positioned in the ventral decubitus position for standard supplemental internal fixation via posterior percutaneous pedicle screw fixation guided by fluoroscopy. In unstable spondylolisthesis, the use of bilateral posterior supplementation is highly recommended to safeguard against the primary fusion achieved by cage insertion.

Neuromonitoring

Given the close proximity of the LLIF pathway and the nerves of the plexus, particularly the femoral nerve, the use of neuromonitoring techniques is mandatory for a safe approach.

Historically, the primary IONM modality used during LLIF has been electromyography (EMG). Both free-run EMG, which provides continuous surveillance for nerve irritation, and triggered EMG, which is used to map the location of nerves relative to dilators and retractors, have been standard practices. However, the use of EMG alone is not sufficient to truly understand nerve health during the procedure. Therefore, the addition of motor-evoked potentials (MEPs) or somatosensory-evoked potentials (SSEPs) provides a more complete assessment of neural pathway integrity. Recent studies underscore that a "one-size-fits-all" approach to neuromonitoring is suboptimal, suggesting that the use of multimodal approaches might be the best framework for improving the safety of the procedure [7, 8].

Tips and Tricks

Approaching L4–L5

Access to L4–L5 requires special attention due to technical challenges. High iliac crests and increases in the anterior position of the lumbar plexus might reduce the working space and increase the risk of neural injury. Detailed preoperative imaging analysis is crucial for success (Table 31.1).

Table 31.1 Tips and tricks to approaching L4–L5, from decision-making to technical advice

Imaging	Dilator and retractor anchorage
Magnetic Resonance Imaging (MRI): Carefully evaluate the psoas major muscle morphology. Amaral et al., 2024 classification system might help in the decision-making process on how to approach L4–L5 [5]. *Anteroposterior (AP) X-rays*: Examine for the presence of transitional vertebrae. *Lateral X-rays*: Assess the relationship between the iliac crest and the L4–L5 disc space.	*Posterior Anchorage*: Avoid placing the initial anchor in a posterior position. This trajectory can bring the surgical corridor too close to the lumbar plexus. *Anterior Anchorage*: While a simple anterior anchorage is safer, it may not provide the optimal angle for a complete discectomy, which is a key step for achieving indirect neural decompression. *Recommended technique*: The preferred approach is to use an anterior anchor point and then rotate the operating table 15°–20°.

To Add or Not Add Posterior Fixation (or the Standalone Dilemma)

The LLIF approach allows the placement of large cages, raising questions about the necessity of posterior fixation in single-level cases to reduce blood loss and muscle damage. However, a stand-alone approach may increase the risk of subsidence, including clinically significant subsidence (Marchi grades II-IV) [6]. Moreover, recent studies have shown that patients who receive posterior fixation alongside LLIF present significantly higher fusion rates and lower rates of subsidence and reoperation [9, 10]. Therefore, currently, the use of stand-alone techniques is rare, and these techniques are rarely applied in very specific scenarios.

Literature

Indirect Decompression

One of the great advantages of the lateral approach is the ability to indirectly decompress neural structures. By restoring the height of the intervertebral disc with the insertion of a large-volume cage, tension is created in the longitudinal ligaments and expansion of the neural foramina and spinal canal in a phenomenon called ligamentotaxis. This strategy provides symptomatic relief without the need for laminectomies or foraminotomies, which considerably reduces the risk of neural injury [11, 12].

LLIF has led to significant clinical improvements in degenerative lumbar spine diseases. Studies have shown significant improvements in the VAS score for back and leg pain and in the ODI. Radiologically, the disc height, foraminal height, and foraminal area increase, and the central canal area also significantly increases during the postoperative period [13, 14]. However, it is important to be aware that factors such as severe central canal stenosis, facet rigidity (blocked facets), and bony stenosis of the lateral recess are the most common causes of failure. Therefore, in those cases, the execution of direct decompression along with LLIF might be beneficial for the patient [15, 16].

Low-Grade Spondylolisthesis

Recent evidence strongly supports the efficacy of LLIF in treating low-grade spondylolisthesis, with favorable clinical and radiographic outcomes. Multiple studies and meta-analyses have shown significant improvements in patient-reported outcomes, including substantial reductions in back and leg pain, as measured by the visual analog scale (VAS), and improvements in functional disability, as measured by the Oswestry Disability Index (ODI) [17, 18].

The principles of LLIF can also be extended to treat Grade II spondylolisthesis. A significant technical challenge in applying LLIF to Grade II spondylolisthesis is the severity of the slip, which can narrow the anteroposterior dimension of the disc space and obstruct the safe insertion of an appropriately sized cage. To overcome this, innovative strategies have been developed that effectively widen the corridor for subsequent cage insertion [19, 20].

Segmental Lordosis

The lateral approach effectively corrects segmental lordosis, which is a key surgical goal for lumbar spine degenerative pathologies. Studies have shown that 20~30% of adult deformity cases stem from poorly treated degenerative diseases due to iatrogenic loss of lordosis, with 90% showing undercorrection of lumbar lordosis, 83% from L1—L4, and 63% from L4—S1 [21].

Comparative retrospective studies provide clear evidence of the impact of LLIF on the correction of segmental lordosis, with several studies showing that LLIF is one of the most capable interbody techniques for restoring segmental lordosis, only behind ALIFs [22]. However, it is important to note that several factors are important for achieving the envisioned segmental lordosis, such as cage positioning, cage angulation, and posterior release [23–25].

Recent Developments

Recent studies have shown that the use of expandable cages might lead to a significant increase in segmental lordosis correction by LLIF and, in some cases, reduced rates of subsidence [26, 27]. However, a recent systematic review and meta-analysis revealed that the use of expandable technology was not able to significantly differ in either radiological outcomes or clinical outcomes, despite several heterogeneities between the studies, which shows that, at present, the use of this technology still needs more standardization in real-world scenarios [28].

Another important advancement in lateral surgery is the use of single-position surgery frameworks. Guiroy et al. (2021) reported in their systematic review that single-position surgery was associated with a reduced operative time and short hospitalization duration, which could lead to a significant cost reduction [29]. Furthermore, recent studies have shown that the single-position lateral decubitus framework does not lead to a loss of radiological correction or worse clinical outcomes than dual-position surgery does [30]. Although significant improvements are being achieved with the use of single-position lateral surgery, one key drawback of this approach lies in the challenges of performing posterior fixation and other posterior maneuvers in a lateral decubitus position, which might present challenges in cases requiring additional direct decompression or facet release [31].

Conflict of Interests Dr. Luiz Pimenta, Dr. Rodrigo Amaral, and Gabriel Pokorny receive consultancy fees from Atec spine.

References

1. Ozgur BM, Aryan HE, Pimenta L, Taylor WR. Extreme lateral Interbody fusion (XLIF): a novel surgical technique for anterior lumbar interbody fusion. Spine J. 2006;6:435–43.
2. Pimenta L, Marchi L, Oliveira L, Fortti F, Coutinho E, Jensen R, Amaral R. History and rationale for the minimally invasive lateral approach. In: Lateral access minimally invasive spine surgery; 2017. p. 3–9.
3. White MD, Uribe JS. Transpsoas approaches to the lumbar spine: lateral and prone. Neurosurg Clin N Am. 2023;34:609–17.
4. Pimenta L, Tohmeh A, Jones D, Amaral R, Marchi L, Oliveira L, Pittman BC Jr, Bae H. Rational decision making in a wide scenario of different minimally invasive lumbar interbody fusion approaches and devices. J Spine Surg. 2018;4:142–55.
5. Amaral R, Pokorny G, Alvernia JE, Pimenta L. L4-L5 anatomy classification system for lateral lumbar interbody fusion. Neurosurg Rev. 2024; https://doi.org/10.1007/S10143-024-02740-2.
6. Marchi L, Abdala N, Oliveira L, Amaral R, Coutinho E, Pimenta L. Radiographic and clinical evaluation of cage subsidence after stand-alone lateral interbody fusion. J Neurosurg Spine. 2013;19:110–8.
7. Alluri RK, Vaishnav AS, Sivaganesan A, Ricci L, Sheha E, Qureshi SA. Multimodality intraoperative neuromonitoring in lateral lumbar Interbody fusion: a review of alerts in 628 patients. Global Spine J. 2021;21925682211000320.
8. Tohmeh A, Somers C, Howell K. Saphenous somatosensory-evoked potentials monitoring of femoral nerve health during prone transpsoas lateral lumbar interbody fusion. Eur Spine J. 2022;31:1658–66.
9. Jiang L, Liu L, Dong L, Xu Z, Zhang X, Qian L. Comparison of instrumented and stand-alone lateral lumbar interbody fusion for lumbar degenerative disease: a systematic review and meta-analysis. BMC Musculoskelet Disord. 2024;25:108. https://doi.org/10.1186/S12891-024-07214-6.

10. Kou N, Zhang R, Liu F, Zhou H, Ren L. Efficacy and safety of lateral lumbar interbody fusion for lumbar degenerative diseases with or without auxiliary posterior fixation: a meta-analysis and systematic review. BMC Musculoskelet Disord. 2025;26:147. https://doi.org/10.1186/S12891-024-08094-6.
11. Elowitz EH, Yanni DS, Chwajol M, Starke RM, Perin NI. Evaluation of indirect decompression of the lumbar spinal canal following minimally invasive lateral transpsoas interbody fusion: radiographic and outcome analysis. Minim Invasive Neurosurg. 2011;54:201–6.
12. Oliveira L, Marchi L, Coutinho E, Pimenta L. A radiographic assessment of the ability of the extreme lateral interbody fusion procedure to indirectly decompress the neural elements. Spine (Phila Pa 1976). 2010; https://doi.org/10.1097/BRS.0B013E3182022DB0.
13. Nikaido T, Konno SI. Usefulness of lateral lumbar Interbody fusion combined with indirect decompression for degenerative lumbar spondylolisthesis: a systematic review. Medicina (Lithuania). 2022; https://doi.org/10.3390/MEDICINA58040492.
14. Kirnaz S, Navarro-Ramirez R, Gu J, et al. Indirect decompression failure after lateral lumbar Interbody fusion—reported failures and predictive factors: systematic review. Global Spine J. 2020;10:8S.
15. Lang G, Perrech M, Navarro-Ramirez R, Hussain I, Pennicooke B, Maryam F, Avila MJ, Härtl R. Potential and limitations of neural decompression in extreme lateral Interbody fusion—a systematic review. World Neurosurg. 2017;101:99–113.
16. Wang TY, Nayar G, Brown CR, Pimenta L, Karikari IO, Isaacs RE. Bony lateral recess stenosis and other radiographic predictors of failed indirect decompression via extreme lateral interbody fusion: multi-institutional analysis of 101 consecutive spinal levels. World Neurosurg. 2017;106:819–26.
17. Ko MJ, Park SW, Kim YB. Correction of spondylolisthesis by lateral lumbar interbody fusion compared with transforaminal lumbar Interbody fusion at L4–5. J Korean Neurosurg Soc. 2019;62:422.
18. Goyal A, Kerezoudis P, Alvi MA, Goncalves S, Bydon M. Outcomes following minimally invasive lateral transpsoas interbody fusion for degenerative low grade lumbar spondylolisthesis: a systematic review. Clin Neurol Neurosurg. 2018;167:122–8.
19. Xu DS, Bach K, Uribe JS. Minimally invasive anterior and lateral transpsoas approaches for closed reduction of grade II spondylolisthesis: initial clinical and radiographic experience. Neurosurg Focus. 2018; https://doi.org/10.3171/2017.10.FOCUS17574.
20. Takami M, Taiji R, Okada M, Minamide A, Hashizume H, Yamada H. Lateral lumbar interbody fusion after reduction using the percutaneous pedicle screw system in the lateral position for Meyerding grade II spondylolisthesis: a preliminary report of a new lumbar reconstruction strategy. BMC Musculoskelet Disord. 2021; https://doi.org/10.1186/S12891-020-03935-6.
21. Diebo BG, Singh M, Balmaceno-Criss M, et al. Defining modern iatrogenic flatback syndrome: examination of segmental lordosis in short lumbar fusion patients undergoing thoracolumbar deformity correction. Eur Spine J. 2024;33:4627–35.
22. Ahlquist S, Park HY, Gatto J, Shamie AN, Park DY. Does approach matter? A comparative radiographic analysis of spinopelvic parameters in single-level lumbar fusion. Spine J. 2018;18:1999–2008.
23. Gambhir S, Wang T, Pelletier MH, Walsh WR, Ball JR. How does cage lordosis influence postoperative segmental lordosis in lumbar Interbody fusion. World Neurosurg. 2019;126:e606–11.
24. Otsuki B, Fujibayashi S, Takemoto M, Kimura H, Shimizu T, Murata K, Matsuda S. Analysis of the factors affecting lumbar segmental lordosis after lateral lumbar interbody fusion. Spine (Phila Pa 1976). 2020;45(14):E839–46. https://doi.org/10.1097/BRS.0000000000003432.
25. Sembrano JN, Horazdovsky RD, Sharma AK, Yson SC, Santos ERG, Polly DW. Do lordotic cages provide better segmental lordosis versus nonlordotic cages in lateral lumbar interbody fusion (LLIF)? Clin Spine Surg. 2017;30:E338–43.
26. Huo CW, Malham GM, Biddau DT, Chung T, Wang YY. Lateral lumbar Interbody fusion using expandable vs static titanium interbody cages: a prospective cohort study of clinical and radiographic outcomes. Int J Spine Surg. 2023;17:265–75.
27. Zakko P, Whaley JD, Preston G, Park DK. Expandable vs static interbody devices for lateral lumbar Interbody fusion. Int J Spine Surg. 2022;16:S53.
28. Beyer RS, Shooshani T, Batista B, Fraipont GM, Pooladzandi O, Brown NJ, Pennington Z, Pham MH. Static versus expandable cages in minimally invasive lateral lumbar interbody fusion. Clin Spine Surg. 2024; https://doi.org/10.1097/BSD.0000000000001737.
29. Guiroy A, Carazzo C, Camino-Willhuber G, Gagliardi M, Fernandes-Joaquim A, Cabrera JP, Menezes C, Asghar J. Single-position surgery versus lateral-then-prone-position circumferential lumbar Interbody fusion: a systematic literature review. World Neurosurg. 2021;151:e379–86.
30. Hiyama A, Katoh H, Sakai D, Sato M, Tanaka M, Watanabe M. Comparison of radiological changes after single- position versus dual- position for lateral interbody fusion and pedicle screw fixation. BMC Musculoskelet Disord. 2019; https://doi.org/10.1186/S12891-019-2992-3.
31. Hiyama A, Katoh H, Sakai D, Sato M, Tanaka M, Watanabe M. Accuracy of percutaneous pedicle screw placement after single-position versus dual-position insertion for lateral Interbody fusion and pedicle screw fixation using fluoroscopy. Asian Spine J. 2022;16:20–7.

Prone Lateral Lumbar Spine Surgery

32

Luiz Pimenta, Gabriel Pokorny, Jullyene Pokorny, Fernando Marcelino, Igor Barreira, Rafael Moriguchi, and Rodrigo Amaral

Introduction

The prone transpsoas (PTP) approach, first formally described by Luiz Pimenta and William Taylor in 2020, emerged as a modification of the traditional lateral lumbar interbody fusion (LLIF) technique. An earlier study in 2019 had already reported radiological outcomes from patients undergoing this approach. The main motivation for transitioning from lateral to prone decubitus was to address two persistent challenges: the limited ability to perform posterior instrumentation in a single position and the restricted capacity to restore lumbar lordosis in the lateral position. This shift in patient positioning also necessitated several technical adjustments to ensure procedural safety and efficacy [1, 2].

Over the past 5 years, literature has increasingly highlighted the advantages of PTP compared to the lateral decubitus technique. Prone positioning, when combined with appropriate surgical tables and supports, has been shown to significantly improve both lumbar and distal lordosis. Additionally, some studies suggest that this position facilitates a posterior shift of the lumbar plexus, potentially expanding the safe working zone, particularly at the L4–L5 level. Beyond positional benefits, recent data indicates that PTP results in greater segmental lordosis restoration than the traditional lateral approach [3–5].

The indications for PTP are largely consistent with those for standard LLIF, including degenerative disc disease, instability, and deformity correction. However, the enhanced access and anatomical modifications in the prone position may broaden indications to include more complex spinal deformities and anatomically challenging cases, such as high iliac crests at L4–L5. Studies by Drossopoulos (2024) and White (2023) support this expanded scope of application. This adaptability places the PTP as a promising option in advanced spinal reconstruction [6, 7].

While most contraindications remain the same as traditional LLIF, such as severe obesity or previous retroperitoneal surgery, PTP introduces additional considerations such as inability to safely place a patient in the prone position, particularly in cases with severe vascular abnormalities, which represents a key limitation. Nonetheless, the use of advanced positioning tables like Jackson or Allen can mitigate these issues.

Interestingly, one traditional contraindication to the traditional lateral access, severe central canal stenosis or bony stenosis, may be less relevant in PTP, as it allows for direct decompression in the same surgical position (Table 32.1) [7–9].

L. Pimenta · G. Pokorny · J. Pokorny (✉) ·
F. Marcelino · I. Barreira · R. Moriguchi · R. Amaral
Instituto de Patologia da Coluna, São Paulo, Brazil
e-mail: lpimenta@patologiadacoluna.com.br

A. A. Baaj et al. (eds.), *Surgery of the Lumbar Spine*, https://doi.org/10.1007/978-3-032-18097-1_32

Table 32.1 Indications and contraindications for the prone lateral interbody fusion technique

Indications	Contraindications (Absolute)
Foraminal and central stenosis	*Absolute contraindications*
Degenerative disc disease	L5–S1 level
Low-grade spondylolisthesis (Grade I and II)	Transitional anatomy (L5–S1-like configuration)
Pseudarthrosis and revision surgeries	
Degenerative scoliosis	Very anterior psoas muscle or excessively high iliac crest (on both access sides)
Adult spinal deformity	
As an adjunct in cases of severe malalignment	
As a primary approach in cases of moderate to mild malalignment (with or without anterior release)	Conditions that prevent prone positioning
Cases where the capacity for adequate indirect decompression via lateral approach in lateral decubitus is uncertain	High-grade fibrosis in both lateral corridors
Discitis	
Fractures	
Tumors	
Relative contraindications (potentially solvable in prone position)	
Very severe central stenosis or posterior element stenosis *(May be addressed with direct decompression in the same prone position, if necessary)*	
Anteriorly positioned psoas/lumbar plexus (in non-transitional anatomy) *(the psoas muscle, and the plexus, may retract posteriorly when the patient is positioned prone)*	
Facet cysts *(may be treated with direct decompression and segmental stabilization in the same position)*	
Bony stenosis of the lateral recess *(Main cause of indirect decompression failure* [10, 11]. Might be treated in the same position with direct decompression*)*	

Preoperative Planning

Preoperative planning and the step-by-step approach for the prone transpsoas (PTP) technique are based on key publications [1, 12, 13], Imaging studies are essential for surgical planning.

Standing X-rays are crucial for evaluating coronal and sagittal alignment and determining the segmental lordosis needed. They also help identify the preferred side for the surgical approach in patients with coronal deformities. Lateral flexion-extension lumbar radiographs are used to assess dynamic instability, potentially indicating the need for circumferential fusion.

MRI provides important information about stenotic levels, psoas morphology, and lumbar plexus position relative to the disc, aiding in predicting the success of indirect decompression and identifying instability signs such as facet joint fluid. MRI is also useful in evaluating tumors, fractures, and infections.

CT scans are particularly valuable in revision cases or when assessing tumors, fractures, or vascular variants, especially when used as angio-CT. These images help refine the surgical approach and assess bone quality and structural changes that may impact implant choice or surgical risk.

Regarding the side of approach, routes with prior fibrosis or altered psoas or vascular anatomy should be avoided. In patients with transitional anatomy or significantly anterior psoas positioning, often seen in deformities associated with hip or lower limb abnormalities, those sides should also be avoided. For degenerative scoliosis, approaching from the concave side is preferred, as it allows better correction of coronal deformity, easier access to multiple levels through a single incision, and more effective foraminal decompression. The concave side typically offers more flexibility due to direct rupture of ipsilateral osteophytes and is more likely to show foraminal narrowing [12, 13].

Surgical Steps

Step 1: Incision Planning

Using intraoperative fluoroscopy, the lateral incision is planned similarly to standard LLIF in lateral decubitus. Posterior incisions (midline or paramedian for percutaneous screws) are also mapped. When using CT-based navigation for pedicle screw placement, the reference is anchored on the posterior superior iliac spine. In these cases, posterior instrumentation is ideally placed before interbody work to preserve navigation accuracy.

Step 2: Retroperitoneal Access

After the flank incision, blunt dissection proceeds through subcutaneous layers and abdominal muscles to reach the retroperitoneal space. In the prone position, reaching the psoas is more challenging due to the greater depth from skin to spine. Letting the abdomen hang freely can reduce intra-abdominal pressure and shorten the working corridor, especially in obese patients. The psoas is accessed by palpating the quadratus lumborum and transverse process; gravity helps shift the peritoneum ventrally, creating a safe path (Fig. 32.1).

Step 3: Dilator and Retractor Placement

With the psoas identified, a dilator is advanced under fluoroscopy toward the disc space, aiming two-thirds from the posterior border. A K-wire is inserted, followed by sequential dilators. Triggered EMG monitors nerve proximity—values <5 mA suggest direct nerve contact, 5–10 mA indicate closeness, and ≥11 mA suggest safe distance. Adjust if thresholds are ≤10 mA. The retractor is inserted and secured, compensating for anterior shift due to gravity. Ensure it is orthogonal to the disc and parallel to the floor (Fig. 32.2).

Step 4: Discectomy

The table may be rotated 10–20° away from the surgeon for ergonomic access, but the C-arm must be adjusted to maintain parallel endplate visualization. The disc is removed using pituitary rongeurs, curettes, and scrapers, avoiding endplate violation to prevent subsidence. Preserve the anterior annulus near the anterior longitudinal ligament (ALL) to minimize rupture risk. Fluoroscopy confirms depth and alignment.

Step 5 and 6: Interbody Device Insertion

Trial implants are used to determine the optimal cage size, beginning conservatively. Oversizing risks subsidence. Once the correct size is chosen,

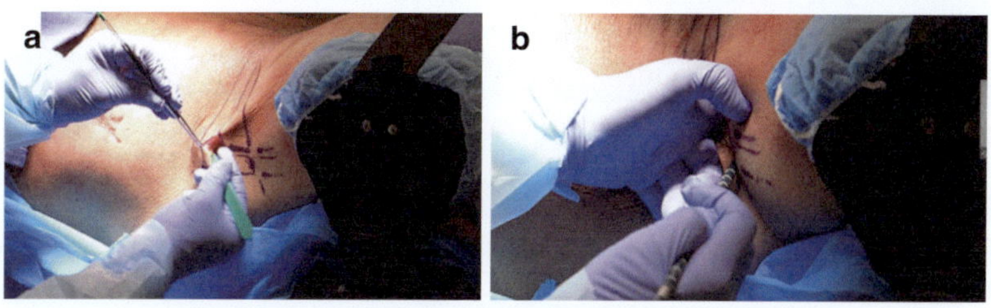

Fig. 32.1 Retroperitoneal access. (**a**) Ample dissection, keep posterior until reaching the *quadratus lumborum*. (**b**) Use of the index finger to guide the first-dilator

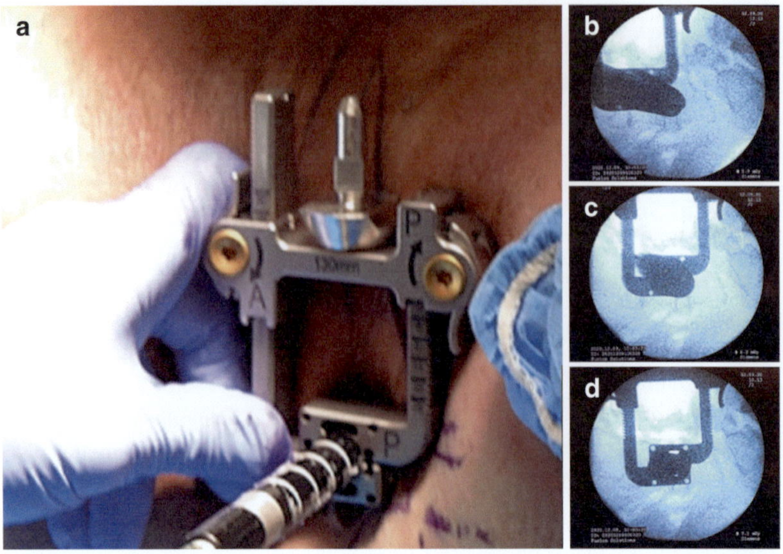

Fig. 32.2 Dilators and retractor placement. (**a**) Retractor placement. (**b** and **c**) Retractor present some angulation. (**d**) Correct orthogonal position

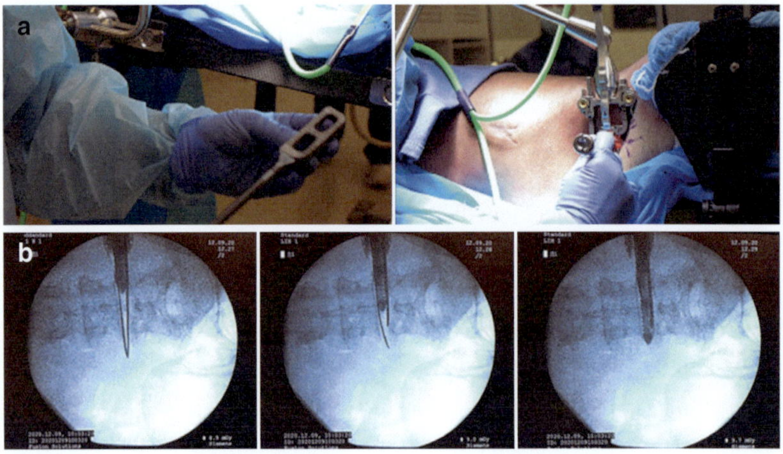

Fig. 32.3 Cage placement steps. (**a**) Cage preparation and placement. (**b**) Fluoroscopy-guidance to evaluate correct position of the cage

the final cage (with graft) is inserted. In prone, mallet force can push the retractor forward; an assistant or strong retractor arms help maintain position. AP fluoroscopy ensures parallel insertion. Larger footprints (22–30 mm) reduce subsidence. For small vertebral bodies, shorter cages may allow better compression and segmental lordosis (Fig. 32.3).

Step 7: Retractor Removal and Wound Closure

After cage placement, the area is irrigated, and the retractor is gently removed. Bipolar cautery is used to manage bleeding. The fascia is closed with 0–0 sutures, subcutaneous tissue with 3–0, and skin with a subcuticular suture and glue. Posterior pedicle screws are then placed percutaneously or via a mini-open Wiltse approach.

Key Technical Considerations

Retractor Time Nerve injury risk, especially femoral nerve at L4-L5, increases with prolonged retraction. Keep retraction time under 15 minutes per level, with periodic releases. However, it is important to notice that neuromonitoring is essential, as deficits can occur even before 20 minutes [14].

Navigation and Robotics While intraoperative navigation and robotics offer promising precision and reduced radiation exposure, their routine use for interbody work remains under evaluation. Fluoroscopy remains the gold standard, though newer platforms are being developed for full procedure assistance [6, 8].

Complications

The complication profile of the prone transpsoas lateral interbody fusion (PTP) technique is similar to that of the traditional lateral decubitus LLIF. The most common adverse events include transient weakness of the psoas muscle or lumbar plexus. Pimenta et al. (2021) demonstrated that early adopters of the PTP approach experienced complication rates comparable to those seen in traditional LLIF. These findings were later supported by Soliman et al. (2023), who confirmed similar complication patterns in their series [15, 16].

Neurological complications are best mitigated through the use of intraoperative neuromonitoring, especially with multimodal strategies, which have shown greater efficacy. Although keeping intrapsoas retraction time under 20 minutes can help reduce nerve injury risk, it does not fully eliminate the possibility of neurological changes [17].

Vascular injuries, while uncommon, are most effectively avoided by preserving the anterior longitudinal ligament (ALL) and exercising caution during discectomy and interbody device insertion, particularly on the contralateral side in lower lumbar levels or when the psoas muscle is anteriorly positioned.

Visceral complications are extremely rare. Ensuring that the dissection remains in the retroperitoneal space is key to preventing injury [16, 18]. Although some studies have raised concerns about intestinal loops potentially being in the surgical path, this risk is largely theoretical. As long as a proper retroperitoneal dissection is performed, the likelihood of visceral injury is negligible—even when loops appear near the access side [19].

Conflict of Interests Dr. Luiz Pimenta, Dr. Rodrigo Amaral, and Gabriel Pokorny receive consultancy fees from Atec spine.

References

1. Pimenta L, Taylor WR, Stone LE, Wali AR, Santiago-Dieppa DR. Prone transpsoas technique for simultaneous single position access to the anterior and posterior spine. Oper Neurosurg. 2020.
2. Smith TG, Joseph SA Jr, Ditty B, Amaral R, Tohmeh A, Taylor WR, et al. Initial multi-centre clinical experience with prone transpsoas lateral interbody fusion: feasibility, perioperative outcomes, and lessons learned. N Am Spine Soc J (NASSJ). 2021;6:100056.
3. Pimenta L, Pokorny G, Amaral R, Ditty B, Batista M, Moriguchi R, et al. Single-position prone transpsoas lateral interbody fusion including L4L5: early postoperative outcomes. World Neurosurg [Internet]. 2021 May 1 [cited 2021 May 24];149. Available from: https://pubmed.ncbi.nlm.nih.gov/33548532/.
4. Smith TG, Pollina J, Joseph SA, Howell KM. Effects of surgical positioning on L4-5 accessibility and lumbar lordosis in lateral transpsoas lumbar interbody fusion: a comparison of prone and lateral decubitus in asymptomatic adults. World Neurosurg. 2021;149:e705–13.
5. McDermott MR, Rogers M, Prior R, Mixa J, Garrett J, Michna R, et al. Analyzing the L4-5 segmental alignment change of two minimally invasive prone-based interbody fusions. Glob Spine J. 2025;15(3):1823–31.
6. Drossopoulos PN, Bardeesi A, Wang TY, Huang CC, Ononogbu-uche FC, Than KD, et al. Advancing prone-transpsoas spine surgery: a narrative review and evolution of indications with representative cases. J Clin Med. 2024;13:1112 [Internet]. 2024 Feb 16 [cited 2024 Oct 17];13(4):1112. Available from: https://www.mdpi.com/2077-0383/13/4/1112/htm.
7. White MD, Uribe JS. Transpsoas approaches to the lumbar spine: lateral and prone. Neurosurg Clin N Am. 2023;34(4):609–17.
8. Giraldo JP, Choy W, Uribe JS. Prone lateral transpsoas approach to the spine: a technical guide for mastery. Int J Spine Surg [Internet]. 2025 Feb 24 [cited 2025 Jun 15];19(S1):S19–27. Available from: http://www.ncbi.nlm.nih.gov/pubmed/39819681.
9. Garg B, Bansal T, Mehta N, Sharan AD. Patient positioning in spine surgery: what spine surgeons should know? Asian Spine J. 2023;17(4):770–81.
10. Wang TY, Nayar G, Brown CR, Pimenta L, Karikari IO, Isaacs RE. Bony lateral recess stenosis and other

radiographic predictors of failed indirect decompression via extreme lateral interbody fusion: multi-institutional analysis of 101 consecutive spinal levels. World Neurosurg. 2017;106:819–26.
11. Kirnaz S, Navarro-Ramirez R, Gu J, Wipplinger C, Hussain I, Adjei J, et al. Indirect decompression failure after lateral lumbar interbody fusion—reported failures and predictive factors: systematic review. Glob Spine J [Internet]. 2020 Apr 1 [cited 2025 Jun 10];10(2 Suppl):8S. Available from: https://pmc.ncbi.nlm.nih.gov/articles/PMC7263336/.
12. Wegner AM, Prior DM, Klineberg EO. Minimally invasive lateral approach for the management of adult degenerative scoliosis. Instr Course Lect. 2017;66:367–77.
13. Castro C, Oliveira L, Amaral R, Marchi L, Pimenta L. Is the lateral transpsoas approach feasible for the treatment of adult degenerative scoliosis? Clin Orthop Relat Res. 2014;472(6):1776–83.
14. Tohmeh A, Somers C, Howell K. Saphenous somatosensory-evoked potentials monitoring of femoral nerve health during prone transpsoas lateral lumbar interbody fusion. Eur Spine J. 2022;31(7):1658–66.
15. Pimenta L, Pokorny G, Pokorny J, Marcelino F, Moriguchi R, Barreira I, et al. Survey of major complications after prone transpsoas surgery: an analysis of early adopters' practice. Neurosurg Rev [Internet]. 2024 Dec 1 [cited 2024 Sep 2];47(1):1–5. Available from: https://link.springer.com/article/10.1007/s10143-024-02500-2.
16. Soliman MAR, Diaz-Aguilar L, Kuo CC, Aguirre AO, Khan A, San Miguel-Ruiz JE, et al. Complications of the prone transpsoas lateral lumbar interbody fusion for degenerative lumbar spine disease: a multicenter study. Neurosurgery [Internet]. 2023 Nov 1 [cited 2024 Mar 19];93(5):1106–11. Available from: https://journals.lww.com/neurosurgery/fulltext/2023/11000/complications_of_the_prone_transpsoas_lateral.19.aspx.
17. Choy W, Serur X, Giraldo JP, Uribe JS. Single-position prone Transpsoas lateral interbody fusion at L4-L5: technical pearls. Neurosurgery. 2025;96(3):S3–8.
18. Farber SH, Valenzuela Cecchi B, O'Neill LK, Chapple KM, Zhou JJ, Alan N, et al. Complications associated with single-position prone lateral lumbar interbody fusion: a systematic review and pooled analysis. J Neurosurg Spine. 2023;39(3):380–6.
19. Wang YY, Pokorny G, Dawes B. Bowel position does not preclude safe access in prone trans-psoas surgery. Neurosurg Rev [Internet]. 2025 Dec 1 [cited 2026 Jan 12];48(1). Available from: https://pubmed.ncbi.nlm.nih.gov/41071387/.

Anterior Lumbar Interbody Fusion (ALIF)

33

Alfredo Guiroy, Matías Orellana, Alfredo Sícoli, and Cristiano Menezes

Introduction

The first articles describing an anterior approach to lumbar spinal fusion were published by Capener [1] in 1932 and Burns [2] in 1933. Both used a transperitoneal approach. It was not until 1944 that Iwahara used the retroperitoneal approach [3]. The next significant milestone in development came in 1992, with the incorporation of instrumentation and cylindrical cages [4].

This approach has the advantages of limiting the need to disrupt the posterior spinal column while allowing broad exposure of the disc space for placing a large interbody graft (reducing the risk of cage subsidence), shorter operating times, less blood loss, indirect decompression of neural tissue, restoration of disc/foraminal height, and correction of sagittal alignment [5, 6].

A. Guiroy (✉) · M. Orellana · A. Sícoli
Clínica de Cuyo, Mendoza, Argentina

C. Menezes
Federal University of Minas Gerais (UFMG), Belo Horizonte, Brazil
e-mail: cristiano@vertebral.com.br

Indications

- Lumbar degenerative disc disease
- Degenerative or lytic spondylolisthesis
- Anterior column support in long fusion constructs
- Restoration of lumbar lordosis
- Pseudoarthrosis following posterior lumbar fusion
- Lumbar fusions with a high risk of pseudoarthrosis
- Trauma
- Tumors
- Spondylodiscitis

Limitations

- Anatomical: location of vascular bifurcation, high pelvic incidence [7].
- Advanced atherosclerosis of major abdominal vessels.
- Morbid obesity: distance to the spine and surgical corridor makes the approach challenging.
- History of abdominal surgery, inflammatory bowel disease, radiotherapy: these conditions create significant scarring, increasing the risk of approach-related complications [8].
- Multilevel disc disease (three levels) (in patients without lumbar spinal deformities) [9].

A. A. Baaj et al. (eds.), *Surgery of the Lumbar Spine*, https://doi.org/10.1007/978-3-032-18097-1_33

- Young male patient: due to the risk of retrograde ejaculation (2–5%) [10].
- Central stenosis without listhesis, with normal disc height.
- Osteopenia, osteoporosis: due to the increased risk of subsidence.

Surgical Technique

Preoperative Evaluation

- Patient: age, BMI, comorbidities, history of abdominal surgeries, previous abdominal radiation, or peritoneal infections.

Imaging

- MRI: evaluation of vascular anatomy (bifurcation level and lateralization of major vessels), psoas muscle.
- X-rays: evaluate the pelvic incidence and whether this angle permits an anterior approach (typically, high pelvic incidence patients are challenging as the pubic symphysis limits the disc access angle).

Positioning

The patient is positioned supine on a radiolucent surgical table.

The patient's arms are either abducted or adducted in a cross-chest position to facilitate lateral fluoroscopy.

A cushion may be placed under the lumbar spine to enhance lordosis.

Lateral fluoroscopic imaging indicates the incision level and the disc angle.

Incision

A Pfannenstiel mini-transverse incision is typically used and planned based on the levels to be treated. For L5-S1, the incision is usually two-thirds of the distance between the navel and the pubic symphysis. For L4-L5, the incision is made just below the navel. A vertical paramedian incision may be utilized for higher lumbar levels and multilevel surgeries.

Step-by-Step Procedure

After the skin incision, the dissection proceeds through the subcutaneous tissue until the anterior rectus fascia is identified.

The rectus fascia is incised longitudinally, and the rectus muscle is mobilized laterally.

An incision is made in the posterior rectus fascia or transversalis fascia and dissected to release it from the parietal peritoneum.

The retroperitoneal cavity is bluntly dissected from lateral to medial, and the peritoneal contents are retracted to expose the spine and major vasculature. The psoas muscle should be identified, and a layer of fat containing the ureter must be displaced medially.

At L5-S1, a functional corridor can be achieved between the iliac vessels below the bifurcation of the inferior vena cava and aorta. See Fig. 33.1.

For higher levels, vascular mobilization of the aorta and iliac vessels is required. Retractors are then placed, centered on the disc space to be addressed. At L4-L5, the aorta and inferior vena cava are retracted from left to right. The iliolumbar vein is a critical structure that must be identified and controlled to avoid venous injury during this maneuver. At L5-S1, the iliac veins are retracted laterally, and the middle sacral artery and vein are ligated/coagulated. See Fig. 33.2.

The target disc space is confirmed with fluoroscopy.

The disc is incised with a long-handled No. 10 scalpel, and a broad annulotomy is performed.

A Cobb elevator cleans the plane between the endplate and cartilaginous plate. Pituitaries remove disc fragments.

Curettes are used to scrape the endplates.

Distraction is applied to the disc space with dilators to restore the appropriate height.

A trial implant is inserted to select the best-fit implant. Anteroposterior and lateral radiographs

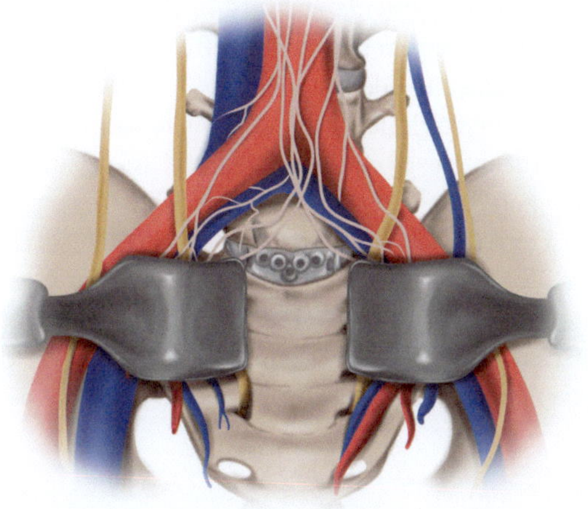

Fig. 33.1 Illustration of the anterior aspect of the spine with the major vessels of the retroperitoneum and the relation with the disc space. Typically, the aorta and cava vein bifurcate at the L4-L5 disc level

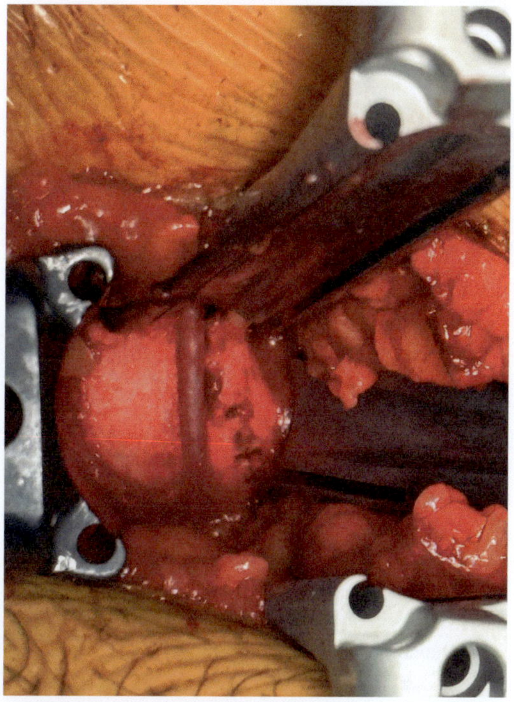

Fig. 33.2 The L5-S1 disc space has been exposed, and the retractors are in place. A prominent anterior sacral artery appears in the midline of the disc space

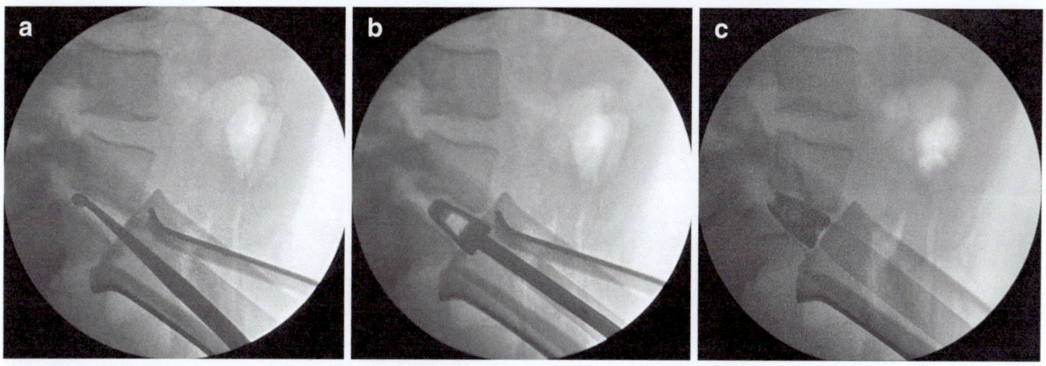

Fig. 33.3 Intraoperative X-rays of an L5-S1 ALIF. (**a**) Disc preparation with curettes to the posterior longitudinal ligament, (**b**) Disc dilation with trial to open the disc space and selection of the proper size implant, and (**c**) Final position of the cage with integrated screws

are taken to confirm depth, position, and lordosis.

The interbody implant is chosen, packed with bone graft, and inserted into the space, guided with fluoroscopy. The implant is secured with screws/plates according to the system used.

After hemostasis, retractors are removed, and the peritoneum is returned to its original position. See Fig. 33.3.

The anterior rectus fascia is closed with thick Vicryl sutures, followed by standard subcutaneous and skin closure.

Results

ALIF fusion rates reach 94.5 ± 5.5% [11].

Significant pain reductions have been reported for various conditions, including spondylosis, spondylolisthesis, and adjacent segment disease [12].

ALIF also achieves excellent restoration of disc height and lumbar lordosis [13].

A debated topic is comparing stand-alone ALIF and ALIF with posterior fixation. Stand-alone ALIFs provide stability in lateral bending and axial rotation but are less effective in flexion and extension. Ideal conditions for stand-alone ALIF are single-level fusions in patients without significant instability or lysis and in relatively low pelvic incidence patients. See Fig. 33.4.

For lythic spondylolisthesis and in high pelvic incidence patients, supplemental posterior fixation offers increased stability, which may not necessarily result in a clinical benefit or detriment [14]. See Fig. 33.5.

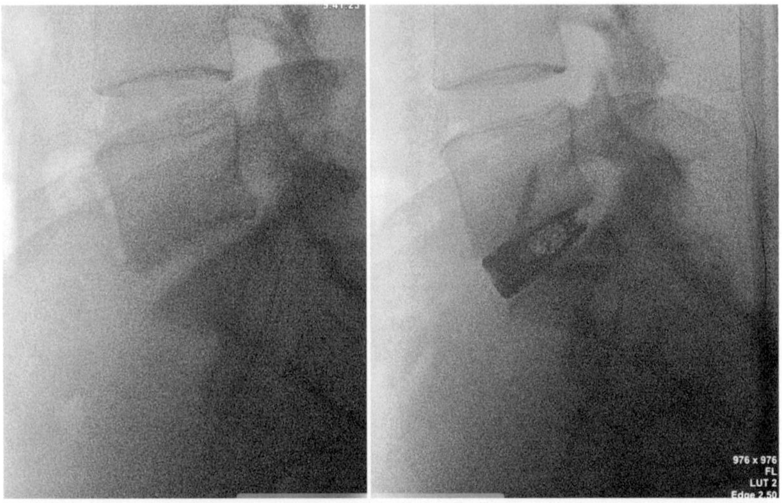

Fig. 33.4 A stand-alone L5-S1 ALIF in a 50-year-old female showed an indirect decompression of the spinal canal and foraminal area and an improvement in segmental lordosis

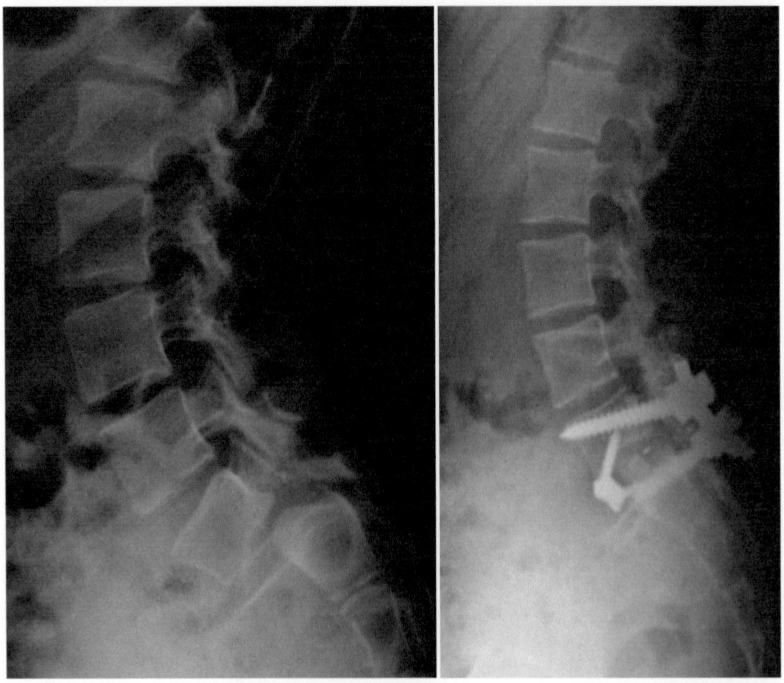

Fig. 33.5 A case example of a high-grade L5-S1 spondylolisthesis in a 15-year-old girl who was treated with segmental circumferential fixation with ALIF and posterior spinal instrumentation. A nice reduction of the slip and the regional kyphosis was obtained

Complications

Predominantly related to surgical access and intra-abdominal exposure [15].

- Retrograde ejaculation (superior hypogastric plexus injury) (2–2.3%).
- Vascular injury (3.03%).
- Deep vein thrombosis (1.4%).
- Hematomas (0.6%).
- Visceral injury (0.37%).
- Incisional hernia (1.3%).
- Wound infection (1.9%).
- Ileus (<5%).
- Dural tears (0.04%).

Postoperative Care

Patients can start drinking clear fluids immediately and rapidly progress with their diet.

They are mobilized on the first postoperative day and then as tolerated.

Hospital stays are usually 2–3 days, depending on the patient's and surgery's specific factors.

Surgical Pearls

- ALIF is the best available strategy for increasing lordosis with high fusion rates.
- Preoperative planning of spinopelvic morphology and vascular anatomy is crucial for minimizing complications.
- Stand-alone ALIF could be a beneficial strategy for certain pathologies, but incorporating posterior pedicle screw fixation provides greater stability.

Contributors' Agreement Alfredo Guiroy: conceptualization, project administration, writing original draft.

Matias Orellana: methodology, writing original draft, review, and editing.

Alfredo Sicoli: review and editing.

Cristiano Menezes: review and editing, supervision.

References

1. Capener N. Spondylolisthesis. Br J Surg. 1932;19(75):374–86.
2. Burns B. An operation for spondylolisthesis. Lancet. 1933;1:1233–9.
3. Iwahara T. A new method of vertebral body fusion. Surg Jpn. 1944;8:271–87.
4. Kuslich SD, Ulstrom CL, Griffith SL, Ahern JW, Dowdle JD. The Bagby and Kuslich method of lumbar interbody fusion. History, techniques, and 2-year follow-up results of a United States prospective, multicenter trial. Spine. 1998;23(11):1267–78.
5. Phan K, Thayaparan GK, Mobbs RJ. Anterior lumbar interbody fusion versus transforaminal lumbar interbody fusion--systematic review and meta-analysis. Br J Neurosurg. 2015;29:705–11.
6. Giang G, Mobbs R, Phan S, et al. Evaluating outcomes of stand-alone anterior lumbar interbody fusion: a systematic review. World Neurosurg. 2017;104:259–71.
7. Inamasu J. Three dimensional computed tomography of the a nal great vessels pertinent to L4-L5 anterior lumbar interbody fusion. Minim Invasive Neurosurg. 2005;48(3):127–31.
8. Osler P, Kim SD, Hess KA, et al. Prior abdominal surgery is associated with an increased risk of postoperative complications after anterior lumbar interbody fusion. Spine. 2014;39(10):E650–6.
9. Mummaneni PV, Haid RW, Rodts GE. Lumbar interbody fusion: state-of-the-art technical advances. Invited submission from the joint section meeting on disorders of the spine and peripheral nerves, March 2004. J Neurosurg Spine. 2004;1(1):24–30.
10. Kuslich SD, Ulstrom CL, Griffith SL, Ahern JW, Dowdle JD. The Bagby and Kuslich method of lumbar interbody fusion. History, techniques, and 2-year follow-up results of a United States prospective, multicenter trial. Spine. 1998;23(11):1267–78; discussion 1279.
11. Formica M, Quarto E, Zanirato A, et al. ALIF in the correction of spinal sagittal misalignment. A systematic review of literature. Eur Spine J. 2021;30(1):50–62.
12. Rao PJ, Loganathan A, Yeung V, et al. Outcomes of anterior lumbar interbody fusion surgery based on indication: a prospective study. Neurosurgery. 2015;76:723; discussion 23–4.
13. Jiang S-D, Chen J-W, Jiang L-S. Which p dure is better for lumbar interbody fusion: anterior lumbar interbody fusion or transforaminal lumbar interbody fusion? Arch Orthop Trauma Surg. 2012;132(9):1259–66.
14. Kiapour A, Massaad E, Joukar A, Hadzipasic M, Shankar GM, Goel VK, et al. Biomechanical analysis of stand-alone lumbar interbody cages versus 360° constructs: an in vitro and finite element investigation. J Neurosurg Spine. 2021;24:1–9.
15. Feeley A, Feeley I, Clesham K, Butler J. Is there a variance in complication types associated with ALIF approaches? A systematic review. Acta Neurochir (Wien). 2021;163(11):2991–3004.

Sacropelvic Fixation Strategies

34

Justin L. Reyes, Prerana Katiyar, Josephine R. Coury, and Zeeshan M. Sardar

Introduction

Sacropelvic fixation has evolved over time with varying techniques to enhance stability and fixation for fusion constructs in spine surgery. For example, the S2-alar-iliac (S2AI) screw technique was just recently described by Dr. Richard E. O'Brien and colleagues in 2007, as a modification of the traditional iliac-only screw. By incorporating the sacrum in pelvic fixation, these screws have improved stability with reduced rates of implant prominence and skin breakdown.

Sacropelvic fixation may be warranted in several scenarios: high-grade spondylolisthesis, sacroiliac (SI) pain or dysfunction, trauma, and long fusion constructs. When sacropelvic fixation is indicated, it is imperative for spinal surgeons to thoroughly assess each patient's bone health, past surgical history, and comorbidities. Additionally, a comprehensive understanding of the patient's individual sacropelvic anatomy, accounting for sacral dysraphism, and spinopelvic alignment is mandatory to maximize the goals of sacropelvic fixation.

In this chapter, we will review the relevant anatomy of the sacrum and pelvis, related biomechanical principles, and principles of lumbopelvic sagittal alignment. Additionally, we will provide an overview of the indications and contraindications related to sacropelvic fixation, relevant instrumentation, and contemporary surgical techniques.

Anatomy and Biomechanics

Transitional anatomy is common at the lumbosacral junction with a sacralized L5 or lumbarized S1 occurring in 25–35% of people [1, 2]. Ankylosis between L5 and S1 can occur at the transverse processes, vertebral bodies, and facet joints [3]. Congenital deformities such as dysraphism of the sacrum are also common. Sacral dysraphism occurs in the event of embryologic failure of closure of the neural tube and can occur as open and closed dysraphism. Open dysraphism exposes neural tissues to the environment via bony anomalies [4]. With closed sacral dysraphism, there is no exposure to the environment because the anomaly is closed by skin.

Additionally, the anatomy of the sacroiliac joint (SIJ) deserves special attention. SIJ pain has been documented to occur in 10–62% of people

J. L. Reyes (✉) · J. R. Coury · Z. M. Sardar
Columbia University Orthopedics,
New York, NY, USA

NewYork-Presbyterian Och Spine Hospital,
New York, NY, USA
e-mail: jlr2268@cumc.columbia.edu;
jrc2243@cumc.columbiaf.edu;
zms2117@cumc.columbia.edu

P. Katiyar
Hospital for Special Surgery, New York, NY, USA
e-mail: katiyarp@hss.edu

A. A. Baaj et al. (eds.), *Surgery of the Lumbar Spine*, https://doi.org/10.1007/978-3-032-18097-1_34

[5]. The SIJ is the largest axial joint in the body with three segments: cranial, middle, and caudal [3, 6]. The S1 (cranial) portion of the SIJ is the largest while the S3 (caudal) segment is the smallest. Anterior and posterior tilt of the SIJ has been shown to affect the L5-S1 facet joints [3]. Additionally, the SIJ has been documented to relieve stress during motion relationships between the axial skeleton and lower limb [3]. SIJ pain tends to be quite common in patients with deformities and degenerative pathologies.

A strong ligamentous complex stabilizes the SIJ ventrally and dorsally. Ventrally, the SIJ is bounded by the thin anterior sacroiliac ligament (ASL) which runs obliquely from the sacral ala to the ilium. Dorsally, the posterior sacroiliac ligament (PSL) runs from the lateral sacrum to the posterior superior iliac spine and the iliac crest. The iliolumbar ligaments run from the transverse processes of L5 to the iliac crest bilaterally. The strong interosseous ligament lies deep to the PSL and connects S1 and S2 to the ilium. The sacrotuberous ligament runs from the sacrum to the ischial tuberosity. The sacrospinous ligament runs posterior to the sacrotuberous ligament and connects the sacrum and coccyx to the ischial spine.

Biomechanically, the lumbosacral junction is subject to high stress forces while the SIJ ligamentous complex acts to transfer large bending moments and compression loads [6]. Dissection of the iliolumbar ligament would disrupt the stability of the L5-S1 segment [6]. The sacrotuberous and sacrospinous ligaments act to prevent anterior sacral tilt which is known as nutation. Anterior sacral tilt is also restricted by the superior portion of the ASL and the inferior aspect of PSL. Most of the PSL acts to resist posterior sacral tilt or counternutation.

Spinopelvic Alignment

Sacropelvic fixation can severely restrict spinopelvic motion and alter postoperative regional and global alignment. In addition to understanding the relevant anatomy of the sacrum and pelvis, appreciation of spinopelvic alignment is paramount. Pelvic incidence (PI) is an important marker of sagittal alignment which is defined as the angle perpendicular to the midpoint of the sacral endplate and the center of the femoral heads [7]. PI is regarded as a static and individualized variable that remains mostly unchanged throughout the lifespan. Two related variables are sacral slope (SS) and pelvic tilt (PT). SS is the angle from the sacral endplate to the horizontal axis, while PT is the angle from the midpoint of the sacrum to the center of the femoral head from the vertical axis. Classically, PI is reported as the summation of both SS and PT. Finally, lumbar lordosis (LL) is an important factor for the surgeon to consider [7]. The relationship between PI and LL has been well documented with the literature highlighting PI-LL “mismatch” greater than ten degrees to be associated with worse health-related quality of life [8]. However, recent literature has challenged this notion with patients who maintain a PI-LL greater than ten degrees having comparable clinical outcomes as those with less than ten degrees [9]. Not only is the total amount of global lordosis important but also the individual segmental lordosis and shape. Recent literature has demonstrated that the distal segments between L4 and S1 encompass the majority of global lordosis [7]. PI has been shown to have a strong correlation with the proximal arc of lordosis [7]. Surgically, key goals related to alignment are to decrease PT, increase SS, and restore lordosis shape both segmentally and globally.

Sacropelvic fixation can alter alignment in several ways depending on the type of fixation. For patients with PI-LL mismatches greater than ten, patients instrumented with S2-alar iliac screws have been shown to compensate through their knees opposed through their pelvis [10]. Additionally, patients with marked PI-LL mismatch, both S2-alar-iliac screws and iliac screws, have been shown to decrease PI-LL significantly [11].

Pelvic Fixation Zones

O'Brien et al. in 2004 created a classification system that is most prominently used today in determining sacropelvic fixation [12]. They described three different zones of fixation. Zone I consists of the S1 body and the cephalad alae. Zone II includes the S2 vertebral body through the coccyx, including the caudal sacral alae. Zone III consists of the bilateral iliacs [12, 13].

The stability of the construct in each zone varies. Zone I rod and/or screw fixation is considered the least biomechanically stable [12, 13]. Typical fixation in this zone includes bicortical pedicle screws placed in the sacral promontory or S1 endplate, converging toward the midline. However, complications of fixation in this zone include high screw pull-out risk as well as high risk of facet fracture [13].

While Zone II would be thought to have more stability, fixations in this zone are not as robust due to low bone density as well as anatomical constraints. Any screws put into the S2 pedicles typically lie dorsal to the biomechanical pivot point, contributing little to stability. More often, fixations in this zone are either augmented with S1 screws or need to be extended further distally into Zone III [13, 14].

Fixation of the iliacs in Zone III is the most biomechanically stable [12, 14]. Instrumentation in this zone allows for fixation anterior to the lumbosacral pivot point, leading to increased stability [15].

Indications and Contraindications

There are various instances in which sacropelvic fixation may be indicated, including fusions extending to the sacrum, correction of pelvic obliquity, grade III or higher spondylolisthesis at the lumbosacral junction (Fig. 34.1), sacral fractures with spinopelvic dissociation, deformities requiring corrective osteotomies (Fig. 34.2), long fusions (>5 levels) including adult degenerative scoliosis, as well as neuromuscular scoliosis (Figs. 34.3 and 34.4) [13, 14, 16]. In deformity surgery, distal sacropelvic fixation has been found to prevent implant failure and pseudarthrosis [16]. In high-grade spondylolisthesis, when reduced, there is increased force on the posteriorly placed implants, and thus sacropelvic fixa-

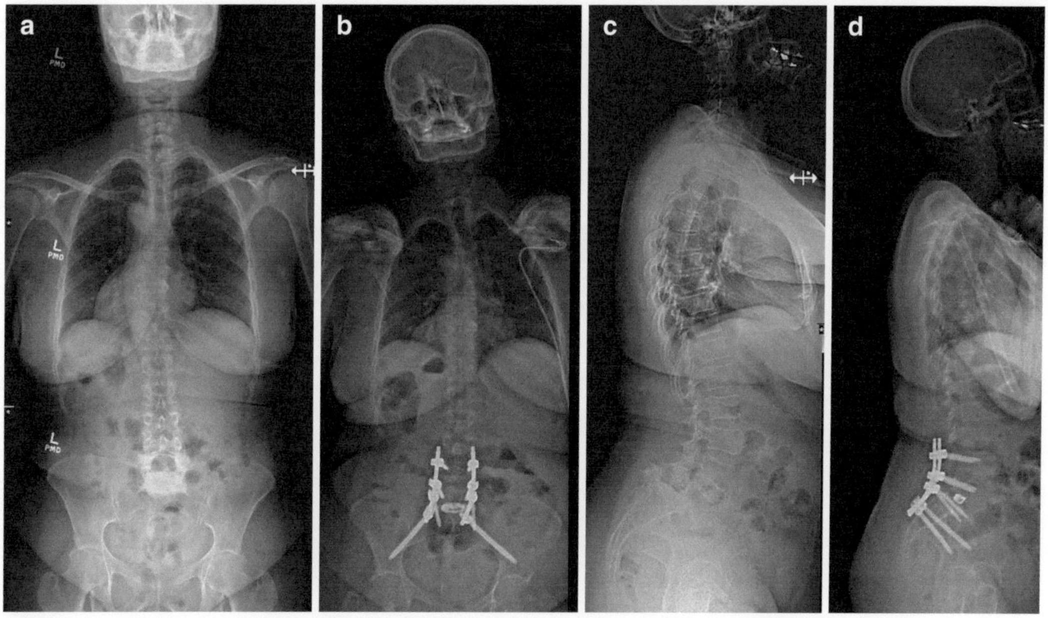

Fig. 34.1 S2AI Screws with High Grade Spondylolisthesis. 58-year-old female with grade 4 spondylolisthesis, s/p reduction and PSIF from L4-Sacrum/Ilium with 1 level TLIF at L5-S1

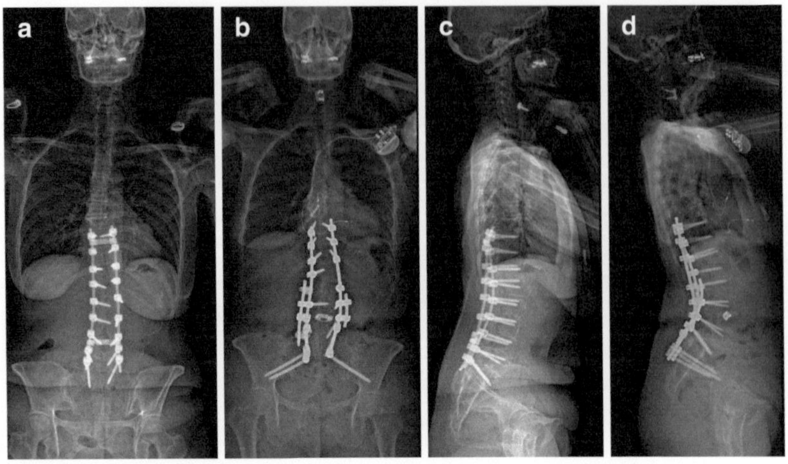

Fig. 34.2 S2AI screws with L3 PSO. A 50 year-old-female with a flatback deformity from prior scoliosis surgery T9-L5 (**a**, **c**). She underwent revision PSIF T9-Sacrum/Ilium with an L3 PSO, with 3 S2AI screws (**b**, **d**)

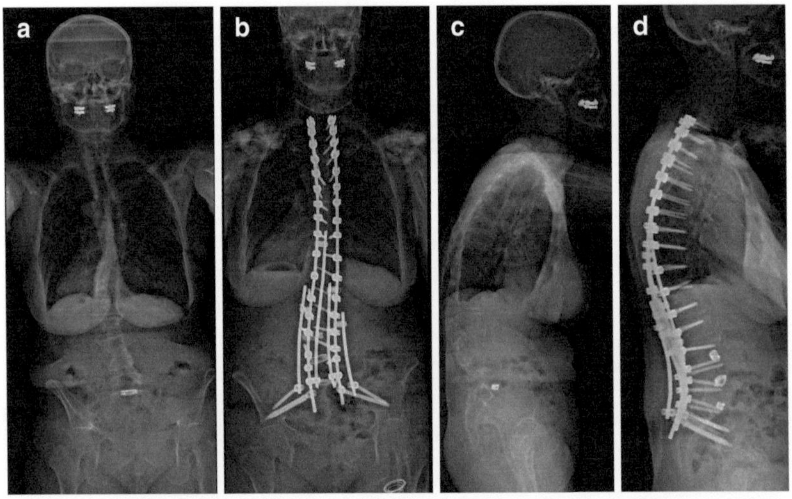

Fig. 34.3 S2AI Screws in Long Constructs. 62 year old female with severe thoracolumbar kyphosis, s/p PSIF T2-Sacrum/Ilium with 4x S2AI Screws, and 6 rods spanning the lumbosacral junction

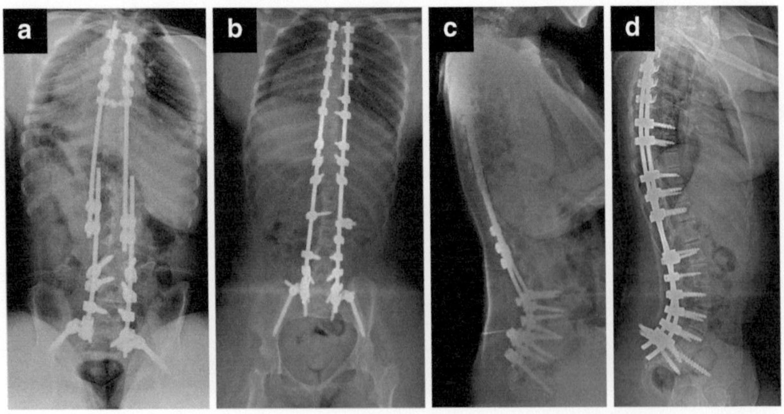

Fig. 34.4 Traditional Iliac Screws. A 14-year-old female with neuromuscular scoliosis with previous history of T3-Sacrum/Ilium spinal arthrodesis (**a**, **c**). She underwent complex revision from T3-Sacrum/ilium with traditional iliac screws (**b**, **d**)

tion is necessary to reduce those forces and stabilize the reduction [14, 16, 17]. Additionally, when constructs terminate at L5 or S1, there is an increased risk of lumbosacral junctional failure [18]. However, sacropelvic fixation with iliac screws can reduce junctional complications at the lumbosacral junction [18]. There is also increased risk of fracture when S1 is the point of fixation of a multi-level fusion construct. In the event of sacral insufficiency fractures, pelvic fixation has been shown to lead to immediate resolution of symptomatology and drastically reduce the likelihood for revision surgery [19].

Long fusions benefit from sacropelvic fixation given the robust flexion and cantilever biomechanics at the lumbosacral junction, requiring a rigid foundation to support the extensive construct [14, 16]. The level at which sacropelvic fixation is indicated is still heavily debated. Some literature suggests fusions extending at or above L2 require sacropelvic fixation for stability [20]. However, other literature argues that sacropelvic fixation is only necessary for fusions extending past the thoracolumbar junction (3–5) [21–23]. Acute pelvic fixation failure can occur for long fusion deformity constructs. Multiple rods and fixation points, at least four points of pelvic fixation, can be used by the surgeon to address pelvic fixation failure [19].

Sacropelvic Screws and Contemporary Fixation Techniques

Spinal instrumentation across the lumbosacral junction has evolved substantially throughout the history of spinal surgery. In the 1960s, Dr. Paul Harrington invented Harrington rod instrumentation to correct post-polio spinal deformities [24]. However, Harrington rods caused flatback deformities and failed to provide adequate support across the lumbosacral junction leading to high rates of pseudarthrosis. Luque and Cotrell-Dubousset instrumentation emerged to address many of the limitations of the Harrington rod but high lumbosacral junctional complications were observed [24]. In 1983, the Galveston technique was the first surgical technique in modern-day spine surgery to include the ilium for lumbosacral fusion [24]. A precontoured L-shape rod was inserted into the posterior superior iliac spine (PSIS) and connected to Luque or Cotrell-Dubousset rod systems [25]. However, high rates of mechanical complications and poor wound healing was associated with this technique [24].

Traditional Iliac Screws

By the late 1990s, sacropelvic fixation changed significantly when Schildhauer introduced traditional iliac screws (IS) to address sacral fractures (Figs. 34.4 and 34.5) [26]. Schildhauer recommended the PSIS as the entry point when placing iliac screws under fluoroscopic guidance [26]. The recommended trajectory for IS placement was from the PSIS to the anterior inferior iliac spine (AIIS). The main advent of the PSIS to AISS trajectory is the possibility to place long screws while mitigating the risk of a breach on the wall of the acetabulum. Iliac screws have remained a prominent fixation tool which is still widely used in contemporary spine surgery.

IS placement is especially useful when a surgeon is considering multiple points of fixation to prevent failure of long constructs. Additionally, iliac screws can be used to supplement "kickstand rod" constructs for patients with severe coronal imbalance (Figs. 34.6 and 34.7) [27]. Makhi et al. described that kickstand rods (KSRs) can be placed in between a thoracolumbar domino and IS [27]. Distraction forces can be applied carefully to secure coronal correction intraoperatively.

There are several known limitations to IS including mechanical complications and damage to anatomical structures related to the sciatic notch, mainly the superior gluteal artery and sciatic nerve [13]. Additionally, due to subperiosteal dissection to insert, there is an increased possibility of infection.

S2-Alar Iliac Screws

S2-alar iliac screws (S2AIs) are another popular form of modern-day sacropelvic fixation. S2AIs arose to address the shortcomings of IS. S2AIs reduce the risk of wound complications and revi-

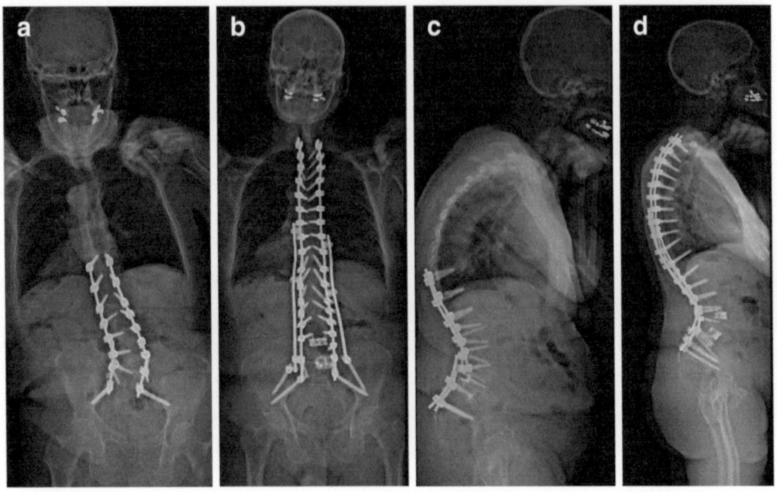

Fig. 34.5 Medial Iliac Screw. A 72-year-old male with previous history of PSF T11-pelvis (**a**, **c**). The patient underwent revision PSIF from T2-S1/ilium. The two proximal pelvic screws are medial iliac screws and the two distal screws are S2AI screws (**b**, **d**)

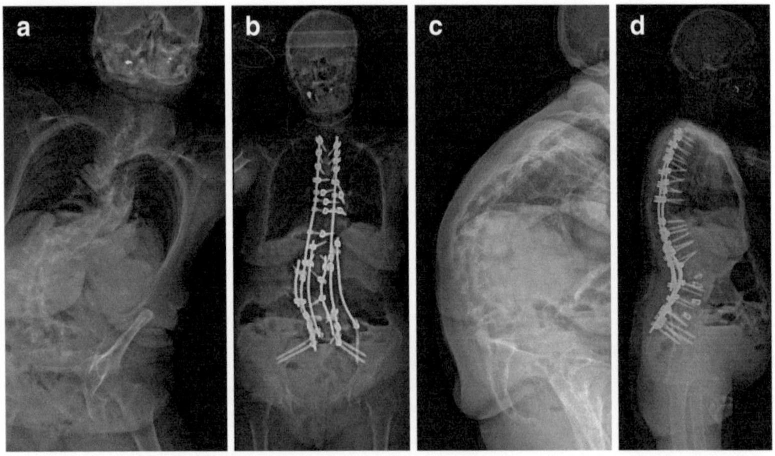

Fig. 34.6 Iliac Screw as Kickstand. A 65-year-old female with adult idiopathic scoliosis, coronal malalignment, and marked thoracic hyperkyphosis (**a**, **c**). The patient underwent PSIF from T2-Sacrum/ilium with an extended L3 PSO (**b**, **d**). She has 4 S2AI screws with 5 rods spanning the lumbosacral junction, in addition to a kickstand iliac screw

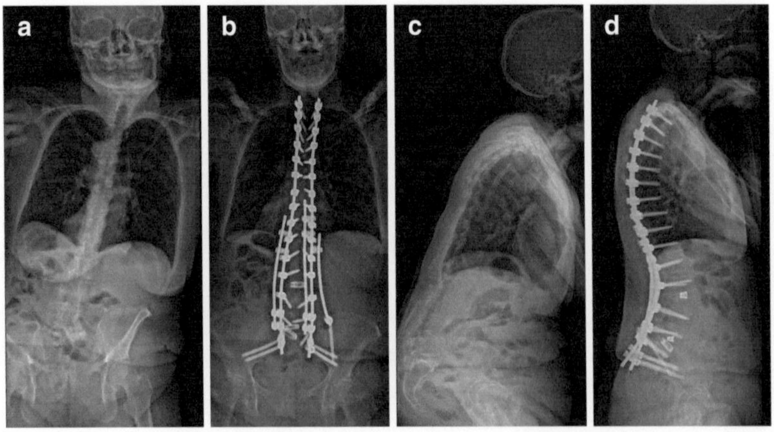

Fig. 34.7 4 S2AI Screws with Kickstand Iliac Screw. A 57-year-old female that underwent PSIF T12-Sacrum/Ilium with 4 iliac screws, with 1 iliac screw used as a kickstand rod

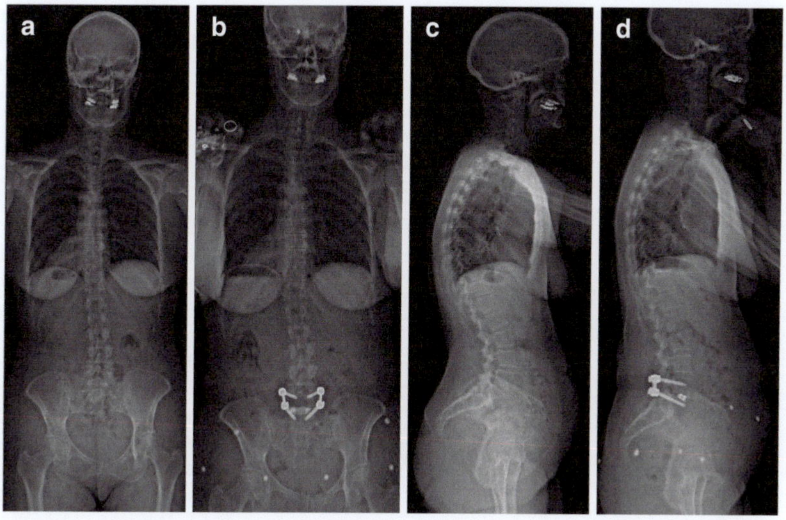

Fig. 34.8 Tricortical S1 Screws. A 54-year-old female with discogenic low back pain (**a**, **c**). She underwent PSIF/TLIF from L5-S1 with tricortical S1 screws (**b**, **d**)

sion rates compared to IS [28, 29]. S2AIs align well with S1 screws allowing for multiple points of fixation in the pelvis for advanced spinal deformities. S1 screws can also be used for single-level cases such as discogenic back pain (Fig. 34.8). S2AIs also align well with multi-rod constructs compared to IS.

S2AIs can be safely instrumented into the pelvis via several entry points—the midpoint between the S1 and S2 dorsal foramen and 1 mm inferolateral to the S1 dorsal foramen [30]. Both freehand techniques and robotic assistance can be used for S2AIs placement.

Robotics and Navigation

Computer-assisted navigation and robotics have been new developments for pedicle screw placement, including placement of Iliac and S2AI screws. While they require pre-operative planning, they have been found to have high accuracy rates and low rates of breaches in the literature.

With navigation, a stereotactic frame is mounted on the spinous process of the lumbar vertebrae and is utilized to find the start point on the CT scan. The CT scan can be obtained preoperatively or intra-operatively and is used to plan the size and trajectory of the screw. However, depth and trajectory must still be free-handed by the surgeon, although the navigation will provide guidance and feedback on the intraoperative depth and trajectory as the screw is being placed [13, 31, 32].

In contrast, robotic pedicle screw placement requires a preoperative CT with 1 mm cuts, as well as intraoperative C-arm x-rays to synchronize positioning with the CT scan. Each vertebra is synchronized individually in case there have been changes in positioning since the preoperative CT. Similar to navigation, the screw size, depth, and trajectory have to be preoperatively planned and registered to the robot. For each screw, the robot arm follows a predetermined plan based on the registration to provide the angle at which the screw needs to be inserted [13, 33–35].

With regard to navigation and robotics, studies have shown anywhere from 95.7% to 100% accuracy in S2AI screw placement [31–36]. Many studies have shown that robotics is as good as, if not more accurate, compared to freehand sacropelvic pedicle screw fixation [33, 36–38]. Compared to freehand techniques though, robotic and navigation-assisted techniques, especially with sacropelvic fixation may decrease operative times as well as radiation exposure [33, 36]. The robot has also been reported to be advantageous in literature to help plan screws relative to each other, to make it easier for the rod to pass through when finalizing constructs (6, 10) [36].

Conflicts/Disclosures None.

References

1. Chiu CK, Chin TF, Chung WH, Chan CYW, Kwan MK. Variations in the number of vertebrae, prevalence of lumbosacral transitional vertebra and prevalence of cervical rib among surgical patients with adolescent idiopathic scoliosis: an analysis of 998 radiographs. Spine (Phila Pa 1976). 2024;49(1):64–70. https://doi.org/10.1097/BRS.0000000000004711.
2. Becker L, Taheri N, Haffer H, et al. Lumbosacral transitional vertebrae influence on acetabular orientation and pelvic tilt. J Clin Med. 2022;11(17):5153. Published 2022 Aug 31. https://doi.org/10.3390/jcm11175153.
3. Vleeming A, Schuenke MD, Masi AT, Carreiro JE, Danneels L, Willard FH. The sacroiliac joint: an overview of its anatomy, function and potential clinical implications. J Anat. 2012;221(6):537–67. https://doi.org/10.1111/j.1469-7580.2012.01564.x.
4. Tortori-Donati P, Rossi A, Cama A. Spinal dysraphism: a review of neuroradiological features with embryological correlations and proposal for a new classification. Neuroradiology. 2000;42(7):471–91. https://doi.org/10.1007/s002340000325.
5. Simopoulos TT, Manchikanti L, Singh V, et al. A systematic evaluation of prevalence and diagnostic accuracy of sacroiliac joint interventions. Pain Physician. 2012;15(3):E305–44.
6. Kiapour A, Joukar A, Elgafy H, Erbulut DU, Agarwal AK, Goel VK. Biomechanics of the sacroiliac joint: anatomy, function, biomechanics, sexual dimorphism, and causes of pain. Int J Spine Surg. 2020;14(Suppl 1):3–13. Published 2020 Feb 10. https://doi.org/10.14444/6077.
7. Le Huec JC, Aunoble S, Philippe L, Nicolas P. Pelvic parameters: origin and significance. Eur Spine J. 2011;20(Suppl 5):564–71. https://doi.org/10.1007/s00586-011-1940-1. Epub 2011 Aug 10. PMID: 21830079; PMCID: PMC3175921.
8. Schwab F, Ungar B, Blondel B, et al. Scoliosis research society—Schwab adult spinal deformity classifcation. Spine. 2012;37:1077–82.
9. Mohanty S, Mikhail C, Lai C, et al. Do adult spinal deformity patients who achieve and maintain PI-LL < 10 have better patient-reported and clinical outcomes compared to patients with PI-LL ≥ 10? A propensity score-matched analysis. Spine Deform. 2024;12(1):209–19. https://doi.org/10.1007/s43390-023-00766-y.
10. Zhi W, Boubez G, Al-Shakfa F, et al. How does Spino-pelvic fixation affect post-operative compensatory mechanisms in adult spinal deformity? Global Spine J. 2025;15(2):548–53. https://doi.org/10.1177/21925682231200832.
11. Rizkallah M, Shen J, Phan P, et al. Can pelvic incidence change after lumbo-pelvic fixation for adult spine deformity, and would the change be affected by the type of pelvic fixation? Spine (Phila Pa 1976). 2024;49(1):E1–7. https://doi.org/10.1097/BRS.0000000000004651.
12. O'Brien MF, Kuklo TR, Lenke LG. Sacropelvic instrumentation: anatomic and biomechanical zones of fixation. Semin Spine Surg. 2004;2(16):76–90.
13. Nanda A, Manghwani J, Kluger PJ. Sacropelvic fixation techniques – Current update [published correction appears in J Clin Orthop Trauma. 2021 Aug 05;21:101558. doi:10.1016/j.jcot.2021.101558]. J Clin Orthop Trauma. 2020;11(5):853–62. https://doi.org/10.1016/j.jcot.2020.07.022.
14. Kebaish KM. Sacropelvic fixation: techniques and complications. Spine (Phila Pa 1976). 2010;35(25):2245–51. https://doi.org/10.1097/BRS.0b013e3181f5cfae.
15. Lombardi JM, Shillingford JN, Lenke LG, Lehman RA. Sacropelvic fixation: when, why, how? Neurosurg Clin N Am. 2018;29(3):389–97. https://doi.org/10.1016/j.nec.2018.02.001.
16. El Dafrawy MH, Raad M, Okafor L, Kebaish KM. Sacropelvic fixation: a comprehensive review. Spine Deform. 2019;7:509–16.
17. Hu SS, Bradford DS, Transfeldt EE, Cohen M. Reduction of high-grade spondylolisthesis using Edwards instrumentation. Spine (Phila Pa 1976). 1996;21(3):367–71. https://doi.org/10.1097/00007632-199602010-00023.
18. Yasuda T, Hasegawa T, Yamato Y, et al. Lumbosacral junctional failures after long spinal fusion for adult spinal deformity-which vertebra is the preferred distal instrumented vertebra? Spine Deform. 2016;4(5):378–84. https://doi.org/10.1016/j.jspd.2016.03.001.
19. Martin CT, Holton KJ, Elder BD, et al. Catastrophic acute failure of pelvic fixation in adult spinal deformity requiring revision surgery: a multicenter review of incidence, failure mechanisms, and risk factors. J Neurosurg Spine. 2022;38(1):98–106. Published 2022 Sep 2. https://doi.org/10.3171/2022.6.SPINE211559.
20. Cunningham BW, Sefter JC, Hu N, Kim SW, Bridwell KH, McAfee PC. Biomechanical comparison of iliac screws versus interbody femoral ring allograft on lumbosacral kinematics and sacral screw strain. Spine (Phila Pa 1976). 2010;35(6):E198–205. https://doi.org/10.1097/BRS.0b013e3181c142bf.
21. Kostuik JP, Errico TJ, Gleason TF. Techniques of internal fixation for degenerative conditions of the lumbar spine. Clin Orthop Relat Res. 1986;203:219–31.
22. Perra JH. Techniques of instrumentation in long fusions to the sacrum. Orthop Clin North Am. 1994;25(2):287–99.
23. VJ, D. Biomechanics and surgical principles of long fusions to the sacrum. Spine State Art Rev. 1996;10:515–44.
24. von Glinski A, Yilmaz E, Godolias P, et al. Historical perspectives on the evolution of Spino-pelvic fixation and its implications on clinical care a narrative review. Global Spine J. 2025;15(1):228–40. https://doi.org/10.1177/21925682241283726.

25. Lonstein JE. The Galveston technique using Luque or Cotrel-Dubousset rods. Orthop Clin North Am. 1994;25(2):311–20.
26. Schildhauer TA, Josten C, Muhr G. Triangular osteosynthesis of vertically unstable sacrum fractures: a new concept allowing early weight-bearing. J Orthop Trauma. 1998;12(5):307–14. https://doi.org/10.1097/00005131-199806000-00002.
27. Makhni MC, Cerpa M, Lin JD, Park PJ, Lenke LG. The "Kickstand Rod" technique for correction of coronal imbalance in patients with adult spinal deformity: theory and technical considerations. J Spine Surg. 2018;4(4):798–802. https://doi.org/10.21037/jss.2018.11.04.
28. Shin HK, Park JH, Jeon SR, et al. Sacropelvic fixation for adult deformity surgery comparing iliac screw and sacral 2 alar-iliac screw fixation: systematic review and updated meta-analysis. Neurospine. 2023;20(4):1469–76. https://doi.org/10.14245/ns.2346654.327.
29. Rahmani R, Stegelmann SD, Andreshak T. S2 alar-iliac screws are superior to traditional iliac screws for spinopelvic fixation in adult spinal deformity: a systematic review and meta-analysis. Spine Deform. 2024;12(3):829–42. https://doi.org/10.1007/s43390-024-00834-x.
30. Yamada K, Abe Y, Satoh S. Safe insertion of S-2 alar iliac screws: radiological comparison between 2 insertion points using computed tomography and 3D analysis software. J Neurosurg Spine. 2018;28(5):536–42. https://doi.org/10.3171/2017.8.SPINE17735.
31. Ray WZ, Ravindra VM, Schmidt MH, Dailey AT. Stereotactic navigation with the O-arm for placement of S-2 alar iliac screws in pelvic lumbar fixation. J Neurosurg Spine. 2013;18(5):490–5. https://doi.org/10.3171/2013.2.SPINE12813.
32. Phan K, Li J, Giang G, et al. A novel technique for placement of sacro-alar-iliac (S2AI) screws by K-wire insertion using intraoperative navigation. J Clin Neurosci. 2017;45:324–7. https://doi.org/10.1016/j.jocn.2017.08.049.
33. Shillingford JN, Laratta JL, Park PJ, et al. Human versus robot: a propensity-matched analysis of the accuracy of free hand versus robotic guidance for placement of S2 alar-iliac (S2AI) screws. Spine (Phila Pa 1976). 2018;43(21):E1297–304. https://doi.org/10.1097/BRS.0000000000002694.
34. Hu X, Lieberman IH. Robotic-guided sacro-pelvic fixation using S2 alar-iliac screws: feasibility and accuracy. Eur Spine J. 2017;26(3):720–5. https://doi.org/10.1007/s00586-016-4639-5.
35. Bederman SS, Hahn P, Colin V, Kiester PD, Bhatia NN. Robotic guidance for S2-alar-iliac screws in spinal deformity correction. Clin Spine Surg. 2017;30(1):E49–53. https://doi.org/10.1097/BSD.0b013e3182a3572b.
36. Khalifeh K, Brown NJ, Pennington Z, Pham MH. Spinal robotics in adult spinal deformity surgery: a systematic review. Neurospine. 2024;21(1):20–9. https://doi.org/10.14245/ns.2347138.569.
37. Naik A, MacInnis BR, Shaffer A, et al. Trends in technology for pedicle screw placement: a temporal meta-analysis. Spine (Phila Pa 1976). 2023;48(11):791–9. https://doi.org/10.1097/BRS.0000000000004604.
38. Matur AV, Palmisciano P, Duah HO, Chilakapati SS, Cheng JS, Adogwa O. Robotic and navigated pedicle screws are safer and more accurate than fluoroscopic freehand screws: a systematic review and meta-analysis. Spine J. 2023;23(2):197–208. https://doi.org/10.1016/j.spinee.2022.10.006.

35 Osteotomies in the Lumbar Spine

Allie Harbert and Cheerag Upadhyaya

Introduction

Spinal deformities in the thoracic and lumbar spine include several disorders resulting in pathologic sagittal and coronal imbalance. Prevalence of spinal deformities continues to increase in adults as the population ages and is estimated to be as high as 68% [1]. This is due to spinal degeneration, poor bone quality, increase in prevalence of comorbidities, and poor posture [2, 3]. Spinal deformities are known to lead to significant pain, neurologic deficits, and have been shown to be associated with a decreased quality of life [2].

A key determination in the workup of spinal deformities is the degree to which they are flexible or rigid. The degree of imbalance, whether the deformity is fixed, and patient-specific spinal anatomy determine the treatment strategy. In rigid deformities, osteotomies are often required for correction and to achieve the goals of deformity correction surgery which include pain reduction and improvement in neurologic deficits when they exist, improved quality of life, and to improve or fully correct spinal curvature and alignment. This chapter will discuss the different types of osteotomies used in the lumbar spine including their indications, technique, and potential complications or pitfalls. The SRS-Schwab classification system is commonly used to describe the types of osteotomies in order of increasing bony removal from 1 to 6 [4]. (Fig. 35.1) Neuromonitoring should be utilized in all cases when performing each osteotomy technique described.

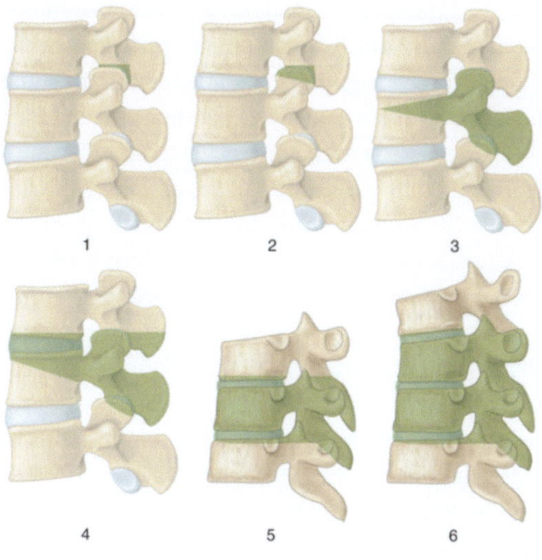

Fig. 35.1 Depiction of the Schwab osteotomy classification. Increasing numbers correlate with increasing amount of bone that is removed [4]

A. Harbert · C. Upadhyaya (✉)
Department of Neurosurgery, University of North Carolina, Chapel Hill, NC, USA
e-mail: allie_harbert@med.unc.edu; Cheerag@unc.edu

A. A. Baaj et al. (eds.), *Surgery of the Lumbar Spine*, https://doi.org/10.1007/978-3-032-18097-1_35

Posterior Column Osteotomies

Posterior column osteotomies (PCO) are indicated in cases of more mild deformity, when the spine is more mobile with intact anterior disc spaces, or when correction is being obtained over many levels to correct gradual kyphotic deformities. Type 1 PCO involves partial resection of the facet (inferior portion) and joint capsule (Fig. 35.1, image 1). The two main types of PCO include the Smith-Peterson osteotomy and Ponte osteotomy. They can also be used in combination with anterior or lateral-based approaches to obtain greater correction and having open/mobile disc spaces is a prerequisite for performing both.

The Smith-Peterson osteotomy (reported as Schwab grade 1 vs. 2 depending on source) was originally used in the lumbar spine when treating patients with ankylosing spondylitis [5]. It involves removing the spinous process, inferior articulating process (IAP) of the chosen level, superior articulating process (SAP) of the level below, and posterior ligaments including supraspinous, interspinous, and ligamentum flavum. This technique corrects sagittal imbalance shortening the posterior column and by expanding the anterior disc space, so a mobile disc is necessary. An anterior graft may be needed in cases of significant correction resulting in significant widening of the disc space [6]. Approximately 10 degrees of correction is obtained per level [7]. Bleeding complications and neurologic deficits are less common than with more extensive osteotomies but there can be neural impingement secondary to foraminal stenosis with significant correction if the facetectomies are not wide enough [5].

The Ponte osteotomy (Schwab grade 2) similarly involves removal of the spinous process, IAP, SAP of the inferior adjacent level, and posterior ligaments, but is performed over multiple consecutive levels to close the posterior elements without opening the anterior disc space (Fig. 35.1, image 2). Mobile discs are necessary. They were traditionally used in treating thoracic kyphosis, specifically Scheuermann's kyphosis [6]. Approximately 5–10 degrees correction can be obtained per level resulting in gradual correction over a longer construct which also results in overall good fusion rates [8]. Success with this technique has been reported using both a combined anterior/posterior approach and posterior only approach [8].

Pedicle Subtraction Osteotomies

Pedicle subtraction osteotomies (PSO) (Schwab grade 3) are three-column osteotomies that involve removal of the spinous processes, lamina, transverse processes, facets, pedicles, and a wedge of vertebral body that does not breach the anterior cortex or disc spaces (Fig. 35.1, image 3). A PSO is most useful in cases of more acute, angled kyphosis rather than more gradual deformities, and most beneficial when performed at the apex of the deformity [6]. They can be utilized in cases where the disc spaces are fused as well as in instances when the patient has already undergone prior fusion [9].

All pedicle screws are placed prior to beginning the osteotomy. The spinous processes, lamina and transverse processes are then removed. Laminectomies are extended to the level above and below the osteotomy to prevent buckling of the spinal cord with correction [9]. Facets are removed to identify and protect existing nerve roots while removing the pedicles. A temporary rod should be placed before removing the wedge of vertebral body using an osteotome, curettes, or rongeurs starting within the cancellous bone, followed by lateral cortex and finally the posterior cortex [9]. After completing the wedge resection, the temporary rod can be loosened to close the created gap by shortening the posterior column. The wedge can be created asymmetrically to achieve correction of coronal deformity as well [6]. Typically, 25–35 degrees of correction can be obtained, and fusion rates are high given the amount of exposed bony surface [7]. A Schwab grade 4 osteotomy is when a PSO is extended to include an endplate of the vertebral body and at least part of the adjacent disc (Fig. 35.1, image 4). This can be advantageous when the apex of the deformity is over the disc space. Anterior support may be necessary depending on the amount of posterior column shortening.

The PSO is associated with higher complication rates in comparison to the PCO. Specifically, there is a high risk of significant blood loss, up to 20% of transient neurologic deficits, and risk of pseudoarthrosis [7, 9, 10].

Vertebral Column Resection

Vertebral column resection (VCR) (Schwab grade 5) includes removing all bone posterior to the posterior longitudinal ligament, the entire vertebral body, and adjacent discs (Fig. 35.1, image 5). A VCR is indicated in cases of severe, rigid multiplanar deformities with significant sagittal and coronal imbalance, cases of spondyloptosis, fixed coronal deformities, and in cases requiring excision of hemivertebra or deformed vertebra secondary to tumor, infection, or congenital anomalies [9]. When the anterior column resection extends past the disc space into an adjacent vertebra it is classified as a Schwab grade 6 (Fig. 35.1, image 6). This can be performed through a posterior-only or combined anterior/posterior approach and anterior reconstruction is often utilized since no bone-on-bone contact is achieved during the procedure. The spine is shortened and translated to improve alignment. Correction of up to 60 degrees can be obtained [11].

The procedure begins with placing all pedicle screws followed by removing the entire posterior column. A temporary rod is placed for stabilization while completing resection of the contralateral pedicle and resecting as much of the vertebral body and adjacent discs as possible using curettes and rongeurs. If necessary, the temporary rod can be moved to the other side to complete resection. The spine can then be mobilized for the desired correction/alignment.

While VCR offers the most correction in the correct clinical scenario, they are associated with significantly longer operative time and larger amounts of blood loss in comparison to the other osteotomies discussed. Additionally rates of neurologic deficits have been reported as high as 17.1% [12], although some deficits have been correctable with appropriate use of neuromonitoring and most neurologic deficits tend to improve over time [13].

References

1. Cerpa M, Lenke LG, Fehlings MG, Shaffrey CI, Cheung KMC, Carreon LY. Evolution and advancement of adult spinal deformity research and clinical care: an overview of the Scoli-RISK-1 Study. Global Spine J. 2019;9:8S–14S. https://doi.org/10.1177/2192568219828729.
2. Diebo BG, Shah NV, Boachie-Adjei O, Zhu F, Rothenfluh DA, Paulino CB, Schwab FJ, Lafage V. Adult spinal deformity. Lancet. 2019;394:160–72.
3. Kim HJ, Yang JH, Chang DG, Lenke LG, Suh SW, Nam Y, Park SC, Suk S-I. Adult spinal deformity: a comprehensive review of current advances and future directions. Asian Spine J. 2022;16(5):776–88. https://doi.org/10.31616/asj.2022.0376.
4. Schwab F, Blondel B, Chay E, et al. The comprehensive anatomical spinal osteotomy classification. Neurosurgery. 2014; https://doi.org/10.1227/NEU.0000000000000182o.
5. Dorward IG, Lenke LG. Osteotomies in the posterior-only treatment of complex adult spinal deformity: a comparative review. Neurosurg Focus. 2010;28(3):E4. https://doi.org/10.3171/2009.12.FOCUS09259.
6. Bridwell KH. Decision making regarding Smith-Petersen vs. pedicle subtraction osteotomy vs. vertebral column resection for spinal deformity. Spine (Phila Pa 1976). 2006;31(19 Suppl):S171–8. https://doi.org/10.1097/01.brs.0000231963.72810.38.
7. Cho KJ, Bridwell KH, Lenke LG, Berra A, Baldus C. Comparison of Smith-Petersen versus pedicle subtraction osteotomy for the correction of fixed sagittal imbalance. Spine (Phila Pa 1976). 2005;30(18):2030–7. https://doi.org/10.1097/01.brs.0000179085.92998.ee.
8. Geck MJ, Macagno A, Ponte A, Shufflebarger HL. The ponte procedure: posterior only treatment of Scheuermann's kyphosis using segmental posterior shortening and pedicle screw instrumentation. J Spinal Disord Tech. 2007;20(8):586–93. https://doi.org/10.1097/BSD.0b013e31803d3b16.
9. Kose KC, Bozduman O, Yenigul AE, Igrek S. Spinal osteotomies: indications, limits and pitfalls. EFORT Open Rev. 2017;2(3):73–82. https://doi.org/10.1302/2058-5241.2.160069.
10. Bridwell KH, Lewis SJ, Edwards C, Lenke LG, Iffrig TM, Berra A, Baldus C, Blanke K. Complications and outcomes of pedicle subtraction osteotomies for fixed sagittal imbalance. Spine (Phila Pa 1976). 2003;28(18):2093–101. https://doi.org/10.1097/01.BRS.0000090891.60232.70.
11. Lenke LG, Sides BA, Koester LA, Hensley M, Blanke KM. Vertebral column resection for the treatment of severe spinal deformity. Clin Orthop Relat

Res. 2010;468(3):687–99. https://doi.org/10.1007/s11999-009-1037-x.

12. Suk S-I, Kim JH, Kim WJ, Lee SM, Chung ER, Nah KH. Posterior vertebral column resection for severe spinal deformities. Spine (Phila Pa 1976). 2002; https://doi.org/10.1097/00007632-200211010-00012.

13. Lenke LG, O'Leary PT, Bridwell KH, Sides BA, Koester LA, Blanke KM. Posterior vertebral column resection for severe pediatric deformity: minimum two-year follow-up of thirty-five consecutive patients. Spine (Phila Pa 1976). 2009;34(20):2213–21. https://doi.org/10.1097/BRS.0b013e3181b53cba.

36 Navigation and Robotics in Lumbar Spine Surgery

Abdurrahman F. Kharbat, Hakeem J. Shakir, Chao Li, and Zachary A. Smith

In recent decades, lumbar spine surgery has co-evolved significantly with the advent of navigation and robotic-assisted surgical techniques. Utilization of novel technology and techniques in both complex and minimally invasive lumbar spine surgery has allowed for improved outcomes. These technological and technical advancements have improved precision, reduced complication rates, and improved patient-reported outcomes for patients of all backgrounds. Lumbar spine surgery has historically consisted of decompression for degenerative claudication or for disk herniations, or fusion in the setting of unstable spinal trauma. With advancements in transpedicular and interbody instrumentation, techniques have emerged with emphasis on minimizing soft-tissue injury through surgical dissection, allowing for complex and minimally invasive reconstruction of the spine and treatment of spinal pathology, which highlights the role of navigation and robotics in the future of lumbar spine surgery. By using navigation systems, tissue-preserving techniques are employed which improves healing, fusion outcomes, and patient-reported outcomes. In this chapter, we will endeavor to highlight the advancements in navigation and robotics in lumbar spine surgery and demonstrate technical success of emerging technologies in an illustrative case.

Much of the foundational knowledge regarding the spine and the medical approach to spinal disorders was practiced by Hippocrates in Greece (460–370 BCE) [1]. His practice of spinal medicine focused around the treatment of back pain, spinal fractures, and spinal deformity. He recognized the connection between the spinal bones' alignment with pathology of the neural elements and implemented treatment of spinal curvature via the Hippocratic ladder, wherein the patient would be tied upside down and shaken to correct spinal curvatures. Another innovation of Hippocrates was the Hippocratic board, wherein spinal curvatures and rigid deformities were manually compressed to release the spine from its deformed curve [1].

A. F. Kharbat (✉) · H. J. Shakir · C. Li · Z. A. Smith
Department of Neurosurgery, University of Oklahoma Health Sciences Center, Oklahoma City, OK, USA
e-mail: Abdurrahman-kharbat@ou.edu; hakeem-shakir@ou.edu; chao-li-1@ou.edu; Zachary-A-Smith@ou.edu

A. A. Baaj et al. (eds.), *Surgery of the Lumbar Spine*, https://doi.org/10.1007/978-3-032-18097-1_36

The first reported surgical treatment of the lumbar spine performed in the United States was in 1829, but the technique gained a foothold in the field of surgery with the seminal work published in 1934 on the treatment of lumbar disk herniations via lumbar laminectomy and diskectomy by Drs. Mixter and Barr [2]. This study ushered in the gold standard for lumbar disk herniations and treatments of lumbar claudication. Interestingly, this iteration of the procedure utilized an intradural approach and extensive diskectomy and remained the standard of treatment for decades. Although this technique became the gold standard of spine surgery, it required extensive tissue dissection, blood loss, exacerbation of cardiopulmonary co-morbidities, and was prone to infection.

In the mid-1960s, Dr. Gazi Yarşargil developed and introduced the operative microscope to neurosurgery, and its use in microsurgical dissection and microsurgery reduced surgical morbidity rates in spine surgery and led to a revolution in the field [3]. Spine surgeons were utilizing smaller approaches with improved visualization, resulting in smaller incisions, tissue dissection, and increased rates of recovery and return to normal activities. The rush to improved surgical precision and minimal tissue dissection led to a revolution in spine surgery that culminated in the introduction of arthroscopic orthopedic techniques to spine surgery via uniportal and biportal visualization utilizing an arthroscope for decompression of neural elements. In 1991, Dr. Obenheim reported the first arthroscopic lumbar diskectomy, and by 1997 Drs. Foley and Smith published their technique for microendoscopic diskectomy via a tubular visualization system which could also be accompanied by improved visualization by using an operative microscope [4]. Lumbar nerve root decompression via minimally invasive modalities became the standard, and this tubular retraction technique allowed for advancements in the treatment of far-lateral disk herniations, as illustrated in 1999 by Foley et al. [5].

The evolution of spine surgery through the early twentieth century was propelled by advancements in laminectomy techniques and technology, and the transition from bracing to surgical fixation of spinal fractures soon took hold with the 1984 publication of Dr. Magerl's experience with external fixation of thoracolumbar spinal fractures with percutaneous pedicle screws [6]. Although this procedure was effective for spinal fixation, it was highly morbid with risks of screw tract infection, pseudoarthrosis, and discomfort whilst in the external fixation apparatus. With advancements in navigation technology, open and percutaneous pedicle screw fixation accuracy improved, and internal fixation techniques advanced. In 1995, the first case demonstrating the use of computer-assisted imaging modalities (computed tomography) was reported, and medical technology companies accelerated their advancements in the field of intraoperative radiographic technologies [7]. A major motivator for improved intraoperative navigation systems was the significant improvement in operative workflow efficiency and reduction in operative times, which translated to improved patient outcomes and reduced healthcare costs [7]. Moreover, many studies were published that proposed that intraoperative navigation reduced screw misplacement rates when compared to free-hand techniques, notably Kotani et al. who showed a reduction from an error rate of 15.3% for 544 screws to 5.4% for 294 screws [8]. The improvement of outcomes for the patient was further compounded by the health benefit to surgeons and surgical staff with the decrease in radiation exposure through navigated procedures when compared to fluoroscopic techniques.

The rise of minimally invasive techniques in spine surgery revolutionized the management of complex spinal disorders, including those requiring decompression, realignment, and fusion. The early twenty-first century witnessed a growing acceptance of minimally invasive lumbar fusion, led by Dr. Foley's seminal work in 2003 on the use of minimally invasive transforaminal lumbar interbody fusion (TLIF) [9]. This approach became a cornerstone for the treatment of various lumbar spine pathologies. Over the subsequent decade, new techniques were refined to allow for interbody fusion through multiple surgical corridors. In 2015, Mobbs et al. described a comprehensive range of interbody fusion techniques—including posterior, transforaminal, oblique, lateral, and anterior approaches—further expanding the indications for minimally invasive spinal fusion [10].

Robotics has also played an increasingly prominent role in spine surgery. The first robotic device for spine surgery, the SpineAssist by Mazor Robotics Ltd., received FDA clearance in 2004. However, its adoption was initially slow due to high costs. Robotic technology gained momentum in the following decades, culminating in studies such as Shahi et al. (2023), which compared robotic-assisted and navigated approaches for minimally invasive lumbar fusion [11]. The study assessed clinical outcomes, patient-reported outcomes (PROMs), screw-related complications, reoperation rates, and more. While robotic assistance did not demonstrate significantly improved clinical outcomes compared to navigation alone, it did offer advantages in reducing radiation exposure, improving screw placement accuracy, and allowing for the use of larger pedicle screws. Furthermore, robotic-assisted surgeries were associated with reduced physical strain for surgeons, enhancing ergonomics in the operating room.

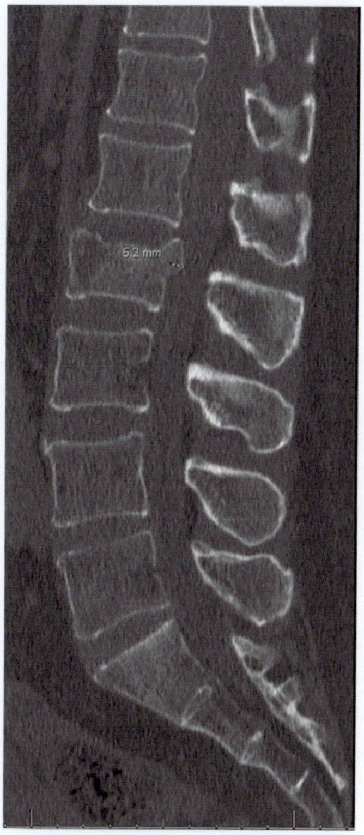

Fig. 36.1 Pre-operative CT Lumbar

Case #1

51-year-old male with past medical history significant for hypertension and depression, as well as chronic lower-back pain, who presents in the trauma bay following motor vehicle collision with intractable back pain and bilateral lower extremity radiculopathy, and otherwise normal motor/sensory neurological examination. CT and MRI Lumbar Spine (Figs. 36.1 and 36.2) demonstrate Chance-fracture at L2 with 30% vertebral body height loss and 5 mm retropulsion with moderate canal stenosis. Patient was placed in TLSO brace pending definitive operative intervention and was planned for T12 to L4 Globus robot-navigated posterior spinal fixation (skipping L2).

Patient was positioned prone and prepped in standard fashion, with midline incision planned to expose T12 to L5, as the L5 spinous process was used for clamping of navigation reference frame. Following subperiosteal surgical exposure of T12 to L4 and exposure of the spinous process of L5, the reference frame was fixed to L5 spinous process and the surgical site was covered and C-arm with Globus drum frame x-rays were taken in AP and lateral views for merging with pre-operative CT scans. The accuracy of navigation was confirmed on bony landmarks and Globus robot was brought into the field with preset trajectory length and size of the screw (Fig. 36.3). Workflow consisted of high-speed drill for pilot hole, navigated low-speed tap, followed by navigated low-speed screw placement, all within the navigation guidance shaft, with ball-tip probe surveillance for bony breech between steps. Following screw placements, O-arm spin confirmed good placement of screws, and patient was debrided, decorticated, and closed in standard fashion. Post-operative day 1 standing thoracolumbar x-rays demonstrated hardware in good position (Fig. 36.4).

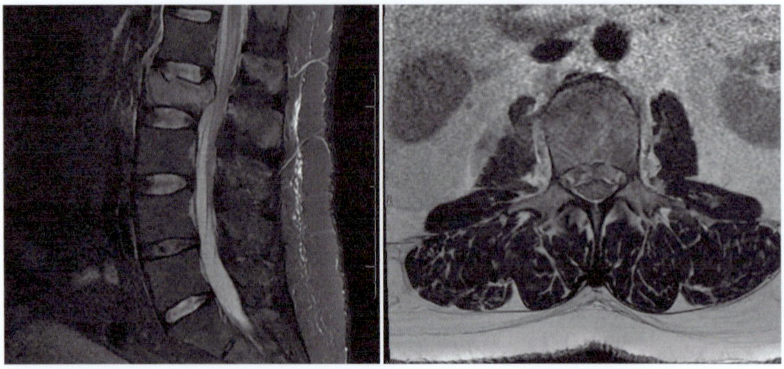

Fig. 36.2 Pre-operative MRI Lumbar sagittal STIR and axial T2 views

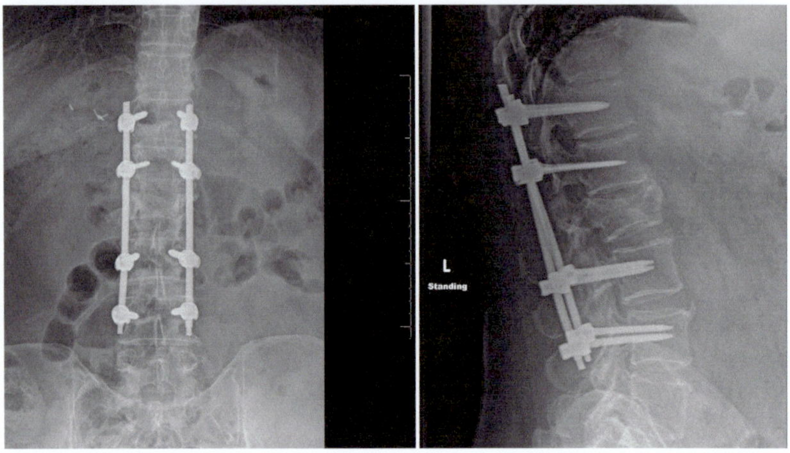

Fig. 36.3 Globus Robot navigated screw trajectory planning

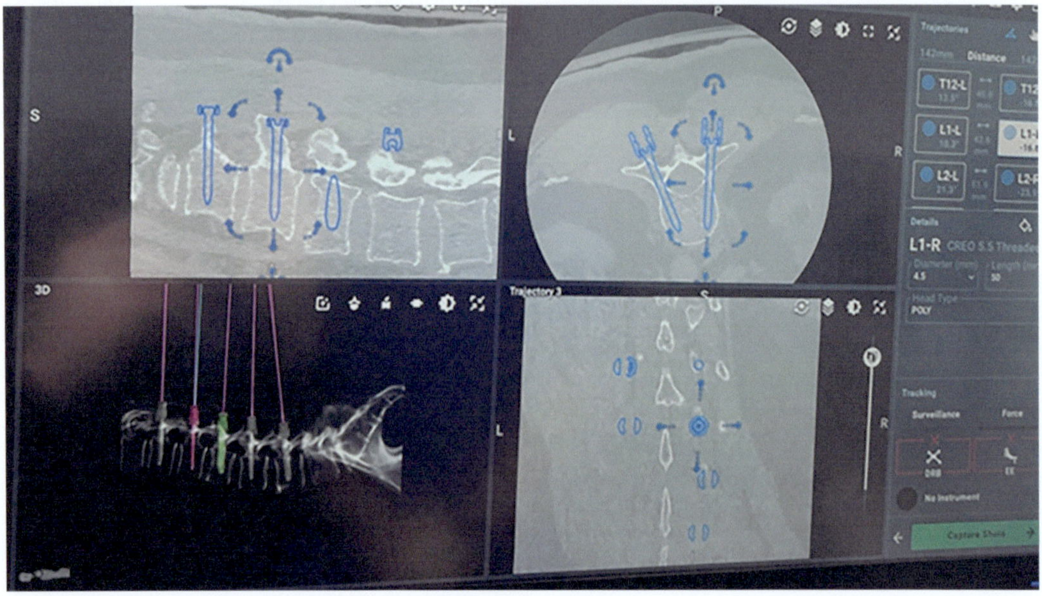

Fig. 36.4 Post-operative thoracolumbar x-ray lateral and AP views

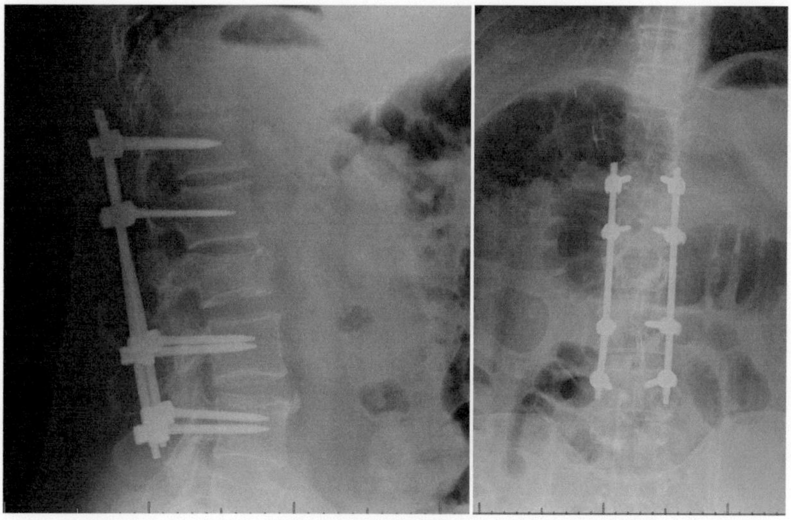

Fig. 36.5 Three-month follow-up thoracolumbar x-ray AP and lateral views

He is doing well on 3-month follow-up with no new neurological deficits, no signs of hardware failure (Fig. 36.5), and improvement in pain. He is cleared for normal activities and has no issues with activities of daily living.

Case #2

47-year-old female who presents with no significant past medical history except for multi-level thoracic and lumbar disc disease with severe T10/T11 central stenosis in the setting of a disc-osteophyte complex and progressive back pain with urinary incontinence (Fig. 36.6). She has had progressive symptoms, the most debilitating of which was her urinary incontinence, which had been present and worsening for 12–15 months. She was counseled extensively regarding the risks of a transpedicular diskectomy with thoracolumbar fusion and elected to proceed with T10–L3 posterior spinal fixation with T11 transpedicular bilateral decompression for diskectomy and L1–2 laminectomies for L1/2 diskectomy under navigation.

Patient was positioned prone and prepped in standard fashion, with midline incision planned to expose T10 to L3, as the L3 spinous process was used for clamping of navigation reference frame. Following subperiosteal surgical exposure of T10 to L3, the reference frame was fixed to L3 spinous process and the surgical site was covered and O-arm scan was performed. The accuracy of navigation was confirmed on bony landmarks and screw placement from T10–L3 (skipping T11) was performed. Workflow consisted of high-speed drill for pilot hole, followed by Lenke pedicle probe, then ball-tip probe feeler to surveil for breech, then low-speed navigated tap, followed by feeler, and finally low-speed navigated screw. Upon screw and rod placement, O-arm spin was conducted to confirm screw positioning and then we proceeded with decompression, diskectomy, and subsequent closure following debridement and arthrodesis.

Patient did well post-operatively with hardware in good position and is pending three-month follow-up (Fig. 36.7).

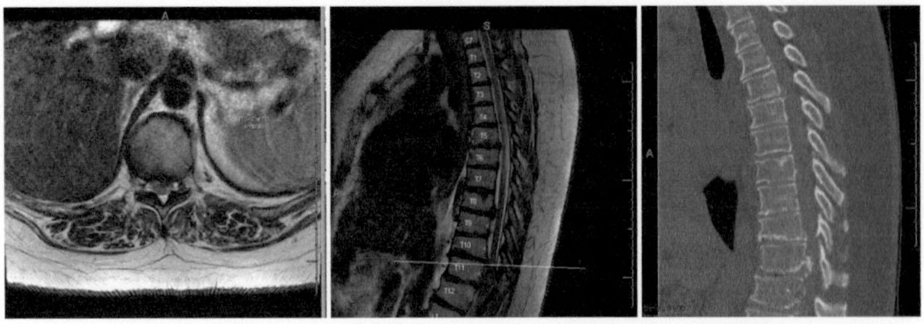

Fig. 36.6 Pre-operative MRI Thoracic axial and sagittal views, with CT Thoracic sagittal view

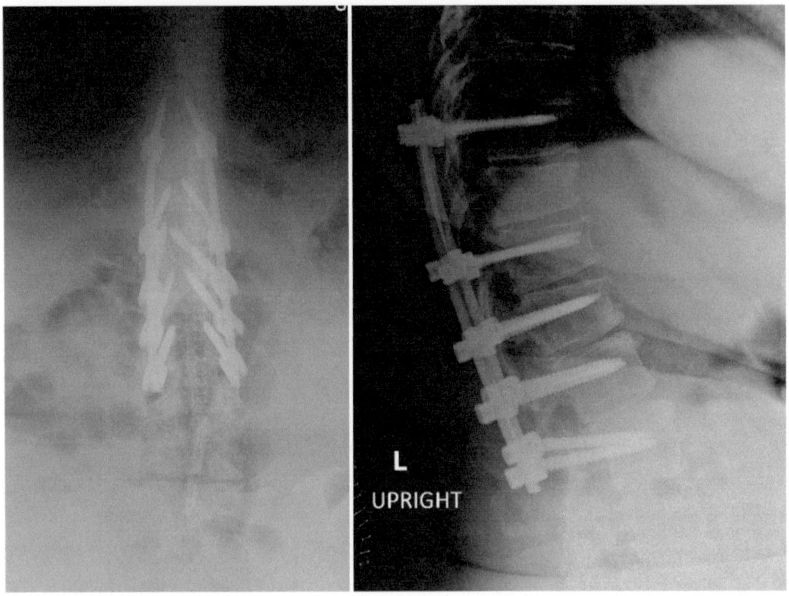

Fig. 36.7 Post-operative standing thoracolumbar x-rays

References

1. Marketos SG, Skiadas P. Hippocrates. The father of spine surgery. Spine (Phila Pa 1976). 1999;24(13):1381–7. https://doi.org/10.1097/00007632-199907010-00018.
2. Mixter WJ, Barr JS. Rupture of the intervertebral disc with involvement of the spinal canal. N Engl J Med. 1934;211:210–5.
3. Yaşargil MG, Krayenbühl H. The use of the binocular microscope in neurosurgery. Bibl Ophthalmol. 1970;81:62–5.
4. Foley KT, Smith MM. Microendoscopic discectomy. Tech Neurosurg. 1997;3:301–7.
5. Foley KT, Smith MM, Rampersaud YR. Microendoscopic approach to far-lateral lumbar disc herniation. Neurosurg Focus. 1999;7(5):e5. https://doi.org/10.3171/foc.1999.7.6.6.
6. Magerl FP. Stabilization of the lower thoracic and lumbar spine with external skeletal fixation. Clin Orthop Relat Res. 1984;189:125–41.
7. Rawicki N, Dowdell JE, Sandhu HS. Current state of navigation in spine surgery. Ann Transl Med. 2021;9(1):85. https://doi.org/10.21037/atm-20-1335.
8. Kotani Y, Abumi K, Ito M, Minami A. Improved accuracy of computer-assisted cervical pedicle screw insertion. J Neurosurg. 2003;99(3 Suppl):257–63. https://doi.org/10.3171/spi.2003.99.3.0257.
9. Foley KT, Holly LT, Schwender JD. Minimally invasive lumbar fusion. Spine (Phila Pa 1976). 2003;28(15 Suppl):S26–35. https://doi.org/10.1097/01.BRS.0000076895.52418.5E.
10. Mobbs RJ, Phan K, Malham G, Seex K, Rao PJ. Lumbar interbody fusion: techniques, indications and comparison of interbody fusion options including PLIF, TLIF, MI-TLIF, OLIF/ATP, LLIF and ALIF. J Spine Surg. 2015;1(1):2–18. https://doi.org/10.3978/j.issn.2414-469X.2015.10.05.
11. Shahi P, Subramanian T, Araghi K, et al. Comparison of robotics and navigation for clinical outcomes after minimally invasive lumbar fusion. Spine (Phila Pa 1976). 2023;48(19):1342–7. https://doi.org/10.1097/BRS.0000000000004721.

Awake Lumbar Spine Surgery

37

Daivik B. Vyas, Brian J. Park, and Michael Y. Wang

Introduction

The ability to perform spine surgery safely requires careful consideration of a patient's overall health status and comorbidities. With the ever-increasing age of the patient population undergoing spine surgery, spine surgeons are faced more and more with the dilemma of operating on sicker and frail patients. General anesthesia has long been the traditionally accepted anesthetic method for spine surgery. Some potential issues associated with general anesthesia include cardiopulmonary complications, long-term cognitive dysfunction, postoperative nausea/vomiting, and delayed discharge [1]. Alternatively, an awake anesthetic technique may be associated with fewer complications, while facilitating faster operative times and reduced length of stay [2]. As spine surgeons become increasingly aware of these benefits, the applications for awake spinal surgery will continue to grow. Careful planning and coordinated teamwork with an expert dedicated anesthesia team to establish key protocols will allow for the successful implementation of awake spinal surgery.

D. B. Vyas · B. J. Park · M. Y. Wang (✉)
Department of Neurological Surgery,
University of Miami, Miami, FL, USA
e-mail: dbv19@miami.edu;
bxp1495@med.miami.edu;
MWang2@med.miami.edu

Perioperative Management and ERAS Protocols

Anesthesia is one key component in the enhanced recovery after surgery (ERAS) concept. ERAS was described by Kehlet as a multimodal approach to implementing various perioperative interventions aimed in reducing surgery-related morbidity and mortality, improving the patient recovery process, and reducing costs [3]. In line with these core philosophies, awake spinal surgery's potential benefits can be utilized as a natural component of a larger ERAS protocol.

The awake spinal surgery patient requires not only intraoperative, but also preoperative and postoperative analgesic considerations. In the immediate preoperative period, administration of various classes of medications has been shown to reduce opioid use and decrease postoperative pain levels [4]. Gabapentinoids and acetaminophen are often given as preoperative adjuncts. NSAIDs are also often utilized in non-fusion decompressive surgery [4]. The preoperative administration of oxymetazoline spray, ondansetron, and glycopyrrolate helps with minimizing secretions and nausea.

Postoperatively, a multimodal pain regimen is important in adequately addressing pain while reducing the need for opioids and its complication profile [4]. This often includes acetaminophen, which can also be given as an IV bolus in the immediate postoperative period. Although contro-

A. A. Baaj et al. (eds.), *Surgery of the Lumbar Spine*, https://doi.org/10.1007/978-3-032-18097-1_37

versial due to concerns of the effects on fusion and postoperative bleeding, NSAIDs can also help in postoperative pain control while reducing the need for opioids. Use of NSAIDs for short durations is unlikely to have significant impact on fusion rates [4]. The goal is to reduce the quantity of opioids needed, but judicious utilization of opioids for postoperative pain control remains an integral component in ERAS protocols.

Surgical Techniques and Patient Selection

A key advantage of awake spinal surgery is the ability to perform surgery on patients who may otherwise be unable to medically tolerate general anesthesia. A case series showed that patients at significantly high risk of complications from general anesthesia were able to tolerate awake spinal anesthesia safely [5]. In addition to decreasing the impact of pre-existing medical comorbidities, awake techniques allow for direct patient feedback for intraoperative monitoring of nerve function [6]. This is useful in endoscopic procedures, especially when utilizing the transforaminal approach, where the dorsal root ganglion is at risk of injury. In general, minimally invasive surgeries that are time-efficient and aim to minimize tissue disruption are ideally suited for awake spinal surgery. Again, in these types of procedures, awake spinal surgery has been shown to promote decreased operative times and blood loss to allow for faster recovery and result in improved postoperative pain scores [2].

There remain significant challenges in awake spine surgery. This includes finding the appropriate balance of sedated and awake status of the patient, controlling a patient's baseline anxiety, and applications in more complex and time-intensive surgeries [2]. The anesthesia team must maintain control of the airway in the prone position without a secured endotracheal tube, while appropriately providing analgesia without eliminating patient responsiveness to certain pain stimuli. The importance of establishing awake protocols in collaboration with an experienced and skilled anesthesia team cannot be stressed enough. Currently, larger operations such as deformity corrections or open procedures with naturally more collateral tissue disruption are not conducive to awake spinal surgery. However, as analgesic techniques continue to evolve, the indications for awake spinal surgery have the potential for continued growth and broader applicability.

Anesthetic Considerations

Approaching a uniform anesthetic protocol for delivery of anesthesia in the awake spine patient requires considering three key factors: (1) mode of sensory blockade; (2) duration of effect; and (3) adjunctive conscious sedation. Regional anesthesia plays a fundamental role in this process [7].

Three major modes of anesthetic delivery are considered with respect to sensory blockade. In the first, intrathecal administration, medication is delivered via lumbar puncture. This modality of regional anesthesia relies upon direct neuronal blockade via the administration of a combination of bupivacaine and fentanyl, followed by thoracolumbar interfascial plane block (TLIP). This provides a high-fidelity blockade, though notable duration of action in the absence of adjunctive anesthesia, i.e., conscious sedation, may limit the duration to 2–4 h [8, 9]. In the second approach, epidural administration, medication is continuously administered via spinal catheter placed into the epidural space. While duration of action can be longer given the continuous infusion of anesthetic, larger dosage of anesthetic is often required to achieve proper efficacy, and the quality of anesthesia achieved may vary secondary to medication dissemination within the epidural space. Finally, local anesthetic administration relies on the delivery of medication, often via image-guidance, across working planes. Most commonly, voltage-gated sodium channel blockers such as bupivacaine are utilized given their short onset and overall long duration of efficacy [10].

The duration of anesthetic required must be framed according to the magnitude of surgery performed. The delivery of local anesthetic alone will provide sufficient short-term anesthesia for small procedures, e.g., on the scale of 30 min–1 h. In contrast, regional anesthesia, especially spinal anesthetic administered in conjunction with paraspinal blockade, may provide up to 4 h of durable anesthetic. This may allow for a greater scope of surgical intervention to be performed, including larger decompression and instrumentation, including interbody fusion. To achieve greater efficacy, light to moderate conscious sedation may be further incorporated. To that end, the use of propofol, ketamine, and midazolam may allow for greater dissociation and relaxation that enables surgery to be performed with a greater degree of comfort.

Conscious sedation techniques are therefore imperative intraoperatively. A nasal cannula is placed, and emergency airway equipment should be readily available. In the authors' institutional experience, a combination of propofol infusion and ketamine infusion is utilized for conscious sedation. Capnography is used to closely monitor the patient's status. Dexmedetomidine may be added if high doses of propofol and ketamine are required. This is a dynamic process and requires the constant communication between surgeon and anesthesia teams to determine appropriate adjustments as necessary. In addition, local anesthetic techniques are a crucial adjunct to sedation. Bupivicaine is often used for local skin and soft tissue infiltration. Liposomal bupivacaine provides longer-lasting local analgesic effects for up to 72 h and can be utilized along percutaneous tracts that may otherwise be a significant source of surgical pain to achieve analgesia during the early course of a brief post-operative hospitalization for more complex procedures.

Limitations to the use of the spinal and regional anesthetic include restrictions related to the route of administration. Spinal anesthesia must be tested sufficiently prior to commencing surgery given the inability to re-dose once surgery has started. Similarly, the use of regional paraspinal blockade may require evaluation of whether interfascial drug administration has occurred within the desired direction; migration of anesthetic to regions beyond the surgeon's scope of interest may result in insufficient blockade. Finally, standard complication profiles and technical proficiency must be considered when evaluating whether patients may receive lumbar puncture, epidural catheter placement, or other perioperative anesthetic interventions before their intended surgery.

Outcomes

Understanding the outcomes of awake lumbar spine surgery requires consideration of the overall trend in non-general anesthetic techniques in spine surgery, healthcare utilization, and patient performance. Since 2005, non-general anesthetic approaches within lumbar spine surgery have demonstrated a steady increase, growing to represent 2% of all spine surgeries performed today [11]. When considered in the context of reimbursements, a similar trend is seen. Ghaith et al. evaluated work relative value units per hour (wRVU/hr) as a function of general and non-general anesthetic spine surgeries performed from 2011 to 2020 and noted that non-general anesthetic spine procedures had higher reported wRVUs/hr. compared to general anesthetic procedures—specifically for lumbar surgery [12]. While limited by between-group differences for patients who receive general and non-general anesthetics, e.g., lower ASA score and comorbidities in the non-GA group, such trends argue for a greater rate of physician compensation—and therefore procedure utilization—as a function of time. Taken together, findings from such studies suggest that greater incorporation of awake lumbar spine surgery may represent a higher, albeit presently small, valuation within the surgical armamentarium for treatment options.

When considering patient performance, early published literature argues that awake procedures are non-inferior to general anesthetic cases. Wahood et al. evaluated 60,222 patients undergoing lumbar decompression and 31,419 patients undergoing posterior lumbar fusion, noting that in both groups, the anesthetic technique demonstrated no differences in readmission rates, length of stay, or complication profiles [13]. Emerging literature has subsequently argued for a more positive influence of non-general anesthetic in the correct patient. Prospective analysis of spinal anesthesia has shown lower self-reported fatigue and improved quality of life when compared to general anesthetic [14]. In their ACS-NSQIP database analysis, Azad et al. note that non-general anesthetic lumbar spine surgery demonstrated lower 30-day complication and readmission rates, as well as overall reduced mean lengths of stay. Finally, polypharmacy, vasopressor needs, and intraoperative episodes of hypotension have been shown to be reduced in lumbar TLIF patients receiving spinal compared to general anesthesia [15].

Conclusions and Further Study

Awake lumbar spine surgery represents a growing, and increasingly valued, component of the spine surgeon's options for lumbar intervention. Successful incorporation of an awake surgery workflow requires close collaboration with a team of surgical technicians, nurses, neuromonitoring technicians, and anesthesiologists for pre-, intra-, and postoperative optimization. Anesthetic technique must ideally combine local analgesia and regional blockade with conscious sedation to achieve durable procedural anesthetic in the context of a multimodal perioperative pain regimen. Overall, awake surgeries offer select patients the opportunity to benefit from shorter hospitalizations and reduced rates of complications and perioperative morbidity.

Future work within awake spine surgery must focus on greater evidence-based characterization of patient-specific characteristics for who would benefit most from such protocols. Additionally, greater focus must be placed on identifying and overcoming barriers to entry for successful awake spine surgery programs, and the specific procedural interventions that benefit the most from non-general anesthetic. Finally, long-term surgical outcomes studies may provide additional clarification regarding the optimal pain management regimen whereby patients can stand to benefit from awake spine surgery.

References

1. Harris M, Chung F. Complications of general anesthesia. Clin Plast Surg. 2013;40(4):503–13. https://doi.org/10.1016/J.CPS.2013.07.001.
2. Perez-Roman RJ, Govindarajan V, Bryant JP, Wang MY. Spinal anesthesia in awake surgical procedures of the lumbar spine: a systematic review and meta-analysis of 3709 patients. Neurosurg Focus. 2021;51(6):E7. https://doi.org/10.3171/2021.9.FOCUS21464.
3. Kehlet H. Multimodal approach to control postoperative pathophysiology and rehabilitation. Br J Anaesth. 1997;78(5):606–17. https://doi.org/10.1093/BJA/78.5.606.
4. Debono B, Wainwright TW, Wang MY, Sigmundsson FG, Yang MMH, Smid-Nanninga H, Bonnal A, le Huec JC, Fawcett WJ, Ljungqvist O, Lonjon G, de Boer HD. Consensus statement for perioperative care in lumbar spinal fusion: Enhanced Recovery After Surgery (ERAS®) Society recommendations. Spine J. 2021;21(5):729–52. https://doi.org/10.1016/J.SPINEE.2021.01.001.
5. Sykes DAW, Tabarestani TQ, Salven DS, Chaudhry NS, Wang TY, Gottfried ON, Shaffrey CI, Guinn NR, Gadsden J, Ayoub CM, Bullock WM, Berger M, Abd-El-Barr MM. Awake spinal anesthesia facilitates spine surgery in poor surgical candidates: a case series. Neuro-Chirurgie. 2023;69(3):101444. https://doi.org/10.1016/J.NEUCHI.2023.101444.
6. Huang M, Brusko GD, Borowsky PA, Kolcun JPG, Heger JA, Epstein RH, Grossman J, Wang MY. The University of Miami spine surgery ERAS protocol: a review of our journey. J Spine Surg. 2020;6(Suppl 1):S29. https://doi.org/10.21037/JSS.2019.11.10.
7. Ní Eochagáin A, Singleton BN, Moorthy A, Buggy DJ. Regional and neuraxial anaesthesia techniques for spinal surgery: a scoping review. Br J Anaesth. 2022;129(4):598–611. https://doi.org/10.1016/J.BJA.2022.05.028.
8. Rizzo P, Hann H, Coombs B, Ali AAH, Stretton A, Sikander M. The hitchhiker's guide to spine awake surgery. The Oxford SAS protocol and early outcomes. World Neurosurg. 2023;176:e289–96. https://doi.org/10.1016/J.WNEU.2023.05.052.
9. Lee JK, Park JH, Hyun SJ, Hodel D, Hausmann ON. Regional anesthesia for lumbar spine surgery: can it be a standard in the future? Neurospine. 2021;18(4):733–40. https://doi.org/10.14245/NS.2142584.292.
10. Wilson JP, Bonin B, Quinones C, Kumbhare D, Guthikonda B, Hoang S. Spinal anesthesia for awake spine surgery: a paradigm shift for enhanced recovery

after surgery. J Clin Med. 2024;13(17):5326. https://doi.org/10.3390/JCM13175326.
11. Azad TD, Alomari S, Khalifeh JM, Ahmed AK, Musharbash FN, Mo K, Lubelski D, Witham TF, Bydon A, Theodore N. Adoption of awake spine surgery – trends from a national registry over 14 years. Spine J. 2022;22(10):1601–9. https://doi.org/10.1016/J.SPINEE.2022.04.012.
12. Ghaith AK, Akinduro OO, El-Hajj VG, de Biase G, Ghanem M, Rajjoub R, Faisal UH, Saad H, Abdulrahim M, Bon Nieves A, Chen SG, Pirris SM, Abode-Iyamah K, Bydon M. General versus nongeneral anesthesia for spinal surgery: a comparative national analysis of reimbursement trends over 10 years. Neurosurgery. 2024;94(2):413–22. https://doi.org/10.1227/NEU.0000000000002670.
13. Wahood W, Yolcu Y, Alvi MA, Goyal A, Long TR, Bydon M. Assessing the differences in outcomes between general and non-general anesthesia in spine surgery: results from a national registry. Clin Neurol Neurosurg. 2019;180:79–86. https://doi.org/10.1016/J.CLINEURO.2019.03.021.
14. de Biase G, Gruenbaum SE, Quiñones-Hinojosa A, Abode-Iyamah KO. Spine surgery under spinal vs general anesthesia: prospective analysis of quality of life, fatigue, and cognition. Neurosurgery. 2022;90(2):186–91. https://doi.org/10.1227/NEU.0000000000001777.
15. Olmos M, Hernandez NS, Kanter M, Liu P, Riesenburger RI, Kryzanski J. Periprocedural polypharmacy in lumbar fusions performed under spinal anesthesia compared with general anesthesia. Neurosurgery. 2023;92(3):632–8. https://doi.org/10.1227/NEU.0000000000002259.

Current Applications of Artificial Intelligence and Machine Learning in Lumbar Spine Surgery

38

Zach Pennington, Karim Rizwan Nathani, and Mohamad Bydon

Background

Artificial intelligence (AI) describes creating computational models capable of performing tasks typically requiring human intelligence, such as decision-making, visual perception, and pattern recognition. Machine learning (ML) is a subset of AI that employs algorithms to identify patterns within extant data for the purposes of making predictions or decisions about novel data without explicit instruction. These technologies have seen increased application across healthcare over the last few decades, with the goal of improving diagnostic efficiency, treatment planning, and clinical decision-making [1–4]. Development of AI applications in healthcare began in the 1970s with systems, such as *MYCIN*, a computerized consultation system designed to facilitate antimicrobial drug selection based upon physician input and pre-programmed clinical decision rules [5, 6]. Though innovative for its time, the success of early AI systems was limited by the complexity of medical data, the need for extensive human input, and the relatively low computational power available [5–7]. As a result, these early systems remained largely experimental and were not widely implemented in clinical practice [5, 7].

Advances toward clinically useful AI applications began in the early 2000s due to increased computing power and the increasing digitization of health data, including the widespread adoption of electronic health records, medical imaging, and genomic sequencing [2, 3, 8]. These models were able to uncover patterns in medical data that were previously undetectable due to sheer volume of data that required analysis. This has led to more accurate predictions, improved risk stratification, and personalized treatment recommendations. Today, AI and ML play a much greater role in various healthcare applications, ranging from interpreting medical data, predicting patient outcomes to supporting clinical decision-making [3, 9, 10].

AI and ML Techniques in Spine Surgery

Exploration of AI and ML in spine surgery has grown significantly in recent years, with much interest paid to its promise to facilitate individualized treatment and improve patient risk stratification [2, 10]. In the preoperative setting, AI-driven tools are increasingly being used to

Z. Pennington · K. R. Nathani · M. Bydon (✉)
Mayo Clinic Neuro-Informatics Laboratory, Department of Neurologic Surgery, Mayo Clinic, Rochester, MN, USA

Department of Neurologic Surgery, Mayo Clinic, Rochester, MN, USA
e-mail: Pennington.Zachary@mayo.edu; Nathani.Karim@mayo.edu; Bydon.Mohamad@mayo.edu

A. A. Baaj et al. (eds.), *Surgery of the Lumbar Spine*, https://doi.org/10.1007/978-3-032-18097-1_38

develop surgical strategies based on patient-specific imaging and data gathered from prior cases suggesting what degree of correction can be achieved with a given surgical maneuver (e.g., pedicle subtraction osteotomy) [9]. Intraoperatively, AI systems are integrated with robotic platforms to provide real-time navigation, increasing surgical accuracy and minimizing human error. Notably, they can merge intraoperatively acquired images with preoperative imaging volumes (e.g., CT) to guide hardware placement. Additionally, AI models are used postoperatively to monitor patient recovery and predict complications, enabling early interventions when needed [2, 9]. ML algorithms enable systems to process vast amounts of data, detect patterns, and generate predictive insights that assist clinicians in decision-making.

Common ML and AI Techniques

- *Supervised Learning* [2, 11]: Supervised learning is one of the most widely used ML techniques in healthcare. In this approach, algorithms are trained on labeled datasets, where the input and corresponding output are known. This allows the model to learn patterns and relationships, which can later be used to predict outcomes in new, unseen data. In lumbar spine surgery, supervised learning is commonly applied to predict surgical outcomes, classify spine conditions based on imaging, and assess patient risk for complications.
- *Unsupervised Learning* [12, 13]: Unsupervised learning is employed when the input data does not have predefined labels or outcomes. Instead, algorithms detect hidden patterns or groupings within the data. This technique is useful for identifying previously unknown relationships or clusters in large datasets, which can provide novel insights into patient subgroups or risk factors in spine surgery.
- *Reinforcement Learning* [12, 14]: Reinforcement learning involves an agent learning to make decisions through trial and error, receiving feedback based on the outcomes of its actions. While less commonly applied in spine surgery than the aforementioned techniques, reinforcement learning holds potential for optimizing surgical procedures, particularly in robotic-assisted surgery. This technique can allow AI-driven surgical systems to continuously improve their accuracy by learning from real-time feedback during operations.
- *Natural Language Processing (NLP)* [3, 9, 15]: NLP techniques are becoming increasingly sophisticated, enabling AI systems to analyze unstructured data such as clinical reports and operative notes.
- *Deep Learning in Image Analysis* [2, 16]: AI models are being further developed to enhance the accuracy of medical imaging interpretation. For spine surgery, this means better detection of spinal abnormalities and more precise 3D reconstructions of the spine for surgical planning and navigation.

AI-Based Preoperative Planning

Surgical Planning

AI-based surgical planning tools are currently one of the most exciting topics in spine surgery as they promise to help individualize surgical plans by identifying at what spinal levels corrective maneuvers should be performed, and how great a correction is required at these levels to achieve the corrective goals of surgery [2, 9, 10, 17]. The first widely applied planning software was SurgiMap, a surgeon-developed tool that helped formulate surgical plans with ideal sagittal alignment metrics, specifically sagittal vertical axis (SVA) and pelvic incidence-lumbar lordosis (PI-LL) mismatch [17].

A similar system—UNiD (formerly Medicrea)—extended the concept of patient-specific surgical plans to the development of patient-specific hardware, specifically customized spinal rods [18]. These rods, which are bent to the planned post-correction curvature and reannealed, have significantly greater fatigue strength relative to conventional intraoperatively contoured rods. Additionally, the UNiD AI-driven software used to design the rods helps surgeons to determine at which spinal levels corrective osteotomies or interbody fusions should be performed. The software can even track surgeon-specific preferences and correction outcomes, potentially tailoring the planning process to individual surgeons.

Predictive Analytics for Surgical Outcomes

Predictive AI models are also increasingly being applied to predict surgical outcomes and complications based upon preoperative clinical and radiographic data [2, 3, 19]. By learning patterns using large volumes of historical data, these models can estimate the likelihood of success for various surgical approaches, allowing surgeons to make data-driven decisions. A growing area of interest in predictive modeling is assessing the risk profiles of different techniques for a particular procedure. For example, Schonfeld and colleagues published on an ML-based model aimed to facilitate the decision of whether to use an anterior or posterior approach to revision cervical spine surgery based on baseline patient characteristics [19].

Multiple other preliminary models have been published, focusing on outcomes including prolonged postoperative opioid use and long-term patient satisfaction [2, 3, 20, 21]. Likewise, AI modeling has been applied to survival prediction for patients undergoing surgery for primary or metastatic spine tumors [20, 21]. These models analyze clinical and demographic data to forecast survival outcomes, helping surgeons make better-informed decisions about the appropriateness and timing of surgery for patients with spinal tumors [20, 21].

AI Intraoperative Assistance

Real-Time Navigation and Robotics

Intraoperative applications of AI and ML to lumbar spine surgery are perhaps the most familiar applications to surgeons and have improved the precision, safety, and efficiency of intraoperative procedures [4, 22, 23]. Two of note are real-time AI-guided navigation and robotic systems, which allow surgeons to perform complex operations with enhanced accuracy and reduced risk of error. An AI-derived tool is LevelCheck, which is designed to assist intraoperative localization by automating the identification of spinal levels, reducing human error in procedures that require precise identification of vertebrae [24]. This technology is particularly helpful for reducing localization errors in cases of distorted anatomy, such as transitional vertebrae, dysmorphic sacrums, or Castellvi joints.

Another example is the 7D Surgical System, also known as machine-vision image-guided surgery, that employs visible light to create a 3D model of the exposed spine intraoperatively [25]. The system shoots beams of visual light at the exposed spine, and the reflections are captured to create a 3D representation, which is then mapped onto preoperative imaging. This can eliminate the need for intraoperative radiation, reducing both surgeon and patient radiation exposure. The system utilizes AI to match the real-time 3D model of the patient's spine with preoperative images, guiding the surgeon with millimeter-level accuracy during hardware placement or corrective procedures [25]. Similarly, AI-powered robotic-assisted surgery systems, such as Mazor X and Excelsius GPS [26–28], use preoperative imaging combined with real-time AI navigation to assist in procedures like spinal fusions and vertebral augmentation. The AI-driven planning software in these systems continuously provides feedback to the surgeon, adjusting surgical trajectories as needed to ensure optimal outcomes [26, 27].

Precision and Reducing Surgical Errors

In complex spine procedures, even small deviations in tool alignment or screw placement can lead to complications such as nerve injury or hardware failure. AI-based systems can mitigate these risks by continuously providing real-time feedback during surgery [25]. The creation of real-time 3D models of the patient's spine ensures that surgical instruments are aligned precisely with anatomical landmarks. AI systems provide continuous feedback to the surgeon during hardware placement, alerting them to deviations or potential issues, such as misalignment or excessive force [25, 27]. The combination of AI-guided navigation, robotic assistance, and machine-vision technology like the 7D Surgical System reduces surgeon-to-surgeon variability and enhances overall procedural accuracy. This may allow surgeons to provide more consistent outcomes with fewer complications, shorter operative times, and improved long-term outcomes.

Postoperative Care and Follow-Up

Predicting Complications

Multiple groups have sought to apply AI and ML to predict complications following lumbar spine surgery [3, 9, 29]. By leveraging preoperative and intraoperative data, surgeons can identify patients at high risk of postoperative complications, which may allow for earlier intervention so as to improve long-term outcomes [9, 10]. A recent review highlighted several studies demonstrating the utility of ML in predicting complications following spine surgery [2]. For example, ML models have been used to predict:

- *Surgical Site Infections (SSI)* [15, 30]—using factors such as diabetes, obesity, and intraoperative blood loss. Early identification of a high-risk patient can guide the surgical team to implement infection control measures, such as recruiting plastic surgery to facilitate closure, employing negative pressure therapy, and more closely monitoring recovery.
- *Deep Vein Thrombosis (DVT)* [31, 32]—based on patient history, operative time, and post-surgical mobility.
- *Chronic Postoperative Pain* [33]—based on factors such as demographics, surgical complexity, and patient pain profiles. These models can assist in identifying those patients who may benefit from inclusion of pain specialists in the care team and who may benefit from increased preoperative counseling about post-operative pain expectations.
- *Hardware Failure* [34]—risk factors such as hardware loosening or rod fractures can be predicted using intraoperative alignment data, surgical techniques, and patient-specific factors. This helps surgeon determine the postoperative imaging schedules and follow-up care.
- *Reoperation Risk* [19, 29]—can be estimated using preoperative risk factors, surgical outcomes, and postoperative recovery data.

The use of predictive ML models helps surgeons to shift from reacting to complications to proactively managing potential risks so as to avoid complications. This shift allows for more personalized follow-up care, tailored specifically to the individual patient's risk profile, thereby improving long-term outcomes and reducing healthcare costs associated with postoperative complications.

Remote Monitoring

One of the most impactful applications of AI in postoperative care is remote monitoring. [35–37] AI systems can analyze data from wearable devices or smartphone applications to continuously assess a patient's recovery progress [35, 36]. AI programs can monitor indicators such as activity levels, pain scores, and heart rate variability, to identify those demonstrating early signs of a complication or clinical decline, allowing physicians to conduct earlier follow-up or order additional studies to diagnose the problem [35–37]. Similarly, AI-equipped digital tools can use patient reports of new symptoms, pain levels, and functional status to provide personalized recommendations and adjustments to rehabilitation protocols or follow-up schedules [37].

Large Datasets and Multi-institutional Registries

The successful application of AI and ML in lumbar spine surgery relies heavily on access to large, high-quality datasets for the development and validation of algorithms. AI and ML models require extensive training on diverse datasets to ensure they are generalizable to multiple patient populations and that their predictions are reliable in the clinical setting [10, 38, 39]. For instance, models used for preoperative planning or postoperative monitoring need to account for a wide range of patient demographics, comorbidities, and surgical variables, which are only possible with large-scale data collection. To achieve this, multi-institutional registries play a critical role [38–40]. These registries collect data from different hospitals and surgical centers, creating comprehensive datasets that reflect a variety of patient populations, surgical techniques, and outcome measures [10, 41]. The availability of such datasets supports the generalizability of AI models, allowing them to be validated across different sites.

Technical Challenges

While AI and ML offer significant improvements in lumbar spine surgery, their integration into clinical practice presents several technical challenges. Addressing these challenges is crucial for ensuring that these technologies are safe, reliable, and beneficial to both patients and healthcare providers. One of the primary technical challenges in developing effective AI and ML models is ensuring the availability of high-quality data [1, 42, 43]. In healthcare, particularly in spine surgery, training data must be comprehensive and accurately labeled, including patient demographics, radiographs, clinical outcomes, and intraoperative details. However, obtaining such data can be difficult due to issues like inconsistent data recording practices and variability in data quality across institutions. Additionally, AI models trained on data from a single institution or region may not generalize well to broader populations [1, 10, 44]. Therefore, multi-institutional databases are needed that allow more robust model training and validation. Without such efforts, models may perform inconsistently across different patient populations, reducing their clinical utility [1, 43].

Another major concern regarding the effectiveness of an AI or ML model is its validation for performance in clinical settings [1, 42]. However, validating these models can be challenging. Many AI models are trained on retrospective data, and while they may show promising results in testing, their performance in real-world clinical scenarios can vary [43, 44]. Additionally, AI models used in spine surgery must be regularly updated to account for new surgical techniques and evolving clinical guidelines [42]. Continuous validation and recalibration of AI models is essential to avoid outdated recommendations that may not reflect the latest standards of care.

Ethical Concerns

In addition to technical challenges, the use of AI and ML in lumbar spine surgery raises important ethical considerations, particularly their use in a way that is fair, transparent, and respectful of patient rights.

- *Patient Privacy and Data Security*: AI models require vast amounts of data, often including sensitive patient information, which can be the target of cyberattacks [2, 45]. Healthcare institutions must implement robust data security protocols, such as encryption and access controls, to protect it from unauthorized access [46]. Additionally, even with de-identification, there is an increasing concern that AI models could inadvertently re-identify individuals through complex data patterns, thereby requiring continuous oversight and ethical review of the AI model application [45, 46].
- *Decision-Making and Potential Biases*: Overreliance on AI can potentially lead to inappropriate clinical decisions in cases where models fail to account for the full complexity of individual patient circumstances [47]. Another

major ethical concern is the potential for algorithmic bias [45]. AI and ML models are only as unbiased as the data they are trained on, and if the underlying data contains biases, those biases may be aggravated by the model. To mitigate these risks, AI programmers must ensure that the training datasets are diverse and representative of the broader patient population.

Future Directions

As AI and ML techniques continue to evolve, their applications in spine surgery are expected to expand, offering new opportunities for improving surgical precision, patient outcomes, and the overall efficiency of care [4, 10, 23]. Some of the most exciting emerging technologies include integration with other technologies, including:

- *Robotic systems*: The integration of AI/ML with robotics can enhance precision and allow for more complex procedures to be performed with greater safety and efficiency [23]. Current robotic-assisted systems, such as Mazor X (Medtronic), are already benefiting from AI-driven planning and real-time navigation capabilities [4, 22].
- *AR/VR*: VR can use AI-analyzed imaging to provide detailed simulations for a surgeon to preoperatively practice a complex procedure in risk-free environment [48, 49]. Similarly, AI-guided AR tools can provide real-time guidance on equipment positioning, implant placement, and the proximity of delicate neural structures.

As these technologies continue to evolve, spine surgery will become increasingly efficient and personalized, improving surgical outcomes [4, 23, 49] (Figs. 38.1 and 38.2).

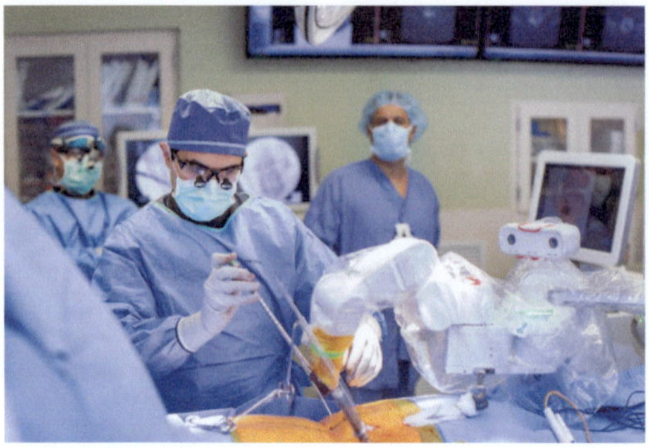

Fig. 38.1 The figure shows a surgeon using an AI-navigated robotic system for screw insertion in lumbar spine surgery. The robotic system assisted the spine surgeon in achieving better precision and control during the procedure

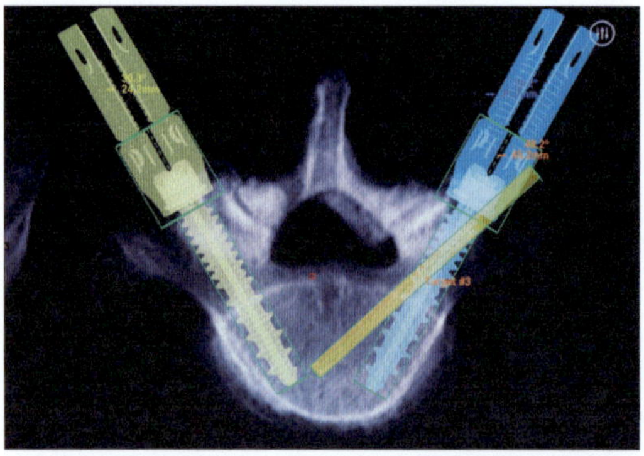

Fig. 38.2 The robot aids in accurately placing screws according to a preoperative plan generated from patient-specific scans. The AI component plays a critical role by analyzing the imaging data to determine precise screw trajectories and guide the surgery

References

1. Warman A, Kalluri AL, Azad TD. Machine learning predictive models in neurosurgery: an appraisal based on the TRIPOD guidelines. Systematic review. Neurosurg Focus. 2023;54(6):E8.
2. DelSole EM, Keck WL, Patel AA. The state of machine learning in spine surgery: a systematic review. Clin Spine Surg. 2022;35(2):80–9.
3. Huang BB, Huang J, Swong KN. Natural language processing in spine surgery: a systematic review of applications, bias, and reporting transparency. World Neurosurg. 2022;167:156–64.e6.
4. Wang J, Miao J, Zhan Y, Duan Y, Wang Y, Hao D, et al. Spine surgical robotics: current status and recent clinical applications. Neurospine. 2023;20(4):1256–71.
5. Shortliffe EH, Davis R, Axline SG, Buchanan BG, Green CC, Cohen SN. Computer-based consultations in clinical therapeutics: explanation and rule acquisition capabilities of the MYCIN system. Comput Biomed Res. 1975;8(4):303–20.
6. Wraith SM, Aikins JS, Buchanan BG, Clancey WJ, Davis R, Fagan LM, et al. Computerized consultation system for selection of antimicrobial therapy. Am J Hosp Pharm. 1976;33(12):1304–8.
7. Amsterdam D. Perspective: limiting antimicrobial resistance with artificial intelligence/machine learning. BME Front. 2023;4:0033.
8. Cho H, Choi J, Lee H. Preoperative nutritional status and postoperative health outcomes in older adults undergoing spine surgery: electronic health records analysis. Geriatr Nurs. 2024;57:103–8.
9. Karhade AV, Bongers MER, Groot OQ, Cha TD, Doorly TP, Fogel HA, et al. Development of machine learning and natural language processing algorithms for preoperative prediction and automated identification of intraoperative vascular injury in anterior lumbar spine surgery. Spine J. 2021;21(10):1635–42.
10. Rodrigues AJ, Schonfeld E, Varshneya K, Stienen MN, Staartjes VE, Jin MC, et al. Comparison of deep learning and classical machine learning algorithms to predict postoperative outcomes for anterior cervical discectomy and fusion procedures with state-of-the-art performance. Spine (Phila Pa 1976). 2022;47(23):1637–44.
11. Baştanlar Y, Ozuysal M. Introduction to machine learning. Methods Mol Biol. 2014;1107:105–28.
12. Hornung AL, Hornung CM, Mallow GM, Barajas JN, Rush A 3rd, Sayari AJ, et al. Artificial intelligence in spine care: current applications and future utility. Eur Spine J. 2022;31(8):2057–81.
13. Traverso A, Dankers F, Osong B, Wee L, van Kuijk SMJ. Diving deeper into models. In: Kubben P, Dumontier M, Dekker A, editors. Fundamentals of clinical data science. Cham: Springer; 2019. p. 121–33.
14. Abdullah Al W, Yun ID. Partial policy-based reinforcement learning for anatomical landmark localization in 3D medical images. IEEE Trans Med Imaging. 2020;39(4):1245–55.
15. Karhade AV, Bongers MER, Groot OQ, Cha TD, Doorly TP, Fogel HA, et al. Can natural language processing provide accurate, automated reporting of wound infection requiring reoperation after lumbar discectomy? Spine J. 2020;20(10):1602–9.
16. Chen T, Su ZH, Liu Z, Wang M, Cui ZF, Zhao L, et al. Automated magnetic resonance image segmentation of spinal structures at the L4-5 level with deep learning: 3D reconstruction of lumbar intervertebral foramen. Orthop Surg. 2022;14(9):2256–64.
17. Elmorsy SEH, Abulnasr HA, Hassan Y, Samra M, Eissa EM. Functional outcome of surgical management of low mid-grade lumbar spondylolisthesis when considering the sagittal balance parameters preoperatively: a prospective study. Chin Neurosurg J. 2022;8(1):35.
18. Ou-Yang D, Burger EL, Kleck CJ. Pre-operative planning in complex deformities and use of patient-specific UNiD(TM) instrumentation. Global Spine J. 2022;12(2_suppl):40s–4s.
19. Schonfeld E, Shah A, Johnstone TM, Rodrigues A, Morris GK, Stienen MN, et al. Deep learning prediction of cervical spine surgery revision outcomes using standard laboratory and operative variables. World Neurosurg. 2024;185:e691–e9.
20. Karhade AV, Thio Q, Ogink PT, Bono CM, Ferrone ML, Oh KS, et al. Predicting 90-day and 1-year mortality in spinal metastatic disease: development and internal validation. Neurosurgery. 2019;85(4):E671–e81.
21. Karhade AV, Thio Q, Ogink PT, Shah AA, Bono CM, Oh KS, et al. Development of machine learning algorithms for prediction of 30-day mortality after surgery for spinal metastasis. Neurosurgery. 2019;85(1):E83–e91.
22. Jiang B, Azad TD, Cottrill E, Zygourakis CC, Zhu AM, Crawford N, et al. New spinal robotic technologies. Front Med. 2019;13(6):723–9.
23. Mualem W, Onyedimma C, Ghaith AK, Durrani S, Jarrah R, Singh R, et al. R2 advances in robotic-assisted spine surgery: comparative analysis of options, future directions, and bibliometric analysis of the literature. Neurosurg Rev. 2022;46(1):18.
24. De Silva T, Lo SL, Aygun N, Aghion DM, Boah A, Petteys R, et al. Utility of the levelcheck algorithm for decision support in vertebral localization. Spine (Phila Pa 1976). 2016;41(20):E1249–e56.
25. Sklar M, Fatemi P, Wadhwa H, Leung C, Zygourakis C. First case report using optical topographic-guided navigation in revision spinal fusion for calcified thoracic disk. J Clin Neurosci. 2021;91:80–3.
26. Buza JA 3rd, Good CR, Lehman RA Jr, Pollina J, Chua RV, Buchholz AL, et al. Robotic-assisted cortical bone trajectory (CBT) screws using the Mazor X Stealth Edition (MXSE) system: workflow and technical tips for safe and efficient use. J Robot Surg. 2021;15(1):13–23.

27. O'Connor TE, O'Hehir MM, Khan A, Mao JZ, Levy LC, Mullin JP, et al. Mazor X stealth robotic technology: a technical note. World Neurosurg. 2021;145:435–42.
28. Zygourakis CC, Ahmed AK, Kalb S, Zhu AM, Bydon A, Crawford NR, et al. Technique: open lumbar decompression and fusion with the Excelsius GPS robot. Neurosurg Focus. 2018;45(VideoSuppl1):V6.
29. Ghaith AK, Ghanem M, Zamanian C, Bon-Nieves AA, Bhandarkar A, Nathani K, et al. Using machine learning to predict 30-day readmission and reoperation following resection of supratentorial high-grade gliomas: an ACS NSQIP study involving 9418 patients. Neurosurg Focus. 2023;54(6):E12.
30. Chen T, Liu C, Zhang Z, Liang T, Zhu J, Zhou C, et al. Using machine learning to predict surgical site infection after lumbar spine surgery. Infect Drug Resist. 2023;16:5197–207.
31. Wang KY, Ikwuezunma I, Puvanesarajah V, Babu J, Margalit A, Raad M, et al. Using predictive modeling and supervised machine learning to identify patients at risk for venous thromboembolism following posterior lumbar fusion. Global Spine J. 2023;13(4):1097–103.
32. Katiyar P, Chase H, Lenke LG, Weidenbaum M, Sardar ZM. Using machine learning (ML) models to predict risk of venous thromboembolism (VTE) following spine surgery. Clin Spine Surg. 2023;36(10):E453–e6.
33. Falla D, Devecchi V, Jiménez-Grande D, Rügamer D, Liew BXW. Machine learning approaches applied in spinal pain research. J Electromyogr Kinesiol. 2021;61:102599.
34. Xiong T, Wang B, Qin W, Yang L, Ou Y. Development and validation of a risk prediction model for cage subsidence after instrumented posterior lumbar fusion based on machine learning: a retrospective observational cohort study. Front Med (Lausanne). 2023;10:1196384.
35. Alhammad N, Al-Dossari H. Recognizing physical activities for spinal cord injury rehabilitation using wearable sensors. Sensors (Basel). 2021;21(16).
36. Heros R, Patterson D, Huygen F, Skaribas I, Schultz D, Wilson D, et al. Objective wearable measures and subjective questionnaires for predicting response to neurostimulation in people with chronic pain. Bioelectron Med. 2023;9(1):13.
37. Li K, Habre R, Deng H, Urman R, Morrison J, Gilliland FD, et al. Applying multivariate segmentation methods to human activity recognition from wearable sensors' data. JMIR Mhealth Uhealth. 2019;7(2):e11201.
38. Flanigan P, Nathani KR, Martini M, Michalopoulos GD, Chen S, Kalani M, et al. Impact of preoperative spinal injections within 30 days of lumbar decompression on surgical outcomes: a matched institutional study. J Neurosurg Spine. 2023;39(5):682–9.
39. Bydon M, Sardar ZM, Michalopoulos GD, El Sammak S, Chan AK, Carreon LY, et al. Representativeness of the American Spine Registry: a comparison of patient characteristics with the National Inpatient Sample. J Neurosurg Spine. 2023;39(2):228–37.
40. Bydon M, Goyal A, Biedermann A, Canoy Illies AJ, Paul T, Ghaith AK, et al. Building and implementing an institutional registry for a data-driven national neurosurgical practice: experience from a multisite medical center. Neurosurg Focus. 2021;51(5):E9.
41. Glassman SD, Carreon LY, Asher AL, De A, Mullen K, Porter KR, et al. Surgeon input can increase the value of registry data: early experience from the American Spine Registry. J Neurosurg Spine. 2023;39(3):404–10.
42. Murphy C, Thomas FP. Generative AI in spinal cord injury research and care: opportunities and challenges ahead. J Spinal Cord Med. 2023;46(3):341–2.
43. Bharadwaj UU, Chin CT, Majumdar S. Practical applications of artificial intelligence in spine imaging: a review. Radiol Clin North Am. 2024;62(2):355–70.
44. Joshi RS, Lau D, Ames CP. Artificial intelligence for adult spinal deformity: current state and future directions. Spine J. 2021;21(10):1626–34.
45. Brahma N, Vimal S. Artificial intelligence in neuroimaging: opportunities and ethical challenges. Brain Spine. 2024;4:102919.
46. Bergeron D, Iorio-Morin C, Bonizzato M, Lajoie G, Orr Gaucher N, Racine É, et al. Use of invasive brain-computer interfaces in pediatric neurosurgery: technical and ethical considerations. J Child Neurol. 2023;38(3–4):223–38.
47. Stengel FC, Stienen MN, Ivanov M, Gandía-González ML, Raffa G, Ganau M, et al. Can AI pass the written European board examination in neurological surgery? – ethical and practical issues. Brain Spine. 2024;4:102765.
48. Ghaednia H, Fourman MS, Lans A, Detels K, Dijkstra H, Lloyd S, et al. Augmented and virtual reality in spine surgery, current applications and future potentials. Spine J. 2021;21(10):1617–25.
49. Judy BF, Menta A, Pak HL, Azad TD, Witham TF. Augmented reality and virtual reality in spine surgery: a comprehensive review. Neurosurg Clin N Am. 2024;35(2):207–16.

Index

A

Abductor sign, 36
ACS-NSQIP database analysis, 310
Acute pelvic fixation failure, 291
Adjacent-level disease, 202
Adjacent segment disease (ASD), 92, 258
Adult degenerative lumbar scoliosis (ADLS)
  classifications, 186, 187
  definition, 185
  etiology/natural history, 185, 186
  nonoperative treatment, 187
  pre-surgical evaluation, 187, 188
  prevalence, 185
  sagittal alignment, 192
  surgical treatment, 188–192
  treatment, 192, 193
Advanced trauma life support (ATLS), 86
Age-related degeneration, 5
All-or-nothing criterion, 51
Ambulatory Surgery Centers (ASCs), 29
American Physical Therapy Association, 77
American Spinal Injury Association (ASIA)
    impairment scale, 86
Amplitude criterion, 51
Anabolic agents, 62
Ankylosing spondylitis (AS), 89–91
Annulus fibrosus (AF), 104
Anterior inferior iliac spine (AIIS), 291
Anterior longitudinal ligament (ALL), 4, 277, 279
Anterior lumbar interbody fusion (ALIF), 180, 259
  advantages of, 281
  complications, 285
  indications, 281
  L5-S1 disc space, 283, 284
  L5-S1 spondylolisthesis, 284
  limitations, 281–282
  postoperative care, 285
  results, 284
  step-by-step procedure, 282, 283
  surgical pearls, 285
  surgical technique
    imaging, 282
    mini-transverse incision, 282
    positioning, 282
    preoperative evaluation, 282
Anterior sacroiliac ligament (ASL), 288
Antiresorptive therapy, 61–63
Areal BMD (aBMD), 58, 59, 61, 62
Artery of Adamkiewicz (AA), 7
Arthrodesis, 20
Artificial intelligence (AI), 46–47, 79
  AR/VR, 318
  complications, 316
  multi-institutional registry, 317
  navigation and robotic systems, 315
  predictive analytics, 315
  remote monitoring, 316
  robot aids, 318
  robotic system, 318
  spine surgery, 313
  surgical errors, 315
  surgical planning, 314
  technical challenges, 317
  techniques, 314
Assessing physical mobility, 78
Astrocytomas, 119
Awake lumbar spine surgery
  anesthetic protocol, 308, 309
  capnography, 309
  challenges in, 308
  ERAS protocols, 307
  limitations of, 309
  liposomal bupivacaine, 309
  multimodal pain regimen, 307
  outcomes of, 309
  spinal surgery patient, 307
  surgical techniques, 308
Axial back pain, 198
Axial low back pain, 70
  BVNA, 71
  compression fractures, 72
  discogenic pain, 72
  facet joint pain, 71
  myofascial pain, 71

A. A. Baaj et al. (eds.), *Surgery of the Lumbar Spine*, https://doi.org/10.1007/978-3-032-18097-1

Axial low back pain (*cont.*)
provocative discography, 72
SCS, 72
TPIs, 71
vertebrogenic low back pain, 71

B
Base of triangle, 7
Basivertebral nerve ablation (BVNA), 71, 72
Biologic therapy, 72
Biomechanical computed tomography (BCT), 60, 61
Biomechanics
biomechanical principles, 15
bone, 14
facet joints, 11
functional spinal unit, 15
fundamental physical concepts, 14, 15
intervertebral disc, 12
kinematic phenomena, 14
lamina and spinal canal, 11–12
ligaments and muscles, 12
pedicles, 12
spinal instability, 16–18
surgical considerations and instrumentation
arthrodesis, 20
decompression procedures, 18–19
segmental alignment, 20–21
spinal fixation procedures, 19–20
transverse and spinous process, 12
vertebral body, 11, 13
Bio-psycho-social approach, 78
Biportal endoscopic spine surgery (BESS), *see* Unilateral biportal endoscopy (UBE)
Bisphosphonates, 61, 63
Bone, 14
bleeding, 249
graft, 265
Bone health optimization
anabolic agents, 62
antiresorptive therapy, 61–63
assessment, 58–61
denosumab, 61
osteoporosis, 57
in vitro data, 58
Bone marrow aspirate concentrate (BMAC), 72
Bone scintigraphy, 44
BONE trial, 61
Bony anatomy
joints, 3
lateral recess, or subarticular zone, 4
mammillary process, 4
transverse processes, 4
vertebral body, 2
vertebral canal, 3
Bowstring sign, 35
Burst fractures (AO Type A3 and A4), 86, 88–89

C
Cancer-related pain, 73
Cement augmentation, 131
Centers for Medicare & Medicaid Services (CMS), 27
Chance fractures, 89
Chronic postoperative pain, 316
Cleaved C-propeptide (CPII), 186
Clinical practice guidelines (CPG), 77, 79
Cobb angle, 17
Cognitive-behavioral therapy (CBT), 79
Compound muscle action potential (CMAP), 51, 52
Compression fractures, 72
Computed tomography (CT), 41–42
COnsensus-based Standards for the selection of health Measurement Instruments (COSMIN) initiative, 78
Conventional-dose radiation therapy (cEBRT), 128
Cram test, 35
C-reactive protein (CRP), 214
Crossed adductors, 36
Cutibacterium acnes, 212

D
Data security protocols, 317
Decompression procedures, 18–19
Deep learning in image analysis, 314
Deep venous thrombosis (DVT), 258, 316
Degenerative disc disease (DDD), 5, 6, 45, 275
Degenerative disorder, 271
Degenerative lumbar spine diseases
physiotherapy assessment, 77–79
biomechanical evaluation, 77
clinical decision-making, 79
functional movement assessments, 77
interdisciplinary collaboration, 79
objective, 78, 79
patient-reported outcome measures, 77
subjective, 77, 78
physiotherapy intervention, 79–81
Degenerative lumbar spondylolisthesis (DLS)
decompression and fusion
clinical assessment, 172
vs. decompression only approach, 178, 179
definition and classifications, 163, 171
indication, 171
lumbar spinal stenosis, 165, 166
nonsurgical treatment, natural history, 173, 174
operative technique, 166, 167
pathophysiology, 172
patient positioning and anesthesia, 166
postoperative care, 167
preoperative imaging, 172, 173
randomized trials, 164, 165
sagittal alignment, 173
surgical techniques, 180, 181
surgical treatment, 174–177
systematic reviews and meta-analysis, 165

Degenerative scoliosis, 276
Degenerative spondylolisthesis, 3
biomechanics, 156
classification, 156
clinical assessment, 157
diagnostic workup, 157, 158
non-operative management, 158
surgical management, 159, 160
Denosumab, 61
Diffuse idiopathic skeletal hyperostosis (DISH), 89–91
Direct corticospinal wave [D-wave] recording, 51
Direct costs, 26
Disc herniation
clinical outcome, 224, 225
complications, 225
indications and patients' selection, 222
open microdiscectomy, 221, 223
postoperative care, 224
tubular microdiscectomy, 221, 224
Discogenic pain, 72
Dual-energy X-ray absorptiometry (DXA), 57–62
Durotomy, 91
D-waves, 53
Dysplastic spondylolisthesis, 197

E
Effective pain management techniques, 80
Electromyography (EMG), 270
Electrophysiology, 121
En bloc spondylectomy, 131
Endoscopic lumbar spine surgery, 53
Endoscopic procedure, 308
Endoscopic spine surgery (ESS)
complications
bleeding, 249, 250
dural tear, 248, 249
infection, 250
instruments, 247, 248
insufficient decompression, 250
interlaminar approach, 250
transforaminal approach, 250, 251
type of anesthesia, 248
wrong site, 248
FESS, 227
features, 227, 228
instrument manipulation, 227
interlaminar approach, 228–230
transforaminal approach, 228, 230–232
operating room set-up, 228, 229
Endplate bone quality (EBQ) score, 60
Enhanced recovery after surgery (ERAS), 307
Enneking-appropriate resection, 140
Ependymoma, 117–118
Epidural abscess, 207
Epidural bleeding, 250
Epidural steroid injections (ESI), 106, 110, 112
Ewing sarcoma, 140
Extreme lateral interbody fusion (XLIF), 216

F
FABER, 36
Facetectomy, 18
Facet joint (FJ), 3, 11
angulation, 3
pain, 71
Fajersztajin's sign, 35
Fear-Avoidance Beliefs Questionnaire (FABQ), 78
Femoral stretch test, 35
Five-repetition sit-to-stand (5R-STS) test, 78
Flexion-distraction injuries, 89
Fracture-dislocation (AO C Type), 89
Fracture risk assessment (FRAX) tool, 57–59
Fragility fracture, 58
Free-run or spontaneous EMG (sEMG), 49, 52–54
Full-endoscopic spine surgery (FESS), 227
features, 227, 228
indications/contraindications, 238
infections, 238, 243
instrument manipulation, 227
interlaminar approach, 228–230
intradural definitive resection, 239–242
intradural lesions, 242
intradural pathologies, 237, 238
overview, 237
spinal oncology, 239, 240
technical insights, 238, 239
tethered cord syndrome, 238, 242, 243
transforaminal approach, 228, 230–232
UBE, 227
interlaminar approach, 228, 232–234
Functional ability, 78
Functional movement screen (FMS), 78
Functional spinal unit (FSU), 15

G
Grade I lumbar spondylolisthesis, 3
Graded exercise, 80

H
Hardware failure, 316
Health-related quality of life (HRQOL), 192
Height of the triangle, 7
Hemangioblastomas, 120
High-energy sacral fractures, 98
High-grade spondylolisthesis, 54
classification, 197, 198
clinical presentation, 198
complications, 202, 203
conservative treatment, 200
epidemiology, 198
imaging strategies, 199, 200
operative treatment
fusion and role of reduction, 201
interbody selection, 201, 202
reduction techniques, 201–202
risk factors, 201

High-grade spondylolisthesis (*cont.*)
spinopelvic parameters and alignment, 198
Hip osteoarthritis, 37
Hooke's Law, 15
Hoover sign, 36
Hounsfield units (HU), 59, 60, 62, 63
Hypotenuse of the triangle, 7

I
Incremental cost-effectiveness ratios (ICER), 29
Indirect costs, 26
Infectious spondylodiscitis (IS)
biology, 206, 207
clinical symptoms, 205
diagnosis, 205
etiology, 205
imaging, 206
medical treatment, 207
surgical treatment, 207, 208
Inferior articular process (IAP), 3, 5, 298
Instantaneous axis of rotation (IAR), 12, 14, 15, 17–19
Interlaminar epidural steroid injections (ILESIs), 70
Internal vertebral venous plexus, 8
International Classification of Functioning, Disability, and Health (ICF) framework, 77
International Society of Clinical Densitometry (ISCD), 57, 58
Interspinous process fixation, 73
Interventional pain management, 72
Intervertebral disc (IVD), 1, 3, 5, 12, 104
Intraarticular facet steroid injections, 71
Intradural lumbar spinal tumors
common tumors
ependymoma, 117–118
myxopapillary ependymomas, 117
rare tumors
hemangioblastomas, 120
meningiomas, 121
metastatic disease, 120
surgical considerations, 121–124
electrophysiology, 121
microscopic technique, 122–123
minimally invasive surgery, 122
standard open technique, 121–122
surgery at filum terminale, 123
surgery at lumbar spinal cord, 123
uncommon tumors
astrocytomas, 119
neurofibroma and malignant nerve sheath tumors, 119–120
paragangliomas, 120
Intraoperative neurophysiology monitoring (IONM)
deformity surgery, 53
degenerative spine conditions, 53
implications, 54
MEPs, 50, 51
oncology surgery, 53
sEMG, 52
SSEPs, 50
tEMG, 52
In vitro data, 58

K
Kambin's prism, 7
Kambin's triangle, 7, 228
Kickstand rods (KSRs), 291

L
Lamartina classification, 189
Lamina and spinal canal, 11–12
Lasègue's sign, 35
Lateral lumbar interbody fusion (LLIF), 53, 180, 275
access to L4-L5, 270
decision-making, 271
decompress neural structures, 271
history of, 269
innovation, 271
low-grade spondylolisthesis, 271
patient's anatomy, 269
posterior fixation, 271
segmental lordosis, 272
technique description
discectomy, 270
EMG, 270
neuromonitoring technique, 270
patient positioning, 269–270
retroperitoneal space, 270
supplementation, 270
Ligamentotaxis, 271
Ligamentous anatomy, 4–5
Ligaments and muscles, 12
Ligamentum flavum, 4, 5
Load-deformation curve, 15
Low back pain (LBP)
economy, 26–30
lost income opportunity, 27–28
treatment costs, 28–29
treatment tradeoffs, 29–30
prevalence, 25, 26
risk factors, 26
L1PA, 192
Lumbar decompression
indication, 110–111
MIS techniques, 111–112
Lumbar deformity, 45
Lumbar disc herniation, 1, 3, 45
anatomy, 104
clinical presentation, 105
diagnostic evaluation, 106
non-operative treatment, 106
pathophysiology, 104–105
prognosis/long-term outcomes, 107
surgery, 107

Lumbar lordosis (LL), 288
Lumbar radiculopathy (LR), 36–37, 79
Lumbar spinal stenosis (LSS), 5, 165, 166
  classification, 109
  clinical presentation, 109
  conservative treatment
    epidural steroid injections, 110
    pharmacological measures, 110
    physiotherapy, 109
    vs. surgical treatment, 110
  definition, 109
  lumbar decompression
    indication, 110–111
    MIS techniques, 111–112
  microtubular decompression, 112–114
  unilateral biportal endoscopy, 114–115
Lumbar spine-related pain
  axial low back pain, 70
    BVNA, 71
    compression fractures, 72
    discogenic pain, 72
    facet joint pain, 71
    myofascial pain, 71
    provocative discography, 72
    SCS, 72
    TPIs, 71
    vertebrogenic low back pain, 71
  cancer-related pain, 73
  interventional pain management, 72
  radicular pain, 70
Lumbar spine trauma
  ankylosing spondylitis, 89, 90
  burst fractures, 88, 89
  chance fracture/flexion distraction (AO Type B1), 89, 90
  classification systems, 87
  clinical evaluation
    ATLS protocol for polytrauma, 86
    history, 86
    physical examination, 86
  complications
    adjacent segment degeneration, 92
    durotomy, 91
    loss of fixation, 91
    neurologic injury, 91
    pseudoarthrosis, 92
    wound complications, 91
  DISH, 90
  epidemiology, 85
  fracture-dislocation injuries, 89
  imaging
    CT, 86, 87
    MRI, 87
    nuclear medicine, 87
    plain films, 86
  outcomes, 92
  surgical indications/contraindications, 88
  vertebral compression fractures, 88
Lumbar stenosis, 5
Lumbopelvic fixation, 99
Lumbopelvic reconstruction, 139
Lumbo-sacral primary tumors
  diagnosis and preoperative workup, 135, 136
  epidemiology, 135
  operative management
    adjuvant therapies, 141
    en bloc resection, 136–139
    lumbopelvic reconstruction, 139
    neurological sequelae and complications, 140, 141
    surveillance, 140, 141
Lytic, 197

M

Machine learning (ML), 46
  AR/VR, 318
  complications, 316
  multi-institutional registry, 317
  navigation and robotic systems, 315
  predictive analytics, 315
  remote monitoring, 316
  robot aids, 318
  robotic system, 318
  spine surgery, 313
  surgical errors, 315
  surgical planning, 314
  technical challenges, 317
  techniques, 314
Machine learning-based gait analysis, 79
Magnetic resonance imaging (MRI), 42–43
Malignant nerve sheath tumors, 119–120
Mammillary process, 4
Meningiomas, 121
Metastatic disease, 120
  conservative treatment, 132
  definition, 127
  localization, 128
  pathophysiology, 127
  scoring systems, 128–130
  surgical modalities, 131, 132
Methicillin-resistant *Staphylococcus aureus* (MRSA) infections, 212
Meyerding classification, 156
Microtubular decompression, 112–114
Minimally invasive surgery (MIS) techniques, 73, 107, 122, 308
Minimally invasive transforaminal lumbar interbody fusion (MIS-TLIF), 29
Morphology criterion, 51
Motor evoked potentials (MEPs), 49–51, 53, 54, 121, 270
Musculoskeletal (MSK) concerns, 25
Myelography, 43, 44
Myofascial pain, 71
Myxopapillary ependymomas, 117

N

National Institute for Health and Care Excellence (NICE), 77
Natural Language Processing, 314
Navigation and robotics, in lumbar spine surgery
  back pain with urinary incontinence, 305
  CT and MRI Lumbar Spine, 303
  laminectomy techniques, 302
  microsurgical dissection, 302
  positioned prone, 305
  pre-operative CT lumbar, 303
  pre-operative MRI lumbar, 304
  rise of minimally invasive techniques, 302, 303
  thoracolumbar x-ray, 305
  treatment of, 302
  x-ray lateral and AP view, 304
Navigation systems, 46
Neural anatomy, 6–7
Neurofibroma, 119–120
Neurogenic claudication, 109, 110, 114
Neurogenic MEPs, 51
Neurologic injury, 91
Newton's Laws of Motion, 15
Novel technology, 301
Nucleus pulposus (NP), 104

O

Objective assessment, 78
  biomechanical assessment, 79
  functional movement screening, 78
  manual and neurological examination, 78
Oblique lumbar interbody fusion (OLIF), 180
Oncologic compression fractures, 72
Osteomyelitis, 216
Osteoporosis, 57
Osteoporosis Index of Risk (OSIRIS), 57
Osteoporosis risk assessment instrument (ORAI), 57, 58
Osteoporosis self-assessment tool (OST), 57
Oswestry disability index (ODI), 78, 271

P

Paradoxical motion, 14
Paragangliomas, 120
Passive intervertebral motion testing (PIVM), 78
Patient reported outcome measures (PROM), 78, 303
Pedicle, 12
  screws, 298
Pedicle subtraction osteotomies (PSO), 298, 299
Pelvic fixation, 189
Pelvic incidence (PI), 288
Percutaneous image-guided lumbar decompression (PILD) procedure, 73
Peripheral nerve stimulation (PNS), 71
Persistent spinal pain syndrome (PSPS), 72
Physical Examination, of lumbar spine
  clinical pearls, 37
  differential diagnosis, 37
  lumbar radiculopathy, 36–37
  motor examination, 35
  palpation, 34
  range of motion, 34
  reflexes, 35
  sensory examination, 34–35
Physiotherapy, 109
Physiotherapy assessment
  biomechanical evaluation, 77
  functional movement assessments, 77
  objective, 78
    biomechanical assessment, 79
    clinical decision-making, 79
    functional movement screening, 78
    interdisciplinary collaboration, 79
    manual and neurological examination, 78
  patient-reported outcome measures, 77
  subjective, 77, 78
Physiotherapy intervention, 79–81
Piriformis syndrome, 37
Plain radiography, 39–40
Platelet-rich plasma (PRP), 72
Ponte osteotomy, 298
Posterior column osteotomies (PCO), 298
Posterior ligamentous complex (PLC), 87–89
Posterior longitudinal ligament (PLL), 4
Posterior lumbar interbody fusion (PLIF), 180
Posterior sacroiliac ligament (PSL), 288
Posterior spinal fusion, 53
Posterolateral lumbar interbody fusion (PLIF), 180
Postoperative spinal infections (PSIs)
  causative bacteria, 212
  classification, 212
  clinical presentation and diagnosis, 213–215
  conservative treatment, 215
  incidence, 211
  risk factors and prevention, 212, 213
  surgical treatment, 215, 216
Pott's disease, 205
Prone transpsoas (PTP) approach
  absolute contraindication, 276
  complication, 279
  CT scans, 276
  indications for, 275
  MRI, 276
  preoperative planning, 276
  surgical technique
    cage placement, 278
    dilators and retractor placement, 278
    discectomy, 277
    incision planning, 277
    posterior pedicle screws, 278
    retroperitoneal access, 277
  vascular injuries, 279
  visceral complications, 279
Provocative discography, 72
Proximal junctional kyphosis (PJK), 191
Pseudoarthrosis, 92, 202

Q

Quality-adjusted life years (QALY), 29, 30
Quality Outcomes Database (QOD), 29

R

Radicular pain, 37, 70
Radiofrequency ablation (RFA), 71
Radiofrequency (RF) probe, 247
Radiological assessment
 bone scintigraphy, 44
 in common pathologies
  degenerative disc disease, 45
  lumbar deformity, 45
  lumbar disc herniation, 45
  spinal stenosis, 45
  spondylolisthesis, 45
 computed tomography, 41–42
 emerging technologies, 46–47
 magnetic resonance imaging, 42–43
 myelography, 43, 44
 plain radiography, 39–40
 postoperative planning, 46
 preoperative planning, 46
 ultrasound, 44
Red flags, 78
Regenerative approaches, 72
Regenerative medicine approaches, 72
Reinforcement learning, 314
Reoperation risk, 316
Roland Morris Disability Questionnaire (RMDQ), 78
Romosozumab, 62, 63

S

Sacral fracture
 anatomy and biomechanics, 95
 classification, 96–97
 examination, 97
 high-energy fractures, 95
 imaging, 98
 low-energy fractures, 95
 nonoperative treatment, 98
 operative treatment, 98
 surgical technique, 99–100
 vertical shear type fracture, 95
Sacral-H fracture, 95
Sacral insufficiency fractures, 97, 98
Sacral slope (SS), 288
Sacral-U fracture, 95
Sacroiliac joint fusion devices, 73
Sacroiliac joint (SIJ) arthritis, 37, 287
Sacropelvic fixation
 contemporary fixation techniques, 291
 high-grade spondylolisthesis, 287
 indications and contraindications, 289–291
 navigation and robotics, 293
 pelvic fixation zones, 289
 SIJ, 288
 spinopelvic motion, 288
Sagittal vertical axis (SVA), 314
S2-alar iliac screws (S2AIs), 291, 293
Scheuermann's kyphosis, 298
Schwab classification, 190
Schwab osteotomy classification, 297
Segmental alignment, 20–21
Selective nerve root blocks (SNRBs), 70
Shared decision-making, 80
Simple Calculated Osteoporosis Risk Estimation (SCORE) tool, 57
Slump Test and Straight Leg Raise (SLR), 79
Smith-Peterson osteotomy, 298
Soft tissue bleeding, 249
Somatosensory evoked potentials (SSEPs), 49, 50, 52–54, 121, 270
Spinal canal stenosis, 255
Spinal cord stimulation (SCS), 72
Spinal deformity, 293
 lumbar spine, 297
 neuromonitoring, 297
 PCO, 298
 PSO, 298, 299
 VCR, 299
Spinal fixation procedures, 19–20
Spinal instability, 16–18
Spinal Instability Neoplastic Score (SINS), 130
Spinal stenosis, 45
Spinopelvic alignment, 288
Spinopelvic fixation, 95
Spinopelvic instability, 96–98
Spondylolisthesis, 45, 155
SRS-Schwab classification system, 297
Stagnara wake-up test, 91
Staphylococcus aureus, 205, 212
Subjective assessment, 77, 78
Superior articular process (SAP), 3–5, 298
Supervised learning, 314
Surgical site infections (SSIs), 316
 See also Post-operative spinal infections (PSIs)
Surveillance, Epidemiology and End Results (SEER) database, 140
Swedish Spinal Stenosis Study (SSSS), 164
Synovial cysts
 clinical presentation, 146
 conservative management, 150
 history, 145
 neurodiagnostics, 146–148
 pathophysiology, 145
 percutaneous aspiration, 151
 steroid injections, 151
 surgical management, 149, 150

T

Tampa Scale of Kinesiophobia (TSK), 78
Teriparatide, 62, 63
Tethered cord syndrome, 238, 242, 243
Therapeutic alliance, 80

Thoracolumbar injury classification and severity score (TLICS), 87, 89, 90
Thoracolumbar interfascial plane block (TLIP), 308
3D imaging, 46
Threshold criterion, 51
Timed Up and Go (TUG) test, 78
T4 pelvic angle (T4PA), 192
Trabecular bone score (TBS), 58, 59
Traditional iliac screws (IS), 291
Transcranial motor evoked potentials (TcMEPs), 51
Transforaminal endoscopic decompression, 54
Transforaminal epidural steroid injections (TFESIs), 70
Transforaminal lumbar interbody fusion (TLIF), 181, 192, 302
  complications, 257, 258
  indications, 254
    lumbar spondylolisthesis, 254
    pseudoarthrosis, 254
    symptomatic degenerative disc disease, 254
  lordosis/kyphosis, 259
  lordosis restoration, 258
  MIS
    ambulatory procedure, 267
    complications and disadvantages, 266, 267
    evidence of, 262
    fusion and bone graft, 265
    indications, 262
    screw insertion, 263
    shape of cages, 266
    small midline incision, 264
    spondylolisthesis, 265
    tips for, 267
    tubular surgery, 262, 263, 265
    types of, 261
  posterolateral fusion, 258
  surgical technique
    closure, 256
    discectomy and endplates preparation, 255
    facetectomy/laminectomy, 255
    interbody fusion, 255, 256
    pedicle screws placement, 254
    posterior lumbar approach and decompression, 254, 255
    preoperative planning, 254
    rods placement, 256, 257
    X-rays, 257
Transverse and spinous process, 12
Transverse processes (TPs), 4
Transverse sacral fracture, 95
Trendelenburg sign, 36
Triggered EMG (tEMG), 49, 52
Trigger point injections (TPIs), 71
Trochanteric fasciitis, 37
Tubular microdiscectomy, 221
Tubular microscopic approaches, 111

U

Ultrasound, 44
Unilateral biportal endoscopy (UBE), 111, 112, 114–115, 227
  interlaminar approach, 228, 232–234
Unsupervised learning, 314

V

Vascular anatomy, 7–8
Venous drainage system, 7
Venous plexus of Batson, 7
Vertebral augmentation procedures, 72
Vertebral body, 11, 13
Vertebral Bone Quality (VBQ) score, 59, 60
Vertebral column resection (VCR), 299
Vertebral Compression Fractures (AO type A1), 88
Vertebral pelvic angles (VPAs), 192
Vertebrogenic low back pain, 71
Vertical shear type fracture, 95
VERT-NA trial, 61
Virtual stress test, 60
Visual analog scale (VAS), 164, 271
Volumetric BMD (vBMD), 58, 60–62

W

Wearable sensors, 79
Weight management, 80
Weinstein-Boriani-Biagini (WBB) system, 136, 137
White blood cell (WBC), 214
Workers Compensation (WC) system, 28
World Health Organization (WHO), 57
Wound complications, 141

Y

Yellow flags, 78

Z

Zygapophysial joint, 3

MIX
Papier aus verantwortungsvollen Quellen
Paper from responsible sources
FSC® C105338

If you have any concerns about our products,
you can contact us on
ProductSafety@springernature.com

In case Publisher is established outside the EU,
the EU authorized representative is:
Springer Nature Customer Service Center GmbH
Europaplatz 3, 69115 Heidelberg, Germany

Printed by Libri Plureos GmbH
in Hamburg, Germany